**Social
and De
Psychop**

Social Cognition and Developmental Psychopathology

Carla Sharp
Assistant Professor,
Director of Training, Clinical Psychology Internship Program,
Menninger Department of Psychiatry and Behavioral
Sciences, USA, Director of Research,
Adolescent Treatment Program,
Menninger Clinic, USA

Peter Fonagy
Freud Memorial Professor of Psychoanalysis,
Head of Department, Research Department of Clinical,
Educational, and Health Psychology,
University College London and
Chief Executive of the Anna Freud Centre, UK

Ian Goodyer
Professor of Child and Adolescent Psychiatry,
University of Cambridge, UK

OXFORD
UNIVERSITY PRESS

OXFORD
UNIVERSITY PRESS

Great Clarendon Street, Oxford OX2 6DP

Oxford University Press is a department of the University of Oxford.
It furthers the University's objective of excellence in research, scholarship,
and education by publishing worldwide in

Oxford New York

Auckland Cape Town Dar es Salaam Hong Kong Karachi
Kuala Lumpur Madrid Melbourne Mexico City Nairobi
New Delhi Shanghai Taipei Toronto

With offices in

Argentina Austria Brazil Chile Czech Republic France Greece
Guatemala Hungary Italy Japan Poland Portugal Singapore
South Korea Switzerland Thailand Turkey Ukraine Vietnam

Oxford is a registered trade mark of Oxford University Press
in the UK and in certain other countries

Published in the United States
by Oxford University Press Inc., New York

© Oxford University Press 2008

The moral rights of the authors have been asserted
Database right Oxford University Press (maker)

First published 2008

All rights reserved. No part of this publication may be reproduced,
stored in a retrieval system, or transmitted, in any form or by any means,
without the prior permission in writing of Oxford University Press,
or as expressly permitted by law, or under terms agreed with the appropriate
reprographics rights organization. Enquiries concerning reproduction
outside the scope of the above should be sent to the Rights Department,
Oxford University Press, at the address above

You must not circulate this book in any other binding or cover
and you must impose this same condition on any acquirer

A catalogue record for this title is available from the British Library
Data available

Library of Congress Cataloguing-in-Publication Data
Data available

Typeset by Cepha Imaging Private Ltd., Bangalore, India
Printed in Great Britain
on acid-free paper by CPI Antony Rowe, Chippenham, Wiltshire

ISBN 978-0-19-856918-3

10 9 8 7 6 5 4 3 2 1

Foreword

Judy Dunn

In the last 30 years there has been a wealth of research on the development of children's understanding of people. The capacity to think about why people behave the way they do—how they think, feel, imagine, remember, what they attribute to others, and how this relates to people's actions—is a core feature of being human. The development of this capacity in the early years of childhood transforms children and their social relationships. But until relatively recently research on this social understanding was chiefly focussed on mapping the normative course of its development. Individual differences in social cognitive abilities—their correlates and sequelae—have had less attention. Yet it is striking that children do differ dramatically in their understanding of others, even within the normal range. Some are, even as two year olds, stars at reading the feelings and intentions of others. Others are simply much less curious about, interested in, or sophisticated in their grasp of others' mental or emotional states or intentions. What are the processes underlying these individual differences within the normal range of children, and can they illuminate the atypical development of some children, and the growth of disorders?

The editors of this timely volume have brought together for the first time chapters that focus on a range of sociocognitive capacities, in a range of different childhood disorders. The aims are ambitious: to examine developments in social understanding within a framework that is oriented around children's psychopathology, to explore how different models and approaches to social cognition and multiple levels of analysis can usefully be combined and integrated, and to show how this helps us to better understand psychopathology in children and adolescents. The heterogeneity of the disorders under scrutiny on the one hand, and the heterogeneity of the aspects of social understanding brought together under the umbrella of 'social cognition' on the other, make this a challenging set of tasks. But the positive, optimistic and integrative approaches evident in this volume are especially welcome and timely. As the editors note in their Introduction, there is a curious anomaly in the field, in that many of the constructs under the heading of social cognition are conceptualized, developed and operationalized as intrapersonal and not interpersonal. Yet, they argue convincingly, the construct of social cognition is essentially interpersonal.

Many of the chapters take such an interactionist approach, yet evidence for a more biologically driven approach is not ignored. The challenges to establishing links between social understanding and childhood disorder are many, and clearly articulated by the editors. For example, many of the measures of social understanding are not truly social. Yet which measures are selected hugely affects the interpretation of findings. The heterogeneity of disorders is notable—as illustrated in the discussion of aggressive behaviour and conduct disorder in several chapters. But by examining the distinctive patterns of social understanding in relation to different patterns of aggression we gain insights into the appropriate grouping of children, and the unique treatment implications for these different patterns are highlighted.

This issue of treatment outcomes is helpfully and thoroughly considered in the final chapter, where the authors take a strictly evidence-based perspective on the causal questions. The evidence that interventions based on the presumed sociocognitive processes implicated in the disorder do affect the outcome is assessed in a hard-headed way. In autism spectrum and psychopathy, for instance, dysfunction in empathizing is seen as an important contributor, yet though behavioural treatment reduces some problems associated with autism, social skills training was not found helpful. Interventions related to specific cognitive deficits have some promising results, but it is not yet clear that these effects generalise to real life situations. In relation to depression and anxiety the findings are also complex. For instance a close connection between treatments focused on social information processing and outcome might be expected. Yet meta-analysis of intervention studies of depression have apparently not shown that treatments involving a change in social cognition were any more effective than noncognitive treatments. Sharp and Fonagy discuss various possible explanations for the findings: one intriguing possibility put forward links the findings to developmental changes in brain maturation—the reorganisation of the brain in adolescence. In anxiety disorders the centrality of problems in social understanding is clear, however again establishing a link between treatments aimed at sociocognitive processes and children's outcome has proved difficult.

Such complexities are evident in each of the disorders discussed. For instance in conduct problems, interventions which have large effect sizes are either non-cognitive in focus—such as parent-training—or focused on only one limited aspect of social information processing. There is clearly much more to be done in developing treatments that link closely to the evidence on social cognitive processes. But the evenhanded discussion of these issues is welcome—as in the consideration of causal questions throughout the volume. Family contexts and attachment relationships are included as influences on social information processes, whether as protective factors (Hughes and Ensor) or as sources of problems in social understanding. It is a stimulating book which provides state of the art summaries about what is known as well as what we need to know.

Acknowledgements

Despite the growing interest in the relationship between social cognition and a developmental perspective on mental disorders which has characterized much of the developmental and child psychiatry literature over the last twenty years, no single volume has integrated findings identifying common trends across disorders and between social cognitive capacities. The idea of compiling this volume was therefore born out of the recognition that such integration would serve several purposes. For researchers it will fill a lacuna and consequently promote a more programmatic approach to future research. For lecturers and students this will enable a more integrated literature in teaching modules of child development and developmental psychopathology. For clinicians this will serve as a useful introduction to the relationship between social cognition and developmental psychopathology.

We are grateful to several people who have made invaluable behind-the-scenes contributions without which this volume would not have been possible. We thank Carolyn Ha, Anna Jarman, Rupal Bhimani, Kari Nixon and Liz Allison for proofreading and help with retrieving references. Many thanks to Carol Maxwell and Kate Wanwimolruk at Oxford University Press in guiding us through the production process as well as Bobbie Nichols for her help.

In addition to the above, Carla Sharp wishes to thank several individuals who supported her development as a clinician-scientist who draws on multiple disciplines to better understand pathologies of human interaction and learning in children. Her mentors in this journey are Ian Goodyer and Tim Croudace at the University of Cambridge, and more recently Peter Fonagy and Don Ross since her move to Baylor College of Medicine. For invaluable intellectual exchanges she wishes to thank Jon Allen, Mike Beauchamp, Efrain Bleiberg, Phil Burton, Marc de Rosnay, Petrus de Vries, Sarah Kine, Read Montague, Brooks King-Casas, Melanie Merricks, Brie Linkenhoker, Donald Skinner, Carol Stott, Gillian Todd, Stephanie van Goozen and Rudy Vuchinich. This book is for her parents, the Sharps in Cape Town, Christian, and Milla.

Peter Fonagy wishes to thank Liz Allison for invaluable intellectual and editorial guidance and a group of brilliant colleagues who have contributed to his understanding of the mysteries of social cognition in children Mary Target, Pasco Fearon, George Gergely, and Linda Mayes, in adults Anthony Bateman, Jon Allen, Efrain Bleiberg, Helen Stein, Jeremy Holmes and Stuart Twemlow, and, more recently, in the brain Lane Strathearn, Brooks King-Casas, and Read Montague. A special thanks is due to Carla Sharp whose creative energy in bringing this volume together has been an inspiration.

Ian Goodyer wishes to thank the clinicians and behavioural scientists who have contributed extensively to the programme of work in Cambridge on emotional and behavioural disorders in children and young people. These include Alison Bacon, Valerie Dunn, Rebecca Park, Paul Wilkinson, Graeme Fairchild, Sarah Kine and Stephanie Van Goozen. A special thanks to Zöe Kyte who first used computerized tests of psychological a function in children and adolescents in our group. The neuropsychological studies of adolescents in Cambridge could not have been conducted without the advice and support of Barbara Sahakian. Carla Sharp has demonstrated first class skills as a researcher, student, colleague and now editor in ensuring a unique place for this volume in the clinical, developmental and behavioural sciences.

Contents

Foreword *v*
Judy Dunn

Acknowledgements *ix*

Abbreviations *xiii*

Contributors *xv*

1 Introduction *1*
   Carla Sharp, Peter Fonagy, and Ian Goodyer

Part I **Developmental disorders**

2 Social cognition and autism spectrum conditions *29*
   Simon Baron-Cohen, Ofer Golan, Bhismadev Chakrabarti, and Matthew K. Belmonte

3 Social cognition in children with learning disabilities *57*
   Michal Shaked and Nurit Yirmiya

4 Language and theory of mind in atypically developing children: evidence from studies of deafness, blindness, and autism *81*
   Michael Siegal and Candida C. Peterson

Part II **Externalizing disorders**

5 Social cognition and disruptive behaviour disorders in young children: families matter *115*
   Claire Hughes and Rosie Ensor

6 Social information processing and the development of conduct problems in children and adolescents: looking beneath the surface *141*
   Jacquelyn Mize and Gregory S. Pettit

7 Empathic dysfunction in psychopathy *175*
   James Blair

Part III **Internalizing disorders**

8 Social cognition in depressed children and adolescents *201*
   Zoë Kyte and Ian Goodyer

9 Social cognition and anxiety in children 239
  Robin Banerjee

10 Social cognition and attachment-related disorders 271
   Carla Sharp and Peter Fonagy

Part IV **Other considerations**

11 Attachment, affect-regulation, and mentalization: the developmental origins of the representational affective self 305
   György Gergely and Zsolt Unoka

12 Emotional understanding and developmental psychopathology in young children 343
   Marc de Rosnay, Paul L. Harris, and Francisco Pons

13 Social cognition and genetics 387
   Thomas G. O'Connor and Cathy Creswell

14 Treatment outcome of childhood disorders: The perspective of social cognition 411
   Peter Fonagy and Carla Sharp

Index 471

Abbreviations

AAI	Adult Attachment Interview
ADHD	attention deficit hyperactivity disorder
APD	antisocial personality disorder
APSD	Antisocial Process Screening Device
AS	Asperger syndrome
ASC	autism spectrum conditions
BPD	borderline personality disorder
CBT	cognitive-behavioural therapy
CD	conduct disorder
CDP	Child Development Project
CU	callous unemotional
DBD	disruptive behaviour disorder
DBT	dialectical behaviour therapy
DLPFC	dorsolateral prefrontal cortex
DMPFC	dorsomedial prefrontal cortex
DZ	dizygotic
EBM	evidence-based medicine
EDA	electrodermal response
EDD	eye direction detector
ES	effect size
EU	emotion understanding
fMRI	functional MRI
FSSC-R	Fear Survey Schedule for Children–Revised
HFA	high-functioning autism
HR	heart rate
ID	Intentionality Detector
IPT-A	interpersonal therapy for adolescents
LCSPT	limbic–cortical–striatal–pallidal–thalamic
LTC	limbic–thalamic–cortical
MAOA	monoamine oxidase A
MASC	Multidimensional Anxiety Scale for Children
MDD	major depressive disorder
MRU	unspecified mental retardation
MST	multisystemic therapy
MZ	monozygotic
OCD	obsessive–compulsive disorder
ODD	oppositional defiant disorder
OFC	orbitofrontal cortex
PARCHISY	Parent–Child Interaction System
PCL	Psychopathy Checklist
PCL-R	Psychopathy Checklist–Revised
PD	personality disorder
PET	positron emission tomography
PFC	prefrontal cortex
PPVT	Peabody Picture Vocabulary Test
PPVT-R	Revised Peabody Picture Vocabulary Test
PSST	problem-solving skills training
PWS	Prader–Willi syndrome
rCBF	regional cerebral blood flow
RCMAS	Revised Children's Manifest Anxiety Scale
RCT	randomized controlled trial
RT	relationship therapy
SAM	Shared Attention Mechanism
SASC-R	Social Anxiety Scale for Children–Revised
SCARED	Screen for Child Anxiety-Related Emotional Disorders
SCAS	Spence Children's Anxiety-Scale
SCIT	Social Cognition and Interaction Training
SDQ	Strengths and Difficulties Questionnaire
SES	socio-economic status

SIP	social information processing
SPAI-C	Social Phobia and Anxiety Inventory for Children
SSRI	selective serotonin reuptake inhibitors
SSRS	Social Skills Rating System
STAIC	State-Trait Anxiety Inventory for Children
STS	superior temporal sulcus
TED	The Emotion Detector
TESS	The Empathizing System
ToM	theory of mind
ToMM	Theory of Mind Mechanism
VIM	Violence Inhibition Mechanism
VLPFC	ventrolateral prefrontal cortex
VMA	verbal mental age
VMPFC	ventromedial prefrontal cortex
WS	Williams syndrome

Contributors

Robin Banerjee
Department of Psychology,
University of Sussex, UK

Simon Baron-Cohen
Autism Research Centre, Section of
Developmental Psychiatry,
Department of Psychiatry,
University of Cambridge,
UK

Matthew K Belmonte
Department of Human Development,
Cornell University,
USA

James Blair
Unit on Affective Cognitive
Neuroscience, Mood and Anxiety
Disorders Programme, National
Institute of Mental Health,
USA

Bhismadev Chakrabarti
Autism Research Centre, Section of
Developmental Psychiatry,
Department of Psychiatry,
University of Cambridge, UK

Cathy Creswell
Winnicot Research Unit
Department of Psychology,
University of Reading, UK

Marc de Rosnay
School of Psychology,
The University of Sydney,
Australia

Rosie Ensor
Centre for Family Research,
University of Cambridge, UK

Peter Fonagy
Research Department of Clinical,
Educational and Health Psychology,
University College London, UK

György Gergely
Central European University,
Budapest, Hungary

Ofer Golan
Department of Psychology,
Bar-Ilan University,
Israel

Ian Goodyer
Section of Developmental Psychiatry,
Department of Psychiatry, University
of Cambridge, UK

Paul Harris
Harvard Graduate School of
Education, Cambridge, USA

Claire Hughes
Centre for Family Research,
University of Cambridge, UK

Zoë Kyte
Section of Developmental Psychiatry,
Department of Psychiatry,
University of Cambridge, UK

Jacquelyn Mize
Human Development and Family
Studies, Auburn University, USA

Thomas O'Connor
Department of Psychiatry, University of Rochester Medical Center, USA

Candida Peterson
School of Psychology, University of Queensland, Australia

Gregory S. Pettit
Human Development and Family Studies, Auburn University, USA

Francisco Pons
Department of Psychology, University of Oslo, Norway

Michal Shaked
Department of Psychology, the Hebrew University of Jerusalem, Israel

Carla Sharp
Menninger Department of Psychiatry and Behavioral Sciences, Baylor College of Medicine, USA

Michael Siegal
Department of Psychology, University of Irieste Italy, and Department of Psychology, University of Sheffield, UK

Zsolt Unoka
Department of Psychiatry and Psychotherapy, Faculty of General Medicine, Semmelweis University, Hungary

Nurit Yirmiya
Department of Psychology and School of Education, The Hebrew University of Jerusalem, Israel

1

Introduction

Carla Sharp, Peter Fonagy, and Ian Goodyer

In the book, *The Siege: A family's journey into the world of an autistic child*, a mother provides a moving account of her autistic daughter's social isolation:

> Another image; she is at the beach, two years old now, walking easily…A bronzed, gold baby of unusual beauty, she walks along the sand. Many people are looking at her because she is so pretty, but she is looking at no one. On she walks, into family groups, by picnic baskets, sand castles, and buckets. She grazes human beings by a quarter of an inch. You would think she did not see them. But she does see them, because no matter how close she comes, her eyes fixed, it seems, on some point beyond them or to one side, she never touches them…She looked through human beings as if they were glass. (Claiborne Park 1967, p. 5)

Accounts such as these highlight the importance of the human capacity to think about people and the social world. This capacity, referred to as social cognition, is already observable in newborn infants (e.g. Franco 1997; Walker-Andrews 1997; see also Gergely and Unoka, Chapter 11, this volume), and can be defined as the processes by which children and adults understand themselves and others in terms of how they think, feel, perceive, imagine, react, attribute, infer, and so on. It is through the capacity to think about others' thoughts, intentions, feelings, attitudes, and perspectives that we are able to engage in the activities that humans value most, such as family, friendship, love, cooperation, play, and community, to name but a few. These processes form such an essential and natural part of our functioning as human beings that it is easy to assume that all humans possess the capacity in equal measure. However, as we observe in the above example, some are very severely disabled in terms of their social cognitive capacity. Clearly, such deficits can have profound negative effects on the lives of children and their families; and also on society.

In contrast, others appear to be outstanding social thinkers. We can think of the skilled politician who holds an audience in the palm of his or her hand during a speech. Or the skilled therapist who knows just when to deliver an empathic response. Or the mind-minded mother who just *knows* how to respond to her child's distress. This variability in social cognitive capacity naturally poses the question as to what may account for individual differences in the capacity for social cognition. What factors may play a role in the uneven development of social understanding?

Over the last 30 years we have seen a growing literature devoted to examining the above question in typically developing children. This literature indicates three classes of factors that contribute to the uneven development of social understanding in normal development (reviewed by Repacholi and Slaughter 2003). First, various *cognitive* constructs are correlated with social cognitive performance. These include most notably language (e.g. Astington and Jenkins 1995; Cutting and Dunn 1999; Perner and Lang 1999) and executive functioning (e.g. Perner and Lang 1999), but also other cognitive factors like creativity (Suddendorf and Fletcher-Flinn 1997) and fantasy (Taylor and Carlson 1997). Secondly, various *family* variables have also been shown to correlate with social cognitive performance (de Rosnay and Hughes 2006). These include, amongst others, family talk about mental states (Dunn et al. 1991), the number of older siblings (Perner et al. 1994), maternal mind-mindedness (Meins 1997), maternal reflective functioning (Fonagy et al. 2002), accurate maternal mentalizing (Sharp et al. 2006), attachment security (Fonagy et al. 1991, 1997), and socio-economic status (Holmes et al. 1996). Finally, a third class of studies explaining individual variability in social cognitive performance have focused on various *social outcome* measures, for instance the quality of children's peer relationships (Sutton 2003) and socially competent behaviour (Wilde-Astington 2003). The data from these studies are, with few exceptions, mostly correlational, and so the direction of influence between these variables and social cognitive functioning remains unclear. Nevertheless, findings suggest a multitude of cognitive and environmental factors which may influence variation in social cognitive performance in typically developing children.

A fourth approach to examining individual differences in social cognitive capacity is by the application of a *developmental psychopathology* framework. Developmental psychopathology is, as its name suggests, concerned with behaviour in children (and adults) which may be considered pathological, i.e. diagnosable using nosological classification systems or symptom checklists. But defining developmental psychopathology merely through its focus on abnormal behaviour would be ignoring most of the distinguishing features of this rapidly growing area of scientific inquiry in child development. First outlined by Sroufe and Rutter (1984), a developmental psychopathology approach refers to an integrative discipline which seeks to unify contributions from multiple fields of inquiry with the goal of understanding psychopathology and its relation to normative adaptation within a developmental lifespan framework (Cicchetti 1990, 1993). It has been described as a 'macroparadigm' (Achenbach 1990) which aims to integrate knowledge across scientific disciplines at multiple levels of analysis and multiple domains, in contrast to using only one theory to account for all developmental phenomena (Cicchetti 1993; Rutter and Sroufe 2000). Therefore a developmental psychopathology approach would include a focus on the following (Cicchetti and Rogosch 2002): the use of interdisciplinary models of development; the factors that may cause continuity or discontinuity of normal and abnormal behaviours across the lifespan; the boundaries and relations between normal and abnormal functioning; the transactions that occur between environmental and more person-specific characteristics, including genes; processes associated with risk and resilience; and, finally, the integration of basic research into the design and provision of prevention and intervention.

In this edited volume our immediate aim was to examine social cognition from within a developmental psychopathology framework. In so doing, we invite the reader to reflect on the lessons learnt about social cognition by investigating it in relation to child and adolescent psychopathology. Other volumes have focused on the normative development of social cognition (e.g. Hala 1997) or on one aspect of social cognition only, most notably theory of mind (Astington *et al.* 1988; Baron-Cohen *et al.* 1993; Repacholi and Slaughter 2003). As of yet, research on disparate social cognitive constructs in the context of developmental psychopathology has not been brought together in one single volume. To this end, the current volume necessarily focuses on a variety of social cognitive capacities across a range of childhood disorders. We have organized the book to cover three classes of abnormal child behaviour: developmental disorders (Part I: Chapters 2–4), externalizing disorders (Part II: Chapters 5–7), and internalizing disorders (Part III: Chapters 8–10). In addition, we have included three chapters in Part IV under the heading of 'Other considerations' which deal with topics that cut across traditional boundaries between classes of childhood disorder. Chapters in this section include a chapter introducing an evolutionary-based social cognitive theory of the early development of social cognition (Chapter 11), a discussion of emotion understanding in relation to developmental psychopathology (Chapter 12), and the value of adding a behavioural genetics perspective to the study of social cognition (Chapter 13). Finally, we conclude the volume with a chapter reviewing the literature on intervention outcome, evaluated from the perspective of social cognition.

A brief description of each chapter follows below. First, we will reflect on some of the unanswered questions that the approach in this volume may elucidate. After all, if there are lessons to be learnt from examining social cognition within a developmental psychopathology framework, there must be questions about social cognition still to be answered in the fields of social, developmental, and cognitive psychology.

1.1 What is social cognition?

A review of the contents page of any social psychology textbook on social cognition will reveal that there exist several social cognitive constructs deemed essential in our attempt to make sense of ourselves and other people. Social psychologists are typically interested in constructs such as attitudes, social schemas, attributions, social identity, social representations, stereotypes, prejudice, judgemental heuristics and intergroup relations. In the child development literature, however, the construct of 'theory of mind' has received most attention over the last two decades. Even so, a review of normative developmental literature reveals several additional social cognitive constructs of interest, some of which overlap with constructs studied in more traditional social psychological approaches. In Figure 1.1 we provide a map of the social cognitive constructs that seem to be most often examined in relation to normative development in children. This map is by no means exhaustive. It is merely intended to give some indication of the social cognitive constructs most commonly investigated in a particular age range over the last 20 years. Thus, whilst a particular social cognitive construct is mapped with a particular developmental phase, it is entirely possible that the social cognitive mechanism is equally important for a different developmental phase, but has not often been examined for that particular age range.

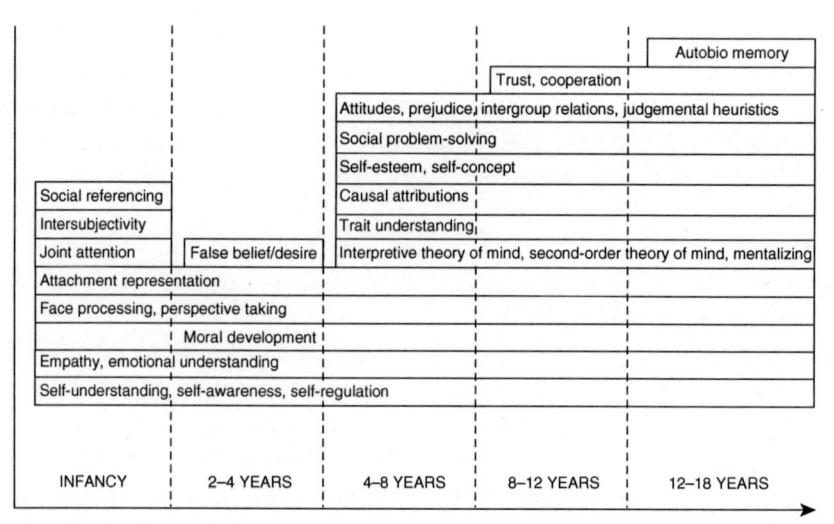

INFANCY	2–4 YEARS	4–8 YEARS	8–12 YEARS	12–18 YEARS
				Autobio memory
			Trust, cooperation	
		Attitudes, prejudice, intergroup relations, judgemental heuristics		
		Social problem-solving		
		Self-esteem, self-concept		
Social referencing		Causal attributions		
Intersubjectivity		Trait understanding		
Joint attention	False belief/desire	Interpretive theory of mind, second-order theory of mind, mentalizing		
Attachment representation				
Face processing, perspective taking				
	Moral development			
Empathy, emotional understanding				
Self-understanding, self-awareness, self-regulation				

Figure 1.1 Social cognitive constructs most commonly studied in relation to normative development.

As Figure 1.1 shows, and as most would agree, social cognition is a polymorphous and heterogeneous construct consisting of multiple concepts. It remains, however, unclear how different social cognitive constructs relate to one another. For instance, should we assume that a child who fails a theory of mind task is also deficient in empathy with limited concern for the well-being of others? That is, should social cognition be regarded as a domain-general or a domain-specific capacity? By studying social cognition within a developmental psychopathology framework we begin to formulate hypotheses about how different aspects of social cognition can be distinguished from one another. Demonstrating dissociable social cognitive capacities (e.g. theory of mind and empathy in Williams' syndrome (Chapter 3, this volume)), which were thought to be all of a piece because of correlations demonstrated in normal development, not only aids clinicians and parents to have realistic expectations of children, but also assists in the scientific refining of the construct of social cognition.

Examining social cognition within a developmental psychopathopathology framework adds to the further delineation of the construct by often requiring the development of new social cognitive constructs and measures. For instance, whereas the false-belief paradigm to measure theory of mind difficulties in children was useful in detecting individual differences in children below the age of four and autistic individuals, it showed ceiling effects in older or conduct-disordered children. By developing new approaches to measure theory of mind associated with conduct problems or psychopathy, the theory of mind construct continues to expand (e.g. O'Connor and Hirsch 1999; Sharp *et al.* 2007), and these approaches can, in turn, be used to study older children and additional clinical populations. Consequently, several other social cognitive constructs can be added to those in Figure 1.1, for example hostile attribution biases (Chapter 6, this volume), intentionality detector, the eye direction detector, shared attention mechanism, theory of mind mechanism and the empathy detector (Chapter 2, this volume), distorted mentalizing (Chapter 10, this volume), and so on.

In bringing together into one volume social cognitive research across different disorders, we also notice an interesting anomaly which relates not only to the definition of social cognition, but also to the ontogeny of social cognition (see below). When considering social cognition in depression (Chapter 8, this volume), anxiety (Chapter 9, this volume), and conduct problems (Chapter 6, this volume), it is often conceptualized as *intra*personal problems of biased attention, encoding, interpretation, or inefficient problem-solving. Thus social cognition in relation to these disorders is neither conceptualized nor operationalized as *inter*personal. In such approaches the only difference between social cognition and non-social cognition is that the former occurs within a social context. The question then arises as to why this should be the case. Why are constructs under the heading of *social* cognition conceptualized, developed, and operationalized as intrapersonal, and not interpersonal?

One answer to this question may lie in the fact that many approaches to social cognition define the latter by its content, i.e. social cognition is any cognition that has social content or that occurs in a social context. It is certainly true that some cognitive processes in human beings may be considered essentially social because they are poorly separated from their social context. For instance, 'catastrophying' is an intrapersonal and typical cognitive distortion considered in both the social cognitive and cognitive literature. However, patients usually tend to catastrophy in the context of social situations. The social phobic may think that everybody will look at him. The depressive may think that she will never be loved. The anxious person may think that her birthday party will end in disaster, and so on.

Whilst we do not feel that we can offer a definitive definition of social cognition, we do feel that we can refine the construct of social cognition by defining it as cognition that is essentially *inter*personal. That is, social cognition is the thing that happens between two (or more) people when they interact, and not merely an intrapersonal characteristic applied to a social situation. In combining social neuroscience approaches with developmental psychopathology we may begin to characterize the critical mental processes in one person socially managing an interaction or relationship with another.

1.2 Deficit or distortion? What about emotions?

Given the heterogeneity of social cognition, how should we conceptualize problems in social cognition when studying atypical development? Throughout this volume, a tension between four approaches to social cognition will emerge: social cognition as deficits, social cognition as distortion, social cognition as the result of an emotional deficit, and social cognition as information processing which contains stepwise components of both deficits and distortions. We believe that these four approaches are not mutually exclusive. Instead, in line with a developmental psychopathology framework, we propose that some approaches may be more relevant than others for some disorders, or aspects of disorders, at particular developmental stages of child development, each with distinct aetiological correlates. For instance, a deficit approach to social cognition may be more relevant in preschool children or in disorders that are more biologically driven. A distortion approach may be more relevant later in development and in disorders that carry a heavier environmental influence. This volume will suggest a myriad of permutations of how different approaches in social cognition can be combined to better understand psychopathology in children.

1.3 The ontogeny of social cognition

A third question in social cognition on which a developmental psychopathology approach can shed light is the question of whether understanding of self and others results from individual cognitive maturation or whether it is better explained by social processes. In short, what drives the development of social cognition? Is it driven by a genetic blueprint that will unfold cognitively in the brain regardless of social experience? Or is it driven by social interaction? Thus, how social is social cognition?

Certain childhood conditions (e.g. Williams' syndrome and autism) are considered more 'biological' than others. Several chapters in this volume show how examining the specific abilities and developmental trajectories of social cognition in one disorder helps to clarify the cognitive, emotional, and perceptual components and the complex interactions between these components underlying certain behaviour or ability in another disorder, as well as the ontogenetic (biological or environmental) basis of these behaviours. Chapters in this volume will put forward equally convincing arguments for a nativist, modular, or biologically driven account of the development of social cognition on the one hand, and a constructivist socially driven account on the other hand. These two accounts are, of course, not mutually exclusive. Indeed, within a developmental psychopathology framework the complex processes by which normal development goes awry to produce psychopathology are acknowledged. Therefore many chapters in this volume will advance an interactionist approach to the role of social cognition in the aetiology of psychopathology in children.

Related to the above, this volume is timely for another reason. Because of the advances in technologies (e.g. functional neuroimaging) that enable us to peer into the living brain, we have seen an explosion of research examining the neurobiological correlates of social behaviour and cognition over the last decade. These advances have been so significant that a new interdisciplinary field called social neuroscience has emerged (e.g. Cacioppo *et al.* 2005). Parallel to these developments, we have seen greater interest in the neurobiological and psychophysiological correlates of abnormal behaviour in children. Now, as we near the end of the first decade of the new century, it is timely to consider the findings of both these developments in tandem. Most of the chapters in this volume will consider the neurobiological correlates of social cognition as it relates to psychopathology. Indeed, a challenge for the next generation of studies at the interface between social neuroscience and developmental psychopathology will be to design studies that simultaneously measure both biological and social variables. As discussed by Mize and Pettit in Chapter 6, such models are already being developed for externalizing behaviour; social experiential factors which have previously been conceptualized to influence social behaviour primarily via cognitive and emotional processes such as modelling, social information processing, and relational schemas are hypothesized to cause neurological structural and functional changes that may mediate later experiences. Such models are truly reflective of a developmental psychopathology approach where multiple levels of explanation are integrated in one explanatory model.

An alternative model to the kind outlined by Mize and Pettit in Chapter 6, but which also takes into account multiple levels of explanation characteristic of the developmental psychopathology approach, is to conceive of social cognition as a special case of interaction between nature and nurture. Along with Sharp and Fonagy (Chapter 10, this volume), Gergely and Unoka (Chapter 11, this volume), and others, we suggest that social cognition is a special case of the interaction between nature and nurture for two reasons. First, social cognition is an example of where 'nature' prepares an individual to be 'in nurture'. By this, we mean that an infant enters the world with a biological preparedness to make use of her social environment through the innate capacity for social cognition. This capacity, which we share with a number of non-human social species such as apes, goats, and avian species including crows, ravens, and scrab-jays (Hare *et al.* 2001; Tomasello *et al.* 2003; Emery and Clayton 2004; Bugnyar and Heinrich 2005; Kaminski *et al.* 2006; Gergely and Unoka, Chapter 11, this volume), enables the infant to enter into her first social relationship. Therefore it enables the infant to make use of 'nurture'.

Secondly, social cognition is a case where nurture is allowed to modify nature. Although some biological preparedness exists in particular forms of 'deep structure' which allows the infant to utilize her social environment, the environment is simultaneously allowed to exert influence on development and maturation. Therefore we conceptualize social cognition similarly to the conceptualization of language espoused by Siegal and Peterson (Chapter 4, this volume). Siegal and Peterson state that the grammar of language is mandatory in that we cannot stop ourselves from acquiring it. Even if all British people speak English, depending on the environment, they have programmed in them ultimate flexibility in terms of the language they acquire. Therefore if a child of British parents is raised in France, she will speak French. However, the fact that she speaks French does not alter the Chomskian (see Siegal and Peterson, Chapter 4, this volume) deep structure of language, which would have enabled her to communicate with others through any kind of language, even sign language.

We believe that we are now starting to understand the 'deep structure' of social cognition, i.e. the grammar of social cognition. Through research on infant social understanding and evolutionary psychology research, we discover that some deep structure is biologically built into the human brain which enables us to identify and read the states of the minds of others. What we may find as this journey continues is that social cognition, like language, is a special case of the interaction between nature and nurture.

1.4 Implicit or explicit?

LeDoux (1989) suggested that most of our cognitive and emotional processing occurs and influences our behaviour outside conscious awareness. Indeed, social understanding often occurs in a blink of an eye, and so it is tempting to explain it in the same way that we can easily explain capacities like knowing when to stop pouring water into a glass to prevent it from spilling over. Yet, social understanding can also occur in a more conscious or explicit way. In fact, by asking a research participant in a laboratory setting to read the mind of another or the expression in the eyes of a photograph, we are asking them to engage in a form of controlled processing.

It is now becoming clear that social cognition, like other cognitive processes, is both implicit and explicit. The distinction between implicit or automatic versus controlled (explicit) processes is well recognized and is hypothesized to be supported by distinct neurocognitive systems (Lieberman 2007). For instance, Lieberman *et al.* (2002) and Satpute and Lieberman (2006) suggest an X-system (refle**x**ive) which is supported by an automatic social cognitive neural system including the amygdala, basal ganglia, ventromedial prefrontal cortex, lateral temporal cortex, and dorsal anterior cingulate cortex. The C-system (refle**c**tive) responds to a controlled social cognitive system and includes the lateral prefrontal cortex, medial prefrontal cortex, lateral parietal cortex, medial parietal cortex, medial temporal lobe, and rostral and anterior cingulate cortex.

Whether the above distinction will emerge as a data-driven finding depends on demonstrating dissociable neural systems for each. Such work is under way (Lieberman 2007). Another way of demonstrating the distinction between explicit (controlled) and implicit (automatic) processes is by investigating these within a developmental psychopathology framework. By discussing how controlled (but not automatic) social cognitive processing is deficient in a disorder, or vice versa, as we do by bringing together research on different disorders in one volume, we believe with Lieberman (2007) and other social psychologists that these two processes are indeed dissociable.

1.5 How do we measure social cognition?

A range of creative measures to tap into social cognitive processing will be reviewed in this volume. We summarize these in Table 1.1.

As is evident from Table 1.1, measures range from observations, the recording of children's responses to social vignettes, experimental tasks (both individual or dyadic), and self-report questionnaire measures. No single approach is ideal for all purposes, and the choice of measurement approach

Table 1.1 Social cognitive tasks and measures referenced in relation to childhood disorders

Chapter Childhood disorder	Measures of social cognition
Chapters 2 and 4 Autism	*Theory of mind tasks* ♦ Several variations of the false-belief (displacement) task ♦ Several variations of the false-belief (unexpected content) task ♦ Understanding of desires tasks ♦ Understanding of deception task ♦ Understanding of lies task ♦ Understanding of jokes task ♦ Second-order theory of mind tasks *Emotion understanding tasks* ♦ Emotion and mental state recognition from ecologically rich social situations containing multimodal sources of information ♦ Emotion recognition task: face (static stimuli) ♦ Emotion recognition task: face (dynamic stimuli) ♦ Emotion recognition from film clips ♦ Emotion recognition: eye region of the face (eyes task) ♦ Emotion recognition: basic vs. complex emotions ♦ Emotion recognition from voices ♦ Identification of emotions from context
Chapter 3 Learning disabilities	*Theory of mind tasks* ♦ Eye gaze direction detection task ♦ Task probing inference of others' intentions and goals from drawings ♦ False-belief task: displacement ♦ False-belief task: unexpected content ♦ Second-order theory of mind task ♦ Complex mental states from the eye region of the face (eyes task) ♦ Explanations of action task ♦ Understanding of metaphor and sarcasm task ♦ Distinction between lies and ironic jokes task ♦ Pretend play ♦ Social referencing

Table 1.1 (continued) Social cognitive tasks and measures referenced in relation to childhood disorders

Chapter Childhood disorder	Measures of social cognition
	Emotion understanding tasks ♦ Emotion matching task ♦ Face recognition tasks of the Rivermead Behavioural Memory Test ♦ Benton Facial Recognition Test ♦ Face-inverted paradigms
Chapter 4 Deaf and blind children	*Theory of mind tasks* ♦ False-belief tasks: displacement ♦ False-belief tasks: unexpected content ♦ False-belief tasks—thought pictures: unexpected outcome ♦ Second-order theory of mind task ♦ Initiation of contact with parents by voice, touch, or posture ♦ Responsivity to parental vocal and facial affective expressions ♦ Mirroring of parents' affectively charged non-verbal postural, facial and vocal cues ♦ Social referencing ♦ Turn taking ♦ Pretend play
Chapter 5 Disruptive preshoolers	*Theory of mind tasks* ♦ Picture-book false belief ♦ Penny-hiding game ♦ Puppet sabotage/deceit task ♦ Deceptive identity: explain, predict ♦ False belief: displacement
	Emotion understanding tasks ♦ Emotion false belief: nice/nasty surprises ♦ Denham Emotional Labelling Task
Chapter 6 Conduct problems	*Encoding* ♦ Recall and recognition of element of social events on videotape, audiotape, or verbal descriptions ♦ Capacity to shift attention away from aggressive stimuli ♦ Response times to words indicative of social threat (hated, loser) vs. neutral words vs. physical threat (murder, hurt)
	Interpretation ♦ Accuracy or valence of attributions about the motives for others' actions in hypothetical ambiguous scenarios ♦ Child decides between multiple hypothetical scenarios whether intention of provocateur was benign or hostile

Table 1.1 (continued) Social cognitive tasks and measures referenced in relation to childhood disorders

Chapter Childhood disorder	Measures of social cognition
	Goal clarification ♦ During hypothetical situation or recall of recent peer encounter child indicates how important a given outcome would be in that situation (e.g. 'How important would it be to you to show the other girl she can't push you around?') or what they wanted to happen or selecting from a list the goal they would pursue ♦ Goal adjustment depending on outcome of different situations *Response generation* ♦ In response to hypothetical social vignettes, children are asked to report how they would respond. Both the number and quality of responses are recorded ♦ Strategies employed during hypothetical dilemmas with puppets *Response evaluation* ♦ Children are asked to judge the appropriateness of aggressive behaviour as response ♦ Children are asked to share their expectancies of the outcome of aggressive behaviour
Chapter 7 Psychopathy	*Theory of mind tasks (cognitive empathy)* ♦ Naming of emotional facial expressions (emotional empathy) ♦ Naming of vocal affect (emotional empathy) ♦ Empathy: autonomic physiological responses to the distress of others through observation of electric shock delivery or video images ♦ Moral/conventional distinction task
Chapter 8 Depression	*Social-cognitive tasks* ♦ Self-schema questionnaire ♦ Attributional style questionnaire ♦ Interpretation of social performance in terms of failure or success ♦ Global self-worth questionnaire ♦ Self-confidence questionnaire ♦ Response style questionnaire: distraction vs. self-focused rumination ♦ Recall of autobiographical events ♦ Decision-making tasks *Emotion processing tasks* ♦ Emotional Stroop tasks ♦ Emotional dot-probe tasks ♦ Emotional go–no-go task

Table 1.1 (continued) Social cognitive tasks and measures referenced in relation to childhood disorders

Chapter Childhood disorder	Measures of social cognition
Chapter 9 Anxiety	*Social-cognitive tasks* ♦ Attention to threatening words vs. neutral words ♦ Dot-probe task: negative vs. neutral faces ♦ Interpretation of homophones (threatening vs. neutral) ♦ Five-sentence stories with themes relating to social anxiety, separation anxiety, generalized anxiety. Guess as quickly as possible whether each story is a scary story which will have a bad ending or a non-scary story which will end well ♦ Social role-play task: social performance ♦ Recall of negative events relevant to public self-image task ♦ Knowledge of social problem-solving strategies task
	Theory of mind tasks ♦ False-belief task: displacement ♦ *Faux pas* theory of mind task ♦ Understanding of self-presentational and pro-social display rules task ♦ Understanding strategies for regulating emotional experiences and expressions task
Chapter 10 Attachment disorders	*Theory of mind/emotion understanding tasks* ♦ Measures of protodeclarative pointing in infants ♦ False-belief tasks ♦ Distorted mentalizing task ♦ Facial emotional processing task ♦ Emotion understanding task ♦ Story stem completion task ♦ Reading the mind in the eyes task
	Measures of parental mentalization ♦ Reflective functioning measure ♦ Quality of parental control ♦ Parental discourse of emotion ♦ Maternal mind-mindedness paradigm ♦ Maternal accuracy task ♦ Still face paradigm

will of course depend on the research question being addressed. Similarly, the interpretation of results will depend strongly on the measurement approach chosen. As will be shown in this volume, a challenge facing social cognitive research in general is the fact that most measures of social cognition are not truly social in nature. An aim of future research would be the design of novel experiments that tap into social cognitive processing in real time. In other words, what are needed are measures of online social cognitive processing as opposed to offline retrospective social reasoning.

1.6 Social cognition and developmental psychopathology: chicken or egg?

So far, we have emphasized the role of social cognition in the aetiology or development of disorder in childhood. Of course, the opposite may also be true. Social cognitive deficits may be the result of psychopathology and not the cause. Thus another aim of this volume is to bring together researchers at the interface between social cognition and developmental psychopathology in order, perhaps, to shed light on this question. Although it is only through longitudinal follow-up studies that such issues can be truly addressed, a developmental psychopathology approach to social cognition would assert that pathology and social cognition are in continuous reciprocal interaction with each other over the course of development.

Related to the above, we have discussed how examining social cognition in relation to childhood disorders emphasizes the heterogeneity of social cognition as a construct. The opposite is also true. Many of the chapters in this volume will show that by investigating social cognition in a developmental psychopathology framework we further refine and describe the heterogeneity of childhood disorders. Chapters 6 (conduct disorders) and 7 (psychopathy) are good examples—it is through studying social cognition in these two disorders that we are better able to define subgroups of aggressive children, each with differential social cognitive correlates and unique treatment implications.

In principle, it will remain a challenge to discover whether psychopathology is caused by social cognition or vice versa. If there is any kind of isomorphism between social cognition and psychopathology we will never know which causes which, because in most instances one is defined by the other due to the fact that many symptoms of most disorders lie in the social domain. Even when independent measures of a disorder (e.g. a biological marker) are discovered, the problem of isomorphism often remains. A possible reformulation of the question of chicken or egg is to ask how social cognition contributes to the endophenotype of a particular disorder. Thus the main contribution of social cognition may lie in characterizing the endophenotype of, for instance, depression. In that case we will state not that depression is caused by a disorder of social processing, but rather that aspects of social processing contribute to describing the endophenotype of depression. Thus we are able to identify subtypes more efficiently and may prevent disorder and intervene in a more specific and targeted way.

1.7 Are social cognitive constructs useful in the treatment or prevention of childhood disorders?

Finally, before we turn to a brief overview of the volume, it is worth emphasizing an additional question that this volume aims to elucidate: How can knowledge about social cognition aid in the treatment and prevention of childhood disorders? Each chapter in Parts I–III includes a section on the clinical applications of the social cognitive construct relevant to the disorder discussed in that chapter. By so doing, we hope to highlight the usefulness of social cognition in clinical practice. In addition, we conclude the volume with Chapter 14, where Fonagy and Sharp reflect on the role of social cognition in the treatment and prevention of childhood disorder.

1.8 A brief overview of the book

In keeping with a developmental psychopathology framework, the chapters focusing on each class of childhood disorder (Parts I–III) are loosely organized around the following structure (not always in this order): (1) description of the disorder; (2) what is known about the normal development of social cognition relevant to the disorder; (3) research on abnormalities of social cognition associated with the disorder with emphasis on developmental aspects; (4) aetiological considerations (what are possible causes of the developmental abnormalities of social cognition including biological and social factors and their interactions); (5) clinical implications (the ways in which new knowledge inform prevention and treatment interventions); (6) expected future directions of research.

Part I. Developmental disorders

Since Baron-Cohen *et al.* (1985) first suggested a theory of mind deficit to lie at the basis of autistic children's social interaction difficulties, there has been an explosion of research investigating social cognitive deficits in relation to autism and developmental disorders. Developmental disorders refer to a class of disorders usually diagnosed in infancy, childhood, and adolescence, characterized by severe deficits and pervasive impairment in multiple areas of development which may be associated with a range of learning difficulties (American Psychiatric Association 2000).

Since the social cognitive deficits associated with this class of disorder have arguably received the most research attention over the last two decades, it is fitting to start our volume with a chapter that presents Baron-Cohen's model of social cognition. Baron-Cohen's model has been tremendously influential in stimulating the most recent wave of social cognitive research in normal and abnormal development through its operationalization of social cognition as a 'mindreading system', and more recently, an 'empathizing system'.

Thus, in Chapter 2, Baron-Cohen, Golan, Chakrabarti, and Belmonte introduce Baron-Cohen's original (Baron-Cohen 1994, 1995) and recently expanded (Baron-Cohen 2005) model for the neurocognitive mechanisms which comprise the 'mindreading' or 'empathizing' system. The chapter presents the model with supporting data and reviews associated neural and genetic abnormalities that are believed to cause the social cognitive deficits associated with autism. The model presented in this chapter is a deficit model of social cognition and is grounded in evolutionary psychology. It provides an explanation of the ontogenesis of a theory of mind and the neurocognitive dissociations that are seen in children with and without autism. In addition to providing the field with dissociable, circumscribed, and measurable social cognitive constructs, the model also charts the normal development of the mindreading system in children, including the developmental precursors to theory of mind understanding before age four.

In Chapter 3, Shaked and Yirmiya review the literature on social cognition in children with learning disabilities, with a specific focus on Williams' syndrome (WS). They chose to focus their review on WS for two reasons. First, since it is a genetic disorder, the study of social cognitive deficits in WS raises important questions about the influence of genes on variability in social cognition. Secondly, in contrast with autistic children, or children with other developmental disorders, children with WS show some relative strengths in the domains of language and social competence. In their review of the literature on theory of mind (ToM) and face-processing in WS, Shaked and Yirmiya show that, despite the sociability of children with WS, these capacities are not spared. In fact, their performance is comparable to that of other populations with mental retardation, and is significantly lower than that expected of age-matched typically developing individuals. However, the interesting profile of strengths and weaknesses found in WS suggests dissociable and multiple constructs underlying social cognitive capacity which may vary across disorders and even individuals with the same disorder. As with the chapter on autism, Chapter 3 demonstrates a deficit approach to the study of social cognition in atypical populations.

One of the most replicated cognitive factors suggested to affect individual differences in social cognitive capacity is language. Therefore examination of how language and social cognition interact in children whose access to verbal and non-verbal input has been limited through physical impediments could shed light on the interactions between language and social cognition. In Chapter 4, Siegal and Peterson present a thorough review of the literature on social cognition (theory of mind) and language acquisition in hearing, deaf, blind, and autistic children. Their chapter hinges on the argument that although children from the latter three groups suffer from relatively similar problems in language and social cognition for very different reasons, the child's early opportunities to share at a very young age in spontaneous family conversation at home and in everyday interactive contexts are limited. Blind children and deaf children of hearing parents are limited by their sensory problems, while children with autism are limited by their inattention to voices and speech. Although Siegal and Peterson also take a deficit approach to social cognition, their understanding of the ontogenesis of social cognitive deficits differ from that espoused in Chapters 2 and 3, in that delayed expression of theory of mind reasoning is suggested to stem from deficits in early social and conversational experience.

Part II. Externalizing disorders

Chapters 2–4 are excellent examples of how the study of atypical populations can aid in understanding how social cognition works in typically developing children, be it by the influence of genes, language ability, social competence, or social and conversational experience. In Chapter 5 the importance of family experiences in the ontogenesis of social cognition is further extended by Hughes and Ensor in their discussion of the interaction between social cognitive deficits associated with disruptive behaviour disorders, family variables (e.g. harsh parenting), and executive functioning in preschool children. Hughes has been one of the pioneers in the application of the deficit approach to theory of mind in preschoolers with externalizing behaviour problems.

Externalizing (or disruptive behaviour) disorders refer to a class of problem behaviours characterized by behaviours directed outwards, often resulting in conflict with both children and adults. For instance, children who are considered to suffer from externalizing disorders may be described by parents and teachers as disruptive, defiant, aggressive, prone to temper tantrums, delinquent, or overactive. Diagnoses grouped under externalizing disorders include conduct disorder, oppositional–defiant disorders, hyperactivity, attention-deficit–hyperactivity disorder, psychopathy, and antisocial personality disorder.

In the work of Hughes and Ensor on externalizing problems in preschoolers, we see examples of two principles of developmental psychopathology applied to social cognition. First, Hughes and Ensor suggest some developmental continuities and discontinuities for explicit and implicit theory of mind from the preschool to school age years. Secondly, Chapter 4 also provides a good example of the boundaries and relations between normal and abnormal functioning by demonstrating how advances in our understanding of normative age-related changes in social cognition may illuminate key mechanisms underlying the development of disruptive behaviour disorders.

Whereas a theory of mind approach to examining the relations between social cognition and externalizing behaviour disorder is a phenomenon of the mid-1990s onwards, the social information processing (SIP) approach of Kenneth Dodge (Dodge and Coie 1987; Dodge and Crick 1990; Dodge 1993) has been the guiding principle of most of the research in this area since the 1980s and continues to exert its influence. In Chapter 6, Mize and Pettit extend Dodge's approach by looking 'beneath the surface' of traditional SIP approaches in two ways. First, they acknowledge SIP to be a proximal mechanism for interpersonal behaviour by outlining several social cognitive constructs (or information processing steps) which associate with aggressive behaviour: encoding social situations, interpretation or representation of others' behaviour, deciding and clarifying goals in social situations, generating responses to social situations or social problem-solving, and response evaluation and social decision-making. Secondly, they discuss a more distal developmental mechanism for conduct problems in the form of schemas as the outcome of an interaction between biological and environmental influences, thereby emphasizing the developmental psychopathology principle of interaction between multiple levels of explanation in the developmental course of social cognition and problem behaviour.

The SIP model is of special interest in the current volume because, by its very nature, it could only have developed in the context of a developmental psychopathology approach precisely because SIP formulations were developed to explain deviations from normal patterns. Although very few formal attempts have been made to create a dialogue between the rich findings derived from SIP research with more recent theory of mind approaches to social cognition, we are beginning to see such dialogues emerging in the literature (Sharp, unpublished manuscript, 2000; Sharp 2006; Sharp *et al.* 2007; Lewis and Carpendale 2002; Banerjee, Chapter 9, this volume).

In Chapter 7, Blair introduces the concept of emotional empathy to describe social cognitive deficits associated with psychopathy in children and adolescents. In contrast with cognitive empathy and motor empathy, emotional empathy refers to emotional responses to the emotional displays of others. While hard-to-manage preschoolers seem to show some theory of mind deficits (Chapter 5), adult psychopaths show no such deficits (Chapter 7). Therefore, in Chapter 7, Blair argues that the social cognitive deficits associated with psychopathy should be conceptualized as deficits in emotional empathy rather than cognitive empathy. He supports his hypothesis with data from neurobiological studies suggesting reduced amygdala activation in adult psychopaths. Blair's contribution to this volume is an excellent example of the application of multiple levels of explanation in the formulation of a developmental psychopathology model of social cognition and psychopathy in youth. He proposes a compelling model of how the effects of the family environment on symptoms of psychopathy (but not other aggressive disorders) may be modulated by the neurobiological mechanisms of emotional empathy. Thus his work illustrates how a focus on social cognition in aetiological research may refine our diagnostic classifications to also reflect causal pathways underlying behavioural phenotypes.

Part III. Internalizing disorders

In contrast with externalizing disorders where problem behaviours are directed 'outwards', internalizing disorders (traditionally referred to as neurotic disorders) refer to that class of emotional problems that appear to be related to problems 'within the self'. Parents or teachers may describe such children as sad, worried, shy, withdrawn, or irritable, with complaints of physical problems like frequent tummy aches or headaches. Diagnoses considered as 'internalizing' include anxiety and depression (Kovacs and Devlin 1988), which often co-occur in the same child (see Chapter 9 for a discussion). Whereas the term 'externalizing disorders' traditionally refers to conditions where the central feature is dysregulated behaviour, the term 'internalizing disorders' traditionally refers to conditions whose central feature is disordered mood.

In the first of the chapters focusing on internalizing disorders (Chapter 8), Kyte and Goodyer suggest (similar to Hughes and Ensor in Chapter 5) that developmental similarities and differences in psychopathology across the lifespan should correlate with socio-cognitive and affective processes embedded in the liability for and outcome of disorder—in this case depression. They use SIP theory (presented in Chapter 6) as a framework to organize literature on social cognition and depression in children to include a discussion of knowledge structures (self-schemas as distal social cognitive mechanism), attention to negative stimuli in the encoding of information, depressiogenic attributional style, cognitive biases in interpretation of social events, over-general autobiographical memory, rumination, and decision-making. They show how these social cognitive constructs may interact with environmental and biological factors, especially in the context of neurodevelopmental accounts of social cognition and depression. By taking this multilevel approach to the study of social cognition in depression, the authors conclude that depression in children and adolescents should be regarded as a disorder of both emotion regulation and social cognition. Therefore this chapter provides an excellent example of emerging models of social cognition and developmental psychopathology in that it takes on the challenge of describing the complex interplay of cognition and emotion.

In Chapter 9, Banerjee starts with a discussion of the phenomenology of anxiety disorder in childhood, including a discussion of the comorbidity between anxiety and depression in childhood. This leads to a discussion of the tripartite model for the overlap between anxiety and depression (Clark and Watson 1991). The overlap and distinction between anxiety and depression is relevant because Banerjee later relates the hyper-arousal which distinguishes anxiety from depression to unique patterns in social cognitive processing in anxious children. He also relates this later in the chapter to how genetics may influence social cognitive processes via negative affectivity, which underlies both depression and anxiety. He then proceeds to a discussion of general social information processing characteristics in anxiety in order to develop an argument that greater threat perception in anxiety is not just specific to social situations but is a domain-general phenomenon. This is an important point, because it highlights a fundamental question in social cognitive literature, namely the debate about domain-general social cognitive abilities versus domain-specific social cognitive abilities. Next, Banerjee discusses social understanding and theory of mind in anxious children and concludes this section with an intriguing model describing how basic social cognitive deficits may result in later cognitive interpretive biases, thus linking the deficit model of social cognition with the cognitive biases approach to social cognition. Finally, Banerjee discusses possible aetiologies of social cognition as it pertains to anxiety, citing both genetic and environmental factors. He concludes with a thorough explication of clinical implications, mostly focusing on cognitive-behavioural models and directions for future research.

Part III on internalizing disorders concludes with Chapter 10 on attachment-related disorders by Sharp and Fonagy. They provide a model for the development of social cognitive capacity which is firmly grounded in attachment theory, thereby providing a view on the ontogeny of social cognition touched upon by Mize and Pettit in Chapter 6, but not fully developed in any of the other preceding chapters. They show why attachment theory is a natural framework for understanding and empirically investigating the social cognitive impairments associated with emerging personality disorder in children and adolescents. They review data that link early attachment experiences with later symptomology through the mechanism of parental mentalization (also referred to as maternal mind-mindedness or reflective function), and discuss a mentalization-based treatment approach that has been developed to address mentalizing problems in children and adolescents.

Part IV. Other considerations

In Parts I–III researchers at the interface between social cognition and developmental psychopathology review some of the most up-to-date and influential models of social cognition as it relates to disorders of childhood. In Part IV we consider complementary themes that need to be considered when approaching social cognition from within a developmental psychopathology framework.

Part IV begins with Chapter 11 by Gergely and Unoka in which an evolutionary-based social cognitive theory of the early development of the representational affective self in humans is presented. Much of the research reviewed in the preceding chapters has referred to the more distal social cognitive mechanisms that may play a role in the development of later psychopathology in children, but none of the authors so far (with the exception of Baron-Cohen and colleagues in Chapter 2) have attempted to describe the exact ontogenetic mechanisms of social cognition in infancy. In a comparable but more detailed vein than Sharp and Fonagy (Chapter 10), Gergely and Unoka do this by showing how the human-specific features of early caregiver–infant interactions provide the necessary input conditions for specialized representation-building and attention socialization mechanisms which form part of the developing mentalizing (social cognitive) system which, in turn, enables the development of emotional self-awareness and affective self-control. Other authors in the current volume (e.g. Hughes and Ensor, and Kyte and Goodyer) have already emphasized the interaction between social cognition and emotional-regulative processes in the development of psychopathology. Gergely and Unoka provide an explanatory model of how such interactive processes may develop or be detected already in infancy. More specifically, they propose that 'when maladaptive patterns of affective parental reactivity become the dominant features of the re-occurring interactive structure of the infant's primary attachment relationships, they can and do play a significant causal role in pathologically *undermining* the developing self's potential to rely on its innate mentalizing capacity as its dominant social cognitive strategy to cope with interpersonal situations and intimate and affiliative relationships during later life' (Chapter 11).

In Chapter 12, de Rosnay, Harris, and Pons offer yet another model of the development of social cognition, this time with an emphasis on one aspect of social cognition, namely emotion understanding. They review a rich but heterogeneous literature on the links between emotion understanding, theory of mind, and children's socio-emotional competence. They synthesize the literature in order to provide a general framework for thinking about socio-emotional competence and the role that emotion understanding may play in this. Their account echoes some of the themes brought forward in chapters on other aspects of social cognitive development. Against this background, they suggest worthwhile avenues for future research that take into account not only children's ability to *understand* emotions, but the effects of *experiencing* emotion, especially in adverse circumstances such as maltreatment.

In most of the preceding chapters there have been some references to the role that genetics may play in the development of social cognitive deficits or distortions associated with childhood disorder. In Chapter 13, O'Connor and Creswell expand on these by first providing a critical review of the basic hypotheses and strategies of a behavioural genetics research approach with respect to addressing questions about gene–environment interplay. Next, they point out that social cognition has received very little research from a behavioural genetic perspective. They proceed to show how a behavioural genetics perspective can elucidate the mechanisms involved in the intergenerational transmission of social cognition and spur research into the neuroscience basis of social cognition. Behavioural genetic research into various social cognitive constructs (theory of mind, attributional style, empathy, and social competence) are reviewed, after which directions of future research in this promising area are suggested.

Finally, in Chapter 14, we conclude the volume with a synthesis of the preceding chapters. In writing the final chapter, Fonagy and Sharp pay special attention to the implications of taking a social cognitive perspective in the treatment of childhood disorder.

References

Achenbach, T. (1990). What is 'developmental' about developmental psychopathology? In *Risk and protective factors in the development of psychopathology* (ed. J. Rolf, A. Masten, D. Cicchetti, K. Nuechterlein, and S. Weintraub), pp. 29–48. New York: Cambridge University Press.

American Psychiatric Association (2000). *Diagnostic and statistical manual of mental disorders* (4th edn). Washington, DC: American Psychiatric Association.

Astington, J.W. and Jenkins, J.M. (1995). Theory of mind development and social understanding. *Cognition and Emotion*, **9**, 151–65.

Astington, J.W., Harris, P.L., and Olson, D.R. (ed.) (1988). *Developing theories of mind*. New York: Cambridge University Press.

Baron-Cohen, S. (1994). The Mindreading System: new directions for research. *Current Psychology of Cognition*, **13**, 724–50.

Baron-Cohen, S. (1995). Mindblindness: an essay on autism and theory of mind. Cambridge, MA: MIT Press.

Baron-Cohen, S. (2005). Autism. In *Cambridge Encyclopaedia of Child Development*. Cambridge University Press.

Baron-Cohen, S., Leslie, A.M., and Frith, U. (1985). Does the autistic child have a 'theory of mind'? *Cognition*, 21, 37–46.

Baron-Cohen, S., Tager-Flusberg, H., and Cohen, D. (ed.) (1993). *Understanding other minds: perspectives from developmental cognitive neuroscience.* Oxford University Press.

Bugnyar, T. and Heinrich, B. (2005). Ravens, *Corvus corax,* differentiate between knowledgeable and ignorant competitors. *Proceedings of the Royal Society of London,* 272, 1641–6.

Cacioppo, J.T., Visser, P.S., and Pickett, C.L. (2005). *People thinking about thinking people.* Cambridge, MA: MIT Press.

Cicchetti, D. (1990). An historical perspective on the discipline of developmental psychopathology. In *Risk and protective factors in the development of psychopathology* (ed. J. Rolf, A. Masten, D. Cicchetti, K. Nuechterlein, and S. Weintraub), pp. 2–28. New York: Cambridge University Press.

Cicchetti, D. (1993). Developmental psychopathology: reactions, reflections, projections. *Developmental Review*, 13, 471–502.

Cicchetti, D. and Rogosch, F.A. (2002). A developmental psychopathology perspective on adolescence. *Journal of Consulting and Clinical Psychology*, 70, 6–20.

Claiborne Park, C. (1967). *The siege: a family's journey into the world of an autistic child.* Harmondsworth: Penguin

Clark, L.A. and Watson, D. (1991). Tripartite model of anxiety and depression: Psychometric evidence and taxonomic implications. *Journal of Abnormal Psychology*, 100, 316–36.

Cutting, A.L. and Dunn, J. (1999). Theory of mind, emotion understanding, language, and family background: individual differences and interrelations. *Child Development*, 70, 853–65.

de Rosnay, M. and Hughes, C. (2006). Conversation and theory of mind. Do children talk their way to socio-cognitive understanding? *British Journal of Developmental Psychology*, 24, 7–37.

Dodge, K.A. (1993). Social-cognitive mechanisms in the development of conduct disorder and depression. *Annual Review of Psychology*, 44, 559–84.

Dodge, K.A. and Coie, J.D. (1987). Social-information-processing factors in reactive and proactive aggression in children's peer groups. *Journal of Personality and Social Psychology*, 53, 1146–58.

Dodge, K.A. and Crick, N.R. (1990). Social information-processing bases of aggressive behavior in children. *Personality and Social Psychology Bulletin*, 16, 8–22.

Dunn, J., Brown, J., and Beardsall. L. (1991). Family talk about feeling states and children's later understanding of others' emotions. *Developmental Psychology*, 27, 448–55.

Emery, N.J. and Clayton, N.S. (2004). The mentality of crows: convergent evolution of intelligence in Corvids and Apes. *Science*, 306, 1903–7.

Fonagy, P., Steele, H., Moran, G., Steele, M., and Higgitt, A. (1991). The capacity for understanding mental states: the reflective self in parent and child and its significance for securtiy of attachment. *Infant Mental Health Journal*, 12, 201–18.

Fonagy, P., Redfern, S., and Charman, T. (1997). The relationship between belief-desire reasoning and a projective measure of attachment security (SAT). *British Journal of Developmental Psychology*, 15, 51–61.

Fonagy, P., Gergely, G., Jurist, E.L., and Target, M. (2002). *Affect regulation, mentalization, and the development of self*. New York: Other Press.

Franco, F. (1997). The development of meaning in infancy: early communication and social understanding. In *The development of social cognition* (ed. S Hala), pp. 95–160. Hove: Psychology Press.

Hala, S. (1997). Introduction. In *The development of social cognition* (ed. S Hala), pp. 3–32. Hove: Psychology Press.

Hare, B., Call, J., and Tomasello, M. (2001). Do chimpanzees know what conspecifics know? *Animal Behavior*, **61**, 139–51.

Holmes, H., Black, C., and Miller, S. (1996). A cross-task comparison of false belief understanding in a Head Start population. *Journal of Experimental Child Psychology*, **63**, 263–85.

Kaminski, J., Call, J., and Tomasello, M. (2006). Goat's behaviour in a competitive food paradigm: evidence for perspective taking? *Behaviour*, **143**, 1341–56.

Kovacs, M. and Devlin, B. (1988). Internalizing disorders in childhood. *Journal of Child Psychology and Psychiatry*, **39**, 47–63.

LeDoux, J.E. (1989). Cognitive-emotional interactions in the brain. *Cognition and Emotion*, **3**, 267–89.

Lewis, C. and Carpendale, J.E.M. (2002). Social cognition. In *Blackwell Handbook of Social Cognition* (ed. P.K. Smith and C. Hart), pp. 375–393. Oxford: Blackwell.

Lieberman, M.D. (2007). Social cognitive neuroscience: a review of core processes. *Annual Review of Psychology*, **58**, 259–89.

Lieberman, M.D., Gaunt, R., Gilbert, D.T., and Trope, Y. (2002). Reflection and relexion: a social cognitive neuroscience approach to attributional inference. *Advances in Experimental Social Psychology*, **34**, 199–249.

Meins, E. (1997). *Security of attachment and the social development of cognition*. Hove: Psychology Press.

O'Connor, T.G. and Hirsch, N. (1999). Intra-individual differences and relationship-specificity of mentalising in early adolescence. *Social Development*, **8**, 256–74.

Perner, J. and Lang, B. (1999). Development of theory of mind and executive control. *Trends in Cognitive Sciences*, **3**, 337–44.

Perner, J., Ruffman, T., and Leekam S.R. (1994). Theory of mind is contagious: you catch it from your sibs. *Child Development*, **65**, 1228–38.

Repacholi, B., and Slaughter, V. (ed.). (2003). *Individual differences in theory of mind*. New York: Psychology Press.

Rutter, M. and Sroufe, L.A. (2000). Developmental psychopathology: concepts and challenges. *Development and Psychopathology*, **12**, 265–96.

Satpute, A.B. and Lieberman, M.D. (2006). Integrating automatic and controlled processing into neurocognitive models of social cognition. *Brain Research*, **1079**, 86–97.

Sharp, C. (2006). Mentalizing problems in childhood disorders. In *Handbook of mentalization-based treatments* (ed. J.G. Allen and P. Fonagy), pp. 101–121. Chichester: John Wiley.

Sharp, C., Fonagy, P., and Goodyer, I.M. (2006). Imagining your child's mind: psychosocial adjustment and mothers' ability to predict their children's attributional response styles. *British Journal of Developmental Psychology*, **24**, 197–214.

Sharp, C., Croudace, T.J., and Goodyer, I.M. (2007). A Latent Class Analysis of a child-focused mentalising task in a community sample of 7–11 year olds. *Social Development*, **16**, 181–202.

Sroufe, L.A. and Rutter, M. (1984). The domain of developmental psychopathology. *Child Development*, **55**, 17–29.

Suddendorf, T. and Fletcher-Flinn, C.M. (1997). Theory of mind and the origins of divergent thinking. *Journal of Creative Behavior*, **31**, 169–79.

Sutton, J. (2003). ToM goes to school: social cognition and social values in bullying. In *Individual differences in theory of mind: implications for typical and atypical development* (ed. B Repacholi and V Slaughter), pp. 99–120. New York: Psychology Press.

Taylor, M. and Carlson, S.M. (1997). The relation between individual differences in fantasy and theory of mind. *Child Development*, **68**, 436–455.

Tomasello, M., Call, J., and Hare, B. (2003). Chimpanzees understand psychological states—the question is which ones and to what extent. *Trends in Cognitive Sciences*, **7**, 153–6.

Walker-Andrews, A.S. (1997). Infants' understanding of affect. In *The development of social cognition* (ed. S Hala), pp. 161–86. Hove: Psychology Press.

Wilde-Astington, J. (2003). Sometimes necessary, never sufficient: false-belief understanding and social competence. In *Individual differences in theory of mind: implications for typical and atypical development* (ed. B Repacholi and V Slaughter), pp. 13–38. New York: Psychology Press.

Part I
Developmental disorders

Chapter 2

Social cognition and autism spectrum conditions

Simon Baron-Cohen, Ofer Golan, Bhismadev Chakrabarti, and Matthew K. Belmonte

2.1 Autism spectrum conditions

Autism is diagnosed when a child or adult has abnormalities in a 'triad' of behavioural domains: social development, communication, and repetitive behaviour/obsessive interests (American Psychiatric Association 1994; World Health Organization 1994). Autism can occur at any point on the IQ continuum, and IQ is a strong predictor of outcome (Rutter 1978). Autism is also invariably accompanied by language delay (no single words before 2 years old). Asperger syndrome (AS) (Asperger 1944) is a subgroup on the autistic spectrum. People with AS share many of the same features seen in autism, but with no history of language delay and with IQ in the average range or above. In this chapter we will use the term autism spectrum conditions (ASC) to describe the whole spectrum of individuals who meet diagnostic criteria for one or other of these subgroups. Because autism is a developmental condition, and because developmental psychopathology is the focus for this volume, we will at times be discussing adults with this diagnosis, even though this book has a focus on childhood conditions. Adult studies are of course relevant not only because the onset of ASC is during early childhood, but also because of how changes across the lifespan throw light on developmental outcomes.

2.2 Typical development of mindreading

In 1994 Baron-Cohen proposed a model to specify the neurocognitive mechanisms that comprise the 'mindreading system' (Baron-Cohen 1994, 1995). Mindreading is defined as the ability to interpret one's own or another agent's actions as driven by mental states. The model was proposed in order to explain (a) the ontogenesis of a theory of mind and (b) neurocognitive dissociations that are seen in children with or without autism. The model is shown in Figure 2.1 and contains four components: the Intentionality Detector (ID),

```
ID            EDD    0–9 m
  \          /
   ↓        ↓
    SAM           9–14 m
     │
     ↓
    ToMM           2–4 years
```

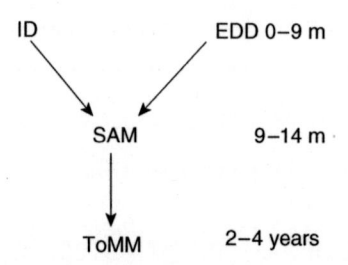

Figure 2.1 Baron-Cohen's model of mindreading (Baron-Cohen 1994): ID, Intentionality Detector; EDD, Eye Direction Detector: SAM, Shared Attention Mechanism; ToMM, Theory of Mind Mechanism.

the Eye Direction Detector (EDD), the Shared Attention Mechanism (SAM), and the Theory of Mind Mechanism (ToMM).

ID and EDD build 'dyadic' representations of simple mental states. ID automatically interprets or represents an agent's self-propelled movement as a desire or goal-directed movement, a sign of its agency, or an entity with volition (Premack 1990). For example, ID interprets an animate-like moving shape as 'it wants x' or 'it has goal y'. EDD automatically interprets or represents eye-like stimuli as 'looking at me' or 'looking at something else', i.e. EDD picks out that an entity with eyes can perceive. Both ID and EDD are developmentally prior to the other two mechanisms, and are active early in infancy.

SAM is developmentally more advanced and comes on line at the end of the first year of life. SAM automatically interprets or represents if the self and another agent are perceiving the same event. It does this by building 'triadic' representations. For example, where ID can build the dyadic representation 'Mother wants the cup' and EDD can build the dyadic representation 'Mother sees the cup', SAM can build the triadic representation 'Mother sees that I see the cup'. As is apparent, triadic representations involve embedding or recursion. (A dyadic representation—'I see a cup'—is embedded within another dyadic representation—'Mum sees the cup') to produce this triadic representation). SAM takes its input from ID and EDD, and triadic representations are made out of dyadic representations. SAM typically functions from 9 to 14 months of age, and allows 'joint attention' behaviours such as protodeclarative pointing and gaze monitoring (Scaife and Bruner 1975).

ToMM allows epistemic mental states to be represented (e.g. 'Mother thinks this cup contains water' or 'Mother pretends this cup contains water'), and it integrates the full set of mental state concepts (including emotions) into a theory. ToMM develops between 2 and 4 years of age, and allows pretend play (Leslie 1987), understanding of false belief (Wimmer and Perner 1983), and understanding of the relationships between mental states (Wellman 1990).

An example of the latter is the seeing-leads-to-knowing principle (Pratt and Bryant 1990), where the typical 3-year-old can infer that if someone has seen an event, then they will know about it.

The model shows the ontogenesis of a theory of mind in the first 4 years of life, and justifies the existence of four components on the basis of developmental competence and neuropsychological dissociation. In terms of developmental competence, joint attention does not appear possible until 9–14 months of age, and joint attention appears to be a necessary but not sufficient condition for understanding epistemic mental states (Baron-Cohen 1991; Baron-Cohen and Swettenham 1996). There appears to be a developmental lag between acquiring SAM and ToMM, suggesting that these two mechanisms are dissociable. In terms of neuropsychological dissociation, congenitally blind children can ultimately develop joint (auditory or tactile) attention using the amodal ID rather than the visual EDD route. Children with autism appear able to represent the dyadic mental states of seeing and wanting, but show delays in shared attention (Baron-Cohen 1989b) and in understanding false belief (Baron-Cohen *et al.* 1985; Baron-Cohen 1989a), i.e. in acquiring SAM and ultimately ToMM. It is this specific developmental delay which suggests that SAM is dissociable from EDD.

The 1994 model of the Mindreading System was revised in 2005 because of certain omissions and too narrow a focus. The key omission is that information about affective states, available to the infant perceptual system, has no dedicated neurocognitive mechanism. The revised model (Baron-Cohen 2005), which now includes a new fifth component, The Emotion Detector (TED), is shown in Figure 2.2. However, the concept of mindreading (or theory of mind) makes no reference to the affective state in the observer

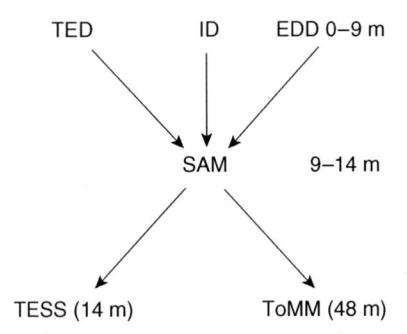

Figure 2.2 Baron-Cohen's model of empathizing (Baron-Cohen 2005): ID, Intentionality Detector; EDD, Eye Direction Detector: SAM, Shared Attention Mechanism; ToMM, Theory of Mind Mechanism; TED, The Emotion Detector; TESS, The Empathizing SyStem.

triggered by recognition of another's mental state. This is a particular problem for any account of the distinction between autism and psychopathy (see also Blair, Chapter 7, this volume). For this reason, the model is no longer of 'mindreading' but is of 'empathizing', and the revised model also includes a new sixth component–The Empathizing SyStem (TESS). Where the 1994 Mindreading System was a model of a passive observer (because all the components had simple decoding functions), the 2005 Empathizing System is a model of an observer impelled towards action (because an emotion is triggered in the observer which typically motivates the observer to respond to the other person).

Like the other infancy perceptual input mechanisms of ID and EDD, the new component of TED can build dyadic representations of a special kind, namely it can represent affective states. An example would be 'Mother – is unhappy', or even 'Mother – is angry – with me'. Formally, we can describe this as an agent-affective state-proposition. We know that infants can represent affective states from as early as 3 months of age (Walker 1982). As with ID, TED is amodal, in that affective information can be picked up from facial expression, or vocal intonation; 'motherese' is a particularly rich source of the latter (Field 1979). Another's affective state is presumably also detectable from their touch (e.g. tense versus relaxed), which implies that congenitally blind infants should find affective information accessible through both auditory and tactile modalities. TED allows the detection of the basic emotions (Ekman and Friesen 1969). The development of TED is probably aided by the simple imitation that is typical of infants (e.g. imitating caregiver's expressions), which in itself would facilitate emotional contagion (Meltzoff and Decety 2003).

When SAM becomes available, at 9–14 months of age, it can receive inputs from any of the three infancy mechanisms, ID, EDD, or TED. Here, we focus on how a dyadic representation of an affective state can be converted into a triadic representation by SAM. An example would be that the dyadic representation 'Mother is unhappy' can be converted into a triadic representation 'I am unhappy that Mother is unhappy', or 'Mother is unhappy that I am unhappy', etc. Again, as with perceptual or volitional states, SAM's triadic representations of affective states have this special embedded, or recursive, property. The phenomenon of social referencing, in which toddlers approach objects towards which their caregiver looks approvingly or avoid those objects towards which the caregiver shows alarm or disapproval, is one index of SAM (Klinnert 1984).

ToMM has been celebrated for the last 20 years in research in developmental psychology (Leslie 1987; Wimmer *et al.* 1988; Whiten 1991). ToMM is of major importance in allowing the child to represent the full range of mental states, including epistemic ones (such as false belief), and is important in allowing the child to pull mentalistic knowledge into a useful theory with which to predict behaviour (Wellman 1990; Baron-Cohen 1995). But TESS allows more than behavioural explanation and prediction (itself a powerful achievement). TESS allows an empathic reaction to another's emotional state. However, this is not to say that these two modules do not interact. Knowledge of mental states of others made possible by ToMM could certainly influence the way in which an emotion is processed and/or expressed by TESS. TESS also allows for sympathy. It is this element of TESS that gives it the adaptive benefit of ensuring that organisms feel a drive to help each other, as seen in a toddler's early comforting behaviour towards those in distress (Harris 1989).

To see the difference between TESS and ToMM, consider this example: 'I see you are in pain'. Here, ToMM is needed to interpret your facial expressions and writhing body movements in terms of your underlying mental state (pain). But now consider this further example: 'I am devastated – that you are in pain'. Here, TESS is needed, since an appropriate affective state has been triggered in the observer by the emotional state identified in the other person. And where ToMM employs M-representations (Leslie 1995) of the form agent–attitude–proposition (e.g. Mother – believes – Johnny – took– the – cookie), TESS employs a new class of representations, which we can call E-representations of the form self-affective state-[self-affective state-proposition] (e.g 'I feel sorry that – Mum feels sad about – the news in the letter') (Baron-Cohen 2003). The critical feature of this E-representation is that the self's affective state is appropriate to and triggered by the other person's affective state. Thus TESS can represent [I am horrified – that you are in pain], or [I am concerned – that you are in pain], or [I want to alleviate – that you are in pain], but it cannot represent [I am happy – that you are in pain]. At least, it cannot do so if TESS is functioning normally. One could imagine an abnormality in TESS leading to such inappropriate emotional states being triggered, or one could imagine them arising from other systems (such as a competition system or a sibling rivalry system), but these would not be evidence of TESS *per se*.

Before moving to review the development of mindreading in autism spectrum conditions, we should mention the literature documenting typical sex differences in empathizing, with females showing greater attention to faces at birth (Connellan *et al.* 2001), more eye contact as toddlers (Lutchmaya *et al.* 2002), greater sensitivity to *faux pas* in childhood (Baron-Cohen *et al.* 1999a), and better ability to decode subtle mental states from facial expressions (Baron-Cohen *et al.* 1997b). Such sex differences are one clear source of evidence for individual differences in empathy. Taking a dimensional approach to empathy as a normally distributed trait in the population leads to the view that autism spectrum conditions may simply be at one end of a spectrum that runs throughout the population. We do not suppose that this is the only relevant dimension along which individuals with autism differ, another one being in 'systemizing', but that literature is reviewed elsewhere (Baron-Cohen 2002, 2006; Goldenfeld *et al.* 2007).

2.3 Mindreading in autism spectrum conditions

Since the first test of mindblindness in children with autism (Baron-Cohen *et al.* 1985), there have been more than 30 experimental tests. The vast majority of these have revealed profound impairments in the development of their empathizing ability. These are reviewed elsewhere (Baron-Cohen *et al.* 1993b; Baron-Cohen 1995). Some children and adults with AS only show their empathizing deficits on age-appropriate tests (Baron-Cohen *et al.* 1997a,b, 2001a). This deficit in their empathizing is thought to underlie the difficulties that such children have in social and communicative development (Baron-Cohen 1988; Tager-Flusberg 1993), and in the imagination of others' minds (Baron-Cohen 1987; Leslie 1987).

The majority of studies of emotion recognition have focused on the face, and tested recognition of six emotions (happiness, sadness, fear, anger, surprise, and disgust). These 'basic emotions' are expressed and recognized universally (Ekman and Friesen 1971; Ekman 1993). Some studies reveal emotion recognition deficits among individuals with ASC, compared with typical or clinical control groups, using both static (MacDonald *et al.* 1989; Celani *et al.* 1999; Deruelle *et al.* 2004) and dynamic (Hobson 1986a,b; Yirmiya *et al.* 1992) stimuli. Other studies have found that children and adults with high-functioning autism (HFA) or AS have no difficulties in recognizing these basic emotions from pictures (Grossman *et al.* 2000; Adolphs *et al.* 2001) or films (Loveland *et al.* 1997). Possible reasons for this apparent lack of consistency are the heterogeneity of symptom severity within the ASC population and the fact that accuracy measures for emotion recognition tasks might not be fine-tuned to pick up subtle differences in measures of perceived task difficulty (e.g. reaction time). It is hoped that correlative designs in future experiments, with quantitative dimensions of 'symptom' severity such as the ADI-R (Lord *et al.* 1994) or AQ (Baron-Cohen *et al.* 2001b), should resolve this issue. The observed deficit in accuracy measures of emotion recognition becomes much more apparent when testing recognition of more 'complex' emotions (such as embarrassment, insincerity, intimacy, etc.) in both adults and children with ASC (Baron-Cohen *et al.* 1997b, 2001a; Golan *et al.* 2006a). These findings suggest that recognition of basic emotions is relatively preserved among high-functioning individuals with ASC, and that they show greater difficulties in recognizing more complex emotional and mental states.

Emotion recognition from voices has been studied less frequently. Here too there are contradictory findings in relation to recognition of basic emotions (Loveland *et al.* 1995, 1997; Boucher *et al.* 2000). Regarding recognition of complex emotions from voices, several studies report a deficit in performance in high-functioning adults with ASC compared with controls (Kleinman *et al.* 2001; Rutherford *et al.* 2002; Golan *et al.* 2006a, 2007).

Studies assessing the ability of individuals with ASC to identify emotions and mental states from context have also shown deficits relative to the general population or to other clinical control groups (Baron-Cohen *et al.* 1986; Fein *et al.* 1992). For example, adolescents and adults with ASC have difficulties in answering questions on the Strange Stories Test (Happé 1994; Jolliffe and Baron-Cohen 1999). This test assesses the ability to provide context-appropriate mental state explanations for non-literal statements made by story characters (e.g. ironic or sarcastic statements).

Studies assessing complex emotion and mental state recognition from ecologically rich social situations containing multimodal sources of information show a deficit in individuals with ASC compared with controls (Heavey *et al.* 2000; Klin *et al.* 2002; Golan *et al.* 2006b). These difficulties may be related to a failure to attend to the right emotional cues, and/or to a failure in integrating them, explained by weak central coherence in the cognitive level (Frith 1989) and under-connectivity between brain regions in the neurobiological level (Belmonte *et al.* 2004a,b; Courchesne and Pierce 2005; McAlonan *et al.* 2005).

To summarize, although emotion recognition deficits in ASC are lifelong, some high-functioning individuals develop compensatory strategies which allow them to recognize basic emotions. However, when recognition of more complex emotions and mental states is required from faces, voices, context, or the integration of these, many find them hard to interpret. It would appear that in autism TED may function, although this may be delayed (Hobson 1986a; Baron-Cohen *et al.* 1993a, 1997b), at least in terms of detecting basic emotions. Even high-functioning people with autism or AS have difficulties in both ToMM (when measured with mental-age-appropriate tests) (Happé 1994; Baron-Cohen *et al.* 1997a, 2001a) and TESS (Attwood 1997; Baron-Cohen *et al.* 1999b, 2003; Baron-Cohen and Wheelwright 2004; Dapretto *et al.* 2006). This suggests that TED and TESS may be fractionated.

In contrast, the psychiatric condition of psychopathy may entail an intact TED and ToMM alongside an impaired TESS. The psychopath (or sociopath) can represent that you are in pain, or that you believe that he is the gas-man so that he can gain access to your house or your credit card. The psychopath can go on to hurt you or cheat you without having the appropriate affective reaction to your affective state. In other words, he or she does not care about your affective state (Mealey 1995; Blair *et al.* 1997). Lack of guilt or shame or compassion in the presence of another's distress is diagnostic of psychopathy (Cleckley 1977; Hare *et al.* 1990). Thus separating TESS and ToMM allows a functional distinction to be drawn between the neurocognitive causes of autism and psychopathy.

2.4 Causes

We can think of causes of the social cognitive deficits in ASC in terms of the brain basis of empathy and mindreading in the typical brain. This is reviewed first.

Neuroimaging experiments have implicated the following different brain areas for performing tasks that tap empathy. Traditional 'theory of mind' (cognitive empathy) tasks have consistently shown activity in medial prefrontal cortex, superior temporal gyrus, and the temporo-parietal junction (Frith and Frith 2003; Saxe *et al.* 2004). This could be equated to the brain basis of ToMM. Studies of emotional contagion have demonstrated involuntary facial mimicry (Dimberg *et al.* 2000) as well as activity in regions of the brain where the existence of 'mirror' neurons has been suggested (Wicker *et al.* 2003; Decety and Jackson 2004; Keysers and Perrett 2004). Sympathy has been relatively less investigated, with one study implicating the left inferior frontal gyrus, among a network of other structures (Decety and Chaminade 2003).

ID has been tested in a PET study in a task involving attribution of intentions to cartoon characters (Brunet *et al.* 2000). Reported activation clusters included the right medial prefrontal (BA 9) and inferior frontal (BA 47) cortices, the superior temporal gyrus (BA 42), and the bilateral anterior cingulate cortex. In an elegant set of experiments that required participants to attribute intentions to animations of simple geometric shapes, it was found that the 'intentionality' score attributed by the participants to individual animations was positively correlated to the activity in superior temporal sulcus, the temporo-parietal junction, and the medial prefrontal cortex (Castelli *et al.* 2000). A subsequent study (Castelli *et al.* 2002) demonstrated a group difference in activity in the same set of structures between people with autism/AS and neurotypical controls.

EDD has been studied in several neuroimaging studies on gaze direction perception (Calder *et al.* 2002; Pelphrey *et al.* 2003), which have implicated the posterior superior temporal sulcus bilaterally. This evidence, taken together with similar findings from primate literature (Perrett and Emery 1994), suggests this area to be a strong candidate for the anatomical equivalent of the EDD.

This fits in with the Haxby model of face-processing, where he suggested a role for this region in processing 'variable' aspects of faces (in contrast with non-varying aspects such as identity) (Haxby et al. 2000). In a recent imaging study, Williams et al. (2005) investigated the neural correlates of SAM and reported bilateral activation in anterior cingulate (BA 32,24) and medial prefrontal cortex (BA 9,10) and the body of caudate nucleus in a joint attention task, when compared with a control task involving non-joint attention (Frith and Frith 2003).

We can now turn to neuroimaging studies of processing facial expressions of emotion in people with ASC. These show less activation in brain regions central to face-processing, such as the fusiform gyrus (Critchley et al. 2000; Pierce et al. 2001; Schultz et al. 2003). Behavioural studies show that children and adults with ASC process faces differently compared with controls: Participants with ASC tend to process faces in a feature-based approach, whereas controls process faces configurally (Hobson et al. 1988; Teunisse and De Gelder 1994; Young and Bruce 1998; Schultz et al. 2003). There is also evidence of reduced activation in brain areas that play a major role in processing of emotion, such as the amygdala, when individuals with ASC process social-emotional information (Baron-Cohen et al. 1999c; McAlonan et al. 2005; Ashwin et al. 2007).

However, a recent study (Dalton et al. 2005) shows that the observed hypoactivation of the amygdala and the fusiform gyrus in response to facial expressions of emotion is related to the lack of fixation on the eye region of the face. In light of this new result, it is essential to re-evaluate existing results from studies that involve emotional stimuli in a non-visual domain. One study measured brain activity of participants with ASC and matched controls whilst listening to theory of mind stories. Activation in the medial frontal area of the brain, whilst judging others' mental states, was less intensive and extensive in the AS group compared with controls (Neiminen-von Wendt et al. 2003). When using a verbal ToM task in a neuroimaging study, reduced activation of the left medial prefrontal cortex was found in people with ASC compared with matched controls (Happé and Frith 1996).

Anatomical abnormalities have been identified in many brain areas in autism. These include the cerebellum (Murakami et al. 1989; Courchesne et al. 1994b,c,d; Hashimoto et al. 1995), the brainstem (Hashimoto et al. 1995; Rodier et al. 1996), the frontal lobes (Carper and Courchesne 2000; Courchesne et al. 2001; Aylward et al. 2002; Sparks et al. 2002), the parietal lobes (Courchesne et al. 1993), the hippocampus (Aylward et al. 1999; Saitoh et al. 2001), and the amygdala (Aylward et al. 1999). Volume deficits have been shown in the cerebellum (Murakami et al. 1989; Courchesne et al. 1988, 1994d;

Hashimoto et al. 1995). However, there has been a report of a subgroup of children with ASC who have an increased cerebellar volume (Courchesne et al. 1994a). Epilepsy also occurs commonly, at least in classic autism (Ballaban-Gil and Tuchman 2000).

In terms of neuropathology, the number of Purkinje cells in the cerebellar cortex is abnormally low (Williams et al. 1980; Bauman and Kemper 1985, 1994; Ritvo et al. 1986). This has been postulated to lead to disinhibition of the cerebellar deep nuclei and consequent over-excitement of the thalamus and cerebral cortex (Courchesne et al. 1994b,c). The brainstem (Hashimoto et al. 1995) and posterior corpus callosum (Egaas et al. 1995) have also been shown to have lower volumes in people with ASC when compared with neurotypical controls. A volume deficit has also been reported in the parietal lobe (Courchesne et al. 1993). Neuropsychology suggests that this is associated with a narrowed spatial focus of attention (Townsend and Courchesne 1994). The results of either MRI volumetric analysis or measures of head circumference show that the autistic brain appears to involve transient postnatal macrocephaly (Courchesne 2002). Neonates later diagnosed with autism or PDD-NOS (pervasive developmental disorder-not otherwise specified) have normal head circumference, but by 2–4 years of age 90 per cent of these have larger than average MRI-based brain volumes (Carper and Courchesne 2000; Courchesne et al. 2001; Aylward et al. 2002; Sparks et al. 2002). This reflects an enlargement of cerebellar and cerebral white matter, and cerebral grey matter (Courchesne et al. 2001; Herbert et al. 2003). Enlargement of superficial white matter tracts containing cortico-cortical fibres may persist abnormally late into development, whilst the internal capsule and corpus callosum are smaller (Herbert et al. 2002). Cerebellar and cerebral white matter volumes, and cerebellar vermis size, can distinguish 95 per cent of toddlers with autism from normal controls, and predict if the child with autism will be high or low functioning (Courchesne et al. 2001). The overgrowth is anterior to posterior (frontal lobes are the largest). This increase in volume of cortical grey matter may reflect a failure of synaptic pruning, an excess of synaptogenesis, or an excess of neurones (Belmonte et al. 2004a).

Abnormalities in the density of packing of neurons in the hippocampus, amygdala, and other parts of the limbic system have also been reported (Bauman and Kemper 1985, 1994; Raymond et al.1996). An abnormally low degree of dendritic branching was also found in a Golgi analysis of the hippocampus of two autistic brains (Raymond et al. 1996), although it remains to be seen if such an abnormality is confirmed in a larger sample. A separate report suggests a reduction in the size of cortical minicolumns and an increase in cell dispersion within these minicolumns. These might indicate an increase in the number of and connectivity between minicolumns (Casanova et al. 2002a,b).

Abnormal levels of arousal have been inferred from physiological and endocrine indices (Tordjman et al. 1997; Hirstein et al. 2001). Functional studies suggest that sensory inputs evoke hyperactivation, resulting in decreased ability to select amongst competing inputs. Thus, on the Embedded Figures Task, people with autism show unusually high activation in ventral occipital areas and abnormally low activation in prefrontal and parietal areas (Ring et al. 1999).

Regarding event-related potential results, the P1 evoked potential is either abnormally heightened in response to stimuli that are the target of attention, or abnormally generalized to stimuli that are outside the target of attention (Townsend and Courchesne 1994). The visual N2 to novel stimuli is also heightened to irrelevant stimuli (Kemner et al. 1994). The P3 in response to auditory stimuli is abnormally generalized to occipital sites in visual cortex (Kemner et al. 1995). Both hemispheres show abnormal activation, indiscriminately, during shifts of attention into either hemifield (Belmonte 2000; Belmonte and Yurgelun-Todd 2003). Regarding attentional research, a deficit has been found in rapid shifting of attention between modalities (Courchesne et al. 1994b,c), between spatial locations (Wainwright-Sharp and Bryson 1993, 1996; Townsend et al. 1996a,b, 1999; Harris et al. 1999; Belmonte 2000), and between object features (Courchesne et al. 1994b,c; Rinehart et al. 2001).

A neural basis of empathy has built on a model first proposed by Brothers (1990). She suggested from animal lesion studies (Kling and Brothers 1992), single-cell recording studies (Brothers et al. 1990), and neurological studies that social intelligence was a function of three regions: the amygdala, the orbito-frontal and medial frontal cortex, and the superior temporal sulcus and gyrus. Together, she called these the 'social brain'. Abnormalities in autism have been found in the amygdala, the orbito-frontal cortex, and the medial frontal cortex.

There is converging evidence from several lines of research on the abnormalities of these 'social brain' structures in ASC. There is evidence for amygdala hypoactivation in an emotion recognition task in autism (Baron-Cohen et al. 2000). We have reported significantly less amygdala activation in adults with HFA/AS during a mentalizing task (Reading the Mind in the Eyes Task) compared with normal subjects (Baron-Cohen et al. 1999c). Reduced activity in these 'social brain' structures has been reported in the left medial frontal cortex (Happé et al. 1996) during an empathizing (theory of mind) task, and also in the orbito-frontal cortex (Baron-Cohen et al. 1994). A neuroanatomical study of autism at post-mortem found microscopic pathology (in the form of increased cell density) in the amygdala in the presence of normal amygdala volume (Bauman and Kemper 1994; Rapin and Katzman 1998). Secondly, patients with autism tend to show a similar pattern of deficits to those seen in patients with amygdala lesions (Adolphs *et al.* 2001). Thirdly, several structural MRI studies of autism have revealed abnormal development of the amygdala (reviewed by Baron-Cohen *et al.* 2005). A recent larger structural study suggests more generalized structural abnormalities in the social brain (McAlonan *et al.* 2005). We have also recently reported a functional dysconnectivity of the amygdala with other brain structures (Welchew *et al.* 2005).

Ultimately, the cognitive and neural abnormalities in autism spectrum conditions are likely to be strongly linked to genetic factors. The sibling risk-rate for autism is approximately 4.5 per cent, or a tenfold increase over general population rates (Jorde *et al.* 1991). Regarding twin studies, in an epidemiological study of same-sex autistic twins, it was found that 60 per cent of monozygotic (MZ) pairs were concordant for autism compared with no dizygotic (DZ) pairs (Bailey *et al.* 1995). When these authors considered a broader phenotype (of related cognitive or social abnormalities), 92 per cent of MZ pairs were concordant compared with 10 per cent of DZ pairs. The high concordance in MZ twins indicated a high degree of genetic influence, and the risk to a co-MZ-twin can be estimated at over 200 times the general population rate. However, genetics cannot be the whole story, since concordance is not 100 per cent and gene–environment interactions can render monozygotic twins strongly discordant for the level of severity of ASC (Belmonte and Carper 2006).

The past few years have seen rapid progress in molecular genetic understanding of autism (O'Roak and State 2008; Abrahams and Geschwind 2008), although there remains a great deal of work to be done in discerning the metabolic and developmental pathways by which identified genetic variants contribute to autistic development. Recent discoveries seem to segregate into four overarching and interacting themes (Belmonte and Bourgeron 2006): (1) anomalies in synaptic formation, maintenance, or signal transduction, (2) imbalance between excitatory and inhibitory tone, (3) abnormal cell number, and (4) abnormal neuromodulation.

Evidence for abnormalities at the synapse comes from rare variants associated with familial autism, as well as from more common variants associated with comorbid syndromes. Autism is comorbid with Fragile X syndrome, caused by transcriptional silencing of FMR1. FMR1 encodes FMRP, an mRNA-binding protein that negatively regulates activity-dependent synaptic modification in response to activation of Group I metabotropic glutamate receptors (Bear *et al.* 2004). Absence of FMRP thus results in runaway synaptic plasticity.

Also relevant to synaptic function, familial variants of the neuroligin genes NLGN3 and NLGN4 segregate with autism (Jamain *et al.* 2003; Laumonnier *et al.* 2004), as do variants of the neuroligin binding partner genes neurexin-1 (NRXN1) (Kim *et al.* 2008) and SHANK3 (Durand *et al.* 2007; Moessner *et al.* 2007), and the neurexin superfamily member contactin-associated protein-like 2 (CNTNAP2) (Alarcón *et al.* 2008; Arking *et al.* 2008). Among other functions, the balance between excitatory and inhibitory synapses is regulated by neuroligins (Chih *et al.* 2005).

Further to excitatory-inhibitory balance, autism has been associated with the ionotropic NMDA receptor gene GRIN2A (Barnby *et al.* 2005) and the ionotropic kainate receptor gene GRIK2 (Jamain *et al.* 2002), and with the GABA receptor subunit gene GABRB3 (Buxbaum *et al.* 2002). GABRB3 in turn is regulated by the methyl-CpG binding protein MeCP2 (Samaco *et al.* 2005), disrupted in Rett syndrome, with which autism is again comorbid.

Regarding cell number, the tumour suppressor genes NF1 and TSC1/TSC2 code for GTPase-activating proteins with widespread effects on cell survival, cell structure and cell function. These, along with the lipid phosphatase tumour suppressor PTEN, negatively regulate the phosphoinositide-3 kinase pathway which spurs cell growth and synaptogenesis and blocks apoptosis. PTEN mutation, in particular, has been associated with cases of autism with macrocephaly (Butler *et al.* 2005), and variations in these three genes may explain autism's comorbidity with neurofibromatosis, tuberous sclerosis, and Cowden syndrome, respectively. Also recently linked to autism is a promoter polymorphism that decreases expression of the MET gene (Campbell *et al.* 2006). MET encodes a receptor tyrosine kinase active not only in brain development but also in immune and gastrointestinal functions—an association that may explain comorbidities in these domains in some cases of autism.

The major result in neuromodulaton and autism concerns the serotonin membrane transporter gene SLC6A4. The short allele of the SLC6A4 promoter is associated with increased volume of cerebral cortical and especially frontal grey matter in autism (Wassink *et al.* 2007), and the division of results between preferential transmission of long and short alleles in autism suggests a gene dosage effect or interaction with other susceptibility and resistance factors (Belmonte and Bourgeron 2006).

Many of these genetic variations may have divergent endophenotypic effects, helping to explain the partial independence of some autistic traits (Ronald *et al.* 2006) as well as the population continuum between autism spectrum conditions and normal cognitive variation (Constantino and Todd 2005), including the subclinical, broader autism phenotype found in some family members (Piven *et al.* 1997; Dawson *et al.* 2002). In addition to this locus and allelic heterogeneity, gene dosage is likely to play a major role, as evidenced by recent findings of copy number variation as a contributing factor especially in sporadic, non-familial cases of autism (Sebat *et al.* 2007). The future of research in this field will be not only to isolate the relevant genes but also to understand the networks within which these genes function, and ultimately the relationships between these different causal levels in autism. It is hoped that during this research endeavour there will also be evaluations of the most promising treatments.

2.5 Clinical implications

Past attempts to teach emotion recognition to adults and children with ASC have either focused on the basic emotions (Hadwin *et al.* 1996; Howlin *et al.* 1999) or have been part of social skills training courses, usually run in groups (Howlin *et al.* 1999; Rydin *et al.* 1999; Barry *et al.* 2003). Typically, these training programmes do not focus specifically on systematically teaching emotion recognition, but instead address other issues, such as conversation, reducing socially inappropriate behaviour, personal hygiene, etc. In such groups it is difficult to target the individual's specific pace of learning. Finally, such groups are socially demanding and therefore might deter more socially anxious participants.

Other attempts to teach individuals with ASC social skills have used computer-based training (Swettenham 1996; Rajendran and Mitchell 2000; Bernard-Opitz *et al.* 2001; Silver and Oakes 2001; Bolte *et al.* 2002; Hetzroni and Tannous 2004). The use of computer software for individuals with autism spectrum conditions has several advantages: First, individuals with ASC favour the computerized environment since it is predictable, consistent, and free from social demands, which they may find stressful. Secondly, users can work at their own pace and level of understanding. Thirdly, lessons can be repeated over and over again until mastery is achieved. Fourthly, interest and motivation can be maintained through different and individually selected computerized rewards (Moore *et al.* 2000; Parsons and Mitchell 2002; Bishop 2003). Previous studies have found that the use of computers can help individuals with autism pass false-belief tasks (Swettenham 1996), recognize basic emotions from cartoons and still photographs (Silver and Oakes 2001; Bolte *et al.* 2002), and solve problems in illustrated social situations (Bernard-Opitz *et al.* 2001). However, participants find it hard to generalize their knowledge from learnt material to related tasks.

The computer-based interventions above used drawings or photographs for training, rather than more life-like stimuli. This might have made generalization harder than if more ecologically valid stimuli were used. In addition, the programs teaching emotion recognition focused on basic emotions, and only on facial expressions. No reported program to date has systematically trained complex emotion recognition in both visual and auditory channels, with life-like faces and voices.

We have recently evaluated *Mind Reading* (Baron-Cohen *et al.* 2004), an interactive guide to emotions and mental states, and its value as a tailored teaching tool for emotion recognition for learners on the autistic spectrum. *Mind Reading* is based on a taxonomic system of 412 emotions and mental states, grouped into 24 emotion groups and six developmental levels (from age 4 to adulthood). The emotions and mental states are organized systematically, according to the emotion groups and developmental levels. Each emotion group is introduced and demonstrated by a short video clip giving some clues for later analysis of the emotions in this group. Each emotion is defined and demonstrated in six silent films of faces, six voice recordings, and six written examples of situations that evoke this emotion. The resulting library of emotional 'assets' (video clips, audio clips, or brief stories) comprises $412 \times 18 = 7416$ units of emotion information to learn to recognize or understand. Therefore this is a rich and systematically organized set of educational material. The software was created for the use of children and adults of various levels of functioning. Vocal and animated helpers give instructions on every screen.

We tested for any improvement in *adults* with HFA/AS in emotion recognition skills following *independent* use of the software, and the extent to which these users can generalize their acquired knowledge. The intervention took place over a period of 10–15 weeks to ensure a meaningful period for training, recognizing that a longer duration might lead to individuals dropping out. Participants were tested before and after the intervention. A no-computer-intervention control group of adults with HFA/AS was matched to the intervention group. This HFA/AS control group was also tested before and after a similar period of time, but had no intervention. The need for a no-intervention HFA/AS group was to assess whether any improvement was related to the intervention or was merely due to taking the tasks twice or to time passing. A third typical control group from the general population was matched to the intervention groups. This group was only tested once, to obtain baseline measures.

Results showed that following 10–20 hours of using the software over a period of 10–15 weeks, users with ASC significantly improved in their ability to recognize complex emotions and mental states from both faces and voices, compared with their performance before the intervention, relative to the control group. This finding is interesting, considering the short usage time and the large number of emotions included in the software, and since participants were not asked to study these particular emotions (Golan and Baron-Cohen 2006).

The above study illustrates one practical teaching method focused on improving mindreading in ASC, but it should be recognized that other approaches (such as preverbal intervention to encourage the development of shared attention) are also being explored.

2.6 Future directions

The area of social cognition in ASC remains important, and in this chapter we have necessarily reviewed research in a range of separate areas (cognitive development, neuroimaging, neuroanatomy, genetics, intervention). The hope is that, in the future, interdisciplinary science will take place so that we can integrate these currently disparate areas and discover which brain regions change as a result of intervention, or are under the control of which genetic mechanisms, in which subgroup on the autistic spectrum.

Acknowledgements

OG was supported by the National Alliance for Autism Research (NAAR) and the Wingate Foundation, SBC was supported by the Medical Research Council, and BC was supported by Trinity College Cambridge. Parts of this chapter are reproduced from elsewhere. (Belmonte *et al.* 2004b; Baron-Cohen 2005; Baron-Cohen and Belmonte 2005; Chakrabarti and Baron-Cohen 2006; Golan and Baron-Cohen 2006).

References

Abrahams, B.S. and Geschwind, D.H. (2008). Advances in autism genetics: on the threshold of a new neurobiology. *Nature Reviews Genetics*, **9**, 341–355.

Alarcón, M., Abrahams, B.S., Stone, J.L., *et al.* (2008). Linkage, association, and gene-expression analyses identify CNTNAP2 as an autism-susceptibility gene. *American Journal of Human Genetics*, **82**, 150–159.

American Psychiatric Association (1994). *Diagnostic and statistical manual of mental disorders*, (4th edn) (DSM-IV). Washington, DC: American Psychiatric Association.

Adolphs, R., Sears, L., and Piven, J. (2001). Abnormal processing of social information from faces in autism. *Journal of Cognitive Neuroscience*, **13**, 232–40.

Arking, D.E., Cutler, D.J., Brune, *et al.* (2008). A common genetic variant in the neurexin superfamily member CNTNAP2 increases familial risk of autism. *American Journal of Human Genetics*, **82**, 160–164.

Ashwin, C., Baron-Cohen, S., Wheelwright, S., O'Riordan, M., and Bullmore, E.T. (2007). Differential activiation of the social brain during fearful face-processing in adults with and without autism. *Neuropsychologia*, **45**, 2–14.

Asperger, H. (1944). Die 'autistischen Psychopathen' im Kindesalter. *Archiv fur Psychiatrie und Nervenkrankheiten*, **117**, 76–136.

Attwood, T. (1997). *Asperger's syndrome*. London: Jessica Kingsley.

Aylward, E.H., Minshew, N.J., Goldstein, G., et al. (1999). MRI volumes of amygdala and hippocampus in non-mentally retarded autistic adolescents and adults. *Neurology*, **53**, 2145–50.

Aylward, E.H., Minshew, N.J., Field, K., Sparks, B.F., and Singh, N. (2002). Effects of age on brain volume and head circumference in autism. *Neurology*, **59**, 175–83.

Bailey, A., Le Couteur, A., Gottesman, I., et al. (1995). Autism as a strongly genetic disorder: evidence from a British twin study. *Psychological Medicine*, **25**, 63–77.

Ballaban-Gil, K. and Tuchman, R. (2000). Epilepsy and epileptiform EEG: association with autism and language disorders. *Mental Retardation and Developmental Disabilties Research Reviews*, **6**, 300–8.

Barnby, G., Abbott, A., Sykes, N., et al. and the International Molecular Genetics Study of Autism Consortium. (2005). Candidate-gene screening and association analysis at the autism-susceptibility locus on chromosome 16p: evidence of association at GRIN2A and ABAT. *American Journal of Human Genetics*, **76**, 950–966.

Baron-Cohen, S. (1987). Autism and symbolic play. *British Journal of Developmental Psychology*, **5**, 139–48.

Baron-Cohen, S. (1988). Social and pragmatic deficits in autism: cognitive or affective? *Journal of Autism and Developmental Disorders*, **18**, 379–402.

Baron-Cohen, S. (1989a). The autistic child's theory of mind: a case of specific developmental delay. *Journal of Child Psychology and Psychiatry*, **30**, 285–98.

Baron-Cohen, S. (1989b). Perceptual role taking and protodeclarative pointing in autism. *British Journal of Developmental Psychology*, **7**, 113–27.

Baron-Cohen, S. (1991). Precursors to a theory of mind: understanding attention in others. In *Natural theories of mind* (ed. A Whiten). Oxford: Basil Blackwell.

Baron-Cohen, S. (1994). The Mindreading System: new directions for research. *Current Psychology of Cognition*, **13**, 724–50.

Baron-Cohen, S. (1995). *Mindblindness: an essay on autism and theory of mind*. Cambridge, MA: MIT Press/Bradford Books.

Baron-Cohen, S. (2002). The extreme male brain theory of autism. *Trends in Cognitive Science*, **6**, 248–54.

Baron-Cohen, S. (2003). *The essential difference: men, women and the extreme male brain*. Harmondsworth: Penguin Books.

Baron-Cohen, S. (2005). Autism. In *Cambridge Encyclopaedia of Child Development*. Cambridge University Press.

Baron-Cohen, S. (2006). Two new theories of autism: hypersystemizing and assortative mating. *Archives of Diseases in Childhood*, **91**, 2–5.

Baron-Cohen, S. and Belmonte, M.K. (2005). Autism: a window onto the development of the social and the analytic brain. *Annual Review of Neuroscience*, **28**, 109–26.

Baron-Cohen, S. and Swettenham, J. (1996). The relationship between SAM and ToMM: the lock and key hypothesis. In *Theories of Theories of Mind* (ed. P. Carruthers and P. Smith). Cambridge University Press.

Baron-Cohen, S. and Wheelwright, S. (2004). The empathy quotient (eq). an investigation of adults with Asperger syndrome or high functioning autism, and normal sex differences. *Journal of Autism and Developmental Disorders*, **34**, 163–75.

Baron-Cohen, S., Leslie, A.M. and Frith, U. (1985). Does the autistic child have a 'theory of mind'? *Cognition*, **21**, 37–46.

Baron-Cohen, S., Leslie, A.M. and Frith, U. (1986). Mechanical, behavioural and Intentional understanding of picture stories in autistic children. *British Journal of Developmental Psychology*, 4, 113–25.

Baron-Cohen, S., Spitz, A., and Cross, P. (1993a). Can children with autism recognize surprise? *Cognition and Emotion*, 7, 507–16.

Baron-Cohen, S., Tager-Flusberg, H., and Cohen, D. (ed.) (1993b). *Understanding other minds: perspectives from autism*. Oxford University Press.

Baron-Cohen, S., Ring, H., Moriarty, J., Shmitz, P., Costa, D., and Ell, P. (1994). Recognition of mental state terms: a clinical study of autism, and a functional neuroimaging study of normal adults. *British Journal of Psychiatry*, 165, 640–9.

Baron-Cohen, S., Jolliffe, T., Mortimore, C., and Robertson, M. (1997a). Another advanced test of theory of mind: evidence from very high functioning adults with autism or Asperger syndrome. *Journal of Child Psychology and Psychiatry*, 38, 813–22.

Baron-Cohen, S., Wheelwright, S., and Jolliffe, T. (1997b). Is there a 'language of the eyes'? Evidence from normal adults and adults with autism or Asperger syndrome. *Visual Cognition*, 4, 311–31.

Baron-Cohen, S., O'Riordan, M., Jones, R., Stone, V., and Plaisted, K. (1999a). A new test of social sensitivity: detection of *faux pas* in normal children and children with Asperger syndrome. *Journal of Autism and Developmental Disorders*, 29, 407–18.

Baron-Cohen, S., Wheelwright, S., Stone, V., and Rutherford, M. (1999b). A mathematician, a physicist, and a computer scientist with Asperger syndrome: performance on folk psychology and folk physics test. *Neurocase*, 5, 475–83.

Baron-Cohen, S., Ring, H., Wheelwright, S., *et al.* (1999c). Social intelligence in the normal and autistic brain: an fMRI study. *European Journal of Neuroscience*, 11, 1891–8.

Baron-Cohen, S., Ring, H., Bullmore, E., Wheelwright, S., Ashwin, C., and Williams, S. (2000). The amygdala theory of autism. *Neuroscience and Behavioural Reviews*, 24, 355–64.

Baron-Cohen, S., Wheelwright, S., Hill, J., Raste, Y., and Plumb, I. (2001a). The 'Reading the Mind in the Eyes' test revised version: a study with normal adults, and adults with Asperger syndrome or high-functioning autism. *Journal of Child Psychology and Psychiatry*, 42, 241–52.

Baron-Cohen, S., Wheelwright, S., Skinner, R., Martin, J., and Clubley, E. (2001b). The Autism Spectrum Quotient (AQ): evidence from Asperger syndrome/high functioning autism, males and females, scientists and mathematicians. *Journal of Autism and Developmental Disorders*, 31, 5–17.

Baron-Cohen, S., Richler, J., Bisarya, D., Gurunathan, N., and Wheelwright, S. (2003). The Systemising Quotient (SQ): an investigation of adults with Asperger syndrome or high functioning autism and normal sex differences. *Philosophical Transactions of the Royal Society of London*, 358, 361–74.

Baron-Cohen, S., Golan, O., Wheelwright, S., and Hill, J.J. (2004). *Mind reading: the interactive guide to emotions*. London: Jessica Kingsley.

Baron-Cohen, S., Knickmeyer, R.C., and Belmonte, M.K. (2005). Sex differences in the brain: implications for explaining autism. *Science*, 310, 819–23.

Barry, T.D., Klinger, L.G., Lee, J.M., Palardy, N., Gilmore, T., and Bodin, S.D. (2003). Examining the effectiveness of an out-patient clinic-based social skills group for high-functioning children with autism. *Journal of Autism and Developmental Disorders*, **33**, 685–701.

Bauman, M. and Kemper, T. (1985). Histoanatomic observation of the brain in early infantile autism. *Neurology*, **35**, 866–74.

Bauman, M. and Kemper, T. (1994). Neuroanatomic observations of the brain in autism. In *The neurobiology of autism* (ed. M.L. Bauman and T.L. Kemper), pp. 119–45. Baltimore, MD: John Hopkins University Press.

Bear, M.F., Huber, K.M. and Warren, S.T. (2004). The mGluR theory of fragile X mental retardation. *Trends in Neurosciences*, **27**, 370–377.

Belmonte, M.K. (2000). Abnormal attention in autism shown by steady-state visual evoked potentials. *Autism*, **4**, 269–85.

Belmonte, M.K. and Bourgeron, T. (2006). Fragile X syndrome and autism at the intersection of genetic and neural networks. *Nature Neuroscience*, **9**, 1221–1225.

Belmonte, M.K. and Carper, R.A. (2006). Monozygotic twins with Asperger syndrome: differences in behaviour reflect variations in brain structure and function. *Brain and Cognition*, **61**, 110–21.

Belmonte, M.K. and Yurgelun-Todd, D.A. (2003). Functional anatomy of impaired selective attention and compensatory processing in autism. *Brain Research. Cognitive Brain Research*, **17**, 651–64.

Belmonte, M.K., Allen, G., Beckel-Mitchener, A., Boulanger, L.M., Carper, R., and Webb, S.J. (2004a). Autism and abnormal development of brain connnectivity. *Journal of Neuroscience*, **24**, 9228–31.

Belmonte, M.K., Cook, E.H., Anderson, G.M., *et al.* (2004b). Autism as a disorder of neural information processing: directions for research and targets for therapy. *Molecular Psychiatry*, **9**, 646–63. Unabridged edition available at: http:// www.cureautism now.org/conferences/summitmeetings.

Bernard-Opitz, V., Sriram, N., and Nakhoda Supuan, S. (2001). Enhancing social problem solving with children with autism and normal children through computer-assisted instruction. *Journal of Autism and Developmental Disorders*, **31**, 377–98.

Bishop, J. (2003). The internet for educating individuals with social impairments. *Journal of Computer Assisted Learning*, **19**, 546–56.

Blair, R.J., Jones, L., Clark, F., and Smith, M. (1997). The psychopathic individual: A lack of responsiveness to distress cues? *Psychophysiology*, **34**, 192–8.

Bolte, S., Feineis-Matthews, S., Leber, S., Dierks, T., Hubl, D., and Poustka, F. (2002). The development and evaluation of a computer-based program to test and to teach the recognition of facial affect. *International Journal of Circumpolar Health*, **61**, 61–8.

Boucher, J., Lewis, V., and Collis, G.M. (2000). Voice processing abilities in children with autism, children with specific language impairments, and young typically developing children. *Journal of Child Psychology and Psychiatry*, **41**, 847–58.

Brothers, L. (1990). The social brain: a project for integrating primate behaviour and neurophysiology in a new domain. *Concepts in Neuroscience*, **1**, 27–51.

Brothers, L., Ring, B., and Kling, A. (1990). Responses of neurons in the macaque amygdala to complex social stimuli. *Behavioural Brain Research*, **41**, 199–213.

Brunet, E., Sarfati, Y., Hardy-Bayle, M.C., and Decety, J. (2000). A PET investigation of the attribution of intentions with a non-verbal task. *NeuroImage*, **11**, 157–66.

Butler, M.G., Dasouki, M.J., Zhou, X.P., et al. (2005). Subset of individuals with autism spectrum disorders and extreme macrocephaly associated with germline PTEN tumour suppressor gene mutations. *Journal of Medical Genetics*, **42**, 318–321.

Buxbaum, J.D., Silverman, J.M., Smith, et al. (2002). Association between a GABRB3 polymorphism and autism. *Molecular Psychiatry*, **7**, 311–316.

Campbell, D.B., Sutcliffe, J.S., Ebert, P.J., et al. (2006). A genetic variant that disrupts MET transcription is associated with autism. *Proceedings of the National Academy of Sciences of the United States of America*, **103**, 16834–16839.

Calder, A.J., Lawrence, A.D., Keane, J., et al. (2002). Reading the mind from eye gaze. *Neuropsychologia*, **40**, 1129–38.

Carper, R.A. and Courchesne, E. (2000). Inverse correlation between frontal lobe and cerebellum sizes in children with autism. *Brain*, **123**, 836–44.

Casanova, M.F., Buxhoeveden, D.P., Switala, A.E., and Roy, E. (2002a). Asperger's syndrome and cortical neuropathology. *Journal of Child Neurology*, **17**, 142–5.

Casanova, M.F., Buxhoeveden, D.P., Switala, A.E., and Roy, E. (2002b). Minicolumnar pathology in autism. *Neurology*, **58**, 428–32.

Castelli, F., Happé, F., Frith, U., and Frith, C. (2000). Movement and mind: a functional imaging study of perception and interpretation of complex intentional movement patterns. *NeuroImage*, **12**, 314–25.

Castelli, F., Frith, C., Happé, F., and Frith, U. (2002). Autism, Asperger syndrome and brain mechanisms for the attribution of mental states to animated shapes. *Brain*, **125**, 1839–49.

Celani, G., Battacchi, M.W., and Arcidiacono, L. (1999). The understanding of the emotional meaning of facial expressions in people with autism. *Journal of Autism and Developmental Disorders*, **29**, 57–66.

Chakrabarti, B. and Baron-Cohen, S. (2006). Empathizing: neurocognitive developmental mechanisms and individual differences. In *Understanding emotions: progress in brain research*, pp. 403–418. Amsterdam: Elsevier.

Chih, B., Engelman, H. and Scheiffele, P. Control of excitatory and inhibitory synapse formation by neuroligins. (2005). *Science*, **307**, 1324–1328.

Cleckley, H.M. (1977). *The mask of sanity: an attempt to clarify some issues about the so-called psychopathic personality.* St Louis, MO: Mosby.

Constantino, J.N. and Todd, R.D. (2005). Intergenerational transmission of subthreshold autistic traits in the general population. *Biological Psychiatry*, **57**, 655–660.

Connellan, J., Baron-Cohen, S., Wheelwright, S., Ba'tki, A., and Ahluwalia, J. (2001). Sex differences in human neonatal social perception. *Infant Behavior and Development*, **23**, 113–18.

Courchesne, E. (2002). Abnormal early brain development in autism. *Molecular Psychiatry*, **7**, 21–3.

Courchesne, E. and Pierce, K. (2005). Why the frontal cortex in autism might be talking only to itself: local over-connectivity but long-distance disconnection. *Current Opinion in Neurobiology*, **15**, 225–30.

Courchesne, E., Yeung-Courchesne, R., Press, G., Hesselink, J., and Jernigan, T. (1988). Hypoplasia of cerebellar vermal lobules VI and VII in infantile autism. *New England Journal of Medicine*, **318**, 1349–54.

Courchesne, E., Press, G.A., and Yeung-Courchesne, R. (1993). Parietal lobe abnormalities detected with MR in patients with infantile autism. *American Journal of Roentgenology*, **160**, 387–93.

Courchesne, E., Saitoh, O., Yeung-Courchesne, R., *et al.* (1994a). Abnormality of cerebellar vermian lobules VI and VII in patients with infantile autism: identification of hypoplastic and hyperplastic subgroups with MR imaging. *American Journal of Roentgenology*, **162**, 123–30.

Courchesne, E., Townsend, J., Akshoomof, N.A., *et al.* (1994b). Impairment in shifting attention in autistic and cerebellar patients. *Behavioural Neuroscience*, **108**, 848–65.

Courchesne, E., Townsend, J., Akshoomoff, N.A., *et al.* (1994c). A new finding: impairment in shifting attention in autistic and cerebellar patients. In *Atypical cognitive deficits in developmental disorders: implications for brain function* (ed. SH Broman and J Grafman). Hillsdale, NJ: Lawrence Erlbaum.

Courchesne, E., Townsend, J., and Saitoh, O. (1994d). The brain in infantile autism: posterior fossa structures are abnormal. *Neurology*, **44**, 214–23.

Courchesne, E., Karns, C.M., Davis, H.R., *et al.* (2001). Unusual brain growth patterns in early life of patients with autistic disorder. *Neurology*, **57**, 245–54.

Critchley, H.D., Daly, E.M., Bullmore, E.T., *et al.* (2000). The functional neuroanatomy of social behaviour: changes in cerebral blood flow when people with autistic disorder process facial expressions. *Brain*, **123**, 2203–12.

Dalton, K.M., Nacewicz, B.M., Johnstone, T., *et al.* (2005). Gaze fixation and the neural circuitry of face processing in autism. *Nature Neuroscience*, **10**, 1–8.

Dapretto, M., Davies, M.S., Pfeifer, J.H., *et al.* (2006). Understanding emotions in others: mirror neuron dysfunction in children with autism spectrum disorders. *Nature Neuroscience*, **9**, 28–30.

Dawson, G., Webb, S., Schellenberg, G.D., Dager, S., Friedman, S., Aylward, E. and Richards, T. (2002). Defining the broader phenotype of autism: genetic, brain, and behavioral perspectives. *Development and Psychopathology*, **14**, 581–611.

Decety, J. and Chaminade, T. (2003). Neural correlates of feeling sympathy. *Neuropsychologia*, **41**, 127–38.

Decety, J. and Jackson, P. (2004). The functional architecture of human empathy. *Behavioural and Cognitive Neuroscience Reviews*, **3**, 71–100.

DeLorey, T.M., Handforth, A., Anagnostaras, S.G., *et al.* (1998). Mice lacking the Beta3 subunit of the GABAa receptor have the epilepsy phenotype and many of the behavioural characteristics of Angelman syndrome. *Journal of Neuroscience*, **18**, 8505–14.

Deruelle, C., Rondan, C., Gepner, B., and Tardif, C. (2004). Spatial frequency and face processing in children with autism and Asperger syndrome. *Journal of Autism and Developmental Disorders*, **34**, 199–210.

Dimberg, U., Thunberg, M., and Elmehed, K. (2000). Unconscious facial reactions to emotional facial expressions. *Psychological Science*, **11**, 86–9.

Durand, C.M., Betancur, C., Boeckers, T.M., Bockmann, J., *et al.* (2007). Mutations in the gene encoding the synaptic scaffolding protein SHANK3 are associated with autism spectrum disorders. *Nature Genetics*, **39**, 25–27.

Egaas, B., Courchesne, E., and Saitoh, O. (1995). Reduced size of corpus callosum in autism. *Archives of Neurology*, **52**, 794–801.

Ekman, P. (1993). Facial expression and emotion. *American Psychologist*, **48**, 384–92.

Ekman, P. and Friesen, W. (1969). The repertoire of non-verbal behavior: categories, origins, usage, and coding. *Semiotica*, **1**, 49–98.

Ekman, P. and Friesen, W. (1971). Constants across cultures in the face and emotion. *Journal of Personality and Social Psychology*, **17**, 124–9.

Fein, D., Lucci, D., Braverman, M., and Waterhouse, L. (1992). Comprehension of affect in context in children with pervasive developmental disorders. *Journal of Child Psychology and Psychiatry*, **33**, 1157–67.

Field, T. (1979). Visual and cardiac responses to animate and inanimate faces by term and preterm infants. *Child Development*, **50**, 188–94.

Frith, U. (1989). *Autism: explaining the enigma*. Oxford: Basil Blackwell.

Frith, U. and Frith, C. (2003). Development and neurophysiology of mentalizing. *Philosophical Transactions of the Royal Society of London*, **358**, 459–73.

Golan, O. and Baron-Cohen, S. (2006). Systemising empathy: teaching adults with Asperger syndrome to recognise complex emotions using interactive multi-media. *Development and Psychopathology*, **18**, 589–615.

Golan, O., Baron-Cohen, S., Hill, J.J. (2006a). The Cambridge Mindreading (CAM) Face–Voice Battery: Testing complex emotion recognition in adults with and without Asperger syndrome. *Journal of Autism and Developmental Disorders*, **36**, 169–183.

Golan, O., Baron-Cohen, S., Hill, J.J., and Golan, Y. (2006b). Reading the Mind in Films – testing recognition of complex emotions and mental states in adults with and without autism spectrum conditions. *Social Neuroscience*, **1**, 111–23.

Golan, O., Baron-Cohen, S., Rutherford, M. D., and Hill, J.J. (2007). Reading the Mind in the Voice – Revised. A study of adults with and without Asperger syndrome. *Journal of Autism and Developmental Disorders*, **37**, 1096–1106.

Goldenfeld, N., Baron-Cohen, S., Wheelwright, S., Ashwin, C., and Chakrabarti, B. (2007). Empathizing and systemizing in males and females, and autism: a test of neural competition theory. In *Empathy and mental illness* (ed. T Farrow and P Woodruff), pp. 322–34. Cambridge University Press.

Grossman, J.B., Klin, A., Carter, A.S., and Volkmar, F.R. (2000). Verbal bias in recognition of facial emotions in children with Asperger syndrome. *Journal of Child Psychology and Psychiatry*, **41**, 369–79.

Hadwin, J., Baron-Cohen, S., Howlin, P., and Hill, K. (1996). Can we teach children with autism to understand emotions, belief, or pretence? *Development and Psychopathology*, **8**, 345–65.

Happé, F. (1994). An advanced test of theory of mind: understanding of story characters' thoughts and feelings by able autistic, mentally handicapped, and normal children and adults. *Journal of Autism and Development Disorders*, **24**, 129–54.

Happé, F. and Frith, U. (1996). Theory of mind and social impairment in children with conduct disorder. *British Journal of Developmental Psychology*, **14**, 385–98.

Happé, F., Ehlers, S., Fletcher, P., *et al.* (1996). Theory of mind in the brain: evidence from a PET scan study of Asperger syndrome. *Neuroreport*, **8**, 197–201.

Hare, R.D., Hakstian, T.J., Ralph, A., *et al.* (1990). The Revised Psychopathy Checklist: reliability and factor structure. *Psychological Assessment*, **2**, 338–41.

Harris, N.S., Courchesne, E., Townsend, J., Carper, R.A., and Lord, C. (1999). Neuroanatomic contributions to slowed orienting of attention in children with autism. *Cognitive Brain Research*, **8**, 61–71.

Harris, P (1989). *Children and emotions*. London: Blackwell.

Hashimoto, T., Tayama, M., Murakawa, K., *et al.* (1995). Development of the brainstem and cerebellum in autistic patients. *Journal of Autism and Developmental Disorders*, **25**, 1–17.

Haxby, J.V., Hoffman, E.A., and Gobbini M.I. (2000). The distributed human neural system for face perception. *Trends in Cognitive Sciences*, **4**, 223–33.

Heavey, L., Phillips, W., Baron-Cohen, S., and Rutter, M. (2000). The awkward moments test. A naturalistic measure of social understanding in autism. *Journal of Autism and Developmental Disorders*, **30**, 225–36.

Herbert, M.R., Zeigler, D.A., Makris, N., *et al.* (2002). White matter increases in autism are largely in superficial radiate regions. Presented at the International Meeting for Autism Research, Orlando, FL.

Herbert, M.R., Zeigler, D.A., Deutsch, C.K., *et al.* (2003). Dissociations of cerebral cortex, subcortical and cerebral white matter volumes in autistic boys. *Brain*, **126**, 1182–92.

Hetzroni, O.E. and Tannous, J. (2004). Effects of a computer-based intervention program on the communicative functionsof children with autism. *Journal of Autism and Developmental Disorders*, **34**, 95–113.

Hirstein, W., Iversen, P., and Ramachandran, V.S. (2001). Autonomic responses of autistic children to people and objects. *Proceedings of the Royal Society of London, Series B*, **268**, 1883–8.

Hobson, R.P. (1986a). The autistic child's appraisal of expressions of emotion. *Journal of Child Psychology and Psychiatry*, **27**, 321–42.

Hobson, R.P. (1986b). The autistic child's appraisal of expression of emotion: a further study. *Journal of Child Psychology and Psychiatry*, **27**, 671–80.

Hobson, R.P., Ouston, J., and Lee, A. (1988). Emotion recognition in autism: coordinating faces and voices. *Psychological Medicine*, **18**, 911–23.

Homanics, G.E., DeLorey, T.M., Firestone, L.L., *et al.* (1997). Mice devoid of gamma-aminobutyrate type A receptor beta3 subunit have epilepsy, cleft palate and hypersensitive behaviour. *Proceedings of the National Academy of Sciences of the USA*, **94**, 4143–8.

Howlin, P., Baron-Cohen, S., and Hadwin, J. (1999). *Teaching children with autism to mindread: a practical guide*. Chichester: John Wiley.

Jamain, S., Betancur, C., Quach, H., Philippe, A., Fellous, M., Giros, B., Gillberg, C., Leboyer, M., Bourgeron, T. and the Paris Autism Research International Sibpair Study. (2002). Linkage and association of the glutamate receptor 6 gene with autism. *Molecular Psychiatry*, **7**, 302–310.

Jamain, S., Quach, H., Betancur, C., *et al.* and the Paris Autism Research International Sibpair Study. (2003). Mutations of the X-linked genes encoding neuroligins NLGN3 and NLGN4 are associated with autism. *Nature Genetics*, **34**, 27–29.

Jolliffe, T. and Baron-Cohen, S. (1999). The Strange Stories Test: a replication with high-functioning adults with autism or Asperger syndrome. *Journal of Autism and Developmental Disorders*, **29**, 395–404.

Jorde, L., Hasstedt, S., Ritvo, E., *et al.* (1991). Complex segregation analysis of autism. *American Journal of Human Genetics*, **49**, 932–38.

Kemner, C., Verbaten, M.N., Cuperus, J.M., Camfferman, G., and van Engeland, H. (1994). Visual and somotosensory event-related brain potentials in autistic children and three different control groups. *EEG Clinical Neurophysiology*, **92**, 225–37.

Kemner, C., Verbaten, M.N., Cuperus, J.M., Camfferman, G., and van Engeland, H. (1995). Auditory event-related brain potentials in autistic children and three different control groups. *Biological Psychiatry*, **38**, 150–65.

Keysers, C. and Perrett, D.I. (2004). Demystifying social cognition: a Hebbian perspective. *Trends in Cognitive Science*, **8**, 501–7.

Kim, H.G., Kishikawa, S., Higgins, *et al.* (2008). Disruption of neurexin 1 associated with autism spectrum disorder. *American Journal of Human Genetics*, **82**, 199–207.

Kleinman, J., Marciano, P.L., and Ault, R.L. (2001). Advanced theory of mind in high-functioning adults with autism. *Journal of Autism and Developmental Disorders*, **31**, 29–36.

Klin, A., Jones, W., Schulz, R., Volkmar, F., and Cohen, D.J. (2002). Visual fixation patterns during viewing of naturalistic social situations as predictors of social competence in individuals with autism. *Archives of General Psychiatry*, **9**, 809–16.

Kling, A. and Brothers, L. (1992). The amygdala and social behavior. In *Neurobiological aspects of emotion, memory, and mental dysfunction* (ed. J. Aggleton). New York: Wiley–Liss.

Klinnert, M.D. (1984). The regulation of infant behaviour by maternal facial expression. *Infant Behaviour and Development*, **7**, 447–65.

Laumonnier, F., Bonnet-Brilhault, F., Gomot, M., *et al.* (2004). X-linked mental retardation and autism are associated with a mutation in the NLGN4 gene, a member of the neuroligin family. *American Journal of Human Genetics*, **74**, 552–557.

Leslie, A.M. (1987). Pretence and representation: the origins of 'theory of mind'. *Psychological Review*, **94**, 412–26.

Leslie, A. (1995). ToMM, ToBy, and Agency: core architecture and domain specificity. In *Domain specificity in cognition and culture* (ed. L Hirschfeld and S Gelman). New York: Cambridge University Press.

Lord, C., Rutter, M., and Le Couteur, A. (1994). Autism Diagnostic Interview—Revised. *Journal of Autism and Developmental Disorders*, **24**, 659–86.

Loveland, K.A., Tunali Kotoski, B., Chen, R., and Brelsford, K.A. (1995). Intermodal perception of affect in persons with autism or Down's syndrome. *Development and Psychopathology*, **7**, 409–18.

Loveland, K.A., Tunali Kotoski, B., Chen, Y.R., *et al.* (1997). Emotion recognition in autism: verbal and non-verbal information. *Development and Psychopathology*, **9**, 579–93.

Lutchmaya, S., Baron-Cohen, S., and Raggatt, P. (2002). Foetal testosterone and eye contact in 12 month old infants. *Infant Behavior and Development*, **25**, 327–35.

McAlonan, G.M., Cheung, V., Suckling, J., *et al.* (2005). Mapping the brain in autism: a voxel based MRI study of volumetric differences and intercorrelations in autism. *Brain*, **128**, 268–76.

MacDonald, H., Rutter, M., Howlin, P., *et al.* (1989). Recognition and expression of emotional cues by autistic and normal adults. *Journal of Child Psychology and Psychiatry*, **30**, 865–77.

Mealey, L. (1995). The sociobiology of sociopathy: an integrated evolutionary model. *Behavioral and Brain Sciences*, **18**, 523–99.

Meltzoff, A.N. and Decety, J. (2003). What imitation tells us about social cognition: a rapproachement between developmental psychology and cognitive neuroscience. *Philosophical Transactions of the Royal Society of London*, **358**, 491–500.

Moessner, R., Marshall, C.R., Sutcliffe, J.S., et al. (2007). Contribution of SHANK3 mutations to autism spectrum disorder. *American Journal of Human Genetics*, **81**, 1289–1297.

Moore, D., McGrath, P., and Thorpe, J. (2000). Computer-aided learning for people with autism—a framework for research and development. *Innovations in Education and Training International*, **37**, 218–28.

Murakami, J., Courchesne, E., Press, G., Yeung-Courchesne, R., and Hesselink, J. (1989). Reduced cerebellar hemisphere size and its relationship to vermal hypoplasia in autism. *Archives of Neurology*, **46**, 689–94.

Neiminen-von Wendt, T.S., Metsahonkala, L., Kulomaki, T.A., et al. (2003). Changes in cerebral blood flow in Asperger syndrome during theory of mind tasks presented by the auditory route. *European Child and Adolescent Psychiatry*, **12**, 172–89.

O'Roak, B.J. and State, M.W. (2008). Autism genetics: strategies, challenges, and opportunities. *Autism Research*, **1**, 4–17.

Parsons, S. and Mitchell, P. (2002). The potential of virtual reality in social skills training for people with autistic spectrum disorders. *Journal of Intellectual Disability Research*, **46**, 430–43.

Pelphrey, K.A., Singerman, J.D., Allison, T., and McCarthy, G. (2003). Brain activation evoked by perception of gaze shifts: the influence of context. *Neuropsychologia*, **41**, 156–70.

Perrett, D.I. and Emery, N. (1994). Understanding the intentions of others from visual signals: neurophysiological evidence. *Current Psychology of Cognition*, **13**, 683–94.

Pierce, K., Muller, R.A., Ambrose, J., Allen, G., and Courchesne, E. (2001). Face processing occurs outside the 'fusiform face area' in autism: evidence from functional MRI. *Brain*, **124**, 2059–73.

Piven, J., Palmer, P., Jacobi, D., Childress, D. and Arndt, S. (1997). Broader autism phenotype: evidence from a family history study of multiple-incidence autism families. *American Journal of Psychiatry*, **154**, 185–190.

Pratt, C. and Bryant, P. (1990). Young children understand that looking leads to knowing (so long as they are looking into a single barrel). *Child Development*, **61**, 973–83.

Premack, D. (1990). The infant's theory of self-propelled objects. *Cognition*, **36**, 1–16.

Rajendran, G. and Mitchell, P. (2000). Computer mediated interaction in Asperger syndrome: the Bubble Dialogue Program. *Computers and Education*, **35**, 189–207.

Rapin, I. and Katzman, R. (1998). Neurobiology of autism. *Annals of Neurology*, **43**, 7–14.

Raymond, G., Bauman, M., and Kemper, T. (1996). Hippocampus in autism: a Golgi analysis. *Acta Neuropathologica*, **91**, 117–19.

Rinehart, N.J., Bradshaw, J.L., Moss, S.A., Brereton, A.V., and Tonge, B.J. (2001). A deficit in shifting attention present in high-functioning autism but not Asperger's disorder. *Autism*, **5**, 67–80.

Ring, H., Baron-Cohen, S., Williams, S., et al. (1999). Cerebral correlates of preserved cognitive skills in autism. a functional MRI study of Embedded Figures task performance. *Brain*, **122**, 1305–15.

Ritvo, E.R., Freeman, B.J., Scheibel, A.B., et al. (1986). Lower Purkinje cell counts in the cerebella of four autistic subjects: initial findings of the UCLA–NSAC autopsy research report. *American Journal of Psychiatry*, **143**, 862–6.

Rodier, P.M., Ingram, J.L., Tisdale, B., Nelson, S.F., and Romano, J. (1996). Embryological origin for autism: developmental anomalies of the cranial nerve motor nuclei. *Journal of Comparative Neurology*, **370**, 247–61.

Ronald, A., Happé, F., Bolton, P., Butcher, et al. (2006). Genetic heterogeneity between the three components of the autism spectrum: a twin study. *Journal of the American Academy of Child Adolescent Psychiatry*, **45**, 691–699.

Rutherford, M., Baron-Cohen, S., and Stone, V. (2002). Reading the mind in the voice: a study with normal adults and adults with Asperger syndrome or high functioning autism. *Journal of Autism and Developmental Disorders*, **32**, 189–94.

Rutter, M. (1978). Language disorder and infantile autism. In *Autism: a reappraisal of concepts and treatment* (ed. M Rutter and E Schopler). New York: Plenum.

Rydin, O.T., Drake, J., and Bratt, A. (1999). The effects of training on emotion recognition skills for adults with an intellectual disability. *Journal of Applied Research in Intellectual Disabilities*, **12**, 253–62.

Saitoh, O., Karns, C.M., and Courchesne, E. (2001). Development of hippocampal formation from 2 to 42 years. *Brain*, **124**, 1317–24.

Samaco, R.C., Hogart, A. and LaSalle, J.M. (2005). Epigenetic overlap in autism-spectrum neurodevelopmental disorders: MECP2 deficiency causes reduced expression of UBE3A and GABRB3. *Human Molecular Genetics*, **14**, 483–492.

Saxe, R., Carey, S., and Kanwisher, N. (2004). Understanding other minds: linking developmental psychology and functional neuroimaging. *Annual Review of Psychology*, **55**, 87–124.

Sebat, J., Lakshmi, B., Malhotra, D., et al. (2007). Strong association of de novo copy number mutations with autism. *Science*, **316**, 445–449.

Scaife, M. and Bruner, J. (1975). The capacity for joint visual attention in the infant. *Nature*, **253**, 265–6.

Schultz, R.T., Grelotti, D.J., Klin, A., et al. (2003). The role of fusiform face area in social cognition: implications for the pathobiology of autism. *Philosophical Transactions of the Royal Society of London*, **358**, 415–27.

Silver, M. and Oakes, P. (2001). Evaluation of a new computer intervention to teach people with autism or Asperger syndrome to recognize and predict emotions in others. *Autism*, **5**, 299–316.

Sparks, B.F., Friedman, S.D., Shaw, D.W., et al. (2002). Brain structural abnormalities in young children with autism spectrum disorder. *Neurology*, **59**, 184–92.

Swettenham, J. (1996). Can children with autism be taught to understand false belief using computers? *Journal of Child Psychology and Psychiatry*, **37**, 157–65.

Tager-Flusberg, H. (1993). What language reveals about the understanding of minds in children with autism. In *Understanding other minds: perspectives from autism* (ed. S. Baron-Cohen, H. Tager-Flusberg and D.J. Cohen). Oxford University Press.

Teunisse, J.P. and De Gelder, B. (1994). Do autistics have a generalised face processing deficit? *International Journal of Neuroscience*, **77**, 1–10.

Tordjman, S., Anderson, G.M., McBride, P.A., *et al.* (1997). Plasma beta-endorphin, adrenocorticotropin hormone and cortisol in autism. *Journal of Child Psychology and Psychiatry*, **38**, 705–15.

Townsend, J. and Courchesne, E. (1994). Parietal damage and narrow 'spotlight' spatial attention. *Journal of Cognitive Neuroscience*, **6**, 220–32.

Townsend, J., Courchesne, E., and Egaas, B. (1996a). Slowed orienting of covert visual-spatial attention in autism: specific deficits associated with cerebellar and parietal abnormality. *Development and Psychopathology*, **8**, 563–84.

Townsend, J., Singer-Harris, N., and Courchesne, E. (1996b). Visual attention abnormalities in autism: delayed orienting to locationi. *Journal of the International Neuropsychology Society*, **2**, 541–50.

Townsend, J., Courchesne, E., Covington, J., *et al.* (1999). Spatial attention deficits in patients with acquired or developmental cerebellar abnormality. *Journal of Neuroscience*, **19**, 5632–43.

Veenstra-Vanderweele, J. and Cook, E.H., Jr (2004). Molecular genetics of autism spectrum disorder. *Molecular Psychiatry*, **9**, 819–32.

Wainwright-Sharp, J.A. and Bryson, S.E. (1993). Visual orienting deficits in high-functioning people with autism. *Journal of Autism and Developmental Disorders*, **23**, 1–13.

Wainwright-Sharp, J.A. and Bryson, S.E. (1996). Visual-spatial orienting in autism. *Journal of Autism and Developmental Disorders*, **26**, 423–38.

Wassink, T.H., Hazlett, H.C., Epping, E.A., *et al.* (2007). Cerebral cortical gray matter overgrowth and functional variation of the serotonin transporter gene in autism. *Archives of General Psychiatry*, **64**, 709–717

Walker, A.S. (1982). Intermodal perception of expressive behaviours by human infants. *Journal of Experimental Child Psychology*, **33**, 514–35.

Welchew, D., Ashwin, C., Berkou, K., *et al.* (2005). Functional disconnectivity of the medial temporal lobe in autism. *Biological Psychiatry*, **57**, 991–8.

Wellman, H. (1990). *Children's theories of mind*. Cambridge, MA: Bradford/MIT Press.

Whiten, A. (1991). *Natural theories of mind*. Oxford: Basil Blackwell.

Wicker, B., Keysers, C., Plailly, J., Royet, J.P., Gallese, V., and Rizzolatti, G. (2003). Both of us disgusted in My insula: the common neural basis of seeing and feeling disgust. *Neuron*, **40**, 655–64.

Williams, J.H.G., Waiter, G.D., Perra, O., Perrett, D.I., and Whiten, A. (2005). An fMRI study of joint attention experience. *NeuroImage*, **25**, 133–40.

Williams, R.S., Hauser SL, Purpura DP, Delong GR and Swisher CN (1980). Autism and mental retardation: neuropathologic studies performed in four retarded persons with autistic behaviour. *Archives of Neurology*, **37**, 749–753.

Wimmer, H. and Perner, J. (1983). Beliefs about beliefs: representation and constraining function of wrong beliefs in young children's understanding of deception. *Cognition*, **13**, 103–28.

Wimmer, H., Hogrefe, J., and Perner, J. (1988). Children's understanding of informational access as a source of knowledge. *Child Development*, **59**, 386–96.

World Health Organization (1994). *International classification of diseases* (10th edn) (ICD-10). Geneva: World Health Organization.

Yirmiya, N., Sigman, M., Kasari, C., and Mundy, P. (1992). Empathy and cognition in high functioning children with autism. *Child Development*, **63**, 150–60.

Young, A. and Bruce, V. (1998). The science of the face. *Psychologist*, **11**, 120–5.

3

Social cognition in children with learning disabilities

Michal Shaked and Nurit Yirmiya

The development of individuals with learning disabilities has been of interest to researchers in various fields of study for many decades. One of the main areas of interest has been the classification of individuals with learning disabilities by aetiology. This refers first to a specification of two groups of learning disabilities: those with familial retardation, and those with organic retardation (Burack 1990). The latter group can further be classified according to one of several hundred pre-, peri-, or postnatal aetiologies that are associated with impairments in cognitive and social functioning (Hodapp et al. 1998). As research develops in these areas, specific developmental and behavioural profiles, termed behavioural phenotypes (Simonoff et al. 1998), are identified for specific aetiological groups. For example, in boys with fragile X syndrome, a specific weakness in sequential processing is found which is not evident in individuals with other aetiologies of learning disabilities such as Down syndrome (Hodapp et al. 1992). These behavioural phenotypes include strengths and weaknesses in areas of social as well as cognitive functioning. For instance, in boys with fragile X syndrome, social and communicative difficulties are also apparent (Simonoff et al. 1998).

In developmental research, studies of typical and atypical development complement each other. Thus an understanding of the sequence of development in communication and social abilities enables a clearer understanding of specific strengths and weakness of individuals with different diagnoses. In addition, tracing the specific abilities and developmental trajectories of certain individuals in one area of development helps to clarify the cognitive, perceptual, and emotional components and the complex interactions between these components in bringing about a certain behaviour or ability, as well as the genetic and environmental basis of these behaviours.

In the area of social cognition, two of the most intensively researched aetiologies are those of autism and Williams syndrome (WS). In this chapter we shall focus on the latter syndrome. Clinical evidence has called attention to a specific behavioural phenotype in individuals with WS, including a profound interest in social interactions, a tendency for social garrulity, and a lack of proper social distinctions in social encounters. This evidence has led to a growing interest in WS, from the perspective of social cognition and development, as an example of the possible effects of genes on social abilities and behaviours. As this research advances, it also serves to exemplify the immense complexity of social understanding and behaviour, in its various perceptual, cognitive, and emotional components.

In what follows, we shall summarize the findings concerning social cognition in individuals with WS, especially as they have been studied using two experimental paradigms—theory of mind and face-processing. These paradigms are the most widely used in social cognition research, tapping both cognitive and perceptual components of this ability. In addition, we shall attempt to contribute to the discussion of this syndrome, emphasizing the need to clarify methodological issues in studies of social cognition, as well as the importance of integrating environmental and genetic data to understand the social abilities of individuals with WS. Finally, we shall discuss the consequences of this debate for intervention with individuals who have WS.

3.1 Description of Williams syndrome

3.1.1 Characteristics of Williams syndrome

WS is a rare genetic disorder, identified in various countries around the world, caused by a microdeletion of somewhere between 16 and 25 genes on chromosome 7q11.23 (Bellugi et al. 1999b). One of the effects of this microdeletion is elastin insufficiency, often resulting in cardiovascular disease in individuals with WS, especially supravalvar aortic stenosis (Ewart et al. 1994). In addition, the syndrome is characterized by musculoskeletal and renal abnormalities as well as distinctive facial features (Pober and Dykens 1996). WS infants are born at below average birth weight and often show no spontaneous sucking, with frequent vomiting during the first few months (Carrasco et al. 2005). They manifest unusual sacral creases, poor muscle tone, and premature ageing of the skin. WS children often suffer from hyperacusis, an abnormal sensitivity to sound (Marriage 1994).

The disorder is associated with mild to moderate mental retardation, with a mean IQ of around 50–60 and a range of IQ scores between 40 and 90 (Karmiloff-Smith et al. 1995; Bellugi et al. 1999b). Individuals with WS present relative weaknesses, including deficits in visuospatial processing, numbers, and problem-solving (e.g. Udwin and Yule 1991; Bellugi et al. 1992). Impulsivity and concentration difficulties are also associated with WS

(Udwin and Yule 1991; Dykens 2003). The WS cognitive profile includes strengths in grammar compared with individuals with mental retardation matched for chronological age, as apparent on formal tests of comprehension and production as well as in their expressive language. Furthermore, individuals with WS show impressive narrating abilities, especially in the use of affective prosody in their conversations and narrations (Bellugi *et al.* 2001). Numerous studies have also confirmed that individuals with WS are more advanced in their language abilities than in their visuospatial constructive abilities such as drawing or pattern construction (e.g. Jarrold *et al.* 1998).

The debate concerning language acquisition and syntactic and morphological abilities in individuals with WS continues, and it would now seem that even if these areas present a relative strength in individuals with WS, they are by no means absolutely intact (reviewed by Dykens *et al.* 2000; Mervis 2003). Thus, although researchers have pinpointed strengths and weaknesses both between and within cognitive domains (Bellugi *et al.* 2001), the extreme view which describes WS as an example of a clear-cut dissociation between intact language abilities and severe cognitive deficits does not hold (Mervis 2003).

3.1.2 Sociability of individuals with Williams syndrome

Aside from the cognitive profile described above, behavioural and personality traits also characterize individuals with WS. Individuals with WS are described as having warm personalities and a keen interest in other people (Dilts *et al.* 1990; Gosch and Pankau 1997). They have been observed to be extremely sociable, charming, outgoing, and highly concerned about the well-being of others (Gosch and Pankau 1994). Young children with WS seem to be drawn to human faces (Mervis and Bertrand 1997), and are highly empathic and responsive to the distress of others (Tager-Flusberg and Sullivan 1999; Klein-Tasman and Mervis 2003).

The sociability of individuals with WS is evidenced not only in observational data but also in clinical experiments. For instance, Bellugi *et al.* (1999a) asked participants with WS to rate the approachability of strangers, i.e. the extent to which they would be willing or interested in approaching these persons from photographs of their faces. Typically developing individuals had previously rated these photographed persons as either positive or negative, i.e. as either highly approachable or inapproachable. Participants with WS exhibited a positive bias in which they expressed a willingness to approach all strangers, although their rank order of these unfamiliar individuals resembled that of the comparison group.

The latter findings coincide with the tendency among individuals with WS to be overly sociable and fearless of strangers, a tendency which causes great concern for parents. Furthermore, despite their interest in others, and despite having good social relationships with adults, research showed that children with WS demonstrated poor relations with peers (Udwin and Yule 1991; Greer et al. 1997) and difficulties in making and sustaining peer friendships (Gosch and Pankau 1994; Sarimski 1997).

Thus, on the one hand, reports have indicated these individuals' relatively intact language abilities, especially strengths in affective prosody in conversations, as well as good eye contact and use of non-verbal gestures such as nodding, smiling, etc. (Semel and Rosner 2003). This, in combination with their strong interest in human beings and social situations, seems to predict a relative strength in social cognition for individuals with WS. On the other hand, evidence exists to suggest that individuals with WS exhibit specific difficulties with the social-pragmatic aspects of language (Laws and Bishop 2004). For instance, they show difficulties in conversational rules such as turn-taking, reliance on contexts, and understanding of double meaning (Sotillo et al. 2002). They also show difficulties in maintaining topic relevance in conversations and in topic closure (Semel and Rosner 2003). Furthermore, WS infants revealed deficient non-verbal predictors of the social aspects of communication such as pointing, as well as specific difficulties in triadic situations, and a lack of the correlation between socio-interactive markers and language that is found in typical development (Laing et al. 2000).

Furthermore, reports have indicated that, by middle childhood, children with WS reveal difficulties interpreting social cues in interpersonal interactions (Gosch and Pankau 1994; Sarimski 1997). Children with WS have often been described as showing a tendency for 'hypersociability', i.e. approaching others without sufficient inhibition or understanding of social norms and possible dangers (Jones et al. 2000; Doyle et al. 2004). All these behaviours suggest that, despite their sociable personalities and interest in other people, individuals with WS may nonetheless experience difficulties in social cognition. In the following two sections, we shall present data concerning two aspects that are central to social cognition: theory of mind and face-processing. In each section, we will first consider the normal development of the social cognitive construct referred to before discussing its manifestation in WS.

3.2 Theory of mind in individuals with Williams syndrome

3.2.1 Theory of mind in typical development

One of the more formal ways of examining social cognition in laboratory conditions, enabling at times an analysis that goes beyond behavioural impressions, is through experiments designed to tap theory of mind abilities. The term 'theory of mind' refers to the ability to attribute mental states, such as thoughts, beliefs, desires, and intentions, to oneself and to others. This ability is important for making sense of behaviours and for predicting actions, and thus is crucial for social interactions.

Since Premack and Woodruff (1978) first raised the issue of examining theory of mind, cognitive and developmental scientists have been involved in the complicated task of tracing the typical as well as the atypical developmental trajectory of theory of mind abilities in children. To this end, researchers developed several different experimental paradigms, including tasks that tap the child's ability to comprehend mental states such as beliefs or false beliefs, desires, deceptions, lies, and jokes. Observational studies of children in their natural environments, as they interact with family members and friends, have identified the first steps in the development of at least some components of theory of mind as early as 2 years of age (e.g. Hala *et al.* 1991; Lewis 1993). Research on infants and toddlers has now begun to include tasks that assess the distinction between human and physical motion, the attribution of intentionality to human action, and talk about mental states (e.g. Bartsch and Wellman 1995; Meltzoff 1995; Woodward 1998; Prinz and Meltzoff 2002; Hughes *et al.* 2005), thus showing the precursors of theory of mind abilities at a very young age.

Formal laboratory testing of theory of mind abilities point to a significant advancement in theory of mind development at around the age of 3–4 years. It is at this age that typically developing children are first able to tackle tasks such as the standard false-belief paradigm (e.g. Wimmer and Perner 1983; Frye and Moore 1991). In this paradigm, children are asked to predict a protagonist's action on the basis of their understanding that he/she is not aware of a change of place or of content that has been conducted in his/her absence. A further development in theory of mind abilities emerges around ages 5–7 years, when children are able to grasp the much harder second-order false-belief paradigm (e.g. Hogrefe *et al.* 1986; Leekam 1990). In these tasks, children must represent what one person thinks about what a second person thinks, reflecting in essence an understanding of social interaction as an interaction of minds, where people are concerned about each other's mental states (Perner 1988).

Research in both typical and atypical development suggests a strong relation between theory of mind development and the development of social skills and the quality of social interactions (Hughes and Leekam 2004). For instance, data from observational research suggested a significant correlation between false-belief performance and both the quality and quantity of children's pretend play with friends (Astington and Jenkins 1995; Youngblade and Dunn 1995;

Hughes and Dunn 1997). Observational studies have also shown a correlation between children's performance on false-belief tasks and the quality of their conversations, specifically the use of mental state terms in conversations (Slomkowski and Dunn 1996; Hughes and Dunn 1997).

3.2.2 Theory of mind in Williams syndrome

Research on children with autism (see Chapter 1) has paved the way for uncovering the deficits in theory of mind abilities associated with learning disabilities. This work has converged on the notion that theory of mind deficits may explain the cardinal features of autism such as impairments in social and communicative functioning. Although it is questionable whether such deficits can indeed be considered the core deficit in autism (Yirmiya *et al.* 1998), it is important to note that in individuals with autism a correlation has also emerged between an ability to pass false-belief tasks and a milder level of diagnostic symptoms, suggesting fewer social interaction impairments. Thus, among individuals who meet the clinical threshold for an autism diagnosis, a relation seems to exist between this aspect of their social cognition and their social skills (Hughes and Leekam 2004).

Several researchers have investigated theory of mind development in individuals with WS. These investigations were first inspired by the contention that individuals with WS may have an intact social ability, a claim that turned out to be overreaching, as mentioned above. The theory of mind studies conducted with this population fully reflect the complexity of the term 'social cognition' in typical as well as atypical development, as the following discussion reveals.

In the first theory of mind study of this population (Karmiloff-Smith *et al.* 1995), 18 participants with WS were enrolled in a series of six theory of mind experiments. These participants ranged in age from 9 to 23 years, and their WISC-R IQ scores ranged from 40 to 65. In the first experiment participants were required to use eye gaze direction, depicted on faces in photographs and in schematic drawings, to infer others' intentions and goals. The participants with WS performed almost at ceiling level on emotional and non-social clues, scoring parallel to typically developing individuals on inferring intentions and goals on the basis of eye gaze direction.

Within that same study, in two experiments utilizing the false-belief paradigm, 94 per cent of the participants with WS were able to predict the protagonist's behaviour on the basis of his/her mental state and to use mental state verbs to explain that behaviour. Thirty-one per cent of the participants with WS passed a second-order belief experiment, and seven of eight participants (88 per cent) passed an easier version of the task. Finally, 50 per cent of the participants with WS succeeded in an experiment measuring their understanding of both metaphor and sarcasm. However, those participants with WS who had difficulties with the task either failed on both the sarcasm and metaphor conditions or found the sarcastic statements easier. The authors emphasized that this pattern of performance contrasts with the pattern found in participants with autism, in which even high-functioning individuals tend to find the sarcastic statements more difficult.

From the six experiments described, the authors concluded that individuals with WS may possess an intact social module despite their difficulties in other cognitive domains such as numerical and visuospatial challenges. Despite methodological limitations (small sample size and lack of a comparison group (Sullivan and Tager-Flusberg 1999)) this work stimulated further investigations into the hypothesis that individuals with WS showed relative strengths in social cognition.

For instance, Tager-Flusberg *et al.* (1998) asked participants to select the correct labels to match photographs of complex mental state expressions in the eye region of the face. Adult participants with WS were compared with adults with Prader–Willi syndrome. Prader–Willi is another genetic syndrome characterized by mental retardation in a similar range to that of WS, but with no distinct cognitive profile except for a relative strength in visuospatial processing (Curfs *et al.* 1991). Participants with WS performed significantly better than adults with Prader–Willi syndrome who were matched for age, IQ, and language ability. Approximately half of the group with WS performed within the same range as the typically developing individuals who were matched for age. These results were again taken as evidence for a relative strength in social cognitive abilities in WS.

In contrast, Tager-Flusberg, Sullivan, and colleagues conducted another series of studies on theory of mind abilities in individuals with WS, and their conclusions seemed to contradict the early claims of an intact theory of mind in this population. In the first of these, Tager-Flusberg *et al.* (1997) demonstrated no significant differences in performance on the standard false-belief task between 14 children with WS and 10 children with Prader–Willi syndrome who were matched on age (5–9 years) and language ability. Moreover, the percentage of children with WS who passed the task was not at ceiling level (43 per cent) and was somewhat lower than that in the Prader–Willi syndrome group (60 per cent).

Next, Sullivan and Tager-Flusberg (1999) examined second-order belief attribution in children with WS compared with two comparison groups, children with Prader–Willi syndrome and children with mental retardation of unknown aetiology, who were matched on age, IQ, and language ability.

Only 45 per cent of the children with WS, 57 per cent of the children with Prader–Willi syndrome, and 13 per cent of those with mental retardation of unknown aetiology were able to pass both second-order belief question trials.

Tager-Flusberg and Sullivan (2000) extended the above findings by a follow-up study with three experiments designed to tap different aspects of theory of mind. The first experiment involved the two standard false-belief tasks, involving location change and unexpected content. Children with WS were again matched on age and language ability to children with Prader–Willi syndrome and children with mental retardation of unknown aetiology. The children with WS performed no better than the children from the two other groups on either task. In fact, a non-parametric analysis for the number of children passing the task revealed that the children with WS performed significantly worse than the control children.

The second experiment involved an explanation of an action task. The experiment included nine stories designed to elicit children's explanations of a person's actions using the mental state categories of desire, emotion, and cognition. On this task, the children with WS performed at the same level as the comparison groups. Overall, children in all three groups provided more emotion and desire terms than cognition terms, a finding that is comparable with the performance of younger typically developing children.

The third experiment involved a task of emotion matching, developed by Hobson et al. (1988). This task asked children to label the emotions depicted on photographed faces of two men and two women, which depicted emotional expressions of happy, sad, angry, and scared. Children with WS emerged as proficient, but no better than the comparison group, in discriminating and matching facial expressions of emotion.

Finally, Sullivan et al. (2003) examined the ability of adolescents with WS to distinguish between different forms of non-literal language, specifically lies and ironic jokes. The performance of these adolescents was compared with that of adolescents with Prader–Willi syndrome or with mental retardation of unknown aetiology, matched for age, IQ, and verbal ability. Results showed that adolescents in all three groups exhibited great difficulties in distinguishing lies from jokes. Almost all the participants in the three groups misclassified the jokes as lies, an error that is comparable to the performance of younger typically developing children.

Taken together, this evidence suggests that the theory of mind abilities of children and adults with WS are not spared, as was first believed. In fact, their performance is comparable to that of other populations with mental retardation, and is significantly lower than that expected of age-matched typically developing individuals. The studies are summarized in Table 3.1.

Table 3.1 Theory of mind studies of Williams syndrome

Study (by year)	WS sample	Task	Comparison group(s)	Matching	Group differences
Karmiloff-Smith et al. 1995	Total $N = 18$ Range CA 9–23 years **Exp. 1**: $N = 12$ **Exp. 2**: $N = 12$ **Exp. 3**: $N = 16$ **Exp. 4**: $N = 14$ **Exp. 5**: $N = 14$ **Exp. 6**: $N = 16$	**Exp. 1** Eye gaze to infer mental states **Exp. 2 & 3** First-order false belief **Exp. 4 & 5** Second-order false belief **Exp. 6** Linguistic utterances: understanding, sarcasm, and metaphor	Only in Exp. 1: (1) TD (2) Autism	None	(1) NS (2) WS > autism
Tager-Flusberg et al. 1997	$N = 14$ Mean CA = 7;5	First-order false belief	PWS $N = 14$, mean CA = 7;7	CA, PPVT-R	NS
Tager-Flusberg et al. 1998	$N = 13$ Mean CA = 27;3	Eyes task	(1) PWS $N = 10$, mean CA = 7;7 (2) TD $N = 25$, mean CA = 26;4	(1) CA, IQ, PPVT (2) CA	(1) WS > PWS (2) TD > WS
Sullivan and Tager-Flusberg 1999	$N = 22$ Mean CA = 11.42	Second-order false belief	(1) PWS $N = 14$, mean CA = 12.08 (2) MRU $N = 13$, mean CA= 11.42	(1) CA, IQ, PPVT (2) CA, IQ, PPVT	(1) NS (2) NS

Table 3.1 (continued) Theory of mind studies of Williams syndrome

Study (by year)	WS sample	Task	Comparison group(s)	Matching	Group differences
Tager-Flusberg and Sullivan 2000	Exp. 1: N = 21 Mean CA = 7;2	**Exp. 1** First-order false belief	(1) PWS $N = 15$, CA = 6;11 (2) MRU $N = 15$, CA = 7;7	(1) CA, IQ, PPVT (2) CA, IQ, PPVT	(1) S (2) NS
	Exp. 2: N = 20	**Exp. 2** Explanation of action (stories)	(1) PWS, $N = 12$ (2) MRU, $N = 12$	(1) CA, IQ, PPVT (2) CA, IQ, PPVT	(1) NS (2) NS
	Exp. 3: N = 22	**Exp. 3** Emotion matching of facial expression	(1) PWS, $N = 15$ (2) MRU, $N = 11$	(1) CA, IQ, PPVT (2) CA, IQ, PPVT	(1) NS (2) NS
Sullivan et al. 2003	N = 16 Mean CA = 12.3	Understanding of non-literal language; lies and jokes	(1) PWS $N = 11$, mean CA = 12.8 (2) MRU $N = 12$, mean CA = 12.0	(1) CA, IQ, PPVT (2) CA, IQ, PPVT	(1) NS (2) NS

CA, chronological age; TD, typical development; NS, non-significant difference; WS, Williams syndrome; PWS, Prader–Willi syndrome; PPVT, Peabody Picture Vocabulary Test; PPVT-R, Revised Peabody Picture Vocabulary Test; MRU, unspecified mental retardation.

Notwithstanding these findings, it may be misleading to conceive of theory of mind as a unified cognitive ability. Possibly, the discrepancies between the different research outcomes may result from an investigation of different aspects of this complex ability. Tager-Flusberg and Sullivan (2000) raised an intriguing possibility that theory of mind may contain two separate components: a social-cognitive component and a social-perceptual component. They suggested that the social-cognition component entails the conceptual understanding of the mind as a representational system, and is revealed in tasks such as the first and second false-belief tasks. This component is related to language acquisition and is thought to rely on the prefrontal cortex. Relying on the data presented above, these authors suggested that it is the social-cognitive component that is deficient in children with WS.

In contrast, the social-perceptual component includes the capacity to distinguish between persons and objects and to recognize people's mental states from their facial and body expressions. This component is related to other cognitive and language abilities, appears earlier than the social-cognitive component, and is thought to rely on the limbic system and, specifically, the amygdala. Perhaps this component is relatively spared in individuals with WS, as evidenced from a study that found emotion recognition to be intact in this population (Tager-Flusberg *et al.* 1998).

A stronger tendency to use the social-perceptual component among individuals with WS may also be evidenced by reports of an immense interest in human faces among infants and young children (Mervis *et al.* 2003) and reports of empathic tendencies among children and adults (Gosch and Pankau 1997). Laing *et al.* (2002) also attributed their findings of relatively intact dyadic interactions and relatively weak triadic joint attention to this distinction between social-perceptual and social-cognitive components in theory of mind.

Further evidence for relative strengths in the social-perceptual sphere among individuals with WS may be found in their face-processing abilities, which were reported to be intact. However, as in the theory of mind research, the exact pattern of success and failure in face-processing tasks in this population continues to be a matter of debate.

3.3 Face-processing in individuals with Williams syndrome

3.3.1 Face-processing in typical development

The ability to recognize and discriminate faces relatively easily represents one of the most remarkable human skills, which relies on specific cognitive and neural mechanisms (Farah *et al.* 1998; Haxby *et al.* 2002). In typical face-processing, faces are encoded globally or configurally, rather than by local features (Farah 1996), even by young children, as can be deduced from studies introducing a disruption in the expected configuration of the face, such as an inverted face (Baenniger 1994; Carey and Diamond 1994; Freire and Lee 2001). Imaging experiments have shown that young infants' brains initially process upright human faces, inverted human faces, and objects in a relatively similar way across both hemispheres (Johnson and de Haan 2001). However, with development, brain processing of human upright faces becomes increasingly specialized and localized, activating the fusiform gyrus in the right hemisphere (Karmiloff-Smith *et al.* 2004). Therefore, for adults, recognition of faces is significantly more difficult when these are presented in inverted form because of the difficulty in recovery of the configuration of inverted faces. The decrement in performance for recognition of inverted as opposed to upright faces is considerably larger than for other objects such as cars or houses (Mills *et al.* 2000).

Face perception *per se*, as well as facial expression processing, is important for social cognition and social interaction. It provides the visual cues to understanding and interpreting others' behaviour.

3.3.2 Face-processing in Williams syndrome

Deficits in face-processing in a variety of clinical populations characterized by difficulties in social interactions, such as autism, have been demonstrated (Phillips 2004). However, there are great variations in performance on face-processing tasks in these populations, raising the possibility that different neurological and cognitive pathways underpin performance on these tasks (Barton *et al.* 2004).

Numerous studies have reported that individuals with WS perform well on face-processing tasks (e.g. Bellugi *et al.* 1990; Udwin and Yule 1991; Rossen *et al.* 1995), despite a significant weakness in other visuospatial tasks such as drawings and block design. For instance, Udwin and Yule (1991) showed that WS children scored significantly higher than children in the comparison group in the face-recognition tasks of the Rivermead Behavioural Memory Test, in which participants attempt to recognize familiar face stimuli among a set of unknown faces. Bellugi *et al.* (1994) found that WS participants achieved higher scores than Down syndrome participants on the Benton Facial Recognition Test (Benton *et al.* 1983) which requires matching one picture of a face (out of either three or six stimuli faces) with an original target photograph. Other authors have emphasized that individuals with WS exhibit an apparent disparity between spatial construction and face-processing skills, whereas individuals with Down syndrome demonstrate equal levels of impairment in the two types of tasks (Paul *et al.* 2002).

Despite this evidence, researchers continue to debate whether this normal or near-normal performance on face-recognition tasks does indeed represent an intact face-processing ability in individuals with WS. A second possibility may be that they achieve this performance level by using different cognitive pathways. For instance, some authors have raised the possibility that individuals with WS may adopt a featural mode of face-processing, and that their high achievements in face-recognition tasks are due to the amount of practice they have acquired with this local mode of analysis (Deruelle *et al.* 1999).

Research conducted by Deruelle *et al.* (2003), who studied children and adolescents with WS, and Tager-Flusberg *et al.* (2003), who studied adolescents and adults with WS, suggests that the pathways used by individuals with WS to achieve their performance on face-recognition tasks resemble those of typically developing individuals. For instance, Tager-Flusberg and colleagues used a part–whole paradigm which involved matching individual face parts in two conditions, either in isolation or in the context of a whole face. These authors also introduced face inversion to assess whether the ability to use the whole-face context was disrupted by inversion. Although findings showed that overall accuracy was better in the chronological age-matched control group than in the WS group, both groups showed the same pattern of performance in that they performed better on the whole-face condition rather than the isolate-part condition for upright faces but not for inverted faces. This seems to suggest that persons with WS process faces holistically, in a similar fashion to typical face-processing.

In contrast, research conducted by Karmiloff-Smith (1997) and Deruelle *et al.* (1999) with face-inverted paradigms seems to indicate that face-processing development is not intact in individuals with WS. This research suggests that face-processing in individuals with WS follows a different pathway, and that they do not process faces holistically but in a piecemeal fashion, much like individuals with autism (see also Karmiloff-Smith *et al.* 2003). Furthermore, Karmiloff-Smith *et al.* (2004) suggested that participants with WS do indeed perform at a comparable level to that of typically developing individuals on holistic face-processing tasks, yet their abnormal face-processing mechanisms emerge in other tasks that require what they term 'second-order configural processing'. One such study (Karmiloff-Smith *et al.* 2004) included tasks that required participants to detect differences in faces with altered contours (i.e. slight changes in the original position of facial features) or altered features. Typically developing individuals significantly outperformed WS participants in detecting differences in the upright configural faces, and showed less sensitivity to face inversion. In a study of facial expression recognition (Gagliardi *et al.* 2003), children with WS performed worse than chronological age-matched participants but as well as mental age-matched participants. The authors proposed that facial expression recognition relies more heavily on configural processing, and that this explains the relative difficulty of participants with WS on this task

Electophysiological studies of face-processing further support the notion that individuals with WS rely on different neural pathways in face-processing than do normal controls. For instance, Mills *et al.* (2000) conducted an experiment requiring participants with WS to match pairs of photographs presented in either upright or inverted form. Previously tested typically developing participants showed electrophysiological differences to matched versus mismatched faces approximately 320 ms after the onset of the second stimulus. In contrast, the mismatch–match effect for inverted faces ranged between 400 and 1000 ms. Participants with WS showed a 320-mismatch effect for both upright and inverted faces. Mobbs *et al.* (2004) compared face and eye-gaze direction processing abilities of individuals with WS with age-matched typically developing individuals. They found that WS individuals showed lower accuracy in determining the direction of gaze and demonstrated significantly longer response latencies. In the WS group, increases in activation were observed in the right fusiform gyrus and several frontal and temporal regions. By comparison, controls showed activation in the bilateral fusiform gyrus and the occipital and temporal lobes. They also found increased frontal activation during face and gaze processing in the WS participants, which may explain the social interests and empathic behaviour associated with WS. Taken together, these findings challenge the findings discussed earlier which suggested a separation between cognitive–perceptual components on the one hand and social–emotional aspects on the other hand.

Therefore the debate concerning face-processing in individuals with WS remains unresolved, as does the connection between these diverging experimental results and observational data concerning the lengthy amount of time that infants and toddlers with WS spend examining human faces (Mervis *et al.* 2003). The observational data suggest an immense interest in humans, but may also indicate a natural tendency for intense 'self-training' in the field of face-processing. Such a tendency may also explain how individuals with WS can achieve high levels of performance on face-processing tasks despite their utilization of different neurological and cognitive pathways (Karmiloff-Smith *et al.* 2004). These questions will need further exploration in future research.

3.4 **Aetiological considerations and future research**

The research review discussed above presents an interesting but complex picture of social cognition abilities in individuals with WS. Early assumptions about intact social abilities in this population seem to have been premature. Subsequent research studies exploring specific components of social cognition, such as theory of mind and face-processing, have yielded both strengths and weaknesses in these areas, highlighting the complexity of the term 'social cognition'. As such, a discussion of the aetiology of the social cognitive deficits associated with WS in children will necessarily be complex and requires several methodological considerations for future research.

First, an accurate phenotypic description is critical to gain an understanding of the genetic basis for the development of social cognition. It is important to define clearly the meaning of relative strengths as opposed to intact abilities. Although certain aspects of social cognition may not be completely intact in individuals with WS, these aspects may represent areas of relative strength compared with other cognitive tasks or with other syndromes with mental retardation. Therefore the selection of comparison groups (both typically developing individuals as well as individuals from clearly defined clinical populations) is crucial for understanding the comparative strengths and weakness of the WS population.

Secondly, in the study of developmental disorders, and especially in studying developmental traits such as social cognition, the matching of groups must be carefully designed so as to reflect possible developmental trajectories (Shaked and Yirmiya 2004). In essence, this requires careful matching procedures between the clinical group and the comparison group. Specifically, mental age must be brought into account, as well as chronological age, gender, and socio-economic status, as these variables are all implicated in the development of social cognition.

Thirdly, careful attention must also be paid to the selection of experimental tasks as the discussion above reflects, different tasks may yield vastly different results, with some pointing to an impressive ability of individuals with WS and some pointing to areas of weakness. Thus individuals with WS may reveal proficiency in one area of theory of mind and not in another, or may achieve high scores on some facial recognition tasks perhaps by using different mechanisms than typically developing individuals. Researchers must unravel the different cognitive mechanisms tapped by specific tasks within the same largely defined domain of social cognition.

Theory of mind performance in children with autism shows significant variation across performance level compared with other atypical populations as well as typically developing individuals (Yirmiya *et al.* 1998). A wider variety of tasks should now be employed in examining theory of mind abilities of individuals with WS, especially tasks that highlight other closely related abilities. For instance, in the theory of mind domain, these may include the

Strange Stories Task (Happé 1994). More naturalistic experiments and observational research may also help further expand understanding of social cognition in WS. Such methods may also promote understanding of the environmental factors involved in the development of social cognition, even in disorders with such a clear genetic basis.

Genes interact with environmental factors from the very beginning. Extensive research on both typical and atypical development has emphasized the significant contribution of social interactions in the development of theory of mind abilities (e.g. Astington and Jenkins 1995; Cutting and Dunn 1999; Peterson *et al.* 2000; Peterson 2004). Although it is tempting to attribute all behavioural findings in WS individuals to their unique genetic profile, this attribution may omit important environmental contributions to these children's development. For example, as mentioned above, infants and toddlers with WS seem to be drawn to the human face as well as to enjoy social interactions from the very beginning. This finding is taken to support the genetic influence on social tendencies, but it is also possible to speculate on how these children's efforts to maintain proximity to people may contribute to the further development of their social cognitive profile.

Several studies have addressed the issue of infant and toddler interest in people and its relationship to language development in WS. For example, Laing *et al.* (2002) found that the tendency among WS infants to fixate on adults led to a failure to disengage from their faces when this would help them learn about the referents of adults' attention. Conversely, Gyori *et al.* (2004) reported that toddlers with WS use social pragmatic cues such as joint attention in learning new words. These studies have begun to explore how these children's language development may or may not benefit from their tendency to be involved in social interactions. These questions are certainly relevant to social development. Given their high interest in people and tendency to be involved in social interactions, perhaps extensive exposure to social situations may give children with WS ample opportunities for improving their social understanding, despite their relative cognitive weaknesses, thus further complicating their strengths and weaknesses profile within this specific domain.

3.5 Clinical applications

The discussion here has attempted to convey the evidence that children, adolescents, and adults with WS encounter specific difficulties in the realm of social cognition. In daily interactions, these difficulties manifest themselves in a tendency to initiate social interactions with strangers or in other inappropriate situations, and in poor peer relationships and a lack of friendships. Children and adults with WS may face an increased risk for exploitation and abuse (Dykens and Hodapp 1997). These issues must be addressed in educational interventions throughout the child's development.

One of the areas where interventions for children with WS have seen relative advances comprises the area of language abilities. Conversational abilities among these children are closely related to their social difficulties and can be addressed within the context of speech and language therapy, as well as in educational settings. Speech and language therapy can be used to help individuals with WS to understand and employ conversational rules including topic relevance, preservation, turn-taking, and closure. WS children need to be taught to read a partner's non-verbal cues such as looking around the room, shifting from foot to foot, losing eye contact, and facial expressions. Discussion of sample conversations, storytelling, role-playing, modelling, and conversation monitoring should all be employed in teaching conversational rules (Semel and Rosner 2003).

One of the major areas of concern for parents is these children's tendency for overfriendliness and a lack of inhibition in social situations. Psychoeducational techniques can be employed to train children with WS to learn socially acceptable ways of interacting as well as methods for self-protection. Such interventions should include a discussion of social role differences between strangers, acquaintances, professionals, friends, family members, and so on, followed by identification of different situations in which children encounter these figures, as well as appropriate greeting behaviours. Mediational strategies such as modelling, role-playing, videotaping, and dramatization can all contribute to this learning process. Specific attention should be paid to the tendency to approach strangers, and clear rules of conduct should be stated and re-stated in this domain (Semel and Rosner 2003).

The social stories technique, designed by Carol Gray (Gray and Gerand 1993; Gray 1998) in working with high-functioning children with autism and Asperger syndrome, may also be a useful tool for working with children with WS. This technique involves creating a story with the child. The story describes a person, skill, event, concept, or social situation and includes appropriate and relevant actions and expressions. The situation is described in terms of relevant social cues, anticipated actions, and information on what is occurring and why. These stories can help make explicit many different nuances that are not always clearly understood by children with WS.

3.6 Conclusions

The case of WS has been explored extensively with reference to the intriguing question of genetic influences on sociability. Clinical observations of children and adults with WS, as well as empirical designs (including questionnaires, observations, and experiments), all point to a significant tendency for socialization in this clinical population. The notion of a distinct social tendency in a genetically based syndrome is intriguing with respect to the possibility of revealing the contribution of genes to the neural systems underlying social behaviour. This connection has been further highlighted by several studies that reported marked differences in social behaviour between individuals with WS who have the typical genetic deletion and those who have a smaller deletion (e.g. Doyle *et al.* 2004).

On the basis of these behavioural observations, in combination with research suggesting an uneven cognitive profile of relative strengths (in language development) and weaknesses (in visuospatial and arithmetic abilities), many researchers have suggested that a relative strength in the social-cognitive domain exists in WS. Research into this question has focused on two components of social cognition: theory of mind abilities and face-processing capacities. As is often the case, initial claims for an intact 'social module', including language, theory of mind, and face-processing abilities, has been proven to represent an over-simplistic view. As is evident in this chapter, the precise abilities and disabilities of individuals with WS in both the theory of mind and face-processing domains still remain unclear. The conflicting results point to the need for further research to highlight both the theoretical and methodological issues raised in this chapter.

References

Astington, J. and Jenkins, J. (1995). Theory of mind development and social understanding. *Cognition and Emotion*, **9**, 151–65.

Baenniger, M. (1994). The development of face recognition: featural or configural processing? *Journal of Experimental Child Psychology*, **57**, 377–96.

Barton, J.S., Cherkasova, M.V., Hefter, R., Cox, T.A., O'Connor, M., and Manoach, D.S. (2004). Are patients with social developmental disorders prosopagnostic? Perceptual heterogeneity in the Asperger and social-emotional processing disorders. *Brain*, **127**, 1706–16.

Bartsch, D. and Wellman, H. (1995). *Children talk about the mind*. Oxford University Press.

Bellugi, U., Birhle, A., Jernigan, T., Trauner, D., and Doherty, S. (1990). Neuropsychological, neurological, and neuroanatomical profile of Williams syndrome. *American Journal of Medical Genetics*, **6**, 115–25.

Bellugi, U., Bihrle, A., Neville, H., Jernigan, T., and Doherty, S. (1992). Language, cognition and brain organization in a neurodevelopmental disorder. In *Developmental behavioral neuroscience* (ed. M. Gunner and C. Nelson), pp. 201–32. Hillsdale, NJ: Lawrence Erlbaum.

Bellugi, U., Wang, P.P., and Jernigan, T.L. (1994). Williams syndrome: an unusual neuropsychological profile. In *Atypical cognitive deficits in developmental disorders: implications for brain function* (ed. S.H. Bronman and J. Grafman), pp. 23–56. Hillsdale, NJ: Lawrence Erlbaum.

Bellugi, U., Adolphs, R., Cassady, C., and Chiles, M. (1999a). Towards the neural basis for hypersociability in a genetic syndrome. *Neuroreport*, **10**, 1653–7.

Bellugi, U., Lichtenberger, L., Mills, D., Galaburda, A., and Korenberg, J.R. (1999b). Bridging cognition, brain, and molecular genetics: evidence from Williams syndrome. *Trends in Neurosciences*, **5**, 197–208.

Bellugi, U., Korenberg, K.R., and Klima, E.S. (2001). Williams syndrome: an exploration of neurocognitive and genetic features. *Clinical Neuroscience Research*, **1**, 217–29.

Benton, A.L., Hamsher, K. de S, Varney, N.R., and Spreen, O. (1983). *Contributions to neuropsychological assessment*. New York: Oxford University Press.

Burack, J.A. (1990). Differentiating mental retardation: the two-group approach and beyond. In *Issues in the developmental approach to mental retardation* (ed. R.M. Hodapp, J.A. Burack, and E. Zigler). New York: Cambridge University Press.

Carey, S. and Diamond, R. (1994). Are faces perceived as configurations more by adults than by children? *Visual Cognition*, **1**, 253–74.

Carrasco, X., Castillo, S., Aravena, T., Rothhammer, P., and Aboitiz, F. (2005). Williams syndrome: pediatric, neurologic, and cognitive development. *Pediatric Neurology*, **32**, 166–72.

Curfs, L.G., Wiegers, A.M., Sommers, R.J., Borghgraef, M., and Fryns, J.P. (1991). Strengths and weaknesses in the cognitive profile of youngsters with Prader–Willi syndrome. *Clinical Genetics*, **40**, 430–4.

Cutting, A. and Dunn, J. (1999). Theory of mind, emotion understanding, language and family background: individual differences and inter-relations. *Child Development*, **70**, 853–65.

Deruelle, C., Mancini, J., Livet, M., Casse-Perrot, C., and de Schonen, S. (1999). Configural and local processing in faces in children with Williams syndrome. *Brain and Cognition*, **41**, 276–98.

Deruelle, C., Rondan, C., Mancini, J., and Livet, M. (2003). Exploring face processing in Williams syndrome. *Cognitie, Creier, Comportament*, **7**, 157–71.

Dilts, C., Morris, C., and Leonard, C. (1990). Hypothesis for development of a behavioral phenotype in Williams syndrome. *American Journal of Medical Genetics*, **6**, 126–31.

Doyle, T.F., Bellugi, U., Korenberg, J.R., and Graham, J. (2004). 'Everybody in the world is my friend': hypersociability in young children with Williams syndrome. *American Journal of Medical Genetics*, **124**, 263–73.

Dykens, D.M. (2003). Anxiety, fears, and phobias in persons with Williams syndrome. *Developmental Neuropsychology*, **23**, 291–316.

Dykens, E.M. and Hodapp, R.M. (1997). Treatment issues in genetic mental retardation syndromes. *Professional Psychology: Research and Practice*, **28**, 263–70.

Dykens, E.M., Hodapp, R.M., and Finucane, B.M. (2000). *Genetics and mental retardation syndromes: a new look at behavior and interventions*. Baltimore, MD: Brookes.

Ewart, A.K., Jin, W., Atkinson, D., Morris, C.A., and Keating, M.T. (1994). Supravalvular aortic stenosis associated with a deletion disrupting the elastin gene. *Journal of Clinical Investigation*, **93**, 1071–7.

Farah, M. (1996). Is face recognition 'special'? Evidence from neuropsychology. *Behavioral Brain Research*, **76**, 181–189.

Farah, M., Wilson, K., Drain, M., and Tanaka, J. (1998). What is 'special' about face perception? *Psychological Review*, **105**, 482–98.

Freire, A. and Lee, K. (2001). Face recognition in 4- to 7-year olds: processing of configural, featural, and paraphernalia information. *Journal of Experimental Child Psychology*, **80**, 347–71.

Frye, D. and Moore, C. (1991). *Children's theories of mind: mental states and social understanding.* Hillsdale, NJ: Lawrence Erlbaum.

Gagliardi, C., Frigario, E., Burt, D., Cazzaniga, I., Perret, D.I., and Borgatti, R. (2003). Facial expression recognition in Williams syndrome. *Neuropsychologia*, **41**, 733–8.

Gosch, A. and Pankau, R. (1994). Social-emotional and behavioral adjustment in children with Williams–Beuren syndrome. *American Journal of Medical Genetics*, **74**, 521–5.

Gosch, A. and Pankau, R. (1997). Personality characteristics and behavior problems in individuals of different ages with Williams syndrome. *Developmental Medicine and Child Neurology*, **39**, 527–33.

Gray, C.A. (1998). Social stories and comic strip conversations with students with Asperger syndrome and high-functioning autism. In *Asperger syndrome or high-functioning autism?* (ed. E. Schopler, G. Mesibov, and L.J. Dunce), pp. 167–98. New York: Plenum Press.

Gray, C.A. and Gerand, J. (1993). Social stories: improving responses of individuals with autism with accurate social information. *Focus on Autistic Behavior*, **8**, 1–10.

Greer, L.K., Brown, F.R., Pai, G.S., Choudry, S.H., and Klein, A.J. (1997). Cognitive, adaptive, and behavioral characteristics of Williams syndrome. *American Journal of Medical Genetics*, **74**, 521–5.

Gyori, M., Lukacs, A., and Pleh, C. (2004). Toward the understanding of the neurogenesis of social cognition: evidence from impaired populations. *Journal of Cultural and Evolutionary Psychology*, **2**, 261–82.

Hala, S., Chandler, M., and Fritz, A.S. (1991). Fledgling theories of mind: deception as a marker of three-year-olds' understanding of false belief. *Child Development*, **62**, 83–97.

Happé, F. (1994). An advanced test of theory of mind: understanding of story characters' thoughts and feelings by able autistic, mentally handicapped, and normal children and adults. *Journal of Autism and Developmental Disorders*, **24**, 129–53.

Haxby, J., Hoffman, E., and Gobbini, M.I. (2002). Human neural systems for face recognition and social communication. *Biological Psychiatry*, **51**, 59–67.

Hobson, R.P., Ouston, J., and Lee, A. (1988). Naming emotion in faces and voices: abilities and disabilities in autism and mental retardation. *British Journal of Developmental Psychology*, **7**, 237–50.

Hodapp, R.M., Leckman, J.F., Dykens, E.M., Sparrow, S., Zelinsky, D., and Ort, S. (1992). K-ABC profiles in children with fragile X syndrome, Down syndrome, and nonspecific mental retardation. *American Journal on Mental Retardation*, **97**, 39–46.

Hodapp, R.M., Burack, J.A., and Zigler, E. (1998). Developmental approaches to mental retardation: a short introduction. In *Handbook of mental retardation and development* (ed. J.A. Burack, R.M. Hodapp, and E. Zigler), pp. 3–19. Cambridge University Press.

Hogrefe, G., Wimmer, H., and Perner, J. (1986). Ignorance versus false belief: a developmental lag in attribution of epistemic states. *Child Development*, **57**, 567–82.

Hughes, C. and Dunn, J. (1997). 'Pretend you didn't know': young children's talk about mental states in the context of pretend play. *Cognitive Development*, **12**, 477–99.

Hughes, C. and Leekam, S. (2004). What are the links between theory of mind and social relations? Review, reflections and new directions for studies of typical and atypical development. *Social Development*, **13**, 590–619.

Hughes, C., Jaffee, S.R., Happé, F., Taylor, A., Caspi, A., and Moffitt, T.E. (2005). Origins of individual differences in theory of mind: from nature to nurture? *Child Development*, **76**, 356–70.

Jarrold, C., Baddeley, A.D., and Hewes, A.K. (1998). Verbal and nonverbal abilities in the Williams syndrome phenotype: evidence for diverging developmental trajectories. *Journal of Child Psychology and Psychiatry*, **39**, 511–23.

Johnson, M.H. and de Haan, M. (2001). Developing cortical specialization for visual-cognitive function: the case of face recognition. In *Mechanisms of cognitive development: behavioral and neural perspectives. Carnegie Mellon Symposia of Cognition* (ed. J.L. McClelland and R.S. Siegler), pp. 253–70. Mahwah, NJ: Lawrence Erlbaum.

Jones, W., Bellugi, U., Lai, Z., Chiles, M., Reilly, J., Lincoln A., and Adolphs R (2000). Hypersociability in Williams syndrome. *Journal of Cognitive Neuroscience*, **12**, 30–46.

Karmiloff-Smith, A. (1997). Crucial differences between developmental cognitive neuroscience and adult neuropsychology. *Developmental Neuropsychology*, **13**, 513–24.

Karmiloff-Smith, A., Klima, E., Bellugi, U., Grant, J., and Baron-Cohen, S. (1995). Is there a social module? Language, face-processing, and theory of mind in individuals with Williams syndrome. *Journal of Cognitive Neuroscience*, **7**, 196–208.

Karmiloff-Smith, A., Brown, J.H., Grice, S., and Peterson, S. (2003). Dethroning the myth: cognitive dissociations and innate modularity in Williams syndrome. *Developmental Neuropsychology*, **23**, 227–42.

Karmiloff-Smith, A., Thomas, M., Annaz, D., *et al.* (2004). Exploring the Williams syndrome face-processing debate: the importance of building developmental trajectories. *Journal of Child Psychology and Psychiatry*, **45**, 1258–74.

Klein-Tasman, B. and Mervis, C.B. (2003). Distinctive personality characteristics of 8-, 9-, and 10-year-olds with Williams syndrome. *Developmental Neuropsychology*, **23**, 269–90.

Laing, E., Butterworth, G., Gsodl, M., Longhi, E., Panagotaki, G., and Karmiloff-Smith, A. (2000). Pre-verbal communication skills in children with WMS. Paper presented at the 8th International WS Professional Meeting, Dearborn, MI.

Laing, E., Butterworth, G., Ansari, D., *et al.* (2002). Atypical development of language and social communication in toddlers with Williams syndrome. *Developmental Science*, **5**, 233–46.

Laws, G. and Bishop, D. (2004). Pragmatic language impairment and social deficits in Williams syndrome: a comparison with Down syndrome and specific language impairment. *International Journal of Language and Communication Disorders*, **39**, 45–64.

Leekam, S. (1990). Jokes and lies: children's understanding of intentional falsehood. In *Natural theories of mind: evolution, development, and simulation of everyday mindreading* (ed. A Whiten), pp. 159–174. Oxford: Basil Blackwell.

Lewis, M. (1993). Commentary on Raver and Leadbeater: The problem of the other in research on theory of mind and social development. *Human Development*, **36**, 146–56.

Marriage, J. (1994). Central hyperacusis in Williams syndrome. Paper presented at the Conference on Building Bridges Across Disciplines: Cognition to Gene, Williams Syndrome Association 6th International Professional Conference, San Diego, CA.

Meltzoff, A.N. (1995). Understanding the intentions of others: re-enactment of intended acts by 18-month-old children. *Developmental Psychology*, 31, 838–50.

Mervis, C.B. (2003). Williams syndrome: 15 years of psychological research. *Developmental Neuropsychology*, 23, 1–12.

Mervis, C.B. and Bertrand, J. (1997). Developmental relations between cognition and language: evidence from Williams syndrome. In *Communication and language acquisition: discoveries from atypical development*, pp. 75–106. Baltimore, MD: Brookes.

Mervis, C.B., Morris, C.A., Klein-Tasman, B.P., *et al.* (2003). Attentional characteristics of infants and toddlers with Williams syndrome during triadic interactions. *Developmental Neuropsychology*, 23, 243–68.

Mills, D.L., Alvarez, T.D., St George, M., Applebaum, L.G., Bellugi, U., and Neville, H. (2000). Electrophysiological studies of face processing in Williams syndrome. *Journal of Cognitive Neuroscience*, 12, 47–64.

Mobbs, D., Garrett, A.A., Menon, V., Rose, F.E., Bellugi, U., and Reiss, A.L. (2004). Anomalous brain activation during face and gaze processing in Williams syndrome. *Neurology*, 62, 1070–6.

Paul, B.M., Stiles, J., Passarotti, A., Bavar, N., and Bellugi, U. (2002). Face and place processing in Williams syndrome: evidence for a dorsal–ventral dissociation. *Cognitive Neuroscience and Neuropsychology*, 13, 1115–19.

Perner, J. (1988). Higher order beliefs and intentions in children's understanding of social interaction. In *Developing theories of mind* (ed. J.W. Astington, P.L. Harris, and D.R. Olson), pp. 271–294. Cambridge University Press.

Peterson, C.C. (2004). Theory of mind development in oral deaf children with cochlear implants or conventional hearing aids. *Journal of Child Psychology and Psychiatry*, 45, 1096–1106.

Peterson, C.C., Peterson, J.L., and Webb, J. (2000). Factors influencing the development of a theory of mind in blind children. *British Journal of Developmental Psychology*, 18, 431–47.

Phillips, M.L. (2004). Facial processing deficits and social dysfunction: how are they related? (Editorial) *Brain*, 127, 1691–2.

Pober, B.R. and Dykens, E.M. (1996). Williams syndrome: an overview of medical, cognitive and behavioral features. *Child and Adolescent Psychiatric Clinics of North America*, 5, 929–43.

Premack, D. and Woodruff, G. (1978). Does the chimpanzee have a 'theory of mind'? *Behavior and Brain Sciences*, 4, 515–26.

Prinz, W. and Meltzoff, A.N. (2002). An introduction to the imitative mind and brain. In *The imitative mind: development, evolution, and brain bases* (ed. A.N. Meltzoff and W. Prinz), pp. 1–18. Cambridge University Press.

Rossen, M., Jones, W., Wang, P.P., and Klima, E.S. (1995). Face processing: remarkable sparing in Williams syndrome. *Genetic Counseling*, 6, 138–40.

Sarimski, K. (1997). Behavioral phenotypes and family stress in three mental retardation syndromes. *European Child and Adolescent Psychiatry*, 63, 26–31.

Semel, E. and Rosner, S.R. (2003). *Understanding Williams syndrome: behavioral patterns and interventions*. Mahwah, NJ: Lawrence Erlbaum.

Shaked, M. and Yirmiya, N. (2004). Matching procedures in autism research: evidence from meta-analytic studies. *Journal of Autism and Developmental Disorders*, **34**, 35–40.

Simonoff, E., Bolton, P., and Rutter, M. (1998). Genetic perspectives on mental retardation. In *Handbook of mental retardation and development* (ed. J.A. Burack, R.M. Hodapp, and E. Zigler), pp. 41–79. Cambridge University Press.

Slomkowski, C. and Dunn, J. (1996). Young children's understanding of other people's beliefs and feelings and their connected communication with friends. *Developmental Psychology*, **32**, 442–7.

Sotillo, M., Campos, R., and Garayzabal, E. (2002). Pragmatic (mis)uses in Williams syndrome: metaphors and other indirect uses of language. Poster presented at IASCL/SRCLD, Madison, WI.

Sullivan, K. and Tager-Flusberg, H. (1999). Second-order belief attribution in Williams syndrome: intact or impaired? *American Journal on Mental Retardation*, **104**, 523–32.

Sullivan, K., Winner, E., and Tager-Flusberg, H. (2003). Can adolescents with Williams syndrome tell the difference between lies and jokes? *Developmental Neuropsychology*, **23**, 85–103.

Tager-Flusberg, H. and Sullivan, K. (1999). Are theory of mind abilities spared in children with Williams syndrome? Paper presented at the meeting of the Society of Research in Child Development, Albuquerque, NM.

Tager-Flusberg, H. and Sullivan, K. (2000). A componential view of theory of mind: evidence from Williams syndrome. *Cognition*, **76**, 59–89.

Tager-Flusberg, H., Sullivan, K., and Boshart, J. (1997). Executive functions and performance on false belief tasks. *Developmental Neuropsychology*, **13**, 487–93.

Tager-Flusberg, H., Boshart, J., and Baron-Cohen, S. (1998). Reading the windows to the soul: evidence of domain-specific sparing in Williams syndrome. *Journal of Cognitive Neuroscience*, **10**, 631–9.

Tager-Flusberg, H., Plesa-Skwerer, D., Faja, S., and Joseph, R.M. (2003). People with Williams syndrome process faces holistically. *Cognition*, **89**, 11–24.

Udwin, O. and Yule, W. (1991). A cognitive and behavioral phenotype in Williams syndrome. *Journal of Clinical and Experimental Neuropsychology*, **13**, 232–44.

Wimmer, H. and Perner, J. (1983). Beliefs about beliefs: representation and constraining function of wrong beliefs in young children's understanding deception. *Cognition*, **13**, 103–28.

Woodward, A.L. (1998). Infants selectively encode the goal object of an actor's reach. *Cognition*, **69**, 1–34.

Yirmiya, N., Erel, O., Shaked, M., and Solomonica-Levi, D. (1998). Meta-analyses comparing theory of mind abilities of individuals with autism, individuals with mental retardation, and normally developing individuals. *Psychological Bulletin*, **124**, 283–307.

Youngblade, L. and Dunn, J. (1995). Individual differences in young children's pretend play with mother and siblings: links to relationships and understanding of other people's feelings and beliefs. *Child Development*, **66**, 1472–92.

4

Language and theory of mind in atypically developing children
Evidence from studies of deafness, blindness, and autism

Michael Siegal and Candida C. Peterson

Language and theory of mind are two essential human capacities that can be considered as the culmination of an evolutionary process. Through language, we converse about our culture and transmit knowledge across generations about the nature of the mental and physical worlds. Communication between people can take place more rapidly when they converse together in a language governed by grammatical rules than through direct observation, facial or bodily signals, pictorial media, or other non-linguistic formats. In this sense, conversation is evolutionarily adaptive as it provides an efficient means to communicate feedback about potentially threatening events that are remote in time and space (Dunbar 1993).

A second essential human characteristic seems inextricably linked to language and conversation (Astington 2000; Harris 2005). This is possession of a theory of mind (ToM) which permits us to reason about the mental states of others—their beliefs, desires, and intentions—and to understand and anticipate how these differ from our own. A lack of ToM would be a formidable obstacle to all sophisticated forms of human social interaction, including family cohesion and close relationships. Without the recognition that beliefs can be true or false, there would exist a constant state of misunderstanding, mistrust, and conflict. Moreover, without ToM reasoning, we would be unable to appreciate many of the hallmarks of human culture. Events portrayed in novels, drama, and song would be meaningless as these often rely on the recognition that persons have been misled by their false beliefs. Indeed, given its importance, ToM has come to dominate the study of social cognition in typically and atypically developing children over the past 20 years (Flavell 2004).

As there are children whose language acquisition is jeopardized because their hearing or vision is impaired, a key issue that arises concerns the effects of disruptions of the typical course of language acquisition on the expression of ToM reasoning. In this chapter, we discuss how sensory impairments can jeopardize the language acquisition and conversational understanding that may play crucial roles for ToM. We examine these issues in relation to the social cognition of typically and atypically developing children, such as children who are deaf or blind or who may be suffering from autism. As such, upon finishing the chapter, the reader will not only be familiar with the role of language in the development of social cognitive deficits associated with deafness, blindness, and autism, but also the role of language in typically developing social cognition.

4.1 The course of language acquisition in hearing and deaf children

Language is typically acquired spontaneously without formal instruction. Indeed, newborns learn sounds for speech even while they are sleeping (Cheour *et al.* 2002) and, in the first few years of human development, virtually all children rapidly acquire the tools of their native language, including that language's lexicon, morphology, and syntactic rules of grammar. In fact, the grammar of language is mandatory in that we cannot stop ourselves from acquiring it.

One influential view of language acquisition is that the manifestation of structure in children's language is triggered even in circumstances where exposure to a linguistic input is highly limited and fragmented—an indication of the fundamental innateness of grammar or syntactic regularity. According to the 'poverty of the stimulus' account (Chomsky 1980; Newport 1990; Pinker 1994; Stromwold 2000; Crain and Pietroski 2001; Laurence and Margolis 2001), the acquisition of grammar proceeds automatically in a modular fashion, largely independently of non-verbal intelligence. Despite wide variations in their language environment, children in different language communities acquire aspects of grammar in a fixed order at about the same time in their development. They make sense of a language input that is compatible not only with the grammar of their own native language but also with the grammar of many other languages. The errors that children make are highly predictable and often reflect what would be grammatical in another language (Crain and Pietroski 2001). Further, it has long been established that children are not corrected for the grammar of what they say but only for the truth value of their utterances (Brown and Hanlon 1970). That children's grammar itself proceeds rapidly and becomes progressively more similar to that of adults largely in the absence of corrective feedback further testifies to the biological foundations of language.

Evidence from deaf children who are cut off from speech input corroborates this account. Petitto and Marentette (1991) found that profoundly deaf infants of deaf parents displayed manual babbling using a reduced set of the phonetic units in American Sign Language. These results support the view that, first, babbling (or the meaningless production of language-like signals devoid of communicative intent) and, later, the meaningful production of symbolically representational word units (either spoken or signed) are both tied to the abstract conceptual structure of language rather than to input specifically from the speech modality. Further analysis reveals that hearing babies who are exposed to the sign language of their deaf parents produce low-frequency hand movements inside a tightly restricted space in front of the body, corresponding to the signing space in most signed languages (Petitto et al. 2001).

Moreover, deaf children from hearing families with no exposure to native users of sign language are found to display similarities to one another in the linguistic structure of their spontaneous iconic gestural communication despite wide variations in the spoken language of their hearing mothers. Furthermore, these children soon outstrip their hearing mothers' limited gestural models in both the versatility and the complexity of the gestures they create in order to communicate meaning. In fact, the spontaneous untutored hand signals of American deaf children from hearing families resemble the signs similarly created by Chinese deaf children more closely than they do the words spoken by their own mothers (Goldin-Meadow and Mylander 1998; Goldin-Meadow 2003).

It would seem that a language model is not necessary in order for 'language-making' skills to be activated. Segmenting words into morphemes, organizing words into syntactically regular sentences, setting up a system of contrasts in morphology, and building up more complex syntactic structures for negation, affirmation, and interrogation can all take place when deaf children without access to speech develop their own system of 'home-sign', or gestural language. Based on a longitudinal observational study of the informal gestural communication schemes that 10 American deaf toddlers from hearing–speaking families created while being exposed only to speech and trained in a purely oral tradition to articulate speech and read lips, Goldin-Meadow (2003, p. 161) concluded that:

> Deaf children's hearing parents are not responsible for their children's gesture systems. Neither the way parents respond to the children's gestures, nor the gestures that parents produce when talking to the children can explain the structure found in the deaf children's gestures.

Even without a model to copy, deaf children create a gestural communicative system that possesses many of the same features as a natural signed or spoken language. As shown in a study of deaf children in Nicaragua exposed initially to a highly degraded language environment (Senghas *et al.* 2004), deaf children can act largely independently of an adult model to create spontaneously a functional scheme of meaningful signs to convey ideas to one another, culminating in the establishment of a mature language (Nicaraguan Sign Language) that has emerged over the past 25 years.

Moreover, research on deaf children in input-deprived language environments points to an optimal or critical period for language acquisition. Persons who become deaf after having already acquired spoken English during childhood are often more proficient at learning a sign language than those born profoundly deaf into a hearing family who received little linguistic experience as infants, toddlers, and preschoolers before exposure to a sign language at school. Deaf persons who are exposed early in childhood to a natural sign language are generally also able to learn a second language, such as spoken English, better than those who have not been exposed to language until later (Mayberry *et al.* 2002). In rare cases when deaf children, throughout the period from birth to the teens, are not exposed to any language whatsoever, whether spoken or signed, nor to any possible human partners in communicative interaction, they do appear to be irreparably impaired in their later language learning as assessed during adulthood (Curtiss 1977; Grimshaw *et al.* 1998; Lenneberg 1967).

While this research highlights the probable important roles of modular human language acquisition capacities and environmental exposure to social, conversational, and linguistic interaction with communication partners from infancy onwards, two important factors complicate the interpretation of many of the empirical studies of language development in the deaf that we have so far examined. These factors are equally central to the studies of social cognition in deaf children to be examined shortly.

The first complication, as we have already seen, relates to the hearing status of the family into which a deaf child is born. If a child has a signing deaf parent, the issue of being deaf versus hearing may play little or no role in that child's rate and manner of language acquisition, even though the language that he/she acquires may be signed rather than spoken. Deaf infants with natively signing deaf parents develop sign language on the same early timetable as hearing infants' acquisition of spoken language (Harris 1992; Bonvillian 1999), but deaf infants with hearing parents are generally delayed in both signed and spoken language mastery (Marschark 1993; de Villiers and de Villiers 2000). Very few hearing parents are able to acquire a command of sign language equal to that of a native user, so that profoundly deaf children who have been exposed to sign language typically do not achieve fluency until they join a community of fluent signers in primary school (Power and Carty 1990).

The homesign that orally trained deaf children often acquire in a hearing family, while containing many of the features of natural language, is not comparable to a fully fledged sign language (Goldin-Meadow 2003). Thus, since most deaf children (about 90 per cent in most contemporary Western populations) are born to hearing parents, language development is typically delayed when the child is severely or profoundly deaf. De Villiers *et al.* (1994, p. 43) remark that there are 'serious shortcomings in the [spoken] English grammars of oral deaf subjects' even when tested during adulthood or the late teens so that 'most deaf children acquiring English develop an incompletely specified grammar'.

A second factor complicating much research on deafness is the level of a child's hearing loss. Research must clearly distinguish among groups of deaf children in terms of the level and nature of their hearing loss, as well as age of onset (e.g. pre-lingual versus post-lingual). Since children with mild hearing losses of 20-40 dB often perceive speech sounds, especially when they are fitted with a hearing aid or a cochlear implant, they do not generally experience substantial interference with their spoken language acquisition. However, severe hearing losses (71–90 dB) and profound deafness (losses of 91 dB or more in the better ear) are associated with delayed language for the vast majority of deaf children of hearing parents. This occurs irrespective of whether these children are given cochlear implants (surgically installed devices which short-circuit the ear to stimulate the auditory nerve electronically) or conventional amplifying hearing aids (Niparko 2000), and irrespective of whether the language they are exposed to, and eventually acquire, is spoken or signed (Marschark 1993). Cochlear implant technology continues to evolve and implants are being fitted earlier and earlier. When the surgery is successful, the implant can drastically improve a deaf child's pure tone perception (Niparko 2000). Yet, typically, many years of intensive and time-demanding speech and hearing therapy is still required in order for the child to learn to perceive and produce speech. Although deaf children who are given cochlear implants early in their development generally perform better on measures of spoken language development by primary school age than those who receive implants later in childhood (Svirsky *et al.* 2000, 2004), language development is generally delayed even for infant-implanted groups during the preschool period. As we shall see, this also has implications for the toddler's capacity to engage in linguistically mediated conversational interaction with peers and adults (Preisler *et al.* 1997) and for the expression of ToM reasoning (Peterson 2004a).

The 'poverty of stimulus' account can make sense of such findings on the basis that some minimal exposure to grammatical language and human social interaction is needed to trigger the maturational unfolding of modularized language growth (Garfield *et al.* 2001). But this account is not the only model of language acquisition to which contemporary researchers and theorists subscribe. Nor does a modular explanation (Fodor 1983) necessarily imply that the emergence of all language-related abilities is best characterized as innate and biological. Fast-acting domain-specific cognitive modules are not necessarily prewired, but can instead be acquired through experiences like acculturation, interaction, and tuition—as in the case of reading, which does not emerge in all cultures (Garfield *et al.* 2001).

Furthermore, there are theorists who emphasize that the social, conversational, and linguistic inputs offered to the child play a more important role than nativist theories of language would suggest (e.g. Cowie 1998; Tomasello 2003). It has been argued that social interaction and successful communication drive language discovery. Some time ago, Bruner (1983) suggested that social, familial, and cultural experiences pave the way for increases in its versatility and lexical and syntactic complexity over development. On this account, language unfolds through social experience, with successful communication providing the reward for prior achievements and the key to future progressive mastery.

Research evidence continues to address these differing accounts. For example, in a recent ingenious series of experiments, Lidz *et al.* (2003a) demonstrated that infants aged 16–18 months could respond to a task in a manner suggesting that they comprehended the syntax of usage of the pronoun 'one' even though their language environment was not yet thought to contain sufficient information to guide unaided learning. Lidz *et al.* (2003a, p. B72; see also Lidz *et al.* 2003b) argued that such results demonstrate that 'innate linguistic structure guides language acquisition' on the grounds that the linguistic input available to infants this young cannot unambiguously support anaphoric representations. However, another possible explanation for these results is that the meaning of the lexical term 'another' had been acquired by 18 months through communication with others (Bruner 1983), in line with a rapid surge in vocabulary development that is noted in the typical hearing child at around this age (Corballis 2002).

Consistent with the view that linguistic structure within the language learner is the main source of grammatical knowledge, Gelman (2005) documents how young children have an understanding that nouns (e.g. 'bird') can be used to refer to generic kinds rather than solely to specific instances and that this understanding is not guided by either perceptual or linguistic cues. Instead, available data suggest that the expression of a system of generic terms appears to be driven by the theoretical assumption on the part of the child that a noun is a generic term unless the context dictates to the contrary. Even deaf children from hearing homes who are without access to spoken or signed models of categorical reference express generic kinds in their gestures (Goldin-Meadow 2003).

4.2 Theory of mind reasoning in hearing and deaf children

Investigations of ToM reasoning have been concerned with children's understanding that beliefs about the world may be true or false and may guide human action even when discrepant from reality. Tasks designed to determine whether young children can identify how a person with a false belief will behave, known collectively as inferential false belief tasks, are used so often to assess ToM development that they have become known as 'litmus tests'. These often involve scenarios in which actors or puppets are given information either about the location of a hidden object, or about the contents of a container, which the child participant comes to discover is obsolete or false. In both cases, task success depends on the child's ability to predict the consequences of a belief that is now discrepant from reality.

Such measures of children's understanding of false beliefs often take the form of the 'Sally–Anne' task involving changed locations for hidden objects (Baron-Cohen *et al.* 1985) and the 'Smarties' task involving unexpected contents of misleadingly labelled containers (Wimmer and Perner 1983). In the Sally–Anne task, children are told about Sally, a story character with a false belief about the location of a marble. The character is described as having placed the marble in a box but, when she is away, another story character called Anne moves it into a different location. The test question concerns where Sally, who has not witnessed the deception and therefore has a false belief, will look for the marble. In the Smarties task, children are shown a Smarties tube (M&M candies in the USA) which, when opened, is revealed to contain pencils. The test question concerns what another person, who again has not witnessed the deception and therefore has a false belief, will think is in the tube. Yet another task takes the form of 'thought pictures' (Custer 1996; Woolfe *et al.* 2002). Here, for example, children are shown a picture of a boy fishing who feels a tug at the end of a fishing line. Unbeknown to the boy, it is a boot rather than a fish. The children are shown four pictures (a fish, a boot, and two distracter objects) and are asked to point to the picture that shows what the boy thinks he has caught and what he has caught in reality.

On such tasks, most typically developing hearing children appear to develop ToM reasoning by about 4–5 years of age (Wellman *et al.* 2001) despite wide cultural variations in their child-rearing circumstances (Avis and Harris 1991) as well as wide variations within the same culture in the extent to which preschoolers from different families are exposed to talk about mental states of others (Dunn 1996; Shatz et al. 2003).

In this sense, the expression of ToM reasoning appears to run parallel to that of the acquisition of the grammar of language, in that ToM, as indexed by false-belief mastery which, as we have noted, emerges on an early timetable in most typical hearing children by about the age of 4–5 years (Wellman et al. 2001) and seems to do so largely independently of variations in social experience. On this basis, Leslie et al. (2004) have argued that the expression of ToM is a manifestation of a dedicated module for mental state reasoning which emerges through the development of a 'selection processor' mechanism. The selection processor involves 'executive functioning' which enables children to inhibit the usual state of affairs in which a person's beliefs correspond to reality and to recognize that beliefs may be true or false, leading children to select the correct alternative on Sally–Anne type ToM tasks.

However, just as children require some minimal access to language in order for grammar to develop, they also require at least some minimal access to conversational and social opportunities in order to display ToM reasoning skills on a normative timetable. For example, Morgan and Kegl (2006) report that Nicaraguan deaf adults without early access to language show persistent difficulties on ToM tasks, although they do display a degree of proficiency in characterizing the mental states of characters in cartoon stories. On this basis, it is conceivable that there is a critical period for access to mentalistic social and conversational input in order to express ToM, at least as shown on some measures to date that have been designed to examine the understanding of others' false beliefs.

As with language development, deaf children from hearing families do not display ToM reasoning as readily as do deaf children from native-signing deaf families (Peterson and Siegal 2000). Furthermore, richer levels of ToM-relevant input during the preschool period are associated with individual advancement in ToM understanding ahead of the norm, both within and between cultures and in both hearing children and deaf children from deaf families (Dunn 1996; Peterson and Slaughter 2003; Ruffman et al. 2003; Woolfe et al. 2003, Slade and Ruffman 2005). Thus children whose families frequently and extensively discuss mental states with them during everyday play, conversation, conflict, emotional outbursts, and disciplinary intervention are usually the first to master concepts of false belief. Moreover, within an age range of 3–5 years, performance on ToM tasks which follow the Sally–Anne or Smarties task procedures is often facilitated when the actual verb used in the test question implies that the actor might have a false belief, as is the case for certain verbs in languages such as Mandarin Chinese, Greek, Turkish, and Puerto Rican Spanish (Lee et al. 1999; Maridaki-Kassotaki et al. 2003; Shatz et al. 2003).

However, children who speak English and are younger than 4 years also succeed for the most part if the tasks are made more pragmatically explicit (Bloom and German 2000). For example, asking 'Where will Sally look first for her marble?' enables most (although not all) 3-year-olds to 'inhibit' the interpretation that the test question in false tasks refers to where Sally will have to look or must look for the desired object. Instead, children are more likely to interpret the question as intended to refer to the consequences of Sally holding an initial false belief about the location of an object (Siegal and Beattie 1991; Joseph 1998; Surian and Leslie 1999; Nelson *et al.* 2003; Yazdi *et al.* 2006).

Vocabulary development may be relevant to ToM mastery, with children needing to have some preliminary understanding of the lexical meaning of words like 'think', 'know', 'want', or 'pretend' in order to reflect upon, and discuss, these inner states with others. Such experiences may play a critical role in developing an awareness of the workings of the human mind. Signing deaf children from hearing families may not acquire words for inner states until school age, with exposure to a sign language and communication with signing teachers and signing deaf peers (Peterson and Slaughter 2006). Orally educated severely and profoundly deaf children from hearing families who are learning to listen and speak with the help of cochlear implants or hearing aids may also be slow to master mental state vocabulary and are often seriously delayed in ToM development. As they typically still fail false-belief tests of ToM at age 7 years or later (Peterson 2004a), they perform similarly to late-signing deaf children from hearing families (Peterson and Siegal 2002). These findings can be interpreted to reflect delayed language development which limits opportunities to converse, in sign or speech, with others about inner mental states.

In addition to simple vocabulary, the development of a grammar adequate to construct propositions about mental states may also underpin children's success in ToM reasoning on false-belief tasks. One view is that acquisition of the grammatical rules for mentalistic discourse is a necessary precursor and prerequisite for ToM mastery of false belief (de Villiers and Pyers 2002). According to this theory, it is a specific feature of the grammar of language, namely mastery of the linguistic rules for embedding tensed complement clauses under verbs of speech or cognition (e.g. 'Sally thinks that the marble is in the basket'), that assists ToM. In embedded complements of this kind, the truth value of the embedded clause (prefaced by 'that …') is independent of that of the main argument ('Sally thinks …'). It is argued that this syntactic feature enables children to conceptualize propositional attitudes. By this account, ToM reasoning is dependent on the possession of syntactic structures such as those that permit the embedding of false propositions within true statements.

In fact, there is a correlation between false-belief test performance and language growth, as shown on measures of vocabulary, in both typically developing children (Astington and Jenkins 1999) and children with autism (Happé 1995). Furthermore, in typically developing children, syntactic skill and semantic word usage, along with receptive vocabulary, predict higher false-belief scores simultaneously and longitudinally (Astington and Jenkins 1999).

However, the interpretation of the correlation between measures of language and measures of ToM remains controversial. The extent to which language influences ToM reasoning, as shown in performance on false-belief tasks, versus the extent to which language growth and conversational sophistication require and reflect emergence of ToM remain open questions (Astington and Baird 2005).

Some researchers have claimed that the grammar of language enables children to entertain propositions that involve the simultaneous representation of alternative states of affairs such as the consequences of behaviour by individuals who hold true or false beliefs (Perner 1991; Astington and Jenkins 1999; Smith *et al.* 2003). In particular, 'sentence complementation' in the grammar of language has been viewed as enabling children to reason out solutions to false beliefs (de Villiers and Pyers 2002). By this account, ToM reasoning is based on the acquisition of syntactic structures such as those that permit the embedding of false propositions within true statements ('Mary knows that John (falsely) thinks chocolates are in the cupboard'). It has also been suggested that conversational exchanges in a language of mental states draws these inner states to children's attention (Astington 2000). Thus better language may help children converse with others and, through conversation, gain insights into others' minds. These insights can then refine their conceptual understanding of vocabulary and syntax (e.g. the meaning of mental state terms and the syntactic point-of-view markers bound up with talk about thinking (de Villiers 2005)) and, via a circular process, these linguistic developments may, in turn, assist conversational exchanges of mental state information and success on standard ToM tests (Nelson *et al.* 2003).

Yet it is likely that none of these hypotheses fully captures the contributions of linguistic and non-linguistic developments to growth of ToM (Harris *et al.* 2005). It may be that a certain level of syntax and semantics is necessary for success on certain ToM tasks but, nevertheless, many young children are adept at syntax and semantics but still do poorly. For example, Woolfe *et al.* (2002) found that late-signing deaf children from hearing families who had achieved the same level of receptive ability in the syntax and morphology of British Sign Language as did native-signing deaf children from deaf families still displayed difficulties on ToM tasks. Although Hale and Tager-Flusberg (2003) and Lohmann and Tomasello (2003) have reported success at training ToM performance with exposure to instruction on sentence complementation, Ruffman *et al.* (2003) found that ToM reasoning was related to general language ability rather than to specific aspects of syntax or semantics. Moreover, as Lohmann *et al.* (2005) recognize, training studies on sentence complementation may in fact involve exposure to discourse that may foster conversational understanding which, in turn, promotes success on false-belief tasks, in line with their finding that general training on appearance–reality contrasts without using any complement clause constructions during the training phase was also beneficial.

As has been previously noted (Custer 1996; Astington and Jenkins 1999; Garfield *et al.* 2001; Woolfe *et al.* 2002), many of the typically developing 3-year-olds who fail ToM tasks are nevertheless able to produce and comprehend sentence complements that take the structure [person]–[pretends]–[that x] (e.g. 'He pretends that his puppy is outside'). More recently, evidence from both Cantonese- and German-speaking children has yielded no support for a link between understanding of sentence complements and ToM reasoning (Perner *et al.* 2003; Cheung *et al.* 2004). Converging evidence comes from studies of adults who have become aphasic and have lost grammar following brain damage despite retaining their ToM reasoning ability (Varley and Siegal 2000; Varley *et al.* 2001). Although such patients have a language-configured mind that could be seen to support ToM development, their performance is consistent with the dissociation between grammar and ToM in childhood. Finally, there are many instances of sign languages and spoken Aboriginal Australian languages in which there is no sentence complementation (M.A. Baker, personal communication). Instead of clausal complements such as 'John told everyone that Mary washed the car', users of such languages instead employ 'clausal adjunct' forms such as 'Mary having washed the car, John told everyone (it)'. If complementation were necessary to instantiate ToM reasoning, no ToM would be possible in these language groups.

A related account of how children come to express ToM reasoning is based on the timing of children's access to language and conversation and has much in common with the poverty of the stimulus account of language acquisition. Just as children acquire syntax without being explicitly taught the concepts of noun, verb, and grammatical subject, they are not usually explicitly taught the concept of belief. Instead, they receive information on the truth value of belief–desire propositions in everyday discourse involving mental state terms while arguing, conversing, or playing pretend with peers and siblings and during everyday interaction with adults. This process may trigger the understanding that the beliefs of others may not correspond to reality.

Deaf children born to hearing parents usually have only very limited access to either a spoken or signed language early in development and this curtails their opportunities for participating in these kinds of conversational social exchanges. As such, their developmental trajectories for language and ToM may throw light on the importance of the timing of access to language and conversation on the expression of ToM reasoning. Using a scaling methodology, Peterson and Slaughter (2006) found that late-signing deaf children from hearing families spontaneously included terms for inner states of desire, affect, and perception ahead of terms for cognition in their signed conversation, whereas spontaneous talk about cognition itself reliably developmentally preceded success on standard false-belief tests of ToM. While some deaf children eventually respond correctly on such tests by middle childhood, many (without any intellectual or social disabilities apart from hearing loss) have been found to have problems with false-belief tests and stories about the mental states of others well into their teens and even adulthood (Morgan and Kegl 2006; Russell et al. 1998), similar to individuals with autism (Happé 1995). For example, only 60 per cent of one sample of late-signing deaf adolescents of hearing parents passed the Sally–Ann false-belief test between age 15 and 18 years (Russell et al. 1998). These difficulties persist even on versions of the tasks in which the test questions are made pragmatically explicit (Peterson and Siegal 1995). A possible contributing factor is a lack of early exposure to family conversation about mental states. In contrast to late signing deaf children, both normal hearing and native signing deaf children appear to enjoy an early conversational access that triggers the expression of reasoning about others' beliefs and their consequences during the preschool period (Woolfe et al. 2002; Courtin and Melot 2005).

This pattern of results supports the importance of early access to language and conversation in the expression of ToM reasoning in normal children, and is consistent with a critical periods hypothesis for which at least some early conversational experience is seen as necessary to alert children to the concept that others' beliefs can differ from their own and be false (Siegal and Varley 2002). Early opportunities for either deaf or hearing children to participate in conversations about mental states with parents and siblings in a sign or spoken language appear to speed up this process of ToM reasoning (Dunn 1994; Peterson 2000; Woolfe et al. 2003). In this way, children come to recognize that speakers are epistemic beings who store and seek to provide information about the world through conversation, thus allowing access to a world of referents and propositions about intangible objects and mental events while creating the potential for imagining the past and future (Harris 1996; Harris et al. 2005). By contrast, as is the case for language, the developmental trajectory of ToM reasoning is adversely affected when the requisite conversational input is not received within an early optimal critical period. Apart from late-signing deaf children, the variable success of deaf children provided with cochlear implants on ToM tasks (Peterson 2004a) may reflect the variable success of implants in permitting deaf children to engage in oral conversation, along with the social participation and peer interaction delays that inevitably arise during post-implant auditory and language mastery. This may also be the case for some non-vocal children with cerebral palsy who, despite normal non-verbal intelligence, are precluded by their motor impairment from mastering the speech that would allow them to engage in conversations with peers, siblings, and parents about mental states (Dahlgren *et al.* 2003; Peterson 2004a).

Based on the attention patterns of preverbal hearing infants, there are demonstrations, albeit controversial, that even hearing 15-month-olds have expectations about the behaviour of persons with a false belief (Onishi and Baillargeon 2005; Perner and Ruffman 2005; Surian *et al.* 2007). Consistent with the position that children display an early sense of ToM reasoning (Scholl and Leslie 1999; Leslie *et al.* 2004), infants by the age of 15 months imitate on the basis of the intentions of an actor rather than on the basis of an actor's actual behaviour (Gergely *et al.* 2002; see also Chapter 11, this volume). They become angry when an actor is unwilling to give them a toy and not when he/she is unableto do so (Behne *et al.* 2005). Information communicating that others are repositories of beliefs that differ from reality is conveyed in infancy, not just from the age of 3–4 years. This input is available for both hearing infants of hearing parents and for deaf children of deaf parents (in sign language). However, as noted in reports describing the difficulties of late-signing deaf children on false-belief tasks (e.g. Woolfe *et al.* 2002), it is largely absent for deaf infants with hearing parents who communicate primarily through speech. Such children with hearing parents show protracted difficulties on false-belief tasks even when they have been specially provided with sign language at the age of 2 years, as is the case in Sweden to comply with government legislation (Falkman *et al.* 2007). These difficulties appear to be specific to the representation of false beliefs and do not generalize to other areas of cognitive development.

4.3 Language development and early communication in blind children

Like deaf children, blind children are a heterogeneous group. Levels of visual loss may vary from legal blindness (defined as a visual acuity of 20/200 or worse—compared with 20/20 vision for a normal eye) through minimal light perception to complete absence of sight. The whole visual field may be affected, or there may be only peripheral, or central, vision. Some visual impairments can be ameliorated with increased illumination and/or magnifying lenses, while others are not susceptible to prosthesis. Age of onset may also vary, although most childhood blindness in the developed world today has its onset either at birth (e.g. hereditary blindness or blindness owing to prenatal rubella virus) or perinatally (e.g. blindness owing to retinopathy of prematurity). These diagnostic variations can all have important implications for individual differences among blind children in social, linguistic, and cognitive development, as well as for variations in their family, peer, and educational experiences.

Blindness is a rare disorder. It is estimated that nine in 10 000 children aged 3–10 years in the USA are legally blind and that two of every three of these children has at least one serious developmental disability besides visual impairment (Centers for Disease Control 2005). In the UK, it is estimated that one preschooler in 1000 has a visual impairment that will necessitate special educational provision and that three in 10 000 are so severely blind that they can perceive light only and will require Braille in order to learn to read (Tirosh *et al.* 1992). The low population prevalence of blindness has resulting in many published studies with very small sample sizes, often based on only two to four children or even single case studies (Lewis 2003). The heterogeneity of visual disorders among blind children as a group, in conjunction with these small sample sizes and the high frequencies of co-diagnoses of additional disabilities (e.g. autism, mental retardation), complicates the interpretation of much ToM and language research, especially when co-diagnosed disabilities may themselves have implications for the child's development. Nevertheless, there are certain consistencies in findings to date, especially those that arise from studies of congenitally or perinatally blind children whose condition is either severe (e.g. 20/400 or less) or profound (e.g. light perception only) without other serious disabilities.

In terms of language development, recent findings largely concur with Fraiberg's (1977) pioneering discovery that the course of language acquisition is both delayed and distinctively different for blind toddlers compared with sighted peers. From birth to 12 months, many important communicative interactions arise between sighted infants and their caregivers that may help to pave the way for language acquisition. Social cues are shared. These include gaze direction, eye contact, pointing at objects of mutual interest, and joint attention such as turning the head to follow the direction of a parent's gaze (Butterworth 1998), as well as imitation of visually perceived facial expressions (Meltzoff and Moore 1977). Late in the first year of life, most sighted infants display social referencing (e.g. consulting a parent's facial expression to discover whether a novel stimulus is threatening or not). At the start of their expressive language, sighted babies witness and learn to copy culturally significant visual signals (e.g. nodding 'yes', waving 'bye-bye'), and parents may initiate a variety of interactive social games and routines like peekaboo, pantomime, and mocking or teasing in the visual modality. These non-verbal social exchanges often resemble conversation in that partners take turns and attend to one another. Thus they prepare children for meaningful spoken exchange and also foster the sharing of perspectives between parent and children who are sighted (whether hearing or deaf). Some have argued (Bruner 1983) that preverbal exchanges like these are crucial for the acquisition of language, while also serving as building blocks for social and conceptual growth (see also Chapter 11, this volume).

As blind infants' access to these experiences is often curtailed, their prelinguistic conversational expressiveness is delayed. For example, in a study comparing blind with sighted 12-month-olds, Tröster and Bambring (1992) found that the blind infants did not initiate much contact with parents by voice, touch, or posture. They tended to maintain blank emotional expressions on their faces and in their voices, even when the parents expressed intense emotion non-verbally. Sighted infants were not only comparatively more responsive to parental vocal and facial affective expressions, but were also inclined to mirror their parents' affectively charged non-verbal postural, facial, and vocal cues by changing the tone, loudness, or pace of their babbled vocalizations and expressing affect, thus setting up responsive sequences of imitative exchange.

Consequently, during this crucial early prelinguistic period, blind infants may miss out on access to parental non-verbal information on inner states of attention, affect, perception, and intention, as well as on the opportunity to learn how to engage in the babbled 'pseudo-conversations' that may foster later semantic and pragmatic language development (Bruner 1983). Similarly, Preisler (1995) reported that social referencing and turn-taking were slow to emerge in infants who were blind. Whereas blind children did eventually develop these behaviours, they did not do so until an average of 21 months of age, compared with 6–9 months for the typical sighted baby.

Dunlea (1989) carried out a naturalistic observational longitudinal study of early language development in four blind children and one typically developing sighted comparison child. She found some important differences in the ways that the blind and sighted children were acquiring their first spoken vocabularies. For example, one striking difference was a lag of comprehension behind speech production for each of the four blind children, in contrast with the sighted toddler whose comprehension far exceeded the words that he could meaningfully produce. In addition, even 'words' that blind children did express were not always comprehended by the same children on a subsequent occasion. For example, if a child said 'rah' when holding a rattle, she would not necessarily select that rattle if an adult said 'rah' while holding it out, nor would a different rattle, or the same rattle handled from a different angle, be labelled 'rah' by the blind child herself. McConachie (1990) also found that word comprehension lagged significantly behind word production for a group of 20 totally blind children (with minimal light perception, or less) aged between 12 and 24 months, and the gap was substantial (up to 13 months). Between age 2 and age 3, this unusual advance of speech over comprehension remained in evidence for about a third of the blind children.

Dunlea (1989) also noted that extension of words to new exemplars and contexts by blind children was very infrequent, even though this over-extension mechanism is one of the main ways in which sighted children communicate meaning and develop new words when their vocabularies are rapidly expanding (Clark 1983). As children develop, they can creatively apply words broadly to conceptually related items beyond the typical range of reference for the same lexical term in adult speech. For example, a child might use the word 'ball' not only for a rubber ball but also for whole beetroot, grapefruit, and marbles (Peterson 2004b). In Dunlea's study, the sighted comparison child, typically of sighted children in general, used 41 per cent of his first 100 words as over-extensions of this kind. The comparable figures for the blind children ranged from only 8 per cent to 13 per cent. Many of the blind children's first words were so restricted in meaning that they appeared to refer to only one restricted instance or personal action. This pattern of results led Dunlea to conclude that blind children are initially not as aware as sighted children of the symbolic function of words to express conceptual meaning and communicate ideas to others. Taken together, these findings indicate that, while blind and sighted children seem to be motivated to acquire words during their second year, the mechanisms that allow sighted children to take an active creative role in vocabulary development and the processes that enable them to recognize and extract information as a basis for deriving word meanings are not functioning at the same level for blind children at the onset of language.

The availability of a sensitive and responsive conversational partner is a crucial ingredient in the child's development (Bruner 1983). When typical sighted children attempt to use language to convey meanings that adult listeners persistently misunderstand, vocabulary development slows markedly (Nelson 1973). Given that blind infants cannot share gaze, pointing, or gestures with conversational partners in order to socially negotiate the meanings conveyed by speech, it is not surprising that the early stages of vocabulary acquisition are delayed. Nor is it surprising that, later on, as individual words are combined into sentences and the rules of syntax are mastered, blind children also have continuing difficulties in aspects of language development. Their language delays are particularly pronounced with the pragmatic and conversational features of speech and with 'areas of language acquisition where visual information can provide input about the world and be a stimulus for forming hypotheses about pertinent aspects of the linguistic system' (Andersen *et al.* 1984, p. 645).

One example concerns the reversal of pronouns, involving the pragmatic rule that the speaker refers to self in the first person and to the listener in the second person, so that the child is 'you' when addressed by an adult, but is 'I' when replying. A number of studies have indicated that blind children are late to master this rule (Fraiberg 1977; Andersen *et al.* 1984; Dunlea 1989), with blind children often persistently referring to themselves as 'you' while in the speaker's role. According to Andersen *et al.*, these errors reflect the more general problem of blind children with lexical, syntactic, and pragmatic features of language that reflect a perspective or point of view, including verbs like 'come' versus 'go', adverbs like 'here' versus 'there', pronouns like 'my/your/his', or articles like 'a' versus' 'the' where the lexical choice depends on the speaker's perspective and the conversational context. Hobson (1993) has linked pronoun reversal with the perspective-taking skills that underpin ToM (see next section) and with visual deprivation of social cues, especially facial expression and pointing in blindness. However, not all blind children have problems with pronouns. Perez-Pereira and Conti-Ramsden (1999) studied three totally blind toddlers aged between 2 and 3.5 years and found that only one of them made frequent reversal errors that showed no tendency to improve over time.

Clearly, there are factors in addition to blindness that influence blind children's mastery of syntactic rules and pragmatic communication. Nevertheless, most researchers have concluded that language development in general is more challenging for blind than for sighted children, and that social uses of language to share meaning with others and to exchange ideas about absent, abstract, intangible, or subjective topics, or contrasting perspectives, are fraught with special difficulties. Thus limited conversational experience, language delays, difficulties in accessing others' non-verbal affective cues, facial expressions and gestures are all likely to limit opportunities for blind children to participate in the kinds of early social interactions with parents, siblings, and peers that are associated with sighted preschoolers' ToM and social cognition (Dunn 1996; Dunn and Brophy 2005).

4.4 Theory of mind reasoning in blind children

As we noted earlier, concepts of pretending are relevant to children's understanding of the mind. Pretend play involves mental representation. Additionally, when children discuss pretend roles, imaginary ideas, and play symbols, they often use embedded syntactic structures ('Let's pretend that [clause]') that are similar, although not identical (de Villiers 2005), to those used for talking about true and false beliefs. Furthermore, a child's social engagement in pretending enables the sharing of others' mental perspectives, conceptualizing alternative worlds and the contrasting of real objects and events with their unreal symbolic representations, all of which are theoretically relevant to the development of successful performance on ToM tasks (Wellman 2002). Children who frequently engage in pretence score high on false-belief tests (Taylor and Carlson 1997), as do preschoolers who have siblings of an age to be partners in fantasy and pretend play (Perner *et al.* 1994; Jenkins and Astington 1996; Peterson 2000). Frequent family and peer conversations are linked with sighted preschoolers' superior performance on ToM tests (Brown *et al.* 1996; Hughes and Dunn 1997), as are discussions of pretend roles and play proposals in preschool (Jenkins and Astington 2000).

Studies of blind preschoolers reveal a dearth of pretend play, coupled with developmental delays in the sophistication, elaboration, versatility, and symbolic abstraction of whatever pretending the blind child does carry out. Limited role play and a lack of private or social imaginative activities have been reported to persist throughout the early primary school period (Fraiberg 1977; Tröster and Bambring 1994). Some research indicates that profoundly blind children may also have problems not only with producing pretend actions but even with comprehending others' pretending or the simple notion of pretend action as distinct from a real act (Hughes *et al.* 1998; Lewis *et al.* 2000).

Although testing a blind child's genuine understanding of pretending in a non-visual modality is tricky, and much of the above research has also been limited by small sample sizes, it is clear that blind children are generally given far fewer opportunities than sighted children to play pretend games in social contexts with peers. Therefore they are less likely to be able to discuss pretence or to negotiate over role assignment and joint pretend enactments in the ways that can prove especially beneficial for the early emergence of ToM (Astington and Jenkins 1995). Blind children spend much of their play time alone, especially in mainstream schools with sighted classmates, further limiting their opportunities for conversations with peers not only about pretending, but also about other subjective inner states of feeling, desire, or belief. Are these restricted experiences linked to delayed development of ToM reasoning in blind children, as measured on false-belief tests?

Several studies have used standard false-belief tests to examine ToM reasoning in children who are blind and all have revealed impaired performance at ages when sighted children typically pass. In the first of these, McAlpine and Moore (1995) tested a group of 16 visually impaired children aged 4–12 years on a pair of misleading container ToM tasks and found that visual acuity predicted ToM performance. Whereas 90 per cent of the partially sighted children (with acuities of 20/300 or better) passed at least one task, those with profound blindness consistently failed both tests up to the age of 9 years. Language ability was also correlated with performance. McAlpine and Moore concluded that, in contrast with sighted children who pass false belief at an average verbal age (VMA) of 5 years, blind children require a VMA of 11 years in order to pass, similar to Happé's (1995) conclusion from studies of children with autism.

Minter *et al.* (1998) (see also Hobson and Bishop 2003) presented a group of totally blind children aged 5–9 years with a single-trial misleading-container false-belief test involving a teapot that contained sand. They found that only 47 per cent passed a test question by predicting a naive 'other would think the pot contained tea', compared with over 90 per cent of an age-matched sighted control group. It is conceivable that this version of the task was unusually difficult for blind children who, for safety reasons, may not have much everyday experience of handling teapots. However, other studies with different types of stimuli have also revealed impaired performance by primary-school-aged blind children on false-belief tasks. Green *et al.* (2004) noted only a 67 per cent pass rate among blind children aged 5–12 years (mean age, 8 years) on three false-belief tests (a Smarties tube with pencils, a Coke can with sand, and a changed location test with textured hiding places). Like McAlpine and Moore, Green *et al.* found that, whereas verbal maturity predicted the blind children's false-belief performance, chronological age did not.

In the most extensive study of blind children's false-belief understanding to date, Peterson *et al.* (2000) administered a battery of four false-belief tests and two tests involving changed hidden locations. The sample consisted of 23 blind children aged 5–13 years who were evenly divided into age groups (5–9 years and 11–13 years). The tasks were carefully designed and pilot-tested with a separate blind sample so as to involve stimuli (e.g. an egg box) that were readily and uniquely identifiable tactually. False-belief performance by blind children aged 5–9 years did not exceed chance and only 23 per cent of this younger group displayed a consistent understanding by passing all four tests—a level similar to those for late-signing deaf children of similar age. Yet, contrary to a strong version of a critical period hypothesis, ToM was expressed in the older group of blind children in Peterson *et al.*'s sample. Seventy per cent of those aged 11–13 years achieved ceiling performance on false-belief tests by passing all four tests, and overall performance by this older group was significantly above chance. In this sense, blind children's difficulties with ToM tests of false belief seem better described as delayed than as reflecting lasting deficits.

4.5 Language and theory of mind in children with autism

In Chapter 2, Baron-Cohen and colleagues presented a compelling discussion of the social-cognitive deficits associated with autism spectrum disorders. What was perhaps less focused on in Chapter 2 is the well-established fact that many children with autism are impaired in their language development. Indeed, classic autism (Kanner 1943) is only diagnosed when serious language and communication problems coincide with impairments of social relatedness and imagination to form a symptomatic triad (Frith 2003). The distribution of autistic symptoms through the population is currently often viewed as a continuum ranging from normal development through conditions such as Asperger's syndrome and high-functioning autism to classic (or Kanner-type) autism (Frith 2004). Classic autism is distinguished by more severe language impairments than are present in Asperger's syndrome (Bailey *et al.* 1996). However, recent evidence suggests that most individuals on the autism spectrum, including those with Asperger's syndrome or high-functioning autism (HFA), do experience language delays and communication problems to at least some degree relative to typical developers (Tager-Flusberg 1994; Joseph *et al.* 2002).

For example, based on a longitudinal study of six boys with HFA who were aged 3–7 years at the start of the study, Tager-Flusberg (1994) found that autistic children had specific language problems in the areas of communicative, conversation, and pragmatic uses of language that did not extend to the mastery of syntax. In fact, their language difficulties across the 2-year observation period were strikingly similar to those that we discussed earlier in relation to the language development of blind children. Specifically, the autistic group was delayed in mastering pronoun reversal, question construction, requests for clarification, and several other functional aspects of language. They had difficulties with speaker–listener roles, tailoring information to listeners' needs and adhering to maxims of effective conversation (Grice 1975; see also Surian *et al.* 1996). However, their syntactic development was relatively unimpaired compared with Down syndrome children of similar age.

Even when syntax is relatively spared, many individuals with autism or autism spectrum disorders have serious and protracted difficulties on ToM tasks (Baron-Cohen *et al.* 1985; Happé 1995; Yirmiya *et al.* 1998; Peterson and

Siegal 1999; see also Chapter 2, this volume)—difficulties that are not ameliorated when the test questions are made more explicit so that these will be interpreted to refer to where a character with a false belief will initially look for a desired object (Surian and Leslie 1999). It has been maintained that problems in the social cognition of children with autism, including the expression of ToM reasoning, reflect the ability to attend to information that is presented in the visual (Baron-Cohen 1995; Milne *et al.* 2002) or auditory (Kuhl *et al.* 2005) modalities. In fact, recent evidence suggests that typically developing children and children with autism differ in their auditory processing, and that such differences are evident in very early development when many cases of autism are first diagnosed (Samson *et al.* 2006).

Typically developing newborns have the perceptual mechanisms necessary to separate the sound sources in their environment, such as distinguishing their mother's voice from other concurrent sounds (Winkler *et al.* 2003). By at least 2 months of age, hearing infants prefer speech to non-speech sounds (Vouloumanos and Werker 2004) By 3 months of age, normal speech, in contrast with reversed speech, activates left-lateralized brain regions that are similar to those in adults (Dehaene-Lambertz *et al.* 2002), and during the first year of life infants display a preference to babble on the right side of the mouth, indicating a preference for left-hemisphere language specialization even before the acquisition of language (Holowka and Petitto 2002).

Given the early maturity of the auditory system compared with the visual system, it is not surprising that before the age of 5 years, stimuli in the auditory modality dominate children's attention whereas adult attention is dominated by a visual preference. In experiments involving typically developing 8-, 12-, and 16-month-old infants, 4-year-old children, and adults, Sloutsky and his coworkers (Napolitano and Sloutsky 2004; Robinson and Sloutsky 2004) found that, unlike adults, for infants aged as young as 8 months and 4-year-olds, new pictures do not attract more attention than familiar pictures when they are paired with familiar sounds. However, infants and 4-year-olds do attend significantly longer to pictures, whether or not these have been previously seen, when these pictures are paired with new sounds. This auditory preference is particularly marked for infants and appears to be automatic rather than under deliberate control. An early auditory dominance is adaptive for language learning and is essential to engage in conversation with others. Whereas visual stimuli are often stationary and do not disappear, language sounds are fleeting and need to be processed rapidly for effective communication.

Neuroimaging and behavioural evidence converge to demonstrate that, compared with typically developing children, individuals with autism often have considerable difficulty in attending to sounds. Up until recently, these studies have involved primarily school-aged children, adolescents, and adults. For example, many individuals with autism have difficulty in detecting speech from noise (Khalfa *et al.* 2001). A wider discrepancy between the frequencies of a signal and a masking sound is required for those with autism than for those without autism to hear the signal (Foxton *et al.* 2003; Plaisted *et al.* 2003). As shown in a study using cortical event-related brain potentials, school-aged children with autism have an attentional deficit in orienting to the 'speechness' quality of sounds as represented by vowels (Ceponiene *et al.* 2003). Moreover, in a functional MRI (fMRI) study, Gervais *et al.* (2004) have established that adult males diagnosed with autism do not show activation in voice-selective STS regions in response to vocal sounds, although they display a normal activation pattern in response to non-vocal sounds.

Since the symptoms of autism are often apparent in preschool children and even in children less than 2 years of age (Osterling *et al.* 2002), auditory processing difficulties in school-aged children, adolescents, and adults may be a consequence, rather than an antecedent, of autism. However, Kuhl *et al.* (2005) have recently reported a study of 29 children aged 32–52 months diagnosed with autistic spectrum disorders (ASD). Compared with typically developing controls, the children with ASD did not show preference for the 'motherese' speech that is commonly used by mothers in their communication with children over non-speech analogues. Moreover, electrophysiological data indicated that the children with autism, unlike the controls, did not show a significant mismatch negativity in ERP responses to a syllable change. The findings of Kuhl *et al.*'s investigation are in keeping with the long-standing observation that preschool children with autism have difficulty in orienting towards human voices and using this information to recognize faces and to attend to speakers in conversation (Klin 1992; Lord 1995; Baranek 2006)—a finding not necessarily characteristic of older children and dependent on the nature of the measures used to examine voice processing (Boucher *et al.* 2000).

Research on childhood autism has taken a large number of directions. However, the neural substrates of auditory processing can be singled out to merit particular attention (Gomot *et al.* 2002; Rubenstein and Merzenich 2003; Siegal and Blades 2003). If children with autism have difficulty attending to speech and voices, they may later show impairment in language and engagement in conversation and conversational understanding, resulting in disproportionate attention to objects at the expense of persons and insight into psychological processes. Difficulties with joint attention, preverbal communication (e.g. pointing), and social reciprocity are also apparent in infants, toddlers, and preschoolers with autism (Mundy *et al.* 1993; Charman 2003), as are deficits and deficiencies in pretend play and comprehension of symbolic pretend acts (Baron-Cohen 1987, 1989). Under these conditions, many children with autism may be persistently impaired in ToM reasoning, with their performance on false-belief and other tasks resembling that of late-signing deaf children (Peterson and Siegal 1999; Peterson *et al.* 2005). They may not easily be able to appreciate that the minds of others contain beliefs that may differ from their own or from reality.

4.6 Clinical implications and concluding remarks

Whereas children with deafness, blindness, and autism could conceivably suffer similar problems in language, ToM, and social cognition for very different reasons, there is a theme that unites the research that we have reviewed in this chapter. This concerns the child's early opportunities to share at a very young age in spontaneous family conversation at home and in everyday interactive contexts. Blind children and deaf children of hearing parents are limited by their sensory problems from full participation in many of these early experiences. Children with autism may also often be cut off from many of these experiences by their inattention to voices and speech.

The seriously delayed expression of ToM reasoning observed in all three of these groups of children appears to stem, at least in part, from deficits in early social and conversational experience, in line with findings showing that frequent spontaneous conversational exchanges of these kinds are linked with advanced ToM in typical children (Dunn 1996; Dunn and Brophy 2005), especially those who have child siblings (Jenkins and Astington 1996; Peterson 2000) or parents who employ a rich vocabulary of mental state terms (Ruffman *et al.* 2002) and frequent elaborations on psychological cognitive themes in their everyday family discourse (Peterson and Slaughter 2003). Similarly, delays in developing language, especially its pragmatic aspects, appear to stem from restricted opportunities to exchange information freely and spontaneously about inner states of emotion, desire, intention, imagination, and belief with child and adult conversational partners. In certain instances, these delays may amount to a long-lasting deficit that is produced by the absence of conversational input about mental states during an early period that is critical to development. In others, however, these may reflect the importance of a sensitive, but not a critical, period for exposure to conversation, the absence of which does not inevitably result in a deficit that persists into adolescence and adulthood. Presumably, an attempt to increase a child's early opportunities for conversational participation in the family context during such a sensitive period could have positive clinical implications for children and their families.

Acknowledgements

Preparation of this chapter was assisted by a Leverhulme Trust International Research Exchange grant. MS is supported by a European Union Sixth Framework Marie Curie Chair and a grant from the Fondazione Benefica Kathleen Foreman-Casali.

References

Andersen, E.S., Dunlea, A., and Kekelis, L.S. (1984). Blind children's language: resolving some differences. *Journal of Child Language*, **11**, 645–64.

Astington, J.W. (2000). Language and metalanguage in children's understanding of mind. In *Minds in the making: essays in honour of David R. Olson* (ed. J.W. Astington), pp. 267–84). Oxford: Blackwell.

Astington, J.W. and Baird, J.A. (2005). *Why language matters for theory of mind*. New York: Oxford University Press.

Astington, J.W. and Jenkins, J.M. (1995). Theory of mind and social understanding. *Emotion and Cognition*, **9**, 151–65.

Astington, J.W. and Jenkins, J.M. (1999). A longitudinal study of the relation between language and theory-of-mind development. *Developmental Psychology*, **35**, 1311–20.

Avis, J. and Harris, P.L. (1991). Belief–desire reasoning among Baka children: evidence for a universal conception of mind. *Child Development*, **62**, 460–7.

Bailey, A., Phillips, W., and Rutter, M. (1996). Autism: towards an integration of clinical, genetic, neuropsychological, and neurobiological perspectives. *Journal of Child Psychology and Psychiatry*, **37**, 89–126.

Baranek, G.T. (2006). Sensory Experiences Questionnaire: discriminating sensory features in young children with autism, developmental delays, and typical development. *Journal of Child Psychology and Psychiatry*, **47**, 591–601.

Baron-Cohen, S. (1987). Autism and symbolic play. *British Journal of Developmental Psychology*, **5**, 139–48.

Baron-Cohen, S. (1989). The autistic child's theory of mind: a case of specific developmental delay. *Journal of Child Psychology and Psychiatry*, **30**, 285–98.

Baron-Cohen, S. (1995). *Mindblindness*. Cambridge, MA: MIT Press.

Baron-Cohen, S., Leslie, A.M., and Frith, U. (1985). Does the autistic child have theory of mind? *Cognition*, **21**, 37–46.

Behne, T.M., Carpenter, M., Call, J., and Tomasello, M. (2005). Unwilling versus unable: infants' understanding of intentional action. *Developmental Psychology*, **41**, 328–37.

Bloom, P. and German, T. (2000). Two reasons to abandon the false belief task as a test of theory of mind. *Cognition*, **77**, B25–31.

Bonvillian, J.D. (1999). Sign language development. In *The development of language* (ed. M Barrett), pp. 277–310. Hove: Psychology Press.

Boucher, J., Lewis, V., and Collis, G. (2000). Voice processing abilities in children with autism, children with specific language impairments, and young typically developing children. *Journal of Child Psychology and Psychiatry*, **41**, 847–57.

Brown, R. and Hanlon, C. (1970). Derivational complexity and order of acquisition in child speech. In *Cognition and the development of language* (ed. J.R. Hayes). New York: John Wiley.

Brown, J.R., Donelan-McCall, N., and Dunn, J. (1996). Why talk about mental states? The significance of children's conversations with friends, siblings and mothers. *Child Development*, **67**, 836–49.

Bruner, J. (1983). *Children's talk*. Oxford University Press.

Butterworth, G. (1998). Origins of joint visual attention in infancy. *Monographs of the Society for Research in Child Development*, **63**, 144–66.

Centers for Disease Control (2005). *Vision impairment*. Available online at: http://www.cdc.gov/ncbddd/dd/ddvi.htm

Ceponiene, R., Lepisto, T., Shestakova, A., *et al.* (2003). Speech–sound-selective auditory impairment in children with autism: they can perceive but do not attend. *Proceedings of the National Academy of Sciencesof the USA*, **100**, 5567–72.

Charman, T. (2003) Why is joint attention a pivotal skill in autism? *Philosophical Transactions of the Royal Society of London, Series B*, **358**, 315–24.

Cheour, M., Martynova, O., Naatanen, R., *et al.* (2002). Speech sounds learned by sleeping newborns. *Nature*, **415**, 599–600.

Cheung, H., Hsuan-Chih, C., Creed, N., Ng, L., Ping Wang, S., and Mo, L. (2004). Relative roles of general and complementation language in theory-of-mind development. *Child Development*, **75**, 1155–70.

Chomsky, N. (1980). *Rules and representations*. Oxford: Blackwell.

Clark, E.V. (1983). Meanings and concepts. In *Handbook of child psychology. Vol. 3: Cognitive development* (ed. J.H. Flavell and E.M. Markman). New York: John Wiley.

Corballis, M.C. (2002). *From hand to mouth: the origins of language*. Princeton University Press.

Courtin, C. and Melot, A.M. (2005). Metacognitive development of deaf children: lessons from the appearance–reality and false belief tasks. *Developmental Science*, **8**,16–25.

Cowie, F. (1998). *What's within: nativism reconsidered*. New York: Oxford University Press.

Crain, S. and Pietroski, P. (2001). Nature, nurture and universal grammar. *Linguistics and Philosophy*, **24**, 139–86.

Curtiss, S. (1977). *Genie: a psycholinguistic study of a modern-day 'wild child.'* New York: Academic Press.

Custer, W.L. (1996). A comparison of young children's understanding of contradictory representations in pretense, memory, and belief. *Child Development*, **67**, 678–88.

Dahlgren, S., Sandberg, A.D., and Hjelmquist, E. (2003). The non-specificity of theory of mind deficits: evidence from children with communicative disabilities. *European Journal of Cognitive Psychology*, **15**, 129–55.

de Villiers, J. (2005). Can language acquisition give children a point of view? In *Why language matters for theory of mind* (ed. J.W. Astington and J.A. Baird), pp. 186–219. New York: Oxford University Press.

de Villiers, J.G. and de Villiers, P. (2000). Linguistic determinism and the understanding of false belief. In *Children's reasoning and the mind* (ed. P. Mitchell and K. Riggs), pp. 191–228. Hove: Psychology Press.

de Villiers, J.G. and Pyers, J.E. (2002). Complements to cognition: a longitudinal study of the relationship between complex syntax and false-belief understanding. *Cognitive Development*, **17**, 1037–60.

de Villiers, J.G., de Villiers, P.A., and Hoban, E. (1994). The central problem of functional categories in the English syntax of oral deaf children. In *Constraints on language acquisition: studies of atypical children* (ed. H. Tager-Flusberg), pp. 9–47. Hillsdale, NJ: Lawrence Erlbaum.

Dehaene-Lambertz, G., Dehaene, S., and Hertz-Pannier, L. (2002). Functional neuroimaging of speech perception in infants. *Science*, **298**, 2013–15.

Dunbar, R.I.M. (1993). Co-evolution of neocortex size, group size and language in humans. *Behavioral and Brain Sciences*, **16**, 681–735.

Dunlea A. (1989). *Vision and the emergence of meaning*. Cambridge University Press.

Dunn, J. (1994). Changing minds and changing relationships. In *Origins of an understanding of mind* (ed. C. Lewis and P. Mitchell), pp. 297–310. Hove: Lawrence Erlbaum.

Dunn, J. (1996). Emanuel Miller Memorial Lecture 1995. Children's relationships: bridging the divide between cognitive and social development. *Journal of Child Psychology and Psychiatry*, **37**, 507–18.

Dunn, J. and Brophy, M. (2005). Communication relationships and individual differences in children's understanding of mind. In *Why language matters for theory of mind* (ed. J.W. Astington and J.A. Baird), pp. 50–69. New York: Oxford University Press.

Falkman, K., Roos, C., and Hjelmquist, E. (2007). Mentalizing skills of non-native, early signers: A longitudinal perspective. *European Journal of Developmental Psychology*, **4**, 178–97.

Flavell, J.H. (2004). Theory-of-mind development: retrospect and prospect. *Merrill-Palmer Quarterly*, **50**, 274–90.

Fodor, J.A. (1983). *The modularity of mind*. Cambridge, MA: Bradford/MIT Press.

Foxton, J.M., Stewart, M.E., Barnard, L., et al. (2003). Absence of auditory 'global interference' in autism. *Brain*, **126**, 2703–9.

Fraiberg, S. (1977). *Insights from the blind*. London: Souvenir Press.

Frith, U. (2003). *Autism: explaining the enigma* (2nd edn). Oxford: Blackwell.

Frith, U. (2004). Emmanuel Miller Memorial Lecture. Confusions and controversies about Asperger's syndrome. *Journal of Child Psychology and Psychiatry*, **45**, 672–86.

Garfield, J., Peterson, C.C., and Perry, T. (2001). Social cognition, language acquisition and the development of the theory of mind. *Mind and Language*, **16**, 494–541.

Gelman, S.A. (2005). Two insights about naming in the preschool child. In *The innate mind: structure and contents* (ed. P. Carruthers, S. Laurence, and S. Stich). New York: Oxford University Press.

Gergely, G., Bekkering, H., and Kiraly, I. (2002). Rational imitation in preverbal infants. *Nature*, **415**, 755.

Gervais, H., Belin, P., Boddaert, N., et al. (2004). Abnormal cortical voice processing in autism. *Nature Neuroscience*, **7**, 801–2.

Goldin-Meadow, S. (2003). *The resilience of language*. New York: Psychology Press.

Goldin-Meadow, S. and Mylander, C. (1998). Spontaneous sign systems created by deaf children in two cultures. *Nature*, **391**, 279–81.

Gomot, M., Giard, M.H., Adrien, J.L., Barthelemy, C., and Bruneau, N. (2002). Hypersensitivity to acoustic change in children with autism: electrophysiological evidence of left frontal cortex dysfunctioning. *Psychophysiology*, **39**, 577–84.

Green, S., Pring, L., and Swettenham, J. (2004). An investigation of first-order false belief understanding of children with congenital visual impairment. *British Journal of Developmental Psychology*, **22**, 1–17.

Grice, H.P. (1975). Logic and conversation. In *Syntax and semantics*. Vol. 3: *Speech acts* (ed. P. Cole and J.L. Morgan), pp. 41–58. New York: Academic Press.

Grimshaw, G.M., Adelstein, A., Bryden, M.P., and MacKinnon, G.E. (1998). First-language acquisition in adolescence: evidence for a critical period for verbal language development. *Brain and Language*, **63**, 237–55.

Hale, C.M. and Tager-Flusberg, H. (2003). The influence of language on theory of mind: a training study. *Developmental Science*, **6**, 346–59.

Happé, F. (1995). The role of age and verbal ability in the theory of mind task performance of subjects with autism. *Child Development*, **66**, 843–55.

Harris, M. (1992). *Language experience and early language development*. Hove: Lawrence Erlbaum.

Harris, P.L. (1996). Desires, beliefs, and language. In *Theories of theory of mind* (ed. P. Carruthers and P.K. Smith). Cambridge University Press.

Harris, P.L. (2005). Conversation, pretence and theory of mind. In *Why language matters for theory of mind* (ed. J.W. Astington and J.A. Baird), pp. 70–83. New York: Oxford University Press.

Harris, P.L., de Rosnay, M., and Pons, F. (2005). Language and children's understanding of mental states. *Current Directions in Psychological Science*, **14**, 69–73.

Hobson, R.P. (1993). *Autism and the development of mind*. Hove: Lawrence Erlbaum.

Hobson, R.P. and Bishop, M. (2003). The pathogenesis of autism: Insights from congenital blindness. *Philosophical Transactions of the Royal Society, Series B* **358**, 335–44.

Holowka, S. and Petitto, L.A. (2002). Left hemisphere cerebral specialization for babies while babbling. *Science*, **297**, 1515.

Hughes, C. and Dunn, J. (1997). 'Pretend you didn't know': young children's talk about mental states in the context of pretend play. *Cognitive Development*, **12**, 477–99.

Hughes, M., Dote-Kwan J., and Dolendo, J. (1998). A closer look at the cognitive play of preschoolers with visual impairments in the home. *Exceptional Children*, **64**, 451–62.

Jenkins, J. and Astington, J.W. (1996). Cognitive factors and family structure associated with ToM development in young children. *Developmental Psychology*, **32**, 70–8.

Jenkins, J. and Astington, J.W. (2000). Theory of mind and social behavior: causal models tested in a longitudinal study. *Merrill-Palmer Quarterly*, **46**, 203–220.

Joseph, R.M. (1998). Intention and knowledge in preschoolers' conception of pretend. *Child Development*, **69**, 966–80.

Joseph, R.M., Tager-Flusberg, H., and Lord, C. (2002). Cognitive profiles and social-communicative functioning in children with autism spectrum disorder. *Journal of Child Psychology and Psychiatry*, **43**, 807–21.

Kanner, L. (1943). Autistic disturbances of affective contact. *Nervous Child*, **2**, 217–50.

Khalfa, S., Bruneau, N., Rogé, B., *et al.* (2001). Peripheral auditory asymmetry in infantile autism. *European Journal of Neuroscience*, **13**, 628–32.

Klin, A. (1992). Listening preferences in regard to speech in 4 children with developmental-disabilities. *Journal of Child Psychology and Psychiatry*, 33, 763–69.

Kuhl, P.K., Coffey-Corina, S., Padden, D., and Wilson, D. (2005). Links between social and linguistic processing of speech in preschool children with autism: behavioral and electrophysiological measures. *Developmental Science*, 8, F1–12.

Laurence, S. and Margolis, E. (2001). The poverty of the stimulus argument. *British Journal for the Philosophy of Science*, 52, 217–76.

Lee, K., Olson, D.R., and Torrance, N. (1999). Chinese children's understanding of false beliefs: the role of language. *Journal of Child Language*, 26, 1–21.

Lenneberg, E.H. (1967). *Biological foundations of language*. New York: John Wiley.

Leslie, A.M., Friedman, O., and German, T.P. (2004). Core mechanisms in 'theory of mind'. *Trends in Cognitive Sciences*, 8, 528–33.

Lewis, V. (2003). *Development and disability* (2nd edn). Oxford: Blackwell.

Lewis, V., Norgate, S., Collis, G., and Reynolds, R. (2000). The consequences of visual impairment for children's symbolic and functional play. *British Journal of Developmental Psychology*, 18, 449–64.

Lidz, J., Waxman, S., and Freedman, J. (2003a). What infants know about syntax but couldn't have learned: Experimental evidence for syntactic structure at 18 months. *Cognition*, 89, B65–73.

Lidz J., Gleitman, H., and Gleitman, L. (2003b). Understanding how input matters: verb learning and the footprint of universal grammar. *Cognition*, 87, 151–78.

Lohmann, H. and Tomasello, M. (2003). The role of language in the development of false belief understanding: a training study. *Child Development*, 74, 1130–44.

Lohmann, H., Tomasello, M., and Meyer, S. (2005). Linguistic communication and social understanding. In *Why language matters for theory of mind* (ed. J.W. Astington and J.A. Baird). New York: Oxford University Press.

Lord, C. (1995). Follow-up of two-year-olds referred for possible autism. *Journal of Child Psychology and Psychiatry*, 36, 1365–82.

McAlpine, L.M. and Moore, C.L. (1995). The development of social understanding in children with visual impairments. *Journal of Visual Impairment and Blindness*, 89, 349–58.

McConachie, H. (1990). Early language development and severe visual impairment. *Child: Care, Health and Development*, 16, 55–61.

Maridaki-Kassotaki, K., Lewis, C., and Freeman, N.H. (2003). Lexical choice can lead to problems: what false belief tests tell us about Greek alternative verbs of agency. *Journal of Child Language*, 30, 1–20.

Marschark, M. (1993). *Psychological development of deaf children*. New York: Oxford University Press.

Mayberry, R.I., Lock, E., and Kazmi, H. (2002). Linguistic ability and early language exposure. *Nature*, 417, 38.

Meltzoff, A. and Moore, M.K. (1977). Imitation of facial and manual gestures by human infants. *Science*, 198, 75–8.

Milne, E., Swettenham, J., Hansen, P., Campbell, R, Jeffries, H., and Plaisted, K. (2002). High motion coherence thresholds in children with autism. *Journal of Child Psychology and Psychiatry*, 43, 255–64.

Minter, M., Hobson, R.P., and Bishop, M. (1998). Congenital visual impairment and 'theory of mind.' *British Journal of Developmental Psychology*, **16**, 183–96.

Morgan, G. and Kegl, J. (2006). Nicaraguan Sign Language and theory of mind: the issue of critical periods and abilities. *Journal of Child Psychology and Psychiatry*, **47**, 811–19.

Mundy, P., Sigman, M., and Kasari, C. (1993). The theory of mind and joint-attention deficits in autism. In *Understanding other minds: perspectives from autism* (ed. S. Baron-Cohen, H. Tager-Flusberg, and D. Cohen), pp. 181–203. Oxford University Press.

Napolitano, A.C. and Sloutsky, V.M. (2004). Is a picture worth a thousand words? Part II: The flexible nature of modality dominance in young children. *Child Development*, **75**, 1850–70.

Nelson, K. (1973). Structure and strategy in learning to talk. *Monographs of the Society for Research in Child Development*, **38** (Serial No. 149).

Nelson, K., Skwerer, D.P., Goldman, S., Henseler, S., Presler, N., and Walkenfeld, F.F. (2003). Entering a community of minds: an experiential approach to 'theory of mind' *Human Development*, **46**, 24–46.

Newport, E.L. (1990). Maturational constraints on language learning. *Cognitive Science*, **14**, 11–28.

Niparko, J. (2000). *Cochlear implants: principles and practices*. Philadelphia, PA: Lippincott.

Onishi, K.H. and Baillargeon, R. (2005). Do 15-month-old infants understand false beliefs? *Science*, **308**, 255–8.

Osterling, J.A., Dawson, G., and Munson, J. (2002) Early recognition of 1-year-old infants with autism spectrum disorder versus mental retardation. *Development and Psychopathology*, **14**, 239–51.

Perez-Pereira, M. and Conti-Ramsden, G. (1999). *Language development and social interaction in blind children*. Hove: Psychology Press.

Perner, J. (1991). *Understanding the representational mind*. Cambridge, MA: MIT Press.

Perner, J. and Ruffman, T. (2005). Infants' insight into the mind. How deep? *Science*, **308**, 214–16.

Perner, J., Ruffman, T., and Leekam, S. (1994). Theory of mind is contagious. You catch it from your sibs. *Child Development*, **65**, 1228–38.

Perner, J., Sprung, M., Zauner, P., and Haider, H. (2003). *Want that* is understood well before *say that, think that*, and false belief: a test of de Villiers's linguistic determinism on German-speaking children. *Child Development*, **74**, 179–88.

Peterson, C.C. (2000). Kindred spirits—influences of siblings' perspectives on theory of mind. *Cognitive Development*, **15**, 435–45.

Peterson, C.C. (2004a). Theory-of-mind development in oral deaf children with cochlear implants or conventional hearing aids. *Journal of Child Psychology and Psychiatry*, **45**, 1–11.

Peterson, C.C. (2004b). *Looking forward through the lifespan* (4th edn). Sydney, Australia: Pearson.

Peterson, C.C. and Siegal, M. (1995). Deafness, conversation, and theory of mind. *Journal of Child Psychology and Psychiatry*, **36**, 459–74.

Peterson, C.C. and Siegal, M. (1999). Representing inner worlds: theory of mind in autistic, deaf, and normal hearing children. *Psychological Science*, **10**, 126–9.

Peterson, C.C. and Siegal, M. (2000). Insights into theory of mind from deafness and autism. *Mind and Language*, **15**, 123–45.

Peterson, C.C. and Siegal, M. (2002). Mindreading and moral awareness in popular and rejected preschoolers. *British Journal of Developmental Psychology*, **20**, 205–24.

Peterson, C.C. and Slaughter, V.P. (2003). Opening windows into the mind: mothers' preferences for mental state explanations and children's theory of mind. *Cognitive Development*, **18**, 399–429.

Peterson, C.C. and Slaughter, V.P. (2006). Telling the story of theory of mind: deaf and hearing children's narratives and mental state understanding. *British Journal of Developmental Psychology*, **24**, 151–79.

Peterson, C.C., Peterson J.L., and Webb, J. (2000). Factors influencing the development of a theory of mind in blind children. *British Journal of Developmental Psychology*, **18**, 431–47.

Peterson, C.C., Wellman, H.M., and Liu, D. (2005). Steps in theory of mind development for children with deafness or autism. *Child Development*, **76**, 502–17.

Petitto, L.A. and Marentette, P.F. (1991). Babbling in the manual mode: evidence for the ontogeny of language. *Science*, **251**, 1493–6.

Petitto, L.A., Holowka, S., Sergio, J.E., and Ostry, D. (2001). Language rhythms in baby hand movements. *Nature*, **413**, 35–6.

Pinker, S. (1994). *The language instinct*. Harmondsworth: Penguin.

Plaisted, K, Saksida, L., Alcantara, J., and Weisblatt, E. (2003) Towards an understanding of the mechanisms of weak central coherence effects: experiments in visual configural learning and auditory perception. *Philosophical Transactions of the Royal Society of London, Series B*, **358**, 375–86.

Power, D. and Carty, B. (1990). Cross-cultural communication and the deaf community in Australia. In *Cross-cultural communication and professional education* (ed. C. Hedrick and R. Holton). Adelaide: Flinders University Centre for Multicultural Studies.

Preisler, G. (1995). The development of communication in blind and deaf infants: similarities and differences. *Child Care, Health and Development*, **21**, 79–110.

Preisler, G., Ahlström, M., and Tvingstedt, A.L. (1997). The development of communication and language in deaf preschool children with cochlear implants. *International Journal of Pediatric Otorhinolaryngology*, **41**, 263–72.

Robinson, C.W. and Sloutsky, V.M. (2004). Auditory dominance and its change in the course of development. *Child Development*, **75**, 1387–1401.

Rubenstein, J.L.R. and Merzenich, M.M. (2003). Model of autism: increased ratio of excitation/inhibition in key neural systems. *Genes, Brain and Behavior*, **2**, 255–67.

Ruffman, T., Slade, L., and Crowe, E. (2002). The relation between children's and mothers' mental state language and theory of mind understanding. *Child Development*, **73**, 734–51.

Ruffman, T., Slade, L., Rowlandson, K., Rumsey, C., and Garnham, A. (2003). How language relates to belief, desire, and emotion understanding. *Cognitive Development*, **18**, 139–58.

Russell, P.A., Hosie, J.A., Gray, C.D., *et al.* (1998). The development of theory of mind in deaf children. *Journal of Child Psychology and Psychiatry*, **39**, 903–10.

Samson, F., Mottron, L., Jemel, B., Belin, P., and Ciocca, V. (2006). Can spectro-temporal complexity explain the autistic pattern of performance on auditory tasks? *Journal of Autism and Developmental Disorders*, **36**, 65–76.

Scholl, B.J. and Leslie, A.M. (1999). Modularity, development and 'theory of mind'. *Mind and Language*, **14**, 131–53.

Senghas, A., Kita, S., and Ozyurek, A. (2004). Children creating core properties of language: evidence from an emerging sign language in Nicaragua. *Science*, **305**, 1779–82.

Shatz, M., Diesendruck, G., Martinez-Beck, I., and Akar, D. (2003). The influence of language and socioeconomic status on children's understanding of false beliefs. *Developmental Psychology*, **39**, 717–29.

Siegal, M. and Beattie, K. (1991). Where to look first for children's knowledge of false beliefs. *Cognition*, **38**, 1–12.

Siegal, M. and Blades, M. (2003). Language and auditory processing in autism. *Trends in Cognitive Sciences*, **7**, 378–80.

Siegal, M. and Varley, R. (2002). Neural systems involved in 'theory of mind'. *Nature Reviews Neuroscience*, **3**, 463–71.

Slade, L. and Ruffman, T. (2005), How language does (and does not) relate to theory of mind: a longitudinal study of syntax, semantics, working memory and false belief. *British Journal of Developmental Psychology*, **23**, 117–41.

Smith, M., Apperly, M., and White, V. (2003). False belief reasoning and the acquisition of relative clauses. *Child Development*, **74**, 1709–19.

Stromwold, K. (2000). The cognitive neuroscience of language acquisition. In *The new cognitive neurosciences* (2nd edn) (ed. M.S. Gazzaniga). Cambridge, MA: MIT Press.

Surian, L. and Leslie, A.M. (1999). Competence and performance in false belief understanding: a comparison of autistic and normal 3-year-old children. *British Journal of Developmental Psychology*, **17**, 141–55.

Surian, L., Baron-Cohen, S., and van der Lely, H. (1996). Are children with autism deaf to Gricean maxims? *Cognitive Neuropsychiatry*, **1**, 55–72.

Surian, L., Caldi, S., and Sperber, D. (2007). Attribution of beliefs by 13-month-old infants. *Psychological Science*, **18**, 580–6.

Svirsky, M.A., Robbins, A.M., Kirk, K.I., Pisoni, D.B., and Miyamoto, R.T. (2000). Language development in profoundly deaf children with cochlear implants. *Psychological Science*, **11**, 153–8.

Svirsky, M.A., Teoh, S.W., and Neuburger, H. (2004). Development of language and speech perception in congenitally, profoundly deaf children as a function of age at cochlear implantation. *Audiology and Neuro-otology*, **9**, 224–33.

Tager-Flusberg, H. (1994). Dissociations in form and function in the acquisition of language by autistic children. In *Constraints on language acquisition: studies of atypical children* (ed. H Tager-Flusberg). Hillsdale, NJ: Lawrence Erlbaum.

Taylor, M. and Carlson, S. (1997). The relation between individual differences in fantasy and theory of mind. *Child Development*, **68**, 436–55.

Tirosh, E., Schnitzer, M.R., Atar S., and Jaffe, M. (1992). Severe visual deficits in infancy in Northern Israel: an epidemiological perspective. *Journal of Pediatric Ophthalmology and Strabismus*, **29**, 366–9.

Tomasello, M. (2003). *Constructing a language: a usage-based theory of language acquisition.* Cambridge, MA: Harvard University Press.

Tröster, H. and Brambring, M. (1992). Early social–emotional development in blind infants. *Child: Care, Health and Development*, **18**, 207–27.

Tröster, H. and Brambring, M. (1994). The play behaviour and play materials of blind and sighted infants and preschoolers. *Journal of Visual Impairment and Blindness*, **88**, 421–32.

Varley, R. and Siegal, M. (2000). Evidence for cognition without grammar from causal reasoning and 'theory of mind' in an agrammatic aphasic patient. *Current Biology*, **10**, 723–6.

Varley, R., Siegal, M., and Want, S.C. (2001). Severe grammatical impairment does not preclude 'theory of mind'. *Neurocase*, **7**, 489–93.

Vouloumanos, A. and Werker, J.F. (2004). Tuned to the signal: the privileged status of speech for young infants. *Developmental Science*, **7**, 270–6.

Wellman, H.M. (2002). Understanding the psychological world: developing a theory of mind. In *Blackwell handbook of childhood cognitive development* (ed. U Goswami), pp. 167–87. Oxford: Blackwell.

Wellman, H.M., Cross, D., and Watson, J. (2001). Meta-analyses of theory-of-mind development. *Child Development*, **72**, 655–84.

Wimmer, H. and Perner, J (1983). Beliefs about beliefs: representation and constraining function of wrong beliefs in young children's understanding of deception. *Cognition*, **13**, 103–28.

Winkler, I., Kushnerenko, E., Horvath, J., *et al.* (2003). Newborn infants can organize the auditory world. *Proceedings of the National Academy of Sciences of the USA*, **100**, 11812–15.

Woolfe, T., Want, S.C., and Siegal, M. (2002). Signposts to development: theory of mind in deaf children. *Child Development*, **73**, 768–78.

Woolfe, T., Want, S.C., and Siegal, M. (2003). Siblings and theory of mind in deaf native signing children. *Journal of Deaf Studies and Deaf Education*, **8**, 340–7.

Yazdi, A.A., German, T.P., Defeyer, M., and Siegal, M. (2006). Competence and contributions to performance in belief-desire reasoning: the truth, the whole truth, and nothing but the truth about false belief? *Cognition*, **100**, 343–68.

Yirmiya, N., Erel, O., Shaked, M., and Solomonica-Levi, D. (1998). Meta-analyses comparing theory of mind abilities of individuals with autism, individuals with mental retardation, and normally developing individuals. *Psychological Bulletin*, **124**, 283–307.

Part II
Externalizing disorders

5

Social cognition and disruptive behaviour disorders in young children: families matter

Claire Hughes and Rosie Ensor

This chapter begins with a description of disruptive behavioural disorder (DBD) and of normal patterns of development in social cognition. We argue that advances in our understanding of age-related changes in social cognition may illuminate key mechanisms underlying the development of DBD. We also summarize recent findings concerning the cognitive and family influences upon social cognition and, by extension, upon possible abnormalities in the development of behavioural regulation. Next, we present findings from two studies that exemplify the kind of research we think will advance understanding social cognition in hard-to-manage preschoolers. Finally, we consider the relevance of the research reviewed in this chapter for interventions aimed at improving problems of DBD and discuss possible future research directions.

5.1 Disruptive behaviour disorders in young children

We use the term disruptive behaviour disorders (DBD) to refer to the broad set of externalizing problems encompassed by diagnoses of attention deficit–hyperactivity disorder (ADHD), conduct disorder (CD), and oppositional defiant disorder (ODD). This general approach is supported by the prevalence of comorbid problems (Hill 2002). The frequency of diagnosed DBD has increased dramatically over recent years (Robison *et al.* 1999). These disorders are linked with numerous negative long-term outcomes, including school failure, substance abuse, criminal activity, and incarceration (Mannuzza *et al.* 1991, 1993; Fergusson and Horwood 1998; Fergusson and Lynskey 1998). Life-course persistent prognoses are especially likely for children with early-onset problem behaviours (Moffitt 1990); therefore targeting early-onset cases maximizes the potential gains of intervention programmes. Although interventions in later years have only limited success (e.g. McNeil *et al.* 1991; Conduct Problems Prevention Research Group 1999), they may be more effective if applied early, when problems are less entrenched and regulatory skills are still emerging. For each of these reasons, understanding the early origins of DBD is an urgent challenge for research.

However, research with young hard-to-manage children presents its own challenges. In particular, great care is needed in identifying 'problem behaviours' amongst preschoolers. Behaviours such as temper tantrums are so common that they may be considered developmentally normative in the early years. This highlights the importance of community-based research, as studies of clinic samples present a restricted picture of normative individual differences in behaviour. As disruptive behaviour is defined in terms of its impact upon others, it is clearly also valuable to use direct observational ratings to facilitate detailed and objective analysis of children's behaviour. For example, while some behaviours (e.g. snatching, hurting) regularly elicit negative responses from peers, other behaviours (e.g. rule-breaking, name-calling) that appear deviant from an adult perspective often elicit amusement and shared enjoyment that may actually provide a foundation for friendship (Hughes *et al.* 2000b). Therefore direct observations are valuable in enabling objective assessments of behaviour that avoid problems of informant effects and transactional influences on questionnaire-based responses (Patterson *et al.* 1993; Briggs-Gowan *et al.* 1996; Hay *et al.* 1999; Masten and Curtis 2000). Observational ratings of child behaviour may be more accurate than either parent or teacher reports in predicting long-term outcomes such as arrest or incarceration (Patterson and Forgatch 1995).

5.2 The typical development of social cognition and executive function in preschoolers

For the past quarter-century, research on the typical development of social cognition in the preschool years has been dominated by experimental studies of children's 'theories of mind', i.e. their growing awareness and understanding of other people's thoughts, feelings, desires, and intentions. The preschool years are also characterized by major improvements in other cognitive domains, especially verbal ability and executive function. Furthermore, as discussed by Siegal and Peterson (Chapter 4, this volume), individual differences in language skills have been shown to be closely related to individual differences in social cognition; likewise, research with typically developing children highlights the synchrony of preschool developmental milestones in social cognition (Wellman *et al.* 2001) and executive function (Gerstadt *et al.* 1994; Zelazo *et al.* 1996). Studies of typically developing children also show consistently strong correlation between these domains, even when the effects of age and IQ are controlled (Frye *et al.* 1995; Hughes 1998a,b; Perner and Lang 1999; Carlson and Moses 2001; Carlson *et al.* 2002). In addition, research with clinical groups has shown widespread pronounced impairments in both executive function and social cognition for individuals with autism (Ozonoff *et al.* 1991), schizophrenia (Corcoran *et al.* 1995), and frontal-lobe pathologies (Channon and Crawford 2000).

At a practical level, a general obstacle to studying social cognition and its correlates (e.g. executive functioning) in preschoolers has been the scarcity of developmentally appropriate cognitive tasks. However, recent research has seen a rapid growth in the number of available suitable tasks (McEvoy *et al.* 1993; Hughes 1998a; Archibald and Kerns 1999; Frye 1999; Griffith *et al.* 1999; Carlson *et al.* 2002; Hughes and Graham 2002). Table 5.1 summarizes some of the tasks that were developed to investigate the relationships between social cognition, verbal ability, executive functioning, and family variables in the development of DBD in two separate community-based studies which form the focus for this chapter: a London study of preschoolers (Hughes *et al.* 1998) and a Cambridge study of 2-year-olds (Hughes and Ensor 2005).

Below, we briefly describe these tasks as examples of novel and creative ways to assess individual differences in early social cognitive and executive functioning abilities.

5.2.1 Theory of mind

Many of these tasks were included in a large-scale epidemiological study of individual differences in theory of mind (ToM) (Hughes *et al.* 2005) and have good test–retest reliability (Hughes *et al.* 2000a). Two tasks were used at all time-points in both studies: a false-belief task (Hughes *et al.* 1998), designed to attract and maintain younger children's attention by using a pop-up peep-through picture-book, and a penny-hiding game (Hughes *et al.* 1998) which capitalizes on children's enjoyment of disappearing objects. The London study also included a second puppet-based deception task (Sodian and Frith 1992), two story-based tasks tapping children's ability to infer an emotion based on a predicted false belief (Harris *et al.* 1989), and two stories involving prototypical boxes (a BandAid box and an egg-box) with deceptive contents (Bartsch and Wellman 1995). The Cambridge study included a task designed to elicit 2-year-olds' pretend play with prototypical and junk objects (Charman and Baron-Cohen 1997), while at ages 3 and 4 years the children completed the two deceptive-contents stories and two standard object-transfer false-belief tasks (Wimmer and Perner 1983).

5.2.2 Executive function

Based on previous studies which demonstrated a fractionated structure for executive function, simple tasks tapping three distinct aspects of executive

Table 5.1 Cognitive measures used in each study

London	Cambridge		
Age 4	**Age 2**	**Age 3**	**Age 4**
Theory of mind			
Picture book FB	Picture book FB	Picture book FB	Picture book FB
Penny-hiding game	Penny-hiding game	Penny-hiding game	Penny-hiding game
Puppet sabotage/ deceit	Elicited pretend play	Object transfer FB	Object transfer FB
Deceptive identity— explain, predict		Deceptive identity— explain, predict	
Emotion FB—nice/nasty			
Emotion understanding			
Denham— labelling: Unambiguous stories Ambiguous stories	Denham— labelling: Unambiguous stories	Denham— labelling: Unambiguous stories Ambiguous stories	Denham— labelling: Unambiguous stories Ambiguous stories
Executive functioning			
Noisy Book (WM)	Bead task (WM)	Bead task (WM)	Bead task (WM)
Teddy card-sort (Rule)	Spin-the-Pots (WM)	Spin-the-Pots (WM)	Spin-the-Pots (WM)
Marbles pattern task (Rule)	Trucks card sort (Rule)	Trucks card sort (Rule)	Trucks card sort (Rule)
Luria's Hand Stroop (Inhib)	Baby Stroop (Inhib)	Luria's Hand Stroop (Inhib)	Day–Night Stroop (Inhib)
Tower of London (Plan)			Tower of London (Plan)
Detour reaching box (Inhib)			

FB, false belief; WM, working memory, Inhib, inhibition.

function (working memory, inhibition, and rule-based action) were included in both studies at all time-points. In addition, a more complex planning task, the Tower of London (Shallice 1982), was included at age 4 in both studies. For working memory, the London study used the Noisy Book task (Hughes *et al.* 1998), which requires children to reproduce an action sequence to activate a series of sounds associated with pictures. The Cambridge study used two working memory tasks at all three time-points: the Stanford–Binet Beads task (Thorndike *et al.* 1986) and the Spin-the-Pots task (Hughes and Ensor 2005), a multi-location subject-ordered search task. For *rule-based action*, the London study used a marbles pattern reproduction task and a teddy card-sorting task (Hughes *et al.* 1998), a simplified version of the Wisconsin Card Sort Test in which the cards (and teddy bears) were changed at each rule-shift to make the demands of the task relevant to young children. The Cambridge study used a further simplified version of this rule-shifting task at all three time-points with picture-pairs that differed in identity rather than dimension. The London study also included the detour reaching task (Hughes and Russell 1993), which required children to perform a rule-guided action to retrieve a marble from a metal apparatus. For *inhibitory control*, both studies used non-verbal Stroop tasks at all three time-points. In the London study (and at age 3 in the Cambridge study), this was Luria's Hand Stroop Game, in which children were asked to execute the opposite action to that shown—fist or finger (Hughes 1996). At age 2 in the Cambridge study, a contextually-supported Stroop task was used: children were asked to identify a baby-cup/spoon or a 'mummy' cup/spoon, and the task was then presented in a topsy-turvy way, so that children had to say the opposite of what was shown (Hughes and Ensor 2005). At age 4 in the Cambridge study, the Day–Night Picture Stroop was used: children had to say 'night' when they saw a sun picture and vice versa (Gerstadt *et al.* 1994).

5.3 Disruptive behaviour disorders in preschoolers: interactive effects of social cognition and parenting

The premise that childhood disorders are best understood as 'normal development gone awry' (Rutter and Quinton 1984) provides a cornerstone for the new discipline of developmental psychopathology. From a clinical perspective the explosion of research into ToM development is exciting as it provides a valuable platform for exploring the onset of problem behaviours in the preschool years, as these may reflect delay or deviance in children's social cognition. Indeed, conduct disorder appears to be associated with a deviant theory of 'nasty minds' (Happé and Frith 1996). In contrast, ring-leader bullies show intact or even superior ToM skills (Sutton *et al.* 1999a,b), and children with ADHD show no clear impairments in ToM (Charman *et al.* 2001; Perner *et al.* 2002). Together, these findings argue against any simple ToM deficit model of disruptive behaviour. In addition, much of the above work has been conducted with school-aged children, and relations between social cognition and problem behaviours may well be developmentally dynamic. In particular, it is plausible that impairments in social cognition will have greatest impact during the preschool years, as this period is characterized by major developmental changes in children's understanding of others.

In asking exactly how developments in social cognition go awry, we need to consider associations between social cognition, verbal ability, and executive functioning. For our purposes, the significance of these findings lies in the fact that young children with elevated levels of problem behaviours have been reported to show poor verbal ability (Speltz *et al.* 1999) and poor executive function (e.g. Moffitt 1993; Pennington and Bennetto 1993; Hughes *et al.* 1998; Seguin *et al.* 1999; Hughes and Dunn 2000). Therefore assessing whether young children's socio-cognitive skills predict unique variance in behavioural problems is an important step towards establishing their primacy in the aetiology of behavioural problems.

Alongside the cognitive correlates described above, individual differences in children's ToM performance have also been linked with a variety of family variables, including family size (e.g. Perner *et al.* 1994), socio-economic status (e.g. Cutting and Dunn 1999), quality of sibling relationships (Hughes and Ensor 2005), maternal disciplinary style (Ruffman *et al.* 1999; Vinden 2001), maternal 'mind-mindedness' (e.g. Meins *et al.* 2003), and family inner-state talk more generally (e.g. Dunn *et al.* 1991). Together with reports of delayed false-belief comprehension among deaf children of hearing parents (e.g. Peterson and Siegal 1995), these findings highlight environmental influences on ToM acquisition. More direct evidence comes from bivariate model-fitting analyses in a recent twin study involving a representative sample of 1116 pairs of same-sex 5-year-old twins (Hughes *et al.* 2005) who each completed a comprehensive battery of ToM tasks. These analyses demonstrated that genetic effects on individual differences in ToM were very modest, with the lion's share of the variance explained by shared environmental factors. Taken alongside the findings linking deficits in ToM to DBD, these twin results suggest that environmental influences upon ToM may also contribute to the onset of DBD. Traditionally, researchers have used direct observational methods to demonstrate that family environments play a key role in the onset and maintenance of early problem behaviours. For example, harsh parenting not only predicts significant variance in children's behavioural problems but also mediates the influence of social disadvantage (Patterson 1981; Conger *et al.* 1994; Morrell and Murray 2003). Positive parental strategies have received much less attention, but pioneering work by Gardner and colleagues has demonstrated that interventions that are effective in promoting pre-emptive parental responses lead to clear improvements in problem behaviours (Gardner *et al.* 2004).

To date, research into the socio-cognitive characteristics of preschoolers with DBD has been conducted almost entirely separately from observational research. What is now needed is research which combines socio-cognitive assessments and family observations, in order to elucidate both their relative independence and their interplay as influences on early behavioural problems. The value of combining child- and family-based research can be seen in the metaphor of the blind sages and the elephant of Indostan: like the elephant, the origins of early problem behaviours can be perceived in many different ways, and only by integrating these distinct research perspectives can they be described with any reasonable accuracy. Interestingly, relatively few studies have adopted this integrative approach. Conceptually, cognitive researchers and observational researchers have been divided by their foci of interest. Cognitive researchers focus on age-related changes in performance; in contrast, observational researchers focus on distinguishing the behaviour of clinical groups from that of controls, to the extent that age-related changes have been relatively neglected (Hartup 2005). However, recent years have seen a rapidly increasing interest in individual differences within both cognitive (Hughes *et al.* 2005) and observational (Hartup 2005) research, such that, for the first time, there is considerable common ground bridging these two fields.

5.4 Combining experimental and observational methods to study disruptive behaviour disorders in preschoolers

As an example of the kind of research we believe is necessary for moving forward the field of social cognition and developmental psychopathology in preschoolers, we present findings from our London and Cambridge studies, which each combined experimental and observational methods to investigate the child and family characteristics of young children at risk of developing DBD (Table 5.2).

Table 5.2 Participant characteristics in each study

	London (4-year-olds)		Cambridge (2-year-olds)	
	H2M	Control	H2M	Control
Male:female ratio	24:16	24:16	26:14	26:14
Ethnic background: Caucasian:Black	22:18	28:12	40:0	40:0
Mean age in years at time 1 (SD)	4.32 (0.39)	4.17 (0.39)	2.34 (0.31)	2.39 (0.33)
Maternal educational qualifications				
<5 at age 16	10	8	19	14
age 18 or 5+ age 16	17	12	15	15
Degree or higher	7	18	6	11
Missing data	6	2	0	0

H2M, hard to manage.

The first study was based in Peckham, a deprived inner-city area of London, and comprised 80 4-year-olds recruited via nurseries, including 40 identified as 'hard to manage' on the basis of parental ratings at or above the 95th percentiles for the ADHD and CD subscales of the Strengths and Difficulties Questionnaire (SDQ) (Goodman and Scott 1999) and 40 age- and gender-matched classmates with SDQ ratings for ADHD and CD that were at or below the 50th percentile (epidemiological data (Golding 1996) were used to identify cut-off scores for these percentiles).

The second study was based in Cambridge (a generally affluent community) and involved 140 families with 2-year-olds, recruited on the basis of family disadvantage. Forty children with the highest SDQ scores for ADHD and CD (i.e. scores above the same cut-offs as used in the London study) were compared with 40 children from the remainder of the sample (with SDQ scores below the sample median) matched for age, gender, and family background. The samples for the two studies, while broadly similar in gender composition and maternal education, differed in neighbourhood characteristics, ethnic diversity, and age. Therefore establishing the extent to which the two studies yielded similar findings provides a strong test of the generalizability of the original findings.

We examined the data from the two studies in relation to four key questions. The first three of these questions hinged on group differences in child behaviour, social cognition, and family characteristics. Specifically, we first asked whether direct observations of the hard-to-manage children in each study indicated elevated levels of problem behaviours. Our second question concerned whether the hard-to-manage children in each study showed impairments in social cognition. Our third question concerned whether the hard-to-manage children in each study showed abnormal patterns of mother–child interactions. In each study, we assessed whether, compared with mothers of control children, mothers of hard-to-manage children showed elevated negative control and reduced positive control. We also examined whether there were group contrasts in the connectedness of conversations between mothers and children. 'Connectedness' reflects the extent to which each member of the dyad is tuned into others, and is defined as speech that relates to the content or theme of another's talk.

Our final question took us beyond group comparisons to assess whether individual differences in behaviour problems were associated with individual differences in child and family characteristics. Although hard-to-manage preschoolers are at a raised risk of pursuing negative developmental trajectories, a significant proportion have shown substantial improvements in behaviour across the early school years (Campbell et al. 2000). In part, this variability in outcome may reflect meaningful variations in social cognition and family relationships within groups of hard-to-manage children.

For example, does a negative response to provocation reflect a problem in 'mindreading', such as the 'hostile attribution bias' that is reported to characterize aggressive children (cf. Dodge and Somberg 1987), or maternal negative control? Distinguishing these alternative (but not mutually exclusive) accounts impacts our understanding of the proximal causes of problem behaviours and is important for constructing interventions that steer children towards positive developmental trajectories.

Before considering the findings from each study in relation to these three questions, we present the observational methods used within each study. Table 5.1 summarizes the experimental measures used in both studies. Verbal ability was assessed via the British Picture Vocabulary Scale (Dunn *et al.* 1982) at age 4 in both studies, and via the verbal subscales of the British Abilities Scale (Elliott *et al.* 1983) at ages 2 and 3 in the Cambridge study.

In the London study, maternal warmth and criticism were coded from a 20-minute audio interview sample of the mothers and their children at ages 4 and 6. Maternal negative and positive control were coded from transcripts of audio-taped observations of the mothers and their children at age 4 at home and from videos of mothers and their children at age 6 playing together using an adapted version of the Parent–Child Interaction System (PARCHISY) (K. Deater-Deckard, M. Pylas, and S. Petrill 1997, unpublished) based on videos. In addition, connected communication, peer-directed antisocial behaviour (e.g. bullying, violent acts/talk), and response to emotion were coded from video-based transcripts of family interaction and peer play, respectively, at age 4, while child non-compliance was coded from videos of mother–child play at age 6.

In the Cambridge study we also used PARCHISY to code videos of laboratory-visit mother–child play for maternal negative and positive control and for child non-compliance. Transcripts of videos of family interaction and sibling play were used to code the connectedness of mother–child conversations and conflict with siblings, respectively.

5.4.1 Do hard-to-manage children show higher rates of problem behaviours?

In the London study, the hard-to-manage group showed no increase in non-compliance with mothers, but did show raised levels of a variety of peer-directed antisocial acts including snatching, hurting, and bullying (Figure 5.1). Interestingly, however, the mean level of refusal to share was significantly higher in the control group than in the hard-to-manage group. Perhaps the simplest explanation for this unexpected finding is that the children in the hard-to-manage group were more likely to flit from toy to toy rather than engage in sustained play with a particular toy, which they therefore relinquished more readily.

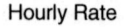

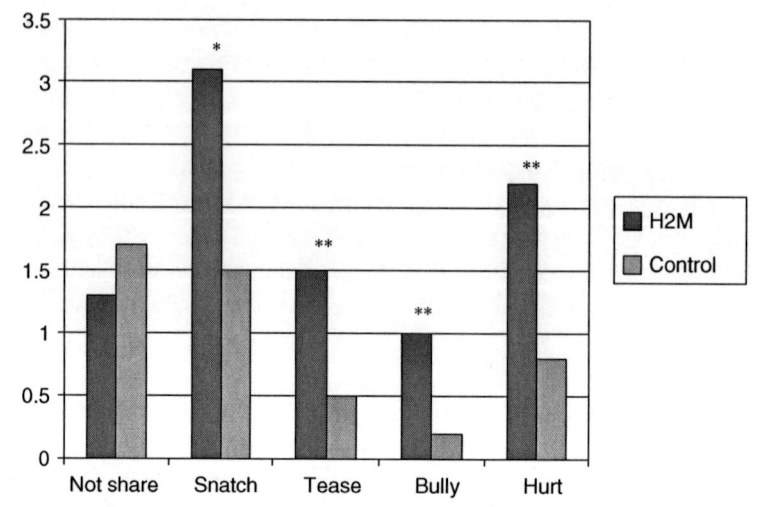

124 | SOCIAL COGNITION AND DISRUPTIVE BEHAVIOUR DISORDERS IN YOUNG CHILDREN

Figure 5.1 Group differences in mean rates of antisocial acts towards peer (London sample of 4-year-olds): H2M, hard to manage.

In the Cambridge study, the hard-to-manage group did show elevated rates of non-compliance with mothers (coded from direct observations in the same way as in the London study). The most plausible explanation of this between-study contrast in findings is that the Cambridge children were 2 years younger; mean levels of non-compliance typically decline sharply

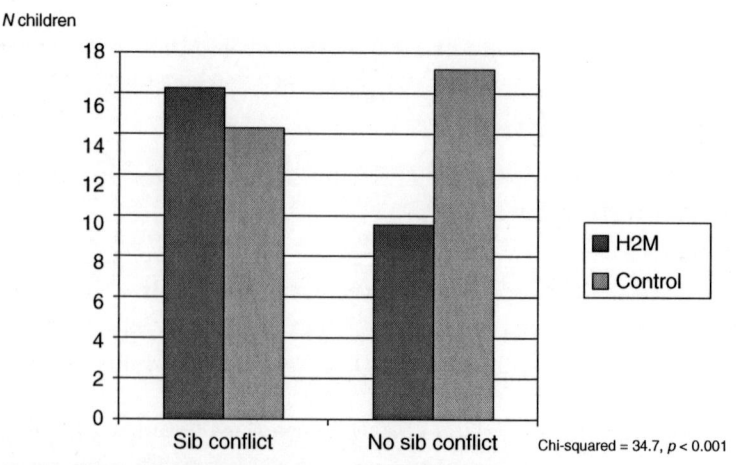

Figure 5.2 Group differences in overt conflict with sibling (Cambridge sample of 2-year-olds): H2M, hard to manage.

between late toddlerhood and the preschool years, such that group differences may be more difficult to detect. Direct observational ratings of children's negative behaviour towards siblings at age 2 reveal that the hard-to-manage group showed elevated rates of overt conflict behaviours with their siblings (Figure 5.2). Overall then, observational findings from the two studies demonstrated significantly higher rates of problem behaviours in the hard-to-manage group than in the control group.

5.4.2 Do hard-to-manage children show impairments in social cognition?

The results from the two studies are summarized in Table 5.3.

In the London study, the Denham emotion-understanding task yielded the strongest group differences, and these differences remained significant even when effects of verbal ability and family background were taken into account. Although the hard-to-manage group also performed more poorly than controls on at least some of the ToM tasks, these group differences were attributable to contrasts in verbal ability. That said, there was some evidence that the children in the hard-to-manage group showed deviance, if not delay, in their understanding of mind. Unlike controls, these children were more likely to be

Table 5.3 Group mean z-scores (and standard deviations) for cognitive performance

Sample	Time	Cognitive domain	H2M (N = 40)	Control (N = 40)	T-value
Cambridge	Age 2	Verbal ability	−0.32 (1.03)	0.32 (0.87)	2.96**
		Executive function	−0.18 (0.65)	0.22 (0.71)	2.57*
		Theory of mind	−0.21 (0.65)	0.30 (0.63)	3.56**
		Emotion understanding	−0.26 (0.80)	0.29 (0.75)	3.14**
Cambridge	Age 3	Verbal ability	−0.24 (1.07)	0.23 (0.89)	2.02*
		Executive function	−0.21 (0.78)	0.22 (0.68)	2.52*
		Theory of mind	−0.09 (0.53)	0.24 (0.74)	2.25*
		Emotion understanding	−0.23 (0.87)	0.29 (0.69)	2.85**
Cambridge	Age 4	Verbal ability	−0.27 (1.00)	0.28 (0.94)	2.41*
		Executive function	−0.17 (.66)	0.22 (0.66)	2.56*
		Theory of mind	−0.14 (.56)	0.02 (0.63)	1.27 (ns)
		Emotion understanding	−0.17 (0.88)	0.34 (0.49)	3.06**
London	Age 4	Verbal ability	−0.35 (0.84)	0.35 (1.04)	3.25**
		Executive function	−0.32 (1.01)	0.32 (0.89)	3.00**
		Theory of Mind	−0.26 (0.63)	0.25 (0.62)	2.88**
		Emotion understanding	−0.01 (1.36)	0.01 (0.39)	0.11 (ns)

H2M, hard to manage; ns, not significant.
*p < .05; ** p < .01

successful in inferring an emotion based on a false belief if the story involved a mean surprise rather than a nice surprise.

At all three time-points of the Cambridge study (i.e. ages 2, 3, and 4), the hard-to-manage group performed more poorly than controls on both the Denham emotion-understanding task and the ToM task battery. When individual differences in verbal ability were taken into account, the group difference in ToM performance was significant at age 2 only, and the group difference in emotion understanding fell just below significance at all three time-points. Indeed, the group difference in ToM performance at age 2 remained significant even when effects of variance in executive function and maternal negative control were taken into account, suggesting a robust and specific contrast between the early mentalizing of the hard-to-manage and control groups. In other words, although effects of verbal ability contributed to group differences in social cognition in both studies, independent group differences in social cognition were also found at age 2. Interestingly, group differences in ToM were clearer in younger children than in older children.

5.4.3 Do hard-to-manage children show abnormal patterns of mother–child interactions?

The results from the two studies are summarized in Table 5.4.

In the London study, mothers of hard-to-manage children showed significantly higher proportions of negative control than mothers of control children at both time-points (Brophy and Dunn 2002) and higher rates of criticism than mothers of control children at age 6 (Hughes and Dunn 2000). At age 4 the hard-to-manage group showed significantly lower proportions of connected conversations than the control group (Brophy and Dunn 2002). At age 6 (but not at age 4), the hard-to-manage group received significantly lower ratings of maternal warmth and positive control than the control group (Brophy and Dunn 2002; Hughes and Dunn 2000).

In the Cambridge study, observational coding of mother–child interaction at the first time-point (age 2) revealed significantly higher levels of negative control among mothers of hard-to-manage children than among mothers of control children. This group contrast remained significant even when individual differences in children's social cognition were taken into account. In contrast, the two groups did not differ in the connectedness of conversations between mothers and children; likewise, mothers in the two groups showed similar levels of positive control.

In sum, across different studies and ages, mothers of hard-to-manage children showed higher levels of negative control than did mothers of control children.

Table 5.4. Group mean scores (standard deviations) for maternal interaction style

	Cambridge sample: age 2			London sample: age 4				London sample: age 6		
	H2M (N = 40)	Control (N = 40)	T-value	H2M (N = 30)	Control (N= 26)	T-value		H2M (N = 29)	Control (N = 29)	T-value
Maternal connectedness (speaker turns/h)	78.76 (75.22)	70.10 (58.82)	0.57 (ns)	32.20 (20.30)	43.90 (15.30)	3.09*		–	–	–
Positive control	3.98 (0.99)	4.21 (0.93)	1.05 (ns)	25.20 (11.30)	18.70 (7.80)	1.49 (ns)		2.77 (0.96)	3.36 (0.50)	4.19*
Negative control	2.12 (0.42)	1.83 (0.47)	2.34*	11.00 (13.20)	4.40 (5.10)	3.34**		2.00 (0.50)	1.54 (0.440)	7.05**

NB. Positive and negative control were rated from video (with a possible range of 0–6 points) in the Cambridge study and at age 6 in the London study, these measures were rated from transcripts in the same way as connectedness, i.e. as a proportion of speaker turns.

H2M, hard to manage; ns, not significant.

In both studies group differences in maternal positive control were *not* found when the children were young (i.e. ages 2 and 4). Early connectedness was also measured in both studies. In the Cambridge study the hard-to-manage and control groups showed similar levels of connected conversation, whereas in the London study the hard-to-manage group showed lower levels of connected conversation.

5.4.4 Do individual differences in social cognition predict variance in social behaviour?

In this section we explore the relationships between the measures of mother–child interaction, social cognition, and child behaviour. First, we consider links between children's social cognition and the maternal interaction measures. In the London study, individual differences in connected conversation and in ToM at age 4 were correlated (Dunn and Brophy 2005). In the Cambridge study, ToM at ages 2, 3, and 4 was correlated (in the expected directions) with maternal positive and negative control. Emotion understanding at all three timepoints was also correlated with positive control, and this relationship was significantly stronger for the hard-to-manage group than for the control group. Overall, individual differences in social cognition were unrelated to connected conversation. However, when the two groups were considered separately, both ToM and emotion understanding at ages 2, 3, and 4 in the hard-to-manage group showed a significant relationship with connectedness.

Next, we consider relations between individual differences in adult-directed problem behaviours and individual differences in child social cognition and mother–child interaction in the Cambridge study. All the cognitive measures showed negative associations with individual differences in non-compliance; however, only deficits in verbal ability showed a significant independent association with non-compliance. Positive and negative maternal control showed significant correlations (in the expected directions) with non-compliance; these relations remained significant once effects of maternal education, child verbal ability, and social cognition were controlled.

Finally, we examine links between child-directed problem behaviours and social cognition. In the London study, when effects of verbal ability were controlled, individual differences in hard-to-manage children's angry and antisocial behaviour towards a peer were related to individual differences in executive function but not to ToM (Hughes *et al.* 2000b). The findings from the Cambridge study regarding negative behaviour towards other children directly parallel those from the London study. Specifically, negative behaviour towards siblings was unrelated to social cognition, but significantly inversely related to executive function. When the two groups were considered separately, the relationship between negative behaviour towards siblings and executive function was marginally significant for the hard-to-manage group only. However, this attenuated association may reflect a diminished sample size—only 25 of these hard-to-manage children had siblings. To address this problem, we also examined associations between cognitive performance and maternal SDQ ratings of peer problems at ages 2, 3, and 4 years. In a nutshell, the pattern that emerged was one of robust independent correlations between poor executive function and peer problems in the hard-to-manage group, concurrent at all three ages and across all time-points. In contrast, associations between social cognition and peer problems were more modest and generally accounted for by underlying effects of verbal ability. Thus across different studies and different approaches to measuring child problem behaviours, our findings provide converging evidence for a close relationship with deficits in executive function rather than social cognition.

5.5 The aetiology of social cognitive problems in hard-to-manage preschoolers

Studies (such as the two described above) that adopt a dual focus on family and child cognitive characteristics highlight three conclusions regarding the early aetiology of DBD.

First, maternal ratings of child behaviour problems show good validity: both studies revealed significant associations between maternal ratings and researchers' detailed observational coding. Secondly, impairments in executive function show a closer link with problem behaviours towards peers than do impairments in social cognition; when effects of verbal ability were controlled, individual differences in problem behaviours at all ages showed significantly stronger associations with executive function than with social cognition. Thirdly, group contrasts showed a number of interesting developmental shifts. For social cognition, group differences were significant at age 2, even with verbal ability controlled, but much less evident at ages 4 and 6. A developmental shift was also found for group differences in positive parenting, which were only significant at age 6. In contrast, mothers in the hard-to-manage group showed elevated rates of negative parenting at all ages.

The first theme in this chapter is the specificity of child and family influences on early problem behaviours. Our findings demonstrate robust group differences and associations between negative parenting and problem behaviours at all ages, even when child cognitive characteristics are taken into account. Likewise, our findings demonstrate that although links between social cognition and behaviour largely overlap with effects of verbal ability, links between poor executive function and problem behaviours are robust and specific. This contrast is intriguing and highlights the importance of including domain-general measures of executive function alongside domain-specific measures of children's ToM when investigating possible cognitive influences upon individual differences in problem behaviours. Currently, developmental relations between executive function and ToM are a topic of lively discussion (Perner and Lang 2000; Carlson et al. 2004); these differential relations with behaviour may provide a fresh perspective upon this debate. In particular, our findings are consistent with the possibility that the link between executive function and ToM is socially mediated: the adverse impact of poor executive control upon children's interactions with siblings and peers limits their experience of sustained cooperative play that may be especially useful for fostering children's growing awareness of others' thoughts and feelings (Dunn 1996). Of course, our present findings only provide evidence for the first half of this chain of associations; further work, which also includes measures of positive interactions, is needed to test this tentative proposal properly.

Note that deficits in executive functions are only more closely linked (than deficits in social cognition) with *child-directed* problem behaviours; adult-directed problem behaviours showed a different pattern of association with children's cognitive performances. Specifically, non-compliance during mother–child interactions showed a strong significant independent association with verbal ability that fully accounted for associations between non-compliance and both executive function and social cognition. One simple explanation for this contrast is that mother–child interactions are typically more verbal than children's interactions with other children. As a result, although deficits in both social cognition and executive function showed significant relations with non-compliance towards mothers, individual differences in verbal ability were more salient. An equally plausible explanation is that young children's limited executive function skills receive much greater scaffolding and support from mothers than from siblings or peers. Each of these explanations points to the importance of attending to the characteristics of children's social partners when exploring links between cognition and behaviour.

The second theme is developmental change: interesting age-related contrasts were found in both studies for both patterns of mother–child interactions and the salience of individual differences in children's early intuitive versus later explicit understanding of mind. With regard to the former, although group differences in negative parenting were consistent across ages, group differences in positive parenting also emerged as the children approached school-age. This developmental shift can be interpreted as reflecting either transactional influences (such that a prolonged history of negative mother–child interactions increasingly limits opportunities for positive interactions) or age-specific societal norms. That is, the approach of the transition to school may make parents more aware of the importance of compliant regulated child behaviour and hence less positive towards their children's problem behaviours. While distinct in their foci, these accounts each highlight processes that may have a common consequence, namely contact with health professionals regarding diagnosis and interventions to address children's problem behaviours.

An additional developmental shift of note in our results was that mean differences in social cognition between the hard-to-manage and control groups were significant at age 2, but became increasingly attenuated at older ages. This shift supports recent theoretical accounts that posit greater social impact for early individual differences in intuitive mentalizing than in children's later explicit understanding of mind (Frith 1989; Tager-Flusberg 2001). This proposal applies to both typically developing children and children with autism. For typically developing children, emotion understanding is linked with individual differences in 2–3-year-olds' prosocial responses to others' distress (Denham 1986), independent of effects of verbal ability (Ensor and Hughes 2005). However, studies of older children (Slaughter *et al.* 2002; Cassidy *et al.* 2003) show no independent association between socio-cognitive skills and social behaviours. Turning to autism research, recent findings suggest that it is the early deficits in 'intuitive mentalizing' which account for the profound social impairments that characterize autism. In particular, Tager-Flusberg (2001) has argued that the delays in language and pragmatic deficits commonly displayed by children with autism are the consequence of earlier impairments in joint attention. Likewise, in a study of 20 verbally able children with autism, Travis *et al.* (2001) reported significant associations between individual differences in intuitive mentalizing and social competence, even when effects of verbal ability were controlled. In contrast, performance on false-belief tasks was unrelated to individual differences in social behaviours.

One plausible interpretation for the lack of association between social competence and false-belief comprehension reported by Travis *et al.* (2001) is that such tasks carry significant linguistic and information-processing demands which may lead younger children to give incorrect responses (Siegal and Beattie 1991; Leslie and Polizzi 1998; Bloom and German 2000) despite having an implicit understanding of mind. Clements and Perner (1994) found that 90 per cent of 3-year-olds who failed a standard false-belief task nevertheless *looked* at the correct location (see also Garnham and Ruffman 2001). Moreover, performance of 3-year-olds (who typically fail standard false-belief tasks) improves when the ecological validity of the standard task is increased (Chandler *et al.* 1989; Hala *et al.* 1991; Cassidy 1998; Carlson *et al.* 2005). In our own work, we have shown that, even at age 2, some children are able to respond correctly to questions about their own and others' false beliefs when these questions are framed within the supportive context provided by a simple picture book in which the false belief is made salient through narrative repetition (Hughes and Ensor 2005). Individual differences in 2-year-olds' performance on such tests of fledgling ToM skills were significantly associated with both frequency of children's references to inner states in their conversations and the quality of their reciprocal play with older siblings (Hughes *et al.* 2006).

The final theme within this chapter is the interplay between child and family influences on early problem behaviours. While our analyses do not directly address this question, we can summarize recent findings (Hughes and Ensor 2006) which speak to this issue. Researchers' home-visit ratings and video-based coding of mother–child dyadic play provided a multi-setting, multi-measure index of harsh parenting, whereas video-based coding of non-compliance, researcher's ratings of emotional dysregulation, and maternal ratings of attention–hyperactivity problems provided a multi-informant, multi-setting, multi-measure index of child problem behaviours. Individual differences in children's scores on this composite index of problem behaviours with adults showed significant independent relations with harsh parenting and with child verbal ability and social cognition. Independent associations with executive function were only marginally significant, supporting our point above regarding the particular salience of executive function for child-directed (rather than adult-directed) problem behaviours. Especially interesting, however, was the significant interplay that was found between harsh parenting and social cognition as predictors of individual differences in problem behaviours. Specifically, effects of harsh parenting were particularly strong for children with poor socio-cognitive skills.

5.6 Clinical implications

In exploring the relevance of the above findings for intervention studies, it is worth noting that the interaction between harsh parenting and social cognition as predictors of problem behaviours can be interpreted in two distinct ways. Early socio-cognitive skills may provide a buffer against the impact of harsh parenting; children who can recognize and anticipate others' feelings and intentions may avoid entering into coercive cycles of violence (Patterson 1981). It follows that interventions aimed at improving young children's social cognition may pre-empt escalating cycles of negative family interactions. Alternatively, children with behavioural problems may be exposed to higher levels of harsh parenting, which in turn limit their developing socio-cognitive skills; maternal disciplinary strategies have been found to influence children's growing understanding of mind (Ruffman *et al.* 1999; Vinden 2001). Thus interventions which provide parents with positive strategies for managing challenging child behaviours may also reap rewards in facilitating children's growing understanding of others, bringing long-term benefits in reducing child problem behaviours. More generally, our findings highlight the need for clinicians to develop multi-pronged interventions that provide support for both children and parents.

In other words, our research findings emphasize the importance of investigating child and family characteristics in tandem in order to achieve a more complete picture of the links between social cognition and problem behaviours. Also clear is the value of including detailed observational measures, both as a bridge between cognitive and family-based approaches to early child problem behaviours and as a means of constructing multi-method, multi-informant ratings that improve the reliability with which individual differences in early problem behaviours can be measured.

5.7 Future research directions

What future research directions appear promising in the light of the research reviewed in this chapter? Clearly, longitudinal analyses are needed for several reasons: to assess the developmental stability of individual differences in problem behaviours, to establish whether children whose problem behaviours persist through to the transition to school can be identified on the basis of their poor performance on fledgling ToM and executive function tasks, to examine developmental change and continuity in atypical patterns of family interactions associated with impairments in both social cognition and behavioural regulation, and to explore transactional mechanisms of interacting child and family influences on DBD. Although challenging, these longitudinal analyses will contribute greatly to the clinical value of cognitive research on early problem behaviours. In this regard, the consistency of the results from these distinct community-based studies and their convergence with current theoretical models gives us reason to be optimistic. Finally, the acid test of the ideas put forward in this chapter hinges on whether interventions that are guided by a twin focus on improving parent–child interactions and children's social cognitions succeed in reducing the impact of DBD upon families, peers, and the children themselves.

References

Archibald, S. and Kerns, K. (1999). Identification and description of new tests of executive functioning in children. *Child Neuropsychology*, **5**, 115–29.

Bartsch, K. and Wellman, H. (1995). *Children talk about the mind.* Oxford University Press.

Bloom, P. and German T. (2000). Two reasons to abandon the false belief task as a test of theory of mind. *Cognition*, **77**, B25–31.

Briggs-Gowan, M., Carter, A., and Schwab-Stone, M. (1996). Discrepancies among mother, child, and teacher reports: examining the contributions of maternal depression and anxiety. *Journal of Abnormal Child Psychology*, **24**, 749–65.

Brophy, M. and Dunn, J. (2002). What did mummy say? Dyadic interactions between young 'hard to manage' children and their mothers. *Journal of Abnormal Child Psychology*, **30**, 103–12.

Campbell, S., Shaw, D., and Gilliom, M. (2000). Early externalizing behavior problems: toddlers and preschoolers at risk for later maladjustment. *Development and Psychopathology*, **12**, 467–88.

Carlson, S. and Moses, L. (2001). Individual differences in inhibitory control and children's theory of mind. *Child Development*, **72**, 1032–53.

Carlson, S., Moses, L., and Breton, C. (2002). How specific is the relation between executive function and theory of mind? Contributions of inhibitory control and working memory. *Infant and Child Development*, **11**, 73–92.

Carlson, S., Mandell D., and Williams, L. (2004). Executive function and theory of mind: Stability and prediction from ages 2 to 3. *Developmental Psychology*, **40**, 1105–22.

Carlson, S., Wong, A., Lemke, M., and Cosser, C., (2005). Gesture as a window on children's beginning understanding of false belief. *Child Development*, **76**, 73–86.

Cassidy, K. (1998). Preschoolers' use of desires to solve theory of mind problems in a pretense context. *Developmental Psychology*, **34**, 503–11.

Cassidy, K., Werner, R., Rourke, M., Zubernis, L., and Balaraman, G. (2003). The relationship between psychological understanding and positive social behaviors. *Social Development*, **12**, 198–221.

Chandler, M., Fritz, A.S., and Hala, S., (1989). Small-scale deceit: deception as a marker of two-, three- and four-year-olds' theories of mind. *Child Development*, **60**, 1263–77.

Channon, S. and Crawford, S. (2000). The effects of anterior lesions on a story comprehension test: left anterior impairment on a theory-of-mind type task. *Neuropsychologia*, **38**, 1006–17.

Charman, A. and Baron-Cohen, S. (1997). Brief report: prompted pretend play in autism. *Journal of Autism and Developmental Disorders*, **27**, 325–32.

Charman, A., Carroll, F., and Sturge, C. (2001). Theory of mind, executive function and social competence in boys with ADHD. *Emotional and Behavioural Difficulties*, **6**, 31–49.

Clements, W. and Perner, J. (1994). Implicit understanding of belief. *Cognitive Development*, **9**, 377–97.

Conduct Problems Prevention Research Group (1999). Initial impact of the fast track prevention trial for conduct problems. I: The high-risk sample. *Journal of Consulting and Clinical Psychology*, **67**, 631–47.

Conger, R., Ge, X., Elder, G., Lorenz, F., and Simons, R. (1994). Economic stress, coercive family processes, and developmental problems of adolescents. *Child Development*, **65**, 541–61.

Corcoran, R., Mercer, G., and Frith, C.D. (1995). Schizophrenia, symptomatology and social influence: investigating 'theory of mind' in people with schizophrenia. *Schizophrenia Research*, **17**, 5–13.

Cutting, A. and Dunn, J. (1999). Theory of mind, emotion understanding, language, and family background: individual differences and interrelations. *Child Development*, 70, 853–65.

Denham, S.A. (1986). Social cognition, prosocial behavior, and emotion in preschoolers: contextual validation. *Child Development*, 57, 194–201.

Dodge, K. and Somberg, D. (1987). Hostile attributional biases among aggressive boys are exacerbated under conditions of threat to the self. *Child Development*, 58, 213–24.

Dunn, J. (1996). The Emanuel Miller Memorial Lecture 1995. Children's relationships: bridging the divide between cognitive and social development. *Journal of Child Psychology and Psychiatry*, 37, 507–18.

Dunn, J. and Brophy, M. (2005). Communication, relationships, and individual differences in children's understanding of mind. In *Why language matters for theory of mind* (ed. J. Astington and J Baird), pp. 50–69. New York: Oxford University Press.

Dunn, J., Brown, J., Slomkowski, C., Tesla, C., and Youngblade, L. (1991). Young children's understanding of other people's feelings and beliefs: individual differences and their antecedents. *Child Development*, 62, 1352–1366.

Dunn, L.M., Dunn, L.M., Whetton, C., and Pintillie, D. (1982). *British Picture Vocabulary Scale*. Windsor: NFER-Nelson.

Elliott, C., Murray, D., and Pearson, L. (1983). *British Abilities Scales*. Windsor: NFER-Nelson.

Ensor, R. and Hughes, C. (2005). More than talk: relations between emotion understanding and positive behaviour in toddlers. *British Journal of Developmental Psychology*, 23, 343–63.

Fergusson, D. and Horwood, L. (1998). Early conduct problems and later life opportunities. *Journal of Child Psychology and Psychiatry*, 39, 1097–1108.

Fergusson, D. and Lynskey, M. (1998). Conduct problems in childhood and psychosocial outcomes in young adulthood: a prospective study. *Journal of Emotional and Behavioural Disorders*, 6, 2–18.

Frith, U. (1989). *Autism: explaining the enigma*. Oxford: Blackwell Scientific.

Frye, D. (1999). Development of intention: the relation of executive function to theory of mind. In *Developing theories of intention: social understanding and self control* (ed. P. Zelazo, J. Astington, and D. Olson), pp. 119–132. Mahwah, NJ: Lawrence Erlbaum.

Frye, D., Zelazo, P.D., and Palfai, T. (1995). Theory of mind and rule-based reasoning. *Cognitive Development*, 10, 483–527.

Gardner F., Hutchings, J., and Lane, E. (2004). 3–8 years: risk and protective factors; effective interventions for preventing antisocial behaviour. In *Support from the start: working with young children and families to reduce risks of crime and antisocial behaviour* (ed. D. Farrington, C. Sutton, and D. Utting), pp. 43–57. London: Department for Education and Science.

Garnham, W. and Ruffman, T (2001). Doesn't see, doesn't know. Is anticipatory looking really related to understanding of belief? *Developmental Science*, 4, 94–100.

Gerstadt, C., Hong, Y., and Diamond, A. (1994). The relationship between cognition and action: performance of children $3^{1}/_{2}$–7 years old on a Stroop-like day–night test. *Cognition*, 53, 129–53.

Golding, J. (1996). Children of the nineties: a resource for assessing the magnitude of long-term effects of prenatal and perinatal events. *Contemporary Reviews in Obstetrics and Gynaecology*, **8**, 89–92.

Goodman, R. and Scott, S. (1999). Comparing the Strengths and Difficulties Questionnaire and the Child Behaviour Checklist. Is small beautiful? *Journal of Abnormal Child Psychology*, **27**, 17–24.

Griffith, E., Pennington, B., Wehner, E., and Rogers, S. (1999). Executive functions in young children with autism. *Child Development*, **70**, 817–32.

Hala, S., Chandler, M., and Fritz, A. (1991). Fledgling theories of mind: deception as a marker of three-year-olds' understanding of false belief. *Child Development*, **62**, 83–97.

Happé, F. and Frith, U. (1996). Theory of mind and social impairment in children with conduct disorder. *British Journal of Developmental Psychology*, **14**, 385–98.

Harris, P., Johnson, C., Hutton, D., Andrews, G., and Cooke, T. (1989). Young children's theory of mind and emotion. *Cognition and Emotion*, **3**, 379–400.

Hartup, W. (2005). Peer interaction. What causes what? *Journal of Abnormal Child Psychology*, **33**, 387–94.

Hay, D., Pawlby, S., Sharp, D., et al. (1999). Parents' judgments about young children's problems: why mothers and fathers might disagree yet still predict later outcomes. *Journal of Child Psychiatry and Psychology*, **40**, 1249–58.

Hill, J. (2002). Biological, psychological and social processes in the conduct disorder. *Journal of Child Psychiatry and Psychology*, **43**, 133–64.

Hughes, C. (1996). Brief Report. Planning problems in autism at the level of motor control. *Journal of Autism and Developmental Disorders*, **26**, 101–9.

Hughes, C. (1998a). Executive function in preschoolers: links with theory of mind and verbal ability. *British Journal of Developmental Psychology*, **16**, 233–53.

Hughes, C. (1998b). Finding your marbles: does preschoolers' strategic behaviour predict later understanding of mind? *Developmental Psychology*, **34**, 1326–39.

Hughes, C. and Dunn, J. (2000). Hedonism or empathy? Hard-to-manage children's moral awareness, and links with cognitive and maternal characteristics. *British Journal of Developmental Psychology*, **18**, 227–45.

Hughes, C. and Ensor, R. (2005). Theory of mind and executive function in 2-year-olds: a family affair? *Developmental Neuropsychology*, **28**, 645–68.

Hughes, C. and Ensor, R. (2006). Behavioral problems in two-year-olds: links with individual differences in theory of mind, executive function and harsh parenting. *Journal of Child Psychology and Psychiatry*, **47**, 488–97.

Hughes, C. and Graham, A (2002). Measuring executive functions in childhood: problems and solutions? *Child and Adolescent Mental Health*, **7**, 131–42.

Hughes, C. and Russell, J. (1993). Autistic children's difficulty with mental disengagement from an object: its implications for theories of autism. *Developmental Psychology*, **29**, 498–510.

Hughes, C., Dunn, J., and White, A. (1998). Trick or treat? Uneven understanding of mind and emotion and executive function among 'hard to manage' preschoolers. *Journal of Child Psychology and Psychiatry*, **39**, 981–94.

Hughes, C., Adlam, A., Happé, F., Jackson, J., Taylor, A., and Caspi, A. (2000a). Good test–retest reliability for standard and advanced false-belief tasks across a wide range of abilities. *Journal of Child Psychology and Psychiatry*, **41**, 483–90.

Hughes, C., White, A., Sharpen, J., and Dunn, J. (2000b). Antisocial, angry and unsympathetic: 'hard to manage' preschoolers' peer problems, and possible social and cognitive influences. *Journal of Child Psychology and Psychiatry*, **41**, 169–79.

Hughes, C., Jaffee, S., Happé, F., Taylor, A., Caspi, A., and Moffitt, T. (2005). Origins of individual differences in theory of mind. From nature to nurture? *Child Development*, **76**, 356–70.

Hughes, C., Fujisawa, K., Ensor, R., Lecce, S., and Marfleet, R. (2006). Cooperation and conversations about the mind: a study of individual differences in two-year-olds and their siblings. *British Journal of Developmental Psychology*, **24**, 53–72.

Leslie, A. and Polizzi, P. (1998). Inhibitory processing in the false-belief task: two conjectures. *Developmental Science*, **1**, 247–54.

McEvoy, R., Rogers, S.J., and Pennington, B.F. (1993). Executive function and social communication deficits in young autistic children. *Journal of Child Psychology and Psychiatry*, **34**, 563–78.

McNeil, C.B., Eyberg, S., Eisenstadt, T.H., Newcomb, K., and Funderburk, B. (1991). Parent–child interaction therapy with behavior problem children: generalization of treatment effects to the school setting. *Journal of Clinical Child Psychology*, **20**, 140–51.

Mannuzza, S., Klein, R.G., Bonagura, N., Malloy, P., Giampino, T.L., and Addalli, K.A. (1991). Hyperactive boys almost grown up. V: Replication of psychiatric status. *Archives of General Psychiatry*, **48**, 77–83.

Mannuzza, S., Klein, R.G., Bessler, A., Malloy, P., and LaPadula, M. (1993). Adult outcome of hyperactive boys: educational achievement, occupational rank, and psychiatric status. *Archives of General Psychiatry*, **50**, 565–76.

Masten, A. and Curtis, W. (2000). Integrating competence and psychopathology: pathways toward a comprehensive science of adaption in development. *Development and Psychopathology*, **12**, 529–50.

Meins, E., Fernyhough, C., Wainwright, R., et al. (2003). Pathways to understanding mind: construct validity and predictive validity of maternal mind-mindedness. *Child Development*, **74**, 1194–1211.

Moffitt, T. (1990). Juvenile delinquency and attention deficit disorder: boys' developmental trajectories from age 3 to age 15. *Child Development*, **61**, 893–910.

Moffitt, T. (1993). The neuropsychology of conduct disorder. *Development and Psychopathology*, **5**, 135–52.

Morrell, J. and Murray, L. (2003). Parenting and the development of conduct disorder and hyperactive symptoms in childhood: a prospective longitudinal study from 2 months to 8 years. *Journal of Child Psychology and Psychiatry*, **44**, 489–508.

Ozonoff, S., Pennington, B.F., and Rogers, S.J. (1991). Executive function deficits in high functioning autistic children: relationship to theory of mind. *Journal of Child Psychology and Psychiatry*, **32**, 1081–1105.

Patterson, G. (1981). *Coercive family process*. Eugene, OR: Castalia Press.

Patterson, G. and Forgatch, M. (1995). Predicting future clinical adjustment from treatment outcome and process variables. *Psychological Assessment*, **7**, 275–85.

Patterson, G., Dishion, T., and Chamberlain, P. (1993). Outcomes and methodological issues relating to treatment of antisocial children. In *Handbook of effective psychotherapy* (ed. T. Giles), pp. 43–88. New York: Plenum Press.

Pennington, B and Bennetto, L. (1993). Main effects or transactions in the neuropsychology of conduct disorder: a commentary on the neuropsychology of conduct disorder. *Development and Psychopathology*, **5**, 153–64.

Perner, J. and Lang, B. (1999). Development of theory of mind and executive control. *Trends in Cognitive Sciences*, **3**, 337–44.

Perner, J. and Lang, B. (2000). Theory of mind and executive function. Is there a developmental relationship? In *Understanding other minds: perspectives from autism and developmental cognitive neuroscience* (ed. S. Baron-Cohen, H. Tager-Flusberg, and D.J. Cohen), pp. 150–81. Oxford University Press.

Perner, J., Ruffman, T., and Leekam, S.R. (1994). Theory of mind is contagious: you catch it from your sibs. *Child Development*, **65**, 1228–38.

Perner, J., Kain, W., and Barchfield, P. (2002). Executive control and higher-order theory of mind in children at risk of ADHD. *Infant and Child Development*, **11**, 141–58.

Peterson, C. and Siegal, M. (1995). Deafness, conversation and theory of mind. *Journal of Child Psychology and Psychiatry*, **36**, 459–74.

Robison, L., Sclar, D., Skaer, T., and Galin, R. (1999). National trends in the prevalence of attention-deficit/hyperactivity disorder and the prescribing of methylphenidate among school-age children. *Clinical Pediatrics*, **38**, 209–17.

Ruffman, T., Perner, J., and Parkin, L. (1999). How parenting style affects false belief understanding. *Social Development*, **8**, 395–411.

Rutter, M. and Quinton, D. (1984). Parental psychiatric disorder: effects on children. *Psychological Medicine*, **14**, 853–80.

Seguin, J.R., Boulerice, B., Harden, P.W., Tremblay, R.E., and Pihl, R.O. (1999). Executive functions and physical aggression after controlling for attention deficit hyperactivity disorder, general memory and IQ. *Journal of Child Psychology and Psychiatry*, **40**, 1197–1208.

Shallice, T. (1982). Specific impairments in planning. *Philosophical Transactions of the Royal Society of London, Series B*, **298**, 199–209.

Siegal, M. and Beattie, K. (1991). Where to look first for children's knowledge of false beliefs. *Cognition*, **38**, 1–12.

Slaughter, V., Dennis, M., and Pritchard, M. (2002). Theory of mind and peer acceptance in preschool children. *British Journal of Developmental Psychology*, **20**, 545–64.

Sodian, B. and Frith, U. (1992). Deception and sabotage in autistic, retarded and normal children. *Journal of Child Psychology and Psychiatry*, **33**, 591–605.

Speltz, M., Deklyen, M., Calderon, R., Greenberg, M., and Fisher, P. (1999). Neuropsychological characteristics and test behaviors of boys with early onset conduct problems. *Journal of Abnormal Psychology*, **108**, 315–25.

Sutton, J., Smith, P., and Swettenham, J. (1999a). Bullying and 'theory of mind': a critique of the 'social skills deficit' view of anti-social behaviour. *Social Development*, **8**, 117–27.

Sutton, J., Smith, P., and Swettenham, J. (1999b). Social cognition and bullying: social inadequacy or skilled manipulation? *British Journal of Developmental Psychology*, **17**, 435–50.

Tager-Flusberg, H. (2001). A re-examination of the theory of mind hypothesis of autism. In *The development of autism: perspectives from theory and research* (ed. J. Burack, T. Charman, N. Yirmiya, and P. Zelazo), pp. 173–94. Mahwah, NJ: Lawrence Erlbaum.

Thorndike, R.L, Hagen, E.P., and Sattler, J.M. (1986). *Stanford–Binet Intelligence Scales*. Chicago, IL: Riverside.

Travis, L., Sigman, M., and Ruskin, E. (2001). Links between social understanding and social behavior in verbally able children with autism. *Journal of Autism and Developmental Disorders*, **31**, 119–30.

Vinden, P. (2001). Parenting attitudes and children's understanding of mind: a comparison of Korean American and Anglo-American families. *Cognitive Development*, **16**, 793–809.

Wellman, H., Cross, D., and Watson, J. (2001). Meta-analysis of theory of mind development: the truth about false belief. *Child Development*, **72**, 655–84.

Wimmer, H. and Perner, J. (1983). Beliefs about beliefs: representation and constraining function of wrong beliefs in young children's understanding of deception. *Cognition*, **13**, 103–28.

Zelazo, P.D., Frye, D., and Rapus, T. (1996). An age-related dissociation between knowing rules and using them. *Cognitive Development*, **11**, 37–63.

6

Social information processing and the development of conduct problems in children and adolescents: looking beneath the surface

Jacquelyn Mize and Gregory S. Pettit

6.1 Disorders of aggression in children

Conduct disorder (CD) and oppositional defiant disorder (ODD) refer to childhood problems defined by a broad array of disruptive antisocial behaviours (American Psychiatric Association 2000). Behaviour disorders are among the most common presenting problems of childhood, and are thought to affect 5–10 per cent of 8- to 16-year-old children (Angold and Costello 2001). Of the wide range of disruptive and destructive behaviours characteristic of the CD–ODD spectrum, persistent aggression is the most predictive of subsequent serious criminality (Stattin and Magnusson 1989; Loeber et al. 1995), and it is aggression on which virtually all studies of social cognition in behaviour-disordered children has focused. Social cognition appears to be crucial in determining the persistence or, conversely, the discontinuity of early aggression problems (Loeber and Coie 2001), and so is of considerable importance both theoretically and practically.

In the past two decades, empirical investigations of social cognition in children with behaviour problems have largely been guided by what has come to be called a social information processing (SIP) model of aggression (Dodge 1993; 2003), also referred to as social cognitive information processing (Huesmann 1998). The focal point of this large and accumulating literature is on how people interpret and respond to challenging and provocative social encounters with others. SIP biases and deficits are thought to underlie maladaptive behaviour—especially aggressive behaviour—in specific social situations. As a fairly mature theoretical model, SIP has had a major impact on the field. In our view, it is useful and timely at this juncture to look somewhat more deeply at the SIP model in relation to its developmental course and its links with distinct forms of aggressive behaviour. We conclude with a discussion of emerging work on psychophysiological processes in aggression that we believe will shed important new light on the role of SIP as an explanatory mechanism in the development of conduct problems. Before turning to a more detailed discussion of these issues, we first present an overview of the SIP framework.

6.2 Social information processing: a proximal mechanism of interpersonal behaviour

The SIP model describes a set of sequential cognitive processing steps that are presumed to function interdependently, in real-time (albeit rapidly), and largely without conscious awareness (Crick and Dodge 1994). In Dodge's SIP model (Dodge 1993; Crick and Dodge 1994), the first two steps can be characterized as the input sequence and the latter steps as the output sequence (Lansford et al. 2006). In step 1, *encoding of cues*, specific bits of information from the multitude that are available in the environment are selected for attention and processing. These cues include stimuli in the external environment (e.g. a jolting push from behind, laughter, the colour of a shirt, a facial expression) and internal sensations (e.g. accelerating heart rate, fear). How much of the potentially relevant information is encoded, how accurately it is encoded, and what specific features are recalled may influence behaviour. Step 2, *interpretation and representation*, involves making inferences about the causes of the event (i.e. attributions), evaluating the meaning of the event for the self, and mentally representing the event in memory. In the aforementioned instance, a child may interpret the jolt as a hostile shove or, alternatively, as a clumsy but benign accident; the event may be seen as constituting a serious threat to his/her reputation or alternatively, as being of little consequence. In step 3, *clarification (or identification) of goals*, a desired outcome for the situation is identified. The child may wish to make a friend, avoid conflict, save face, or instill fear in other children, for example. Goals may serve as motivation for step 4, *response generation* (also called *response access or construction*), which involves scanning memory for possible responses or developing a new response. Possible responses are evaluated in terms of likely results, confidence in enacting the strategy, or its appropriateness in step 5, *response decision (or response selection)*. Finally, in step 6, *behavioural enactment*, the selected response is carried out. Although step 6 clearly is necessary for aggression to occur, research on individual differences in enacting aggressive behaviour has not been central to studies of childhood aggression, and will not be considered in this review. Clearly, what occurs at each step affects processing at subsequent steps, such that, for example, interpretation of another's actions as hostile makes selection of a retaliatory goal and an angry response more likely.

The SIP model assumes that a knowledge base derived from an individual's experiences in prior and current relationships guides social information processing at each step (Crick and Dodge 1994). This knowledge base has been referred to as a set of relational schemas (Baldwin 1992), scripts (Schank and Abelson 1977), latent knowledge structures (Burks *et al.* 1999), and working models of relationships (Bowlby 1969). Relationship schemas form through interactions with other people, particularly significant others such as parents, peers, and teachers. It is through schemas that prior events and relationships influence online processing, and ultimately behaviour, according to SIP theory and several other influential developmental models (e.g. attachment theory (Bretherton 1985)). That is, based on experiences, particularly interactions with significant others, individuals largely unconsciously construct schemas that are made up of scripts for expected patterns of interaction, images of the self and others (Baldwin 1992), and socially relevant constructs such as memories, expectations, attitudes, and beliefs (Huesmann 1998). These schemas then influence information processing in future social encounters including which stimuli elicit attention and are encoded and recalled, how stimuli are interpreted, individuals' goals in relationships, the store of strategies on which an individual can draw, evaluation of the likely result of each possible course of action and the desirability of that result, and presumably even the ability to enact the selected strategy.

6.3 Normative developmental changes in social information processing

Developmental research has yielded rich descriptions of changes from infancy to adolescence in many aspects of social and non-social cognition, including attention, memory, theory of mind, and moral reasoning (Flavell *et al.* 1993). However, perhaps because the goal of SIP formulations is to explain deviations from normal patterns, there have been few theoretical or empirical attempts to describe normative developmental changes in SIP (Orobio de Castro 2004) or to integrate theories or data from cognitive and social cognitive developmental research. Even in longitudinal or cross-sectional studies of SIP, typically no hypotheses concerning developmental changes in SIP are posed (Orobio de Castro 2004) and often developmental differences are not described. Data from studies of different age groups are not easily compared and often present inconsistent patterns (Orobio de Castro *et al.* 2002). Because typical assessments of SIP rely on children's verbal responses to interviewer prompts, verbal skills undoubtedly influence performance, but are rarely measured or controlled. These and other methodological issues complicate the ability to infer developmental changes in SIP. With these caveats in mind, it still is possible to draw some tentative conclusions about developmental changes in SIP.

Encoding typically, but not always (see Gouze 1987; Schippell *et al.* 2003), is operationalized in SIP research as the accuracy and completeness of children's recall (i.e. descriptions) or recognition (i.e. correct selection from a set of options) of elements of social exchanges that they have witnessed or heard about (e.g. Dodge and Frame 1982; Milich and Dodge 1984; Dodge and Tomlin 1987; Slaby and Guerra 1988; Lochman and Dodge 1994). Judging by what they typically can describe verbally, preschool children notice and encode at most a few key elements of social interactions, but by middle childhood children report more details about social exchanges (Dodge *et al.* 1984; Dodge and Price 1994). However, assessments based on what children can describe may underestimate what they perceive, and this may be particularly the case for young children. Enactive assessments using dolls or puppets (Nelson 1981; Getz *et al.* 1984; Mize and Ladd 1988) reveal that young children possess (and thus presumably have encoded from experiences) considerably more knowledge of past events than they can describe verbally.

What children encode certainly appears to change with age. Young children are more likely to recall descriptions of peer aggression than descriptions of withdrawn behaviours, but by age 10 or 11 children recall withdrawn behaviour and aggressive behaviour equally well (Younger and Piccinin 1989). Together with data indicating that children recall information about withdrawn girls or aggressive boys better than they recall information about aggressive girls or withdrawn boys (Bukowski 1990), these data emphasize the role of schemas in guiding information processing. Specifically, information consistent with, or relevant to, an existing schema is more likely to be encoded and recalled. Even young children appear to have well-developed schemas for aggression, but they do not develop schemas for withdrawal until middle childhood (Younger and Boyko 1987).

Accuracy in interpreting events (step 2) seems to improve with age when others' intentions are clear (Dodge *et al.* 1984; Dodge and Price 1994), but normative changes in the tendency to assign culpability when intentions are ambiguous are less well understood. Both theory (Damon 1983; Dodge 2006) and some data (Pettit *et al.* 1988) suggest that young children universally assume a correlation between the effects of an action and the motivation for the action, i.e. bad things happen because someone intended to cause harm. Conversely, some researchers report that even in ambiguous situations preschool children assume hostile intent only about a quarter of the time

(Webster-Stratton and Lindsay 1999). The pattern of normative developmental changes among older children is similarly unclear. Some studies (e.g. Dodge and Price (1994), studying first- to third-graders) report that older elementary children make more hostile attributions in ambiguous situations than do younger children, whereas other data indicate the opposite pattern—that it is the younger children who are more likely to assume hostile intent (Crick and Dodge (1996), studying third- to sixth graders). As children approach adolescence, they often become less forgiving and harsher judges of deviant behaviour, attributing it to permanent personality or character flaws (Coie and Pennington 1976; Boxer and Tisak 2003). Children appear to be equally biased at all ages studied towards interpreting behaviour of liked peers positively and behaviour of disliked peers negatively (Hymel 1986; Burgess *et al.* 2006).

It is not surprising that as children mature beyond the preschool years, they are able to think of a wider range of things to do in the face of a social challenge, more strategies are active (as opposed to passive or withdrawing) (Mayeux and Cillessen 2003), and strategies become more sophisticated (Dodge and Price 1994; Mayeux and Cillessen 2003) and competent (Feldman and Dodge 1987). Older children also are more competent than younger children when they are asked to act out, or demonstrate, a behavioural strategy (Dodge and Price 1994).

Developmental improvements in strategically directing attention (Vurpillot 1968; DeMarie-Dreblow and Miller 1988; Posner and Rothbart 2000) and in basic information-processing capacity or speed (Kail 1984) probably largely underlie apparent gains in how much information about social interactions children encode, and perhaps permit encoding of more subtle cues, as children mature. The ability to generate more, and more sophisticated, active, and prosocial strategies may be driven by growth in verbal skills and understanding of persons and emotions, direct teaching and modelling by adults (Mize and Pettit 1997), and accumulation of experiences with peers.

It is more difficult to explain developmental differences in causal attributions, generation of aggressive responses, and evaluation of aggressive responses because patterns are not consistent across studies and because some studies suggest that children become more tolerant of aggression in middle childhood. Inconsistencies across studies may be partially a result of methodological differences in how children are asked to evaluate aggression—sometimes as to whether it would be justified (Huesmann and Guerra 1997), sometimes as to whether it would be effective (Dodge and Price 1994), and sometimes as to self-efficacy for performing aggression (Crick and Dodge 1996). The fact that the hypothetical situations presented to children (teasing, other provocation, group entry) also vary across studies and that younger children appear to be less able to tailor strategies to particulars of situations could also account for some apparent inconsistencies. Alternatively, inconsistencies may reflect real, but non-linear, developmental changes in SIP that arise from changes in the relative influence of parents and peers and in peer norms (Fine 1987). Although children value relationships with peers more highly as they grow older (Rubin *et al.* 1998), they simultaneously become more concerned with saving face, and different goals probably take precedence in different situations. During the preschool and early elementary years, children learn to think in increasingly complex ways about others' behaviour and to suppress aggressive impulses. Then, as they move through elementary and into high school, children become more concerned about the opinions of age-mates and at the same time more aware of the power of aggression and intimidation (Cillessen and Mayeux 2004). This could produce a U-shaped curve in children's perceptions and approval of aggression.

Most intriguing is the possibility that, because socialization pressures, school characteristics, and peer behaviour and norms differ across ethnic groups, neighbourhoods, and peer groups (Parke and Buriel 2006), patterns of developmental change in attributions, responses to social situations, and evaluation of responses may be moderated by community and peer-group norms. If this were the case, consistency in patterns of change across studies and samples in these aspects of SIP would not be expected. Longitudinal studies make it clear that children's social and emotional competence and behaviour undergo change consistent with characteristics of the settings they frequent (Ladd 1990; Kellam *et al.* 1998; Hoglund and Leadbeater 2004). For instance, Hoglund and Leadbeater (2004) found that, over children's first grade year, school disadvantage independently predicted increases in children's behaviour problems, and low levels of prosocial behaviour and high levels of victimization in classrooms predicted increases in emotional problems. Systematic investigation of SIP as a function of ecological context is rare (but see Schultz and Shaw 2003), and we know of no studies of developmental changes in SIP in different sociocultural contexts.

Another developmental issue concerns the extent to which individual differences in SIP are stable over time. Problem aggression is remarkably stable; Olweus (1979) estimated that the correlation over 10 years from childhood to adulthood is around 0.60. If anomalies in SIP underlie problem aggression, it would seem reasonable to expect stability in SIP patterns. Over short periods of time (up to a year or so), modest to moderate continuity has been demonstrated in each of the SIP steps, with older children evidencing greater stability than younger children. Dodge and colleagues report moderate stability for each of the SIP steps for early elementary age children in two separate samples over 1-year (Dodge et al. 1995) and 3-year (Dodge et al. 2003) periods. However, little stability in specific SIP steps has been detected over longer periods (Keltikangas-Järvinen 2001; Lansford et al. 2006). In an analysis of Child Development Project (CDP) data in which SIP was examined across childhood, Lansford et al. (2006) report no stability before eighth grade, but moderate stability from eighth to eleventh grades (i.e. about ages 13–16) for a dichotomous categorization based on presence (one or more) or absence of SIP problems. Stability in terms of specific SIP steps was below chance levels. The modest stability in SIP over long periods, particularly for younger children, does not necessarily undermine SIP theory. Dodge and colleagues (Crick and Dodge 1994; Dodge 2003) suggest that relationship schemas and SIP patterns become stable only in middle childhood when cognitive processes become less malleable.

Measurement issues may also limit the ability to detect stability in SIP patterns, particularly in comparison with aggression. Assessments of children's aggression are typically based on numerous sampling points, either observations over several days or ratings by adults or peers who have observed the child over long periods of time; these are highly reliable and thus have considerable sensitivity for detecting stability. In contrast, SIP assessments typically take place in a single session. SIP is powerfully influenced by recent encounters, emotions, and activities, factors that are rarely manipulated or controlled in SIP assessments. Thus children's responses on standard SIP assessments probably reflect stable individual differences as well as the effects of more transient circumstances.

Clearly, there is a need for research with typically developing children on whether and how changes in SIP underpin or parallel the transformation from the reactive emotional outbursts characteristic of frustrated toddlers to the normally more restrained and reflective style of competent adolescents. To our knowledge, no such studies exist. As noted by Orobio de Castro (2004), analytical techniques are available to evaluate whether or not SIP and aggression trajectories develop in parallel (Nagin 1999).

6.4 Social information processing patterns of aggressive children

According to SIP models, problem aggression is a result, at least partially, of biased or deficient processing at one or more of the information processing steps. The effects of maladaptive processing are considered cumulative, such that aggression becomes more likely with each additional aggressogenic cognition. Scores of studies have examined social information processing in aggressive children and youths, with findings largely supportive of the model.

A meta-analysis incorporating studies of four SIP steps (encoding, interpretation, response generation, and response evaluation and selection) concluded that each was moderately associated with children's aggressive behaviour, and reported average effect sizes in the 'medium' range (0.39–0.44) (Yoon et al. 1999). Collectively, the processing steps have been found to account for 9–11 per cent of the variance in aggression (Dodge et al. 1995).

Aggression is a heterogeneous construct, and researchers have drawn distinctions along several dimensions, such as time of onset and course (early onset versus adolescent limited (Moffitt 1993a)), form (relational versus overt (Crick and Grotpeter 1995)), and motivation or function (reactive versus proactive (Dodge and Coie 1987; Atkins and Stoff 1993; Crick and Dodge 1996; Dodge et al. 1997; Vitaro et al. 2002; Vitaro and Brendgen 2005; Card and Little 2006). Of particular relevance here, SIP models (Crick and Dodge 1994) suggest that reactive and proactive aggression should be related differentially to individual SIP steps. Reactive aggression (also referred to as angry, defensive, emotional, or hot-blooded aggression) refers to aggressive acts motivated by anger, frustration, or retaliation (Berkowitz 1993); reactive aggression often appears to be an emotionally dysregulated response to a perceived offense (Card and Little 2006). Proactive aggression (also called instrumental or cold-blooded aggression) is motivated by a desire to obtain valued outcomes or resources (Bandura 1983). Although the two types of aggression are moderately to highly correlated (e.g. Dodge and Coie 1987; Dodge et al. 2003), there is considerable evidence that the distinction is valid and useful (Dodge and Coie 1987; Vitaro et al. 2002; Card and Little 2006; Raine et al. 2006). Based on neurobiological analyses, Blair et al. (2006) (see also Chapter 7, this volume) argue that children high in proactive aggression are almost always also at risk for reactive aggression; thus there should be few purely proactively aggressive children, whereas there should be a population of children who present almost exclusively with reactive aggression. SIP models suggest that reactive aggression should be predicted by early-stage SIP problems (i.e. deficits in encoding and biased attributions), whereas proactive aggression should be predicted by later-stage processing anomalies (competitive goals, generation of aggressive responses, and evaluation of aggression as appropriate or effective). The extent to which empirical evidence supports differential patterns of SIP anomalies in reactively and proactively aggressive children will be considered in subsequent sections of this chapter.

6.4.1 Encoding in aggressive children

According to SIP theory, aggressive children are likely to have deficiencies in attending to and accurately encoding relevant social cues, and may selectively notice and recall cues consistent with hostility or threat. Encoding is among the least studied of the SIP steps and is the process for which research findings remain most ambiguous. Most studies have operationalized encoding as children's ability to describe or recognize details of social events observed on videotape (e.g. Dodge and Frame 1982; Dodge *et al.* 1990a, 1997; Weiss *et al.* 1992; Lochman and Dodge 1994), heard about on audiotape (e.g. Milich and Dodge 1984; Dodge and Tomlin 1987), or which have been described to them (Dodge 1980). Most published studies support the model's claims, reporting that aggressive children seek and use less information about social situations before drawing conclusions (Dodge and Newman 1981; Milich and Dodge 1984; Dodge and Tomlin 1987; Slaby and Guerra 1988), describe fewer relevant details of an interaction accurately (Dodge *et al.* 1990a; Weiss *et al.* 1992; Mize *et al.* 1995), make more errors of omission (failing to recall events that did occur) and commission (endorsing as having occurred events that did not occur) than do their non-aggressive peers (Dodge and Frame 1982; Milich and Dodge 1984; Lochman and Dodge 1994), and recall more information indicative of guilt or hostility (Dodge and Newman 1981). Deficiencies in cue encoding and utilization appear to be characteristic particularly of reactively aggressive children (Dodge and Coie 1987; Dodge *et al.* 1997) and of children who are both aggressive and hyperactive (Milich and Dodge 1984). Dodge *et al.* (1997) report that in two samples, one a large sample of elementary children and the second a group of seriously violent boys with psychiatric diagnoses, reactively aggressive children had more cue-encoding problems than did either proactively aggressive children or non-aggressive children.

To encode others' behaviour accurately and thoroughly, and then use it to guide one's own, requires attentional skills, the ability to inhibit responding for an appropriate interval, and sufficient processing capacity to hold the information in the memory and act on it. To describe in the context of an SIP assessment what has been seen and heard requires, additionally, adequate verbal ability. It is not clear whether encoding deficiencies, particularly in what Yoon *et al.* (1999) refer to quantitative subprocesses (i.e. how much is encoded), are uniquely social–perceptual, or whether they reflect more general neurocognitive or language deficits that are correlated with antisocial behaviour (Moffitt 1993b; van Nieuwenhuijzen *et al.* 2004; Raine *et al.* 2005). Some efforts have been made in the SIP literature to control for individual differences in intelligence (Dodge *et al.* 1990b), discrimination abilities (Dodge *et al.* 1984), attention and inhibitory control (Waldman 1996), and verbal skill (Dodge *et al.* 1984; Mize *et al.* 1995). In a recent meta-analysis, Orobio de Castro *et al.* (2002) determined that when intellectual abilities are controlled, effect sizes for the association between SIP and behaviour problems are weaker than when they are not controlled. However, few of these studies specifically assess encoding. In one that did so, Meece and Mize (in press) adapted a measure from Dodge *et al.* (1990a) to operationalize encoding as the extent to which preschool children were able to describe the relevant events in a series of brief videotaped vignettes of children engaged in potentially conflictual situations. Encoding scores independently predicted boys', but not girls', aggression after controlling for receptive vocabulary. Thus far, then, there is modest evidence of discriminant validity for the encoding construct, at least as measured through children's verbal reports.

Many models of social behaviour suggest that stimuli encoded out of conscious awareness have powerful effects on cognition and behaviour, perhaps more powerful effects than do consciously encoded stimuli (Bargh and Pietromonaco 1982; LeDoux 1996; Todorov and Bargh 2002). To date, neither the notion of unconscious encoding nor methods for measuring unconscious encoding have been incorporated widely into SIP studies with children. A few studies have used selective attention tasks, which may capture out-of-awareness encoding, to compare children's attention to aggressive versus non-aggressive behaviour (Gouze 1987), faces with positive, negative, and neutral affective expressions (Pollack and Tolley-Shell 2003), and social-threat-relevant versus neutral words (Schippell *et al.* 2003). Aggressive children appear to differ from non-aggressive children on selective attention measures, but the differences do not always fit what would be expected based on SIP theory. Consistent with SIP models, aggressive preschool children are less able to shift their attention away from aggressive stimuli in videotaped puppet shows and cartoons (Gouze 1987). Contrary to theory, however, Schippell *et al.* (2003) found that 11- to 16-year-old highly reactively aggressive children (but not proactively aggressive or moderately reactively aggressive children) showed suppressed attention (as indicated by slower responses), rather than heightened attention, to words indicative of social threat (hated, loser) compard with neutral words and words indicative of physical threat (murder, hurt). Schippell and colleagues suggest that highly reactively aggressive children deploy attention defensively: Following an initial unconscious recognition of a threat, aggressive children suppress attention to it, thus shielding themselves from information about others' reactions to their inappropriate behaviour.

It would appear that aggressive children, particularly reactively aggressive children, show anomalies in encoding social information. Moreover, anomalies may take several forms: being tuned out and encoding relatively little relevant information, being hypersensitive to threat, or defensively avoiding threatening information. It would be useful in future research to employ multiple measures of encoding and to control for neuropsychological and cognitive deficits. Certainly more attention should be given to unconscious attentional and encoding processes that cannot be articulated by research participants but nonetheless undoubtedly influence other SIP steps, and ultimately behaviour.

6.4.2 Interpretation/representation in aggressive children

The second step, referred to in the SIP literature as representation or interpretation, has largely been studied in terms of the accuracy or valence of one's attributions about the motives for others' actions. Studies assessing attributions typically present to children one or more hypothetical scenarios in which the participant is to imagine that he/she comes to some harm at the hands of peers (whose intentions are often ambiguous) and is asked whether the peer's motive was hostile (e.g. 'The kid was being mean') or not (e.g. 'It was an accident') (Dodge et al. 1984, 1990b; Crick and Dodge 1996). Another approach is to show children multiple scenarios, one of which differs in the intent of the provocateur (e.g. two with benign intent and one with hostile intent), and ask the participant to identify which differs from the others (Dodge et al. 1984; Waldman 1996). In both types of measure, hostile bias is reflected in the relative tendency to identify non-hostile intentions as hostile. Although both aggressive and non-aggressive children justifiably assume that another person was acting with hostility when that person's actions are clearly intended to cause harm, aggressive children are much more likely to infer hostility when another person's intentions are not clear (Dodge 1980; Dodge et al. 1990a; Weiss et al. 1992; Crick and Dodge 1996), and sometimes infer hostility even when the other person's intentions are clearly not hostile (Nasby et al. 1980; Dodge et al. 1984, 1986; Waldman 1996). A recent meta-analysis of this literature (Orobio de Castro et al. 2002) concluded that hostile bias was robustly associated with aggressive behaviour, with an average weighted effect size of 0.17. Stronger effect sizes were found for studies involving more severely aggressive children, for studies whose participants were both aggressive and also rejected by peers, and for studies using staged provocation situations which probably elicit more real-world reactions than do situations presented via pictures, verbal descriptions, or video.

Dodge (2006) has argued that a hostile attributional bias is normative early in life, and indeed that it is universal, because young children tend to presume that causes match outcomes. However, by about age 4, the age of the youngest participants in studies of SIP, attributional style usually (Mize et al. 1995; Katsurada and Sugawara 1998; Webster-Stratton and Lindsay 1999), but not always (Pettit et al. 1988), differentiates aggressive from non-aggressive children. Still, consistent with Dodge's suggestion, associations between hostile attributional bias and aggression appear to be stronger for older children (8–12-year olds) than for younger children (Orobio de Castro *et al.* 2002).

As noted previously, it has been argued (Dodge and Coie 1987; Crick and Dodge 1994; Dodge *et al.* 1997) that hostile bias should be more characteristic of reactive aggression than of proactive aggression. There is mixed support for this proposition. The meta-analysis conducted by Orobio de Castro *et al.* (2002) revealed, contrary to the model, larger effect sizes for the hostile attribution–aggression link when proactively aggressive children were included in analyses. However, some individual studies do support the claim. Dodge and Coie (1987) found that reactively aggressive and reactively–proactively aggressive first- and third-grade boys attributed hostility to a peer in 83 per cent and 68 per cent, respectively, of ambiguous provocation scenarios. In contrast, boys who were rated as solely proactively aggressive made hostile attributions in only 38 per cent of ambiguous situations, a figure comparable to the 41 per cent of ambiguous situations in which non-aggressive average status boys made hostile attributions in the study. The mixed findings may reflect the difficulty of distinguishing between reactively and proactively aggressive children, particularly when teacher or parent reports are the basis for the distinction (Card and Little 2006).

Although associations between hostile interpretations and aggressive behaviour are replicable, the magnitude of associations is not large (Dodge and Somberg 1987; Orobio de Castro *et al.* 2002). One possible explanation for the modest associations is that, although hostile attributional bias is often thought of as an all-or-none phenomenon (aggressive children assume hostility and non-aggressive children do not), there appears to be considerable variation within persons across different situations in inferences about others' motivations. That is, even highly aggressive children probably do not infer hostile intent every time they are harmed by a peer, whereas even passive children may sometimes takes unwarranted offence. Developing a clear understanding of the conditions or situations that moderate the likelihood that a child will infer hostility is of considerable theoretical and practical interest. Experimental manipulations have been most helpful in this regard, and suggest that the interactant, recent experiences, the child's mood, and recent exposure to, or priming of, constructs consistent with hostility, aggression, or blame influence the tendency to infer hostility.

The identity of the other child has powerful effects on children's assumptions and inferences about that child's motives and behaviour. Children are more likely to infer hostility when a disliked or unknown peer is the provocateur, and more likely to assume benign intent when a friend is involved (Hymel 1986; Burgess *et al.* 2006). When the other child is known to be aggressive, children are five times more likely to attribute hostility than when the other child is a cooperative classmate (Dodge 1980). In a study of boys' playgroups, Coie *et al.* (1999) found that relationship factors explained more of the variance in boys' reactive aggression toward other boys than did either characteristics of the aggressor or characteristics of the victim. In particular, boys who had mutually aggressive relationships (i.e. frequently fought) were highly likely to attribute hostile intent to each other. These data are a reminder that assumptions of hostility are sometimes rational, based on a history of victimization or mutual aggression.

In one of the first studies to systematically investigate conditions that might exacerbate children's tendency to infer hostile intent, Dodge and Somberg (1987) demonstrated that the experience of feeling threatened heightens the hostile bias of aggressive boys. These investigators first determined that, under relaxed conditions, there was no significant difference between aggressive and non-aggressive boys' attributions for hypothetical provocations. Following the baseline assessment of attributions, boys were exposed to a threat of potential conflict from a peer whom they believed was in an adjacent room. Following exposure to the simulated peer threat, aggressive, but not non-aggressive, boys made significantly more hostile attributions in response to another set of hypothetical ambiguous provocations. Thus social threat appears to make hostile attributions more likely, and aggressive children appear to be particularly sensitive to such threats. Dodge and Somberg (1987) suggest that the perceived threat was cognitively, emotionally, or physiologically arousing for the aggressive boys and that the arousal triggered rapid pre-emptive processing that bypassed rational analysis (Costanzo and Dix 1983). Situations that arouse negative emotions, even those not caused by a social threat (see Orobio de Castro *et al.* 2003), that involve competition (Lochman and Dodge 1998), or that expose children to fantasy violence (Kirsh 1998) have similar effects, increasing aggressive children's attributions of hostile intent. Moreover, for aggressive more than for non-aggressive children, these effects seem to carry over into subsequent situations (e.g. a non-competitive game) in which hostile attributions are even less appropriate (Lochman and Dodge 1998).

It is important to note that recent experience need not be physiologically or emotionally arousing, and individuals need not be aware of an experience for there to be an effect on subsequent attributions (Bargh and Pietromonaco 1982; Todorov and Bargh 2002). Even brief exposure to words that are congruent with the idea of causing intentional harm can make hostile attributions more likely. Graham and Hudley (1994) randomly assigned aggressive and non-aggressive African American boys to one of three conditions. In an 'intentional prime' condition, boys read sentences in which a negative event occurred for which the target child was responsible (e.g. a boy had no money to help his friends buy pizza because he had spent all his money). In an 'unintentional prime' condition, boys read sentences in which a negative event occurred, but the target in the story was not responsible (e.g. a boy had no money to help his friends pay for pizza because his wallet had been stolen). Boys in a control condition read sentences about neutral events with no causal information. Following the priming activity, the participants' attributions about an ambiguous provocation were probed. Regardless of priming condition, aggressive boys tended to assume that the peer in the ambiguous story had acted with malicious intent. In contrast, non-aggressive boys tended to assume benign intentions, unless they had received the intentional prime, in which case they judged the provocateur in the ambiguous stories to be as mean and blameworthy and said they would be as angry as did the aggressive boys. Graham and Hudley (1994) suggest that exposure to the construct of intentionality primed the related construct of blame or hostility for the non-aggressive boys, making it easier to access. For aggressive boys, however, hostility may have been a chronically accessible construct that brief exposure to the construct of unintentional harm could not trump (Graham and Hudley 1994).

6.4.3 Goals and aggressive behaviour

The third step in the Dodge SIP model (Crick and Dodge 1994) involves deciding on and clarifying goals for the current situation. According to the model, once children have made sense of a situation by encoding and representing it, their interpretation prompts a desire, wish, or hope for some outcome. Because the SIP model focuses on online processing, the term goal clarification refers to the transient and dynamically constructed aims and intentions within a given situation, or what Erdley and Asher (1996) call situated goals. Although children possess more global goal orientations, or what might be called values, situated goals have proved to be better predictors of behaviour in a given situation than are values (Renshaw and Asher 1983; Erdley and Asher 1996). The literature on aggressive children's situated goals is modest, but the findings are robust, with some studies reporting that goals were the most powerful predictors of aggression from among several SIP measures (Hughes *et al.* 2004). Murphy and Eisenberg (2002) report that children's goals made unique contributions to behaviour even after controlling for their anger, the specific conflict event, the friendship status of the partner, age, and sex.

Goals typically are assessed by asking children to imagine a hypothetical situation or recall a recent peer encounter and indicate how important a given outcome would be in that situation (e.g. 'How important would it be to you to show the other girl she can't push you around?' (Hughes *et al.* 2004, p. 296)), to describe what they were trying to accomplish in the situation (e.g. 'What were you trying to do, what did you want to happen?' (Murphy and Eisenberg 2002, p. 541)), or to select from a list the goal they would pursue (e.g. 'I would be trying to stay fair,' or 'get back at my friend' (Rose and Asher 1999, p. 71)). Aggressive children tend to endorse more instrumental goals (dominance or control of others) (Boldizar et al. 1989; Egan et al. 1998; Hughes et al. 2004), and care less about whether or not others suffer, retaliate, or reject them (Boldizar et al. 1989). Instrumental goals appear to be particularly characteristic of proactively aggressive children (Crick and Dodge 1996), as suggested by the SIP model. Social goals are reliably associated with the strategies children say they would use in hypothetical social encounters: Hostile goals are more likely to lead to aggression, whereas goals to get along with peers are more likely to lead to positive problem-solving (Erdley and Asher 1996). Moreover, hostile goals predict increases in aggressive behaviour over time, particularly for boys who already are above average in aggression (Egan et al. 1998).

Individuals may approach a situation with one goal in mind, but modify that goal as the situation evolves (Crick and Dodge 1994). To determine whether aggressive and non-aggressive children differ when their first attempt to resolve a conflict is thwarted, Troop-Gordon and Asher (2005) asked children to suggest strategies and motives in hypothetical conflict situations. The experimenter then asked what the child would do if the first strategy was unsuccessful and why. Aggressive rejected children became more focused on retaliation and were less willing to relinquish their instrumental aims after their first attempts to resolve the conflict failed, whereas non-aggressive well-liked children became less focused on instrumental goals (Troop-Gordon and Asher 2005).

As has already been suggested for other aspects of SIP, research on children's goals may be limited to the extent that it is based on children's conscious understanding of their own motivation. Although children undoubtedly sometimes consciously construct and pursue social goals, there are probably many situations in which they act without awareness of their motives. Social psychology research has shown that people often pursue goals of which they are not aware, and then attribute their actions to motives that fit their own theories about what causes that sort of behaviour (Todorov and Bargh 2002). Moreover, as is the case with attributions, recent experiences and characteristics of the situation can prime goals out of conscious awareness, and unconscious goals are often more strongly related to behaviour than are goals of which an individual is aware (Fitzsimons and Bargh 2004). That is, children's explanations (and, for that matter, adults' explanations) for their behaviour may sometimes be post hoc, and may not always accurately reflect the true motivation.

6.4.4 Response generation

There is a large literature on children's generation of responses (also called solutions or strategies) to social interaction situations. Response generation, like other aspects of SIP, is typically assessed by presentation of hypothetical vignettes; children are asked to report what they would do if they were involved in the events. In many early studies, the number, or quantity, of strategies children could generate was of primary interest (Shure and Spivack 1980; Pettit *et al.*1988; Mize and Cox 1989). This approach reflects early models of social problem-solving that focused on children's ability to reflect on social situations, generate a range of possible responses, and select an effective approach. In fact, although more competent and less aggressive children can generate more responses (Shure and Spivack 1980; Slaby and Guerra 1988; Mize and Cox 1989; Webster-Stratton and Lindsay 1999), it is not clear that the quantity of strategies predicts social behaviour after controlling for age and verbal ability.

More recently, research has been guided by models of response generation that focus on the quality of strategies children generate in social situations. As would be expected, and consistent with SIP models, aggressive children, from preschool to adolescence, tend to generate strategies that are more physically aggressive (Mize and Ladd 1988; Mize and Cox 1989; Mize *et al.* 1995; Waldman 1996; Keltikangas-Järvinen 2001; Dodge *et al.* 2003), more manipulative and coercive (Rubin *et al.* 1987), and less friendly (Mize and Cox 1989; Mize and Ladd 1990). Some aggressive children tend to generate idiosyncratic, vague, irrelevant, and ineffective strategies (Ladd and Oden 1979; Asher and Renshaw 1981; Pettit *et al.*1988), a pattern that may reflect neurocognitive deficits common among aggressive children (Moffitt 1993b; Raine *et al.* 2005).

As with other SIP steps, a concern about response generation assessments is that they typically permit, or even encourage in the case of quantitative measures, reflective thinking that may or may not correspond to how children approach real-life social situations (Orobio de Castro 2004). Mize and Ladd (1988) argued that children's verbal responses to hypothetical dilemmas may 'pull for thinking', particularly for children's notions of socially desirable responses. They found that strategies that preschool children enacted with puppets and props while role-playing hypothetical dilemmas were better predictors of classroom aggression than were the strategies they described verbally in response to the same set of dilemmas. Regression analyses indicated that children's verbal responses to hypothetical situations contributed 4 per cent, and their enactive strategies contributed an additional unique 19 per cent, to the prediction of teacher ratings of aggression. A similar pattern was obtained in the prediction of children's peer aggression as judged by classroom observers. Presumably, enacted responses are more similar to the strategies that children automatically access during peer interaction. Enactive assessments are probably more emotionally and behaviourally engaging, particularly for children, than are requests to describe what one would do in a hypothetical situation (Mize and Ladd 1988).

6.4.5 Response evaluation and decision

In the fifth step in the SIP model, children evaluate the strategies they have generated and make a decision about which strategy to use based on, among other possibilities, anticipated gains, possible punishment, feelings of self-efficacy for performing a strategy, beliefs about the appropriateness of the approach, and moral or ethical judgements. Crick and Dodge (1994) identified four subprocesses involved in this step: response evaluation (e.g. whether a specified response is 'good'), outcome expectations (what would happen if the response were actually used), self-efficacy for performing the behaviour (how confident the child feels), and response selection (deciding what to do based on evaluation of alternatives). Goals probably influence the extent to which individuals evaluate a given response as acceptable. For instance, a child who does not care about peers' opinions, pain, or possible retaliation will be undeterred from being aggressive by an expectation that it will lead to peers' suffering and rejection. Preference for or aversion to particular outcomes has been referred to as 'outcome values' (Boldizar *et al.* 1989; Egan *et al.* 1998).

Most research on aggressive children's response evaluation has focused on their judgements and expectancies regarding aggressive behaviour. Aggressive children and adolescents tend to view aggressive responses as being acceptable or even good (Deluty 1983; Bandura *et al.* 1996) and likely to lead to valued outcomes such as gaining possession of a toy (Perry *et al.* 1986; Egan *et al.* 1998), making others stop unpleasant behaviour (Perry *et al.* 1986), and positive evaluations of the self (Slaby and Guerra 1988). One of the most consistent findings in the SIP literature is that aggressive children feel more confident in their ability to carry out aggressive behaviour than do non-aggressive children (Perry *et al.* 1986; Quiggle *et al.* 1992; Crick and Dodge 1994; Erdley and Asher 1996). Finally, during the last subprocess of response evaluation, aggressive children are more likely to say that they actually would use aggression (Quiggle *et al.* 1992).

Subprocesses in the evaluation and decision step are internally consistent, with moderate to high intercorrelations among them (Egan *et al.* 1998; Fontaine *et al.* 2008). Individual differences in response evaluation and decision are moderately stable over periods ranging from several months (Egan *et al.* 1998) to 3 years (Fontaine *et al.* 2008). Importantly, positive evaluations of aggressive strategies are associated with aggressive behaviour not only concurrently, but also predictively. Aggressive elementary school children who evaluate aggression more positively in the autumn tend to become more aggressive by spring (Egan *et al.* 1998), and children who evaluate aggression more positively in the eighth grade tend to become more aggressive by the eleventh grade (Fontaine *et al.* 2008).

SIP models suggest that positive evaluation of aggression should be characteristic particularly of proactively aggressive children, whereas acting without evaluating consequences is often considered a hallmark of reactive aggression (Dodge and Coie 1987; Crick and Dodge 1994, 1996; Card and Little 2006). Support for differences between reactively and proactively aggressive children in response evaluation has been mixed. Some studies report that proactively aggressive children (Crick and Dodge 1996; Smithmeyer *et al.* 2000) and aggressive children with callous–unemotional traits (Pardini *et al.* 2003), but not reactively aggressive children, evaluate aggressive responses more positively, whereas other studies have found few differences in response evaluation between proactively and reactively aggressive children (Dodge *et al.* 1997). The fact that reactively aggressive children reduce aggression as much as do proactively aggressive children in response to clearly defined contingencies (Phillips and Lochman 2003) suggests that, at least under some conditions (perhaps when sanctions are highly salient (Budhani and Blair 2005)), the behaviour of reactively and proactively aggressive children can be influenced by the evaluation of costs and benefits.

For most children, the costs of aggression—in terms of possible punishment, victim's pain, and damage to their own self-image—outweigh the benefits. However, some children may morally disengage and justify, minimize, disregard, or deny the harm caused to others by aggressive behaviour; this may be the case particularly for children who have experienced abuse, neglect, rejection, discrimination, or poverty (Bandura *et al.* 1996; Dodge *et al.* 2006). Children with callous–unemotional traits may be temperamentally (Loney *et al.* 2003) or neurologically (Blair 2001; Blair *et al.* 2006; see also Chapter 7, this volume) predisposed toward this sort of moral and emotional disengagement.

As is the case for other steps of SIP, the most significant limitation of research on response evaluation and decision is probably that assessments are based on children's reports of their own conscious thoughts and motivations. It is not clear to what extent or how often children engage in rational response evaluation processes during social encounters. As many others have pointed out, some aggressive behaviour is impulsive, presumably giving individuals no time to weigh the costs and benefits of their options (e.g. Mize and Ladd 1988; Rabiner *et al.* 1990; Fontaine *et al.* 2002; Todorov and Bargh 2002). In fact, neuroscientists suggest that most cognitive and emotional processing occurs and influences behaviour outside of conscious awareness (LeDoux 1989).

Psychophysiological methods provide one window into non-conscious mental processing. For instance, studies of the psychophysiology of aggressive children may address issues of whether, as has been proposed, heightened arousal in provocation situations predicts hostile attributional biases among aggressive children. We now turn to a discussion of biological processes that have been linked to problem aggression and to the small body of research that integrates psychophysiological and SIP methods in the study of aggressive children.

6.5 Aetiological considerations

6.5.1 Social information processing and the biology of aggression

The last decade has witnessed a dramatic increase in research on biological processes underlying individual differences in social–emotional development (Eisenberg 2006). In the study of antisocial behaviour, findings from biologically based research are sufficiently robust for knowledgeable observers to conclude that serious problems of aggression derive partly from biological dysfunction (Scarpa and Raine 2006). Researchers have identified risk factors for aggression in genetic, endocrine, neurotransmitter, and autonomic and central nervous system functioning of animals and humans (Nelson 2006). In this section we focus on psychophysiological correlates of aggression and conduct problems because this probably represents the largest body of research on the biology of aggression in children, and it is the only area of biological research that has begun to be integrated into SIP formulations. Following a brief description of major findings regarding the psychophysiology of aggression, we summarize the small body of research that integrates psychophysiological and SIP data in studies of aggressive children.

Perhaps the best-known and most replicated psychophysiological correlate of aggression in children is low resting heart rate (HR) (Oritz and Raine 2004). Low resting heart rate has been interpreted as an indicator of low autonomic arousal, although consensus is lacking on the meaning of this phenomenon. Recent meta-analyses report moderate to strong effect sizes for this association in children and adolescents (Lorber 2004; Oritz and Raine 2004). Other indices that seem to reflect low autonomic arousal, such as low resting and task electrodermal response (EDA) (Lorber 2004; van Bokhoven *et al.* 2004) and low baseline cortisol (McBurnett *et al.* 1991; van Goozen *et al.* 1998; Smider *et al.* 2002; Shirtcliff *et al.* 2005; Loney *et al.* 2006; Mize *et al.* 2007), have also been linked to aggression. Low autonomic arousal as indexed by resting HR and EDA is associated with antisocial behaviour not only concurrently, but also predictively (Raine *et al.* 1997; van Bokhoven *et al.* 2005). The most frequently offered explanation for these associations (Eysenck 1964; Raine 1993; Scarpa and Raine

2006) is that low autonomic arousal reflects fearlessness, or even a dysfunction in the fear system, which eliminates the normal deterrent value of potential punishment and danger and makes children difficult to socialize because punishment is ineffective (see also Kochanska 1997). In addition, low autonomic arousal is hypothesized to be unpleasant, a condition that makes thrill-seeking and risk-taking reinforcing (see Raine (2002) for a discussion of these related hypotheses). Data indicating that individuals with antisocial personality disorders show poor classical conditioning to punishment, do not exhibit the normal augmentation of the startle–blink response to threatening stimuli, and show poor reversal learning (Blair and Frith 2000) have been interpreted as offering support for the fear–dysfunction hypothesis. Further support for the stimulation-seeking hypothesis comes from data indicating that boys with low resting HRs prefer to watch videos depicting intense (as opposed to mild) conflict (El-Sheikh *et al.* 1994) and evidence that symptoms of conduct disorder are reduced by administration of stimulant medication (Klein *et al.* 1997).

The fear–dysfunction and stimulation-seeking hypotheses have been criticized on several grounds (Blair and Frith 2000), most notably for assuming that problems of aggression have the same root cause and are mediated by the same neural circuitry (Blair 2001; Blair *et al.* 2006). A model proposed by Blair and colleagues (Blair *et al.* 2006; see also Chapter 7, current volume) rests on the assumption that reactive and proactive aggression are mediated by partially separable systems and provides a starting point for developing more comprehensive models incorporating social cognition, psychophysiology, and antisocial behaviour processes. In short, reactive aggression can be seen as a response to a perceived severe threat (Blair *et al.* 2006), although the perception may be unconscious and erroneous. The perception of threat stimulates release of hormones and neurotransmitters that increase activity of the sympathetic nervous system, resulting in increased HR, blood pressure, and skin conductance (Sapolsky 2004). A high level of proactive aggression, in contrast, is seen as one manifestation of the callous unemotional traits characteristic of psychopathy (Frick *et al.* 2003). This form of emotional dysfunction also manifests as a deficit in the ability to learn from punishment and modify responses as a function of changed contingencies (Birbaumer *et al.* 2005; Budhani and Blair 2005). Of interest here, hostile attributional bias appears to be absent in conduct-disordered boys with callous–unemotional traits (Frick *et al.* 2003).

Differences in how reactively and proactively aggressive children respond physiologically to threat was evaluated in a study by Hubbard *et al.* (2002) using a peer provocation methodology similar to that used in studies of SIP. Although reactive aggression and proactive aggression were highly correlated, they had dissimilar associations with both physiology measures and measures of children's anger. Specifically, HR reactivity and anger were positively associated with reactive, but not proactive, aggression.

The proposal by Blair *et al.* (2006) that heightened sensitivity of the neural circuitry involved in threat perception causes high levels of reactive aggression can be seen to correspond, in social information processing terms, to increased hostile attributions observed when reactively aggressive children are provoked. The failure to learn from negative reinforcement and punishment may translate, at the psychological level, into characteristics of proactively aggressive and psychopathic individuals, in particular a callous disregard for others' pain and a discounting of potentially disastrous consequences for the self that are frequent outcomes of inappropriate aggression.

There have been few efforts to investigate SIP–aggression–physiology links, and only one published study that did so could be located. Williams *et al.* (2003) measured the hostile attributions and HR of fifth- and sixth-grade boys (about 11–12 years old) before and after a simulated peer provocation. More aggressive boys had lower HR both pre- and post-threat, but had greater HR increases (i.e. reactivity) in response to the threat. Hostile attributions were not related to aggression prior to the threat, but, consistent with previous SIP research, after the threat more aggressive boys made more hostile attributions. Of particular interest here, the boys' HR changes were correlated with changes in attributions. Specifically, HR acceleration after threat was accompanied by increasingly hostile attributions, whereas HR deceleration after threat was associated with declining hostility in attributions.

6.5.2 Socialization and experiential influences

There is a large literature on sources of individual differences in antisocial behaviour and SIP. This research, which has generally focused on socialization and experiential influences, can now be integrated with some of the biological approaches described above. Harsh parenting and exposure to aggressive peers are robust predictors of worsening antisocial behaviour and anomalous patterns of SIP. A detailed review of this literature is beyond the scope of this chapter (see Dodge and Pettit (2003) and Dodge *et al.* (2006) for excellent reviews). As mentioned previously, theoretical models suggest that early experiences in the family foster the development of individual differences in social cognition, which then guide children's interactions with peers. It is of interest that, although each pair of constructs (experience–SIP, experience–aggression, and SIP–aggression) in this hypothesized chain is reliably associated, with only a few exceptions (e.g. Dodge *et al.* 1990a), evidence of statistical mediation has been surprisingly weak (Mize *et al.* 2000). Mize and colleagues suggest numerous reasons why evidence of mediation is not stronger (Mize *et al.* 2000).

Of most interest here is their proposal that mediational linkages are probably moderated by biological predispositions. The finding that, for callous–unemotional youths, the quality of parenting does not predict antisocial behaviour (Wooten et al. 1999) provides one example of moderated effects that probably have a basis in biology. A documented instance of biological moderation comes from recent research on gene–environment interactions. Physically maltreated children are protected from developing antisocial behaviour problems if they have inherited the version of the monoamine oxidase A (*MAOA*) gene that results in high levels of MAOA (Caspi et al. 2002).

Increasingly, then, biological factors, of both genetic and environmental origin, are being identified as risk or protective factors for behaviour problems. Environmental factors linked directly to risk for disruptive behaviour problems include malnutrition (Liu et al. 2004), prenatal exposure to nicotine (Wakschlag et al. 2006) and alcohol (Barr et al. 2006; Olson et al. 1997), and pre- and postnatal exposure to neurotoxicants such as lead (Needleman et al. 1996, 2002; Bellinger 2004), polychlorinated biphenyls (Stein et al. 2002), and methylmercury (Newland and Rasmussen 2003). Each of these substances, at levels to which significant portions of developing children are exposed (Stein et al. 2002), modifies neural circuitry or neural functioning, and thus may modify cognitive processes that are integral to SIP.

Simultaneously, social experiential factors that previously have been conceptualized to influence social behaviour primarily via cognitive and emotional processes, such as modelling, SIP, and relational schemas, cause neurological structural and functional changes that may mediate the experience–aggression linkage. For instance, interactions between young organisms and caretakers sculpt neuroendocrine response to stress, brain structure, neurochemistry, and gene expression, making offspring more or less susceptible to stressful circumstances throughout life (Sanchez et al. 2001; Maestripieri et al. 2006).

6.6 Clinical implications

SIP models are based on the notion that deficits in social cognitive processing skills underlie aggressive behaviour; thus these models have clear implications for prevention and treatment. A number of interventions have demonstrated efficacy in both modifying specific SIP components that were targeted and decreasing aggressive behaviour, suggesting that changes in SIP mediated the effects of the interventions. Hudley and Graham (1993) found that aggressive African American boys who received attribution retraining complained less, were less insulting, and made fewer hostile attributions in a provocation situation than did aggressive boys in control conditions. Boys who participated in the intervention were also perceived as less aggressive by teachers after the intervention.

A number of programmes targeting social-problem-solving strategies have proved effective in increasing use of specific trained behaviours during peer interaction and also in improving children's peer acceptance (Oden and Asher 1977; Ladd 1981; Mize and Ladd 1990). Mize and Ladd (1990) showed that increases in preschool children's use of positive strategies in classroom peer interaction was correlated with improvements in their performance on a response generation assessment, providing strong evidence that the ability to generate more appropriate strategies was at least partially responsible for the observed behavioural change. The Coping Power Program (Lochman and Wells 2004) and Problem-Solving Skills Training (Kazdin 2003) target several SIP components including goals, attribution retraining, and generating constructive strategies. These efforts have resulted in lasting positive effects on aggressive boys' delinquency and school behaviour. SIP components have also been included in comprehensive prevention approaches, such as Fast Track (Conduct Problems Prevention Research Group 1999). Although comprehensive interventions are probably more powerful, they are less able to provide evidence of the role of SIP in problem behaviour than are programmes that target and document changes in a single component.

6.7 Conclusion and future research

For the past two decades, SIP has been the most influential model guiding research on social cognition among conduct-disordered children. Dozens of studies document anomalous patterns of perceiving and thinking about social interaction among aggressive children, and interventions based on the SIP model have demonstrated efficacy in reducing antisocial behaviour. Future research could benefit from greater attention to normative developmental patterns of social information processing, to the role of non-conscious mental processes in social interaction, and to examination of how biological processes implicated in aggressive behaviour may be associated with social information processing patterns.

There is an astonishing lack of normative developmental data on SIP across childhood and adolescence. Moreover, patterns of normative change may vary as a function of the cultural and peer contexts in which children live. Yet data bearing on these issues are virtually non-existent. Clinical applications of the SIP model would be facilitated by knowledge of normative patterns within cultural niches. Such knowledge would reduce the risk of promoting SIP that is developmentally inappropriate, adult-centric, or contrary to local norms.

SIP assessments have largely relied on what children are able to report about their cognitive processing. This limits what can be learned about SIP in two ways. First, SIP and language ability are confounded and few studies control for verbal ability. Secondly, we have argued that much of the mental activity that guides social behaviour is not accessible to conscious reflection. Understanding links between mental processes that occur within conscious awareness and processes that occur outside of awareness will require integrating new methods into traditional SIP studies. Procedures adopted from social psychological research, such as priming (Graham and Hudley 1994) and reaction-time tasks (Schippell *et al.* 2003), have already contributed to refinements in SIP models, and should continue to do so.

As described in a preceding section of this chapter, there is a substantial literature on biological factors that are associated with conduct problems. Although SIP models acknowledge the role of biological factors in the development of aggression and information processing anomalies, efforts to integrate neurological and SIP explanations are lacking. Virtually none of the many biological risk factors for aggression have been investigated in relation to social cognitive mechanisms. To further advance understanding of the role of SIP in antisocial behaviour problems, it will be necessary to integrate models of biological mechanisms and non-conscious mental processes more fully and to do so in a developmental framework.

Acknowledgements

Preparation of this chapter was supported by research grants from the National Science Foundation (BCS 0126584) and the National Institutes of Mental Health (R01 MH 57095).

References

American Psychiatric Association (2000). *Diagnostic and statistical manual of mental disorders* (4th edn). Washington, DC: American Psychiatric Association.

Angold, A. and Costello, E.J. (2001). The epidemiology of disorders of conduct: nosological issues and comorbidity. In *Conduct disorders in childhood and adolescence* (ed. J. Hill and B. Maughan), pp. 126–68, New York: Cambridge University Press.

Asher, S.R. and Renshaw, P.D. (1981). Children without friends: social knowledge and social skill training. In *The development of children's friendships* (ed. S.R Asher and J.M. Gottman), pp. 273–96. Cambridge University Press.

Atkins, M.S. and Stoff, D.M. (1993). Instrumental and hostile aggression in childhood disruptive behavior disorders. *Journal of Abnormal Child Psychology,* 21, 165–78.

Baldwin, M.W. (1992). Relational schemas and the processing of social information. *Psychological Bulletin,* 112, 461–84.

Bandura, A. (1983). Psychological mechanisms of aggression. In *Aggression: theoretical and empirical reviews.* Vol. 1: *Theoretical and methodological issues* (ed. R. Geen and E. Donnerstein), pp. 1–40. New York: Academic Press.

Bandura, A., Barbaranelli, C., Caprara, G.V., and Pastorelli, C. (1996). Mechanisms of moral disengagement in the exercise of moral agency. *Journal of Personality and Social Psychology*, **71**, 364–74.

Bargh, J.A. and Pietromonaco, P. (1982). Automatic information processing and social perception: the influence of trait information presented outside of conscious awareness on impression formation. *Journal of Personality and Social Psychology*, **43**, 437–49.

Barr, H.M., Bookstein, F.L., O'Malley, K.D., Connor, P.D., Huggins, J.E., and Streissguth, A.P. (2006). Binge drinking during pregnancy as a predictor of psychiatric disorders on the Structured Clinical Interview for DSM-IV in young adult offspring. *American Journal of Psychiatry*, **163**, 1061–5.

Bellinger, D.C. (2004). Lead. *Pediatrics*, **113**, 1016–22.

Berkowitz, L. (1993). *Aggression: its causes, consequences, and control*. New York: McGraw-Hill.

Birbaumer, N., Veit, R., Lotze, M., et al. (2005). Deficient fear conditioning in psychopathy: a functional magnetic resonance imaging study. *Archives of General Psychiatry*, **62**, 799–805.

Blair, J.R.J. (2001). Neurocognitive models of aggression, the antisocial personality disorders, and psychopathy. *Journal of Neurology, Neurosurgery and Psychiatry*, **71**, 727–31.

Blair, J.R.J. and Frith, U. (2000). Neurocognitive explanations of the antisocial personality disorders. *Criminal Behaviour and Mental Health*, **10**, S66–81.

Blair, J.R.J., Peschardt, K.S., Budhani, S., and Pine, D.S. (2006). Neurobiology of aggression in children. In *The biology of aggression* (ed. R.J. Nelson), pp. 351–68. New York: Oxford University Press.

Boldizar, J.P., Perry, D.G., and Perry, L.C. (1989). Outcome values and aggression. *Child Development*, **60**, 571–79.

Bowlby, J. (1969). *Attachment and loss*. Vol. 1: *Attachment*. New York: Basic Books.

Boxer, P. and Tisak, M.S. (2003). Adolescents' attributions about aggression: an initial investigation. *Journal of Adolescence*, **26**, 559–73.

Bretherton, I. (1985). Attachment theory: retrospect and prospect. *Monographs of the Society for Research in Child Development*, **50**, 3–35.

Budhani, S. and Blair, R.J.R. (2005). Response reversal and children with psychopathic tendencies: success is a function of salience of contingency change. *Journal of Child Psychology and Psychiatry*, **46**, 972–81.

Bukowski, W.M. (1990). Age differences in children's memory of information about aggressive, socially withdrawn, and prosociable boys and girls. *Child Development*, **61**, 1326–34.

Burgess, K.B., Wojslawowicz, J.C., Rubin, K.H., Rose-Krasnor, L., and Booth-LaForce, C. (2006). Social information processing and coping strategies of shy/withdrawn and aggressive children. Does friendship matter? *Child Development*, **77**, 371–83.

Burks, V.S., Laird, R.D., Dodge, K.A., Pettit, G.S., and Bates, J.E. (1999). Knowledge structures, social information processing and children's aggressive behavior. *Social Development*, **8**, 220–36.

Card, N.A. and Little, T.D. (2006). Proactive and reactive aggression in childhood and adolescence: a meta-analysis of differential relations with psychosocial adjustment. *International Journal of Behavioral Development*, **30**, 466–80.

Caspi, A., McClay, J., Moffitt, T.E., *et al.* (2002). Role of genotype in the cycle of violence in maltreated children. *Science*, **297**, 851–4.

Cillessen, A.H.N. and Mayeux, L. (2004). From censure to reinforcement: developmental changes in the association between aggression ad social status. *Child Development*, **75**, 147–63.

Coie, J.D. and Pennington, B.F. (1976). Children's perceptions of deviance and disorder. *Child Development*, **47**, 407–13.

Coie, J.D., Cillessen, A., Dodge, K.A., *et al.* (1999). It takes two to fight: a test of relational factors and a method for assessing aggressive dyads. *Developmental Psychology*, **35**, 1179–88.

Conduct Problems Prevention Research Group (1999). Initial impact of the Fast Track prevention trial for conduct problems. 1: The high risk sample. *Journal of Consulting and Clinical Psychology*, **67**, 631–47.

Costanzo, P.R. and Dix, T.H. (1983). Beyond the information processed: socialization in the development of attributional processes. In *Social cognition and social development: a sociocultural perspective* (ed. E.T. Higgins, D.N. Ruble, and W.W. Hartup), pp. 63–81. New York: Cambridge University Press.

Crick, N.R. and Dodge, K.A. (1994). A review and reformulation of social information-processing mechanisms in children's social adjustment. *Psychological Bulletin*, **115**, 74–101.

Crick, N.R. and Dodge, K.A. (1996). Social information-processing mechanisms on reactive and proactive aggression. *Child Development*, **67**, 993–1002.

Crick, N.R. and Grotpeter, J.K. (1995). Relational aggression, gender, and social-psychological adjustment. *Child Development*, **66**, 710–22.

Damon, W. (1983). The nature of social-cognitive change in the developing child. In *The relationship between social and cognitive development* (ed. W.F. Overton), pp. 103–42. Hillsdale, NJ: Lawrence Erlbaum.

Deluty, R.H. (1983). Children's evaluations of aggressive, assertive, and submissive responses. *Journal of Clinical Child Psychology*, **12**, 124–9.

DeMarie-Dreblow, D. and Miller, P.H. (1988). The development of children's strategies for selective attention: evidence for a transitional period. *Child Development*, **59**, 1504–13.

Dodge, K.A. (1980). Social cognition and children's aggressive behavior. *Child Development*, **51**, 162–70.

Dodge, K.A. (1993). Social-cognitive mechanisms in the development of conduct disorder and depression. *Annual Review of Psychology*, **44**, 559–84.

Dodge, K.A. (2003). Do social information-processing patterns mediate aggressive behavior? In *Causes of conduct disorder and juvenile delinquency* (ed. B.B. Lahey, T.E. Moffitt, and A. Caspi), pp. 254–74. New York: Guilford Press.

Dodge, K.A. (2006). Translational science in action: hostile attributional style and the development of aggressive behavior problems. *Development and Psychopathology*, **18**, 791–814.

Dodge, K.A. and Coie, J.D., (1987). Social-information-processing factors in reactive and proactive aggression in children's peer groups. *Journal of Personality and Social Psychology*, **53**, 1146–58.

Dodge, K.A. and Frame, C.L. (1982). Social cognitive biases and deficits in aggressive boys. *Child Development*, **53**, 620–35.

Dodge, K.A. and Newman, J. (1981). Biased decision-making processes in aggressive boys. *Journal of Abnormal Psychology*, **90**, 375–9.

Dodge, K.A. and Pettit, G.S. (2003). A biopsychosocial model of the development of chronic conduct problems in adolescence. *Developmental Psychology*, **39**, 349–71.

Dodge, K.A. and Price, J.M. (1994). On the relation between social information processing and socially competent behavior in early school-aged children. *Child Development*, **65**, 1385–97.

Dodge, K.A. and Somberg, D.R. (1987). Hostile attributional biases among aggressive boys are exacerbated under conditions of threats to the self. *Child Development*, **58**, 213–24.

Dodge, K.A. and Tomlin, A.M. (1987). Utilization of self-schemas as a mechanism of interpretational bias in aggressive children. *Social Cognition*, **5**, 280–300.

Dodge, K.A., Murphy, R.R., and Buchsbaum, K. (1984). The assessment of intention-cue detection skills in children: implications for developmental psychopathology. *Child Development*, **55**, 163–73.

Dodge, K.A., Pettit, G.S., McClaskey, C.L., and Brown, M.M (1986). Social competence in children. *Monographs of the Society for Research in Child Development*, **51**, 1–85.

Dodge, K.A., Bates, J.E., and Pettit, G.S. (1990a). Mechanisms in the cycle of violence. *Science*, **250**, 1678–83.

Dodge, K.A., Price, J.M., Bachorowski, J., and Newman, J.P (1990b). Hostile attributional biases in severely aggressive adolescents. *Journal of Abnormal Psychology*, **99**, 385–92.

Dodge, K.A., Pettit, G.S., Bates, J.E., and Valente, E. (1995). Social information processing patterns partially mediate the effect of early physical abuse on later conduct problems. *Journal of Abnormal Psychology*, **104**, 632–43.

Dodge, K.A., Lochman, J.E., Harnish, J.D., Bates, J.E., and Pettit, G.S. (1997). Reactive and proactive aggression in school children and psychiatrically impaired chronically assaultive youth. *Journal of Abnormal Psychology*, **106**, 37–51.

Dodge, K.A., Lansford, J.E., Burks, V.S., *et al.* (2003). Peer rejection and social information-processing factors in the development of aggressive behavior problems in children. *Child Development*, **74**, 374–93.

Dodge, K.A., Coie, J.D., and Lynam, D. (2006). Aggression and antisocial behavior in youth. In *Handbook of Child Psychology* (6th edn). Vol 3: *Social, emotional, and personality development* (ed. N. Eisenberg), pp. 719–88. New York: John Wiley.

Egan, S.K., Monson, T.C., and Perry, D.G. (1998). Social-cognitive influences on change in aggression over time. *Developmental Psychology*, **34**, 996–1006.

Eisenberg, N. (2006). Introduction. In *Handbook of Child Psychology* (6th edn). Vol 3: *Social, emotional, and personality development* (ed. N. Eisenberg), pp. 1–23. New York: John Wiley.

El-Sheikh, M., Ballard, M., and Cummings, E.M. (1994). Individual differences in preschoolers' physiological and verbal responses to videotaped angry interactions. *Journal of Abnormal Child Psychology*, **22**, 303–20.

Erdley, C.A. and Asher, S.R. (1996). Children's social goals and self-efficacy perceptions as influences on their responses to ambiguous provocation. *Child Development*, **67**, 1329–44.

Eysenck, H.J. (1964). *Crime and personality*. London: Routledge and Kegan Paul.

Feldman, E. and Dodge, K.A. (1987). Social information processing and sociometric status: sex, age, and situational effects. *Journal of Abnormal Child Psychology*, 15, 211–27.

Fine, G.A. (1987). *With the boys: Little League baseball and preadolescent culture*. University of Chicago Press.

Fitzsimons, G.M. and Bargh, J.A. (2004). Automatic self regulation. In *Handbook of self-regulation: research, theory, and applications* (ed. R.F. Baumeister and K.D. Vohs), pp.151–70. New York: Guilford Press.

Flavell, J.H., Miller P.H., and Miller, S.A. (1993). *Cognitive development* (3rd edn). Upper Saddle River, NJ: Prentice-Hall.

Fontaine, R.G., Burks, V.S., and Dodge, K.A. (2002). Response decision processes and externalizing behavior problems in adolescents. *Development and Psychopathology*, 14, 107–22.

Fontaine, R.G., Yang, C., Dodge, K.A., Bates, J.E., and Pettit, G.S. (2008) Testing an individual systems model of response evaluation and decision (RED) and antisocial behavior across adolescence. *Child Development*, 79, 462–75.

Frick, P.J., Cornell, A.J., Bodin, D.S., Dane, H.E., and Loney, B.R. (2003). Callous–unemotional traits and developmental pathways to severe conduct problems. *Developmental Psychology*, 39, 246–60.

Getz, J.A., Goldman, J.A., and Corsini, D.A. (1984). Interpersonal problem solving in preschool children: a comparison of assessment procedures using two dimensional versus three-dimensional stimuli. *Journal of Applied Developmental Psychology*, 5, 293–304.

Gouze, K.R. (1987). Attention and social problem solving as correlates of aggression in preschool males. *Journal of Abnormal Child Psychology*, 15, 181–97.

Graham, S. and Hudley, C. (1994). Attributions of aggressive and nonaggressive African American male early adolescents: a study of construct accessibility. *Developmental Psychology*, 30, 365–73.

Hoglund, W.L. and Leadbeater, B.J. (2004). The effects of family, school, and classroom ecologies on changes in children's social competence and emotional and behavioral problems in first grade. *Developmental Psychology*, 40, 533–44.

Hubbard, J.A., Smithmeyer, C.M., Ramsden, S.R., *et al.* (2002). Observational, physiological, and self-report measures of children's anger: relations to reactive versus proactive aggression. *Child Development*, 73, 1101–18.

Hudley, C.A. and Graham, S. (1993). An attributional intervention to reduce peer-directed aggression among African-American boys. *Child Development*, 64, 124–38.

Huesmann, L.R. (1998). The role of social information processing and cognitive schema in the acquisition and maintenance of habitual aggressive behavior. In *Human aggression: theories, research, and implications for social policy* (ed. R.G. Geen and E. Donnerstein), pp. 73–109. San Diego, CA: Academic Press.

Huesmann, L.R. and Guerra, N.G. (1997). Children's normative beliefs about aggression and aggressive behavior. *Journal of Personality and Social Psychology*, 72, 408–19.

Hughes, J.N., Mehan, B.T., and Cavell, T.A. (2004). Development and validation of a gender-balanced measure of aggression-relevant social cognition. *Journal of Clinical Child and Adolescent Psychology*, 33, 292–302.

Hymel, S. (1986). Interpretation of peer behavior: affective bias in childhood and adolescence. *Child Development*, 57, 431–45.

Kail, R. (1984). *The development of memory in children* (2nd ed.). New York: Freeman.

Katsurada, E. and Sugawara, A.I. (1998). The relationship between hostile attributional bias and aggressive behavior in preschoolers. *Early Childhood Research Quarterly*, **13**, 623–36.

Kazdin, A.E. (2003). Problem-solving skills training and paraent management training for conduct disorder. In *Evidence-based psychotherapies for children and adolescents* (ed. A.E. Kazdin and J.R. Weisz), pp. 241–62. New York: Guilford Press.

Kellam, S.G., Ling, X., Merisca, R., Brown, C.H., and Ialongo, N. (1998). The effect of the level of aggression in the first grade classroom on the course and malleability of aggressive behavior into middle school. *Development and Psychopathology*, **10**, 165–85.

Keltikangas-Järvinen, L. (2001). Aggressive behavior and social problem-solving strategies: a review of the findings of a seven-year follow-up from childhood to late adolescence. *Criminal Behavior and Mental Health*, **11**, 236–50.

Kirsh, S.J. (1998). Seeing the world through Mortal Kombat colored glasses: violent video games and the development of a short-term hostile attribution bias. *Childhood*, **5**, 177–84.

Klein, R.G., Abikoff, H., Klass, E., Ganeles, D., Seese, L.M., and Pollack, S. (1997). Clinical efficacy of methylphenidate in conduct disorder with and without attention deficit hyperactivity disorder. *Archives of General Psychiatry*, **54**, 1073–80.

Kochanska, G. (1997). Multiple pathways to conscience for children with different temperaments: from toddlerhood to age 5. *Developmental Psychology*, **33**, 228–40.

Ladd, G.W. (1981). Effectiveness of a social learning method for enhancing children's social interaction and peer acceptance. *Child Development*, **52**, 171–8.

Ladd, G.W. (1990). Having friends, keeping friends, making friends, and being liked by peers in the classroom: Predictors of children's early school adjustment. *Child Development*, **61**, 312–31.

Ladd, G.W. and Oden, S. (1979). The relationship between peer acceptance and children's ideas about helpfulness. *Child Development*, **50**, 402–8.

Lansford, J.E., Malone, P.S., Dodge, K.A., Crozier, J.C., Pettit, G.S., and Bates, J.E. (2006). A 12-year prospective study of patterns of social information processing problems and externalizing behaviors. *Journal of Abnormal Child Psychology*, **34**, 715–24.

LeDoux, J.E. (1989). Cognitive–emotional interactions in the brain. *Cognition and Emotion*, **3**, 267–89.

LeDoux, J.E. (1996). *The emotional brain: the mysterious underpinnings of emotional life*. New York: Simon & Schuster.

Liu, J.H., Raine, A., Venables, P.H., and Mednick, S.A. (2004). Malnutrition at age 3 years and externalizing behavior problems at ages 8, 11, and 17 years. *American Journal of Psychiatry*, **161**, 2005–13.

Lochman, J.E. and Dodge, K.A. (1994). Social-cognitive processes of severely violent, moderately aggressive, and nonaggressive boys. *Journal of Consulting and Clinical Psychology*, **62**, 366–74.

Lochman, J.E. and Dodge, K.A. (1998). Distorted perceptions in dyadic interactions of aggressive and nonaggressive boys: effects of prior expectations, context, and boys' age. *Development and Psychopathology*, **10**, 495–512.

Lochman, J.E. and Wells KC (2004). The Coping Power Program for preadolescent boys and their parents: outcome effects at the 1-year follow-up. *Journal of Consulting and Clinical Psychology*, **72**, 571–8.

Loeber, R. and Coie, J. (2001). Continuities and discontinuities of development, with particular emphasis on emotional and cognitive components of disruptive behaviour. In *Conduct disorders in childhood and adolescence* (ed. J. Hill and B. Maughan), pp. 379–407. New York: Cambridge University Press.

Loeber, R., Green, S.M., Keenan, K., and Lahey, B.B. (1995). Which boys will fare worse? Early predictors of the onset of conduct disorder in a six-year longitudinal study. *Journal of the American Academy of Child and Adolescent Psychiatry*, **34**, 499–509.

Loney, B.R., Frick, P.J., Clements, C.B., Ellis, M.E., and Kerlin, K. (2003). Callous–unemotional traits, impulsivity, and emotional processing in adolescents with antisocial behavior problems. *Journal of Clinical Child and Adolescent Psychology*, **32**, 66–80.

Loney, B.R., Butler, M.A., Lima, E.N., Counts, C.A., and Eckel, L.A. (2006). The relation between salivary cortisol, callous–unemotional traits, and conduct problems in an adolescent non-referred sample. *Journal of Child Psychology and Psychiatry*, **47**, 30–6.

Lorber, M.F. (2004). Psychophysiology of aggression, psychopathy, and conduct problems: a meta-analysis. *Psychological Bulletin*, **130**, 531–52.

McBurnett, K., Lahey, B.B., Frick, P.J., *et al.* (1991). Anxiety, inhibition, and conduct disorder in children. II: Relation to salivary cortisol. *Journal of the American Academy of Child and Adolescent Psychiatry*, **30**, 192–6.

Maestripieri, D., Higley, J.D., Lindell, S.G., Newman, T.K., McCormack, K.M., and Sanchez, M.M. (2006). Early maternal rejection affects the development of monoaminergic systems and adult abusive parenting in rhesus macaques (*Macaca mulatta*). Behavioral *Neuroscience*, **120**, 1017–24.

Mayeux, L. and Cillessen, A. (2003). Development of social problem solving in early childhood: stability, change, and associations with social competence. *Journal of Genetic Psychology*, **164**, 153–73.

Meece, P. and Mize, J. (in press). Multiple aspects of preschool children's social cognition: relations with peer acceptance and peer interaction style. *Early Child Development and Care*.

Milich, R. and Dodge, K.A. (1984). Social information processing in child psychiatric populations. *Journal of Abnormal Child Psychology*, **12**, 471–89.

Mize, J. and Cox, R.A. (1989). Social knowledge and social competence: number and quality of strategies as predictors of peer behavior. *Journal of Genetic Psychology*, **15**, 117–27.

Mize, J. and Ladd, G.W. (1988). Predicting preschoolers' peer behavior and status from their interpersonal strategies: a comparison of verbal and enactive responses to hypothetical social dilemmas. *Developmental Psychology*, **24**, 782–8.

Mize, J. and Ladd, G.W. (1990). Toward the development of successful social skills training for preschool children. In *Peer rejection in childhood* (ed. S.R. Asher and J.D. Coie), pp. 338–61. New York: Cambridge University Press.

Mize, J. and Pettit, G.S. (1997). Mothers' social coaching, mother–child relationship style, and children's peer competence: Is the medium the message? *Child Development*, **68**, 312–32.

Mize, J., Pettit, G.S. and Meece, D.W. (2000). Explaining the link between parenting behavior and children's peer competence: a critical examination of the 'mediating process' hypothesis. In *Family and peers: linking two social worlds* (ed. K. Kerns, J. Contreras, and A.M. Neal-Barnett), pp. 137–68. New York: Greenwood–Praeger.

Mize, J., Lisonbee, J.A., Lapp, P.A., Parrett, E., and Lin, M. (2007). Cortisol in child care predicts kindergarten adjustment after controlling for earlier adjustment. Paper presented at the biennial meeting of the Society for Research in Child Development, Boston, MA.

Moffitt, T.E. (1993a). Adolescence-limited and life-course persistent antisocial behavior: a developmental taxonomy. *Psychological Review*, **100**, 674–701.

Moffitt, T.E. (1993b). The neuropsychology of conduct disorder. *Development and Psychopathology*, **5**, 135–51.

Murphy, B.C. and Eisenberg, N. (2002). An integrative examination of peer conflict: children's reported goals, emotions and behaviors. *Social Development*, **11**, 534–557.

Nagin, D.S. (1999). Analyzing developmental trajectories: a semiparametric, group-based approach. *Psychological Methods*, **4**, 139–57.

Nasby, W., Hayden, B., and DePaulo, B.M. (1980). Attributional bias among aggressive boys to interpret unambiguous social stimuli as displays of hostility. *Journal of Abnormal Psychology*, **89**, 459–68.

Needleman, H.L., Riess, J.A., Tobin, M.J., Biesecker, G.E., and Greenhouse, J.B. (1996). Bone lead levels and delinquent behavior. *Journal of the American Medical Association*, **275**, 363–9.

Needleman, H.L., McFarland, C., Ness, R.B., Fienberg, S.E., and Tobin, M.J. (2002). Bone lead levels in adjudicated delinquents: a case control study. *Neurotoxicology and Teratology*, **24**, 711–17.

Nelson, K. (1981). Social cognition in a script framework. In Social-cognitive development (ed. J.H. Flavel and L. Ross), pp. 97–118. New York: Cambridge University Press.

Nelson, R.J. (2006). Preface. In *The biology of aggression* (ed. R.J. Nelson), pp. v–ix. New York: Oxford University Press.

Newland, M.C. and Rasmussen, E.B. (2003). Behavior in adulthood and during aging is affected by contaminant exposure *in utero*. *Current Directions in Psychological Science*, **12**, 212–17.

Oden, S. and Asher, S.R. (1977). Coaching children in skills for friendship making. *Child Development*, **48**, 495–506.

Olson, H.C., Streissguth, A.P., Sampson, P.D., Barr, H.M., Bookstein, F.L., and Thiede, K. (1997). Association of prenatal alcohol exposure with behavioral and learning problems in early adolescence. *Journal of the American Academy of Child and Adolescent Psychiatry*, **36**, 1187–94.

Olweus, D. (1979). Stability of aggressive reaction patterns in males: a review. *Psychological Bulletin*, **86**, 852–75.

Oritz, J. and Raine, A. (2004). Heart rate level and antisocial behavior in children and adolescents: a meta-analysis. *Journal of the American Academy of Child and Adolescent Psychiatry*, **43**, 154–62.

Orobio de Castro, B. (2004). The development of social information processing and aggressive behavior: current issues. *European Journal of Developmental Psychology*, **1**, 87–102.

Orobio de Castro, B., Veerman, J.W., Koops, W., Bosch, J.D., and Monshouwer, H.J. (2002). Hostile attribution of intent and aggressive behavior: a meta-analysis. *Child Development*, **73**, 916–34.

Orobio de Castro, B., Slot, N.W., Bosch, J.D., Koops, W., and Veerman, J.W. (2003). Negative feelings exacerbate hostile attributions of intent in highly aggressive boys. *Journal of Clinical Child and Adolescent Psychology*, **32**, 56–65.

Pardini, D.A., Lochman, J.E., and Frick, P.J. (2003). Callous/unemotional traits and sociocognitive processes in adjudicated youth. *Journal of the American Academy of Child and Adolescent Psychiatry*, **42**, 364–71.

Parke, R.D. and Buriel, R. (2006). Socialization in the context of the family: ethnic and ecological perspectives. In *Handbook of Child Psychology* (6th edn). Vol 3: *Social, emotional, and personality development* (ed. N Eisenberg), pp. 429–504. New York: John Wiley.

Perry, D.J., Perry, L.C., and Rasmussen, P. (1986). Cognitive and social learning mediators of aggression. *Child Development*, **57**, 700–11.

Pettit, G.S., Dodge, K.A., and Brown, M. (1988). Early family experience, social problem solving patterns, and children's social competence. *Child Development*, **5**, 107–20.

Phillips, N.C. and Lochman, J.E. (2003). Experimentally manipulated change in children's proactive and reactive aggressive behavior. *Aggressive Behavior*, **29**, 215–27.

Pollack, S.D. and Tolley-Shell, S.A. (2003). Selective attention to facial emotion in physically abused children. *Journal of Abnormal Psychology*, **112**, 323–38.

Posner, M.I. and Rothbart, M.K. (2000). Developing mechanisms of self-regulation. *Development and Psychopathology*, **12**, 427–41.

Quiggle, N., Panak, W.F., Garber, J., and Dodge, K.A. (1992). Social information processing in aggressive and depressed children. *Child Development*, **63**, 1305–20.

Rabiner, D.L., Lenhart, L., and Lochman, J.E. (1990). Automatic versus reflective social problem solving in relation to children's sociometric status. *Developmental Psychology*, **26**, 1010–16.

Raine, A. (1993). *The psychopathology of crime: criminal behavior as a clinical disorder*. San Diego, CA: Academic Press.

Raine, A. (2002). Annotation: the role of prefrontal deficits, low autonomic arousal, and early health factors in the development of antisocial and aggressive behavior in children. *Journal of Child Psychology and Psychiatry*, **43**, 417–34.

Raine, A., Venables, P.H., and Mednick, S.A. (1997). Low resting heart rate at age 3 years predisposes to aggression at age 11 years: findings from the Mauritius Joint Child Health Project. *Journal of the American Academy of Child and Adolescent Psychiatry*, **36**, 254–66.

Raine, A., Moffitt, T.E., Caspi, A., Loeber, R., Stouthamer-Loeber, M., and Lynam, D. (2005). Neurocognitive impairments in boys on the life-course persistent antisocial path. *Journal of Abnormal Psychology*, **114**, 38–49.

Raine, A., Dodge, K., Loeber, R., *et al.* (2006). The reactive–proactive aggression questionnaire: differential correlates of reactive and proactive aggression in adolescent boys. *Aggressive Behavior*, **32**, 159–71.

Renshaw, P.D. and Asher, S.R. (1983). Children's goals and strategies for social interaction. *Merrill-Palmer Quarterly*, **29**, 353–74.

Rose, A.J and Asher, S.R. (1999). Children's goals and strategies in response to conflicts within a friendship. *Developmental Psychology*, 35, 69–79.

Rubin, K.H., Moller, L., and Emptage, A. (1987). The Preschool Behaviour Questionnaire: a useful index of behaviour problems in elementary school-age children? *Canadian Journal of Behavioral Science*, 19, 86–100.

Rubin, K.H., Bukowski, W., and Parker, J.G. (1998). Peer interactions, relationships, and groups. In *Handbook of Child Psychology* (6th edn). Vol. 3: *Social, emotional, and personality development* (ed. N Eisenberg), pp. 619–700. New York: John Wiley.

Sanchez, M.M., Ladd, C.O., and Plotsky, PM. (2001). Early adverse experience as a developmental risk factor for later psychopathology: evidence from rodent and primate models. *Development and Psychopathology*, 13, 419–49.

Sapolsky, R.M. (2004). *Why zebras don't get ulcers* (3rd edn). New York: Henry Holt.

Scarpa, A. and Raine, A. (2006). The psychophysiology of human antisocial behavior. In *The biology of aggression* (ed. R.J. Nelson), pp. 447–61. New York: Oxford University Press.

Schank, R.C. and Abelson, R.C. (1977). Scripts, plans, goals, and understanding: an inquiry into human knowledge structures. Hillsdale, NJ: Lawrence Erlbaum.

Schippell, P.L., Vasey, M.W., Cravens-Brown, L.M., and Bretveld, R.A. (2003). Suppressed attention to rejection, ridicule, and failure cues: a unique correlate of reactive but not proactive aggression in youth. *Journal of Child and Adolescent Psychology*, 32, 40–55.

Schultz, D. and Shaw, D.S. (2003). Boys' maladaptive social information processing, family emotional climate, and pathways to early conduct problems. *Social Development*, 12, 440–60.

Shirtcliff, E.A., Granger, D.A, Booth, A., and Johnson, D. (2005). Low salivary cortisol levels and externalizing behavior problems in youth. *Development and Psychopathology*, 17, 167–84.

Shure, M.B. and Spivack, G. (1980). Interpersonal problem-solving as a mediator of behavioral adjustment in preschool and kindergarten children. *Journal of Applied Developmental Psychology*, 1, 29–44.

Slaby, R.G. and Guerra, N.G. (1988). Cognitive mediators of aggression in adolescent offenders. I: Assessment. *Developmental Psychology*, 24, 580–8.

Smider, N.A., Essex, M.J., Kalin, N.H., et al. (2002). Salivary cortisol as a predictor of socioemotional adjustment during kindergarten: a prospective study. *Child Development*, 73, 75–92.

Smithmyer, C.M., Hubbard, J.A., and Simons, R.F. (2000). Proactive and reactive aggression in delinquent adolescents: relations to aggression outcome expectancies. *Journal of Clinical Child Psychology*, 29, 86–93.

Stattin, H. and Magnusson, D. (1989). The role of early aggressive behavior in the frequency, seriousness, and types of later crime. *Journal of Consulting and Clinical Psychology*, 57, 710–18.

Stein, J., Schettler, T., Wallinga, D., and Valenti, M. (2002). In harm's way: toxic threats to child development. *Journal of Developmental and Behavioral Pediatrics*, 23, S13–22.

Todorov, A. and Bargh, J.A. (2002). Automatic sources of aggression. *Aggression and Violent Behavior*, 7, 53–68.

Troop-Gordon, W. and Asher, S.R. (2005). Modifications in children's goals when encountering obstacles to conflict resolution. *Child Development*, **76**, 568–82.

van Bokhoven, I., Matthys, W., van Goozen, S.H.M., and van Engeland, H. (2004). Prediction of adolescent outcome in children with disruptive behavior disorders: a study of neurobiological, psychological, and family factors. *European Child and Adolescent Psychiatry*, **14**, 153–63.

van Goozen, S.H.M., Matthys, W., Coehn-Kettenis, P.T., Gispen-de Wied, C., Wiegant, V.M., and van Engeland, H. (1998). Salivary cortisol and cardiovascular activity during stress in oppositional-defiant disorder boys and normal controls. *Biological Psychiatry*, **43**, 531–9.

van Nieuwenhuijzen, M., Orobio de Castro, B., Wijnroks, L., Vermeer, A., and Matthys, W. (2004). The relations between intellectual disabilities, social information processing, and behavrioural problems. *European Journal of Developmental Psychology*, **1**, 215–29.

Vitaro, F. and Brendgen, M. (2005). Proactive and reactive aggression: a developmental perspective. In *Developmental origins of aggression* (ed. R.E. Tremblay, W.W. Hartup, and J. Archer), pp. 178–201. New York: Guilford Press.

Vitaro, F., Brendgen, M., and Tremblay, R.E. (2002). Reactively and proactively aggressive children: antecedent and subsequent characteristics. *Journal of Child Psychology and Psychiatry*, **43**, 495–506.

Vurpillot, E. (1968). The development of scanning strategies and their relation to visual differentiation. *Journal of Experimental Child Psychology*, **6**, 632–50.

Wakschlag, L.S., Leventhal, B.L., and Pine, D.S. (2006). Elucidating early mechanisms of developmental psychopathology: the case of prenatal smoking and disruptive behavior. *Child Development*, **77**, 893–906.

Waldman, I.D. (1996). Aggressive boys' hostile perceptual and response biases: the role of attention in impulsivity. *Child Development*, **67**, 1015–33.

Webster-Stratton, C. and Lindsay, D.W. (1999). Social competence and conduct problems in young children: issues in assessment. *Journal of Clinical Child Psychology*, **28**, 25–43.

Weiss, B., Dodge, K.A., Bates, J.E., and Pettit, G.S. (1992). Some consequences of early harsh discipline: child aggression and a maladaptive social information processing style. *Child Development*, **63**, 1321–35.

Williams, S.C., Lochman, J.E., Phillips, N.C., and Barry, T.D. (2003). Aggressive and nonaggressive boys= physiological and cognitive processes in response to peer provocation. *Journal of Clinical Child and Adolescent Psychology*, **32**, 568–76.

Wooten, J.M., Frick, P.J., Shelton, K.K., and Silverthorn, P. (1999). Ineffective parenting and childhood conduct problems: the moderating role of callous–unemotional traits. *Journal of Consulting and Clinical Psychology*, **65**, 301–8.

Yoon, J., Hughes, J., and Gaur, A. (1999). Social cognition in aggressive children: a meta-analytic review. *Cognitive and Behavioral Practice*, **6**, 320–31.

Younger, A.J. and Boyko, K.A. (1987). Aggression and withdrawal as social schemas underlying children's peer perceptions, *Child Development*, **58**, 1094–1100.

Younger, A.J. and Piccinin, A.M. (1989). Children's recall of aggressive and withdrawn behaviors: recognition memory and likability judgments. *Child Development*, **60**, 580–90.

7

Empathic dysfunction in psychopathy

James Blair

7.1 Introduction

The goal of the current chapter is to consider the social cognitive impairment associated with psychopathy in children and adolescents. The chapter will begin with a brief description of the disorder, touching on the core feature of psychopathy—the impairment in emotional processing including specific forms of empathy (section 7.2). Section 7.3 will consider what empathy is, how it develops in typical individuals, and what its developmental implications are for those same individuals (i.e. its role in care-based socialization and reasoning). Section 7.4 will describe the nature of the empathic impairment seen in individuals with psychopathy and the corresponding dysfunction in care-based socialization and reasoning. Section 7.5 will consider the aetiological origins of this disorder and will conclude that there probably is a genetic basis to the empathic dysfunction. Social etiological factors will also be considered. Section 7.5 will consider the clinical implications of this work. It will be concluded that these are currently primarily in assessment given the absence of viable potential treatments for psychopathy. The chapter concludes with a section considering the core in targets for research.

7.2 The disorder of psychopathy

The principles of the current description of psychopathy were defined by Cleckley in his book *The mask of sanity* (Cleckley 1976). From the anecdotal criteria delineated by Cleckley and his own clinical impressions, Robert Hare developed the original Psychopathy Checklist (PCL) (Hare 1980). Importantly, this was an empirically determined formalized tool for the assessment of psychopathy in adults. On the basis of empirical work, it was revised first in 1991 (the Psychopathy Checklist–Revised (PCL-R) (Hare 1991)), and then again in 2003 (Hare 2003). Empirically validated assessment tools for the assessment of psychopathy in childhood and adolescence have also been developed.

These include the Psychopathy Checklist: Youth Version (Kosson et al. 2002a; Forth et al. 2007) and the Antisocial Process Screening Device (APSD) (Frick and Hare 2001). See Sharp and Kine (2008) for a review of child psychopathy measures.

Psychopathy involves two core components: emotional dysfunction and antisocial behaviour. The emotional dysfunction involves reduced guilt and empathy, callous and unemotional (CU) traits, and reduced attachment to significant others. The antisocial behaviour component involves a predisposition to antisocial behaviour from an early age. This two-component structure was identified through factor analysis (Harpur et al. 1988; Hart et al. 1990; Frick et al. 1994; Frick 1995; Hobson and Shine 1998). Some recent work has questioned the two-factor description of psychopathy in favour of a three-factor solution where, effectively, the emotional dysfunction factor is split into two subcategories: the callous–unemotional dimension (concentrating on the lack of guilt/empathy/attachment to significant others) and a narcissism dimension (concentrating on grandiose feelings of self-worth) (Cooke and Michie 2001; Frick and Hare 2001).

With respect to epidemiological issues, preliminary work conducted by Paul Frick using the APSD, and using a cut-off for psychopathy commonly used in the literature, results in a prevalence rate of psychopathic tendencies (psychopathy in childhood) of around 1–3.5 per cent (Frick, personal communication). Very little is known with respect to incidence and gender. Work on psychopathy has been conducted largely on males, and relatively little is known about psychopathy in females (reviewed by Cale and Lilienfeld 2002).

An important feature of the clinical description of psychopathy is that it considers emotion (Blair et al. 2005b). This is important because the emotional dysfunction has causal significance for the emergence of the disorder (see section 7.4). This is in marked contrast to the descriptive strategy adopted for childhood conduct disorder (CD/adult antisocial personality disorder (APD)). CD and APD, indexed by the *Diagnostic and Statistical Manual of Mental Disorders* (4th edition) (DSM-IV), are the main psychiatric disorders associated with antisocial behaviour. Unfortunately, DSM-IV diagnoses focus on antisocial behaviour and do not differentiate between potential causes for its development. This leads to a situation where different individuals may be given this diagnosis even though their pathophysiology is very different. Thus the antisocial behaviour of some children with CD/adults with APD is associated with the reduced emotional responsiveness of psychopathy, while that of others is associated with heightened emotional responsiveness or dysregulated emotional responding. In short, while individuals with psychopathic tendencies share a common aetiology—a specific dysfunction in emotional processing—individuals identified as showing CD or APD do not.

A classification system is only as good as its usefulness. One of the major strengths of the PCL-R has been its utility in risk assessment. This is in rather striking contrast to the diagnoses of CD and ASPD. Considerable work has shown the predictive power of scores on the PCL-R with respect to recidivism (Hart *et al.* 1988; Hare *et al.* 2000; Kawasaki *et al.* 2001). Moreover, this work has shown that the correlation between recidivism and psychopathy is significantly higher than that of the DSM diagnoses (Hemphill *et al.* 1998).

In recent work with children, Hawes and Dadds (2005) found that amongst boys referred for conduct problems to a 10-week behavioural parent-training intervention, CU traits uniquely predicted clinical outcomes when analysed in relation to conduct-problem severity, other predictors of antisocial behaviour, and parents' implementation of treatment. Specifically, they found that boys with high CU traits were less responsive to discipline with time-out than boys with low CU traits (Hawes and Dadds 2005).

7.3 The development of (emotional) empathy

Psychopathy has been related to a core deficit in empathy since its earliest classification (Cleckley 1976; Hare 1980, 2003). However, empathy remains a rather nebulous term with a variety of definitions. Three main divisions can be made: cognitive, motor, and emotional empathy (see Blair (2005) for a discussion of the neurocognitive basis of differing forms of empathy). The term 'cognitive empathy' has been used where the individual represents the internal mental state of another individual, i.e. theory of mind (ToM) (Leslie 1987; Frith and Frith 2003; see also Chapter 2, this volume). Motor empathy occurs when the individual mirrors the motor responses of the observed actor. More recently this notion of 'motor' empathy has been incorporated within the perception–action model of emotional empathy (Preston and de Waal 2002). Emotional empathy reflects an emotional response to the emotional displays of others (their facial and vocal expressions and body movements) or other emotional stimuli (e.g. a phrase such as 'Adam just lost his house') (see Blair 2005).

There are no indications of ToM impairment in individuals with psychopathy (Widom 1978; Blair *et al.* 1996; Richell *et al.* 2003). In contrast, there have been suggestions that antisocial children, or at least 'hard-to-manage' preschoolers, show ToM impairment (Hughes *et al.* 1998; Hughes and Ensor 2006). However, studies of children with emotional and behavioural difficulties (Happé and Frith 1996), school bullies (Sutton *et al.* 1999), and children with 'disruptive behaviour disorder' (Sutton *et al.* 2000) have, like those with adults with psychopathy, failed to find any relationship between ToM functioning and antisocial behaviour. Given this, cognitive empathy/ToM will not be considered in this chapter. In addition, there is also no reason to believe that individuals with psychopathy show motor empathy impairment. This form of empathy will also not be considered in this chapter.

In contrast, there is every reason to believe that 'emotional empathy' is dysfunctional in individuals with psychopathy (Blair 2005). Thus deficits in empathy for the victims of their antisocial behaviour have been noted since the earliest clinical descriptions of the disorder (Cleckley 1941; Hare 1970; Hare 1980). In this section of the chapter, we will briefly consider the development of empathy and the implications of its development for moral socialization.

7.3.1 Emotional empathy: the functional architecture

The first goal is to consider the functional process of empathy in order to consider what develops and how. One common type of view of the empathic process makes considerable reference to mirror neurons (Preston and de Waal 2002; Carr *et al.* 2003; Decety and Jackson 2004). Mirror neurons are neurons which show activity during the execution and also the observation of an action (Rizzolatti *et al.* 2001). Within the account, the perception of another individual's emotional state activates the observer's corresponding representations, which in turn activate an emotional response. This approach was perhaps best specified at the anatomical level by Carr *et al* (2003). They argued that superior temporal cortex codes an early visual description of the action and sends this information to posterior parietal mirror neurons (codes the precise kinesthetic aspect of the movement) which then sends this information to inferior frontal (BA 44/45) mirror neurons (codes the goal of the action). According to this position, connections from superior temporal, parietal, and inferior frontal cortices to the insula and from there to the amygdala generate the empathic emotional response (Carr *et al.* 2003).

A main prediction of such a position is that there is a unitary empathic response recruiting all of the above regions. This is a popular viewpoint among some researchers (e.g. Ochsner 2004). Moreover, some data have suggested that, for example, the amygdala does respond to all expressions (Winston *et al.* 2003; Fitzgerald *et al.* 2006). However, it should be noted that the studies suggesting this have been underpowered with respect to the identification of the necessary interaction ($n = 11$; Winston *et al.* 2003) or found, effectively, that the amygdala responds to faces rather than emotional expressions (Fitzgerald *et al.* 2006). Moreover, there is almost overwhelming evidence that, for example, the amygdala shows greater responses to, and is more important for the recognition of, some expressions, particularly fear, than others (Morris *et al.* 1996; Phillips *et al.* 1998; Whalen *et al.* 2001; Adolphs 2002; Blair 2003a). This is not to suggest that the cortical processing implicated in the mirror neuron approach to empathy does not occur. It only suggests that the emotional empathic response does not necessarily rely on this particular cortical route or this type of functional processing.

An alternative approach considers that emotional expressions act like other elicitors of emotional responses—they are conditioned/unconditioned stimuli. This approach assumes that emotional expressions have specific communicatory functions and impart specific information to the observer (Blair 2003a). From this view, empathy, at least to facial and vocal emotional expressions, is the 'translation' of the communication by the observer. This translation occurs in several separable systems because of the different implications of these communicatory signals (see Blair 2003a).

For example, fearfulness, sadness, and happiness are reinforcers that modulate the probability that a particular behaviour will be performed in the future (Mineka and Cook 1993; Blair 1995; Matthews and Wells 1999). The amygdala is crucially involved in aversive and appetitive conditioning, i.e. the use of reinforcement information in emotional learning (LeDoux 1998; Baxter and Murray 2002; Everitt et al. 2003). In line with the suggested role of fearful, sad, and happy expressions as reinforcers, neuroimaging studies have generally found that fearful, sad, and happy expressions all activate the amygdala relative to other expressions (Morris et al. 1996; Phillips et al. 1998; Blair et al. 1999; Drevets et al. 2000; Whalen et al. 2001; Adolphs 2002; Blair 2003a).

In contrast, disgusted expressions are also reinforcers, but reinforcers that most frequently provide valence information about foods (Rozin et al. 1993). Disgusted expressions are particularly important for the rapid transmission of taste aversions; the observer is warned not to approach the food to which the emoter is displaying the disgust reaction. Neuropsychological work has shown the importance of the insula for taste aversion learning (Cubero et al. 1999). In line with the notion that disgusted expressions are important cues for initiating taste aversion learning, neuroimaging work shows that they also recruit the insula (Phillips et al. 1998; Wicker et al. 2003), while neuropsychological work shows that patients with damage to the insula present with selective impairment for the recognition of disgusted expressions (Sprengelmeyer et al. 1996; Calder et al. 2000).

There appear to be two pathways to the amygdala: one from visual cortex via temporal cortex and onto limbic areas (the cortical pathway: retinogeniculostriate–extrastriate–fusiform), and a second subcortical pathway (retinocollicular–pulvinar–amygdalar) following the earlier claims of others (e.g. de Gelder et al. 1999; Morris et al. 1999; Adolphs 2002). The existence of a subcortical pathway in non-human animals is not debated (Armony et al. 1997; LeDoux 2000). However, whether a subcortical pathway conveys information to the amygdala in humans remains unclear. Part of this is because of inconsistencies in the literature.

Early data supporting the existence of the subcortical pathway suggested, surprisingly, that it could provide sufficiently fine-grained stimulus encoding to allow discrimination learning (Morris *et al.* 1999). This was in sharp contrast with the animal literature (Armony *et al.* 1997; LeDoux 2000). Moreover, later work by the same group has not supported the claim (Vuilleumier *et al.* 2003). Despite this, on the basis of the available literature, we assume that the subcortical route exists and that it conveys coarse-grained low-frequency information to the amygdala (cf. Vuilleumier *et al.* 2003). This occurs very rapidly (Luo *et al.* 2007). This information is sufficient to allow basic stimulus-reinforcement learning to occur and may also allow the orientation of attention (the priming of active representations in temporal cortex) (see below).

Information is also conveyed to the amygdala through the cortical route. In this conception, the empathic response involves the representation of the expression in temporal cortex, in the same way that any other conditioned stimulus is represented (i.e. it does not require the involvement of parietal or frontal mirror neurons), and the subsequent activation of the amygdala. It is then argued that the amygdala feeds information on the valence of the expression to middle frontal cortex which can use this information in decisions of approach/avoidance (Blair 2004).

7.3.2 The development of emotional empathy

The two-route model, when extended, has clear similarities with the work of Morton and Johnson on early face recognition (Johnson and Morton 1991; Morton and Johnson 1991). They proposed a two-system model of face recognition. CONSPEC was considered to be an innately specified, subcortically mediated system which provides information about biologically relevant objects and directs attention towards the cues which activated it. CONLERN stands for a variety of mechanisms that could mediate learning of particular members of one's species (Johnson and Morton 1991; Morton and Johnson 1991).

With respect to emotional empathy, it can be speculated that there is an innately specified subcortically mediated system, the subcortical route, which responds to coarse-grained representations of expressions (cf. Vuilleumier *et al.* 2003), primes an attentional response, and may also provide valence information to the amygdala; that is, fearful/sad expressions are aversive, and happy expressions appetitive. The cortical route allows detailed learning about the parameters of expressive faces and more detailed coding for familiar individuals, thus enhancing empathic responses to familiar individuals (cf. Krebs 1975). It would be this route that mediates empathic responses to emotional stimuli such as phrases like 'Adam just lost his house' (see Blair 2005). Prior pairings of representations associated with this phrase with the distress of others will result in these representations also activating the amygdala and generating an emotional empathic response.

Of course, the above is speculative. However, it is clear that, even in the first days of life, infants can detect emotional expression information (reviewed by de Haan 2001). For example, 2-day-old infants can distinguish—and even imitate—happy, sad, and surprised facial expressions (Field *et al.* 1982). By 7 months, they appear to perceive emotional expressions as discrete categories (Kotsoni *et al.* 2001; reviewed by Herba and Phillips 2004).

7.3.3 Developmental consequences of the emergence of emotional empathy: the development of care-based morality

Considerable developmental literature indicates that moral socialization is achieved through the induction and fostering of empathy (Hoffman 1984). For example, studies have shown that moral socialization is better achieved through the use of induction (reasoning that draws children's attention to the effects of their transgressions on others and increases empathy) than through harsh authoritarian or power-assertive parenting practices which rely on the use of punishment (Hoffman and Saltzstein 1967; Baumrind 1971, 1983).

The importance of empathy for moral socialization was one of the reasons for the development of the original Violence Inhibition Mechanism (VIM) model of psychopathy (Blair 1995, 1997). This model has now been expanded into the Integrated Emotion Systems model (Blair 2004; Blair *et al.* 2005b).

The position rests on the phenomenon that many social animals, including humans, find the experience of the distress of conspecifics aversive (Blair 1995; Blair *et al.* 1997). Thus, both rats and monkeys will learn to make instrumental responses (press levers/pulling chains) which terminate unpleasant occurrences to conspecifics (Church 1959; Rice and Gainer 1962; Masserman *et al.* 1964; Rice 1965). Similarly, humans are 'punished' by signals of another human's sadness or fear. This will reduce their probability of engaging in actions that gave rise to another individual's distress or increase their probability of engaging in actions that remove another individual's distress. The distress of another individual is considered aversive by most humans (Bandura and Rosenthal 1966). The presentation of cues indicating another individual's sadness or fear reduces the probability of future physical aggression (Perry and Perry 1974), disputes over property ownership (Camras 1977), and aggressive sexual activity (Chaplin *et al.* 1995). Moreover, the accuracy with which a perceiver is able to identify the fear expression is positively associated with the perceiver's experience of sympathy and willingness to help others (Marsh and Ambady 2007; Marsh and Ambady, 2007).

According to the model, moral socialization occurs through the pairing of the activation of the mechanism by distress cues with representations of the acts that caused the distress cues (i.e. moral transgressions; e.g. hitting another individual) (Blair 1995; Blair et al. 2005b). Through association these representations of moral transgressions become triggers for the mechanism. The appropriately developing child thus initially finds the pain of other individuals aversive and then, through socialization, thoughts of acts that cause pain to others also become aversive. It is for this reason that children and adults distinguish between care-based moral transgressions and social-disorder-based conventional transgressions (e.g. Turiel et al. 1987; Smetana 1993). Only care-based moral transgressions are associated with the emotional reaction to a potential or actual victim's distress.

Work has also suggested that fearfulness is an important temperamental factor with respect to the development of morality/conscience (Kochanska 1993, 1997; Fowles and Kochanska 2000). Thus Kochanska and others have found fearful children to show higher levels of moral development/conscience using a variety of measures (Asendorpf and Nunner-Winkler 1992; Kochanska 1993, 1997; Rothbart et al. 1994; Fowles and Kochanska 2000). However, the temperamental variable 'fearfulness' can be understood as an index of the functional integrity of the amygdala (Blair 2003b; Blair et al. 2005b, 2006). The amygdala is a crucial neural structure with respect to emotional empathy (see above and Blair 2005).

7.4 Abnormalities in empathy and moral socialization/reasoning in psychopathy

7.4.1 Impairment in emotional empathy

There are very clear indications of impairment in emotional empathy in psychopathy.

1. A series of studies have investigated the ability of children with psychopathic tendencies and adult individuals with psychopathy to name the emotional expressions of others. These studies have revealed an impairment in the naming of fearful expressions (Blair and Coles 2000; Blair et al. 2001a; Stevens et al. 2001), although there has also been one report of impaired disgust recognition (Kosson et al. 2002b). In addition, there have been reports of impairment in the naming of sad expressions in the children with psychopathic tendencies. A recent meta-analysis examining the relationship between expression recognition ability and antisocial

behaviour showed that antisocial behaviour was selectively associated with impairment in the recognition of fearful expressions (Marsh and Blair, 2008). Three studies have also examined the naming of vocal affect, where it has been revealed that children with psychopathic tendencies and adults with psychopathy show impairment in recognizing fearful vocal affect and, although less consistently, sad vocal affect (Stevens *et al.* 2001; Blair *et al.* 2002, 2005a).

2. A second series of studies has examined autonomic responses to the distress of others (Sutker 1970; House and Milligan 1976; Aniskiewicz 1979; Blair *et al.* 1997; Blair 1999). Two out of three studies examining the skin conductance responses of participants while they observed confederates whom they believed were being administered electric shocks reported reduced autonomic responsiveness in individuals with psychopathy relative to comparison individuals (House and Milligan 1976; Aniskiewicz 1979). Moreover, two studies recorded skin conductance responses whilst participants simply watched images on a screen and reported that both children with psychopathic tendencies and adults with psychopathy showed reduced autonomic responsiveness to the distress of others relative to comparison individuals (Blair *et al.* 1997; Blair 1999).

3. Recent work has examined BOLD responses to emotional expressions in adults with psychopathic tendencies. These studies have revealed reduced BOLD responses within the amygdala to fearful expression in adults with subclinical psychopathic tendencies (Gordon *et al.* 2004).

7.4.2 Impairment in moral socialization/reasoning

If, as was argued above, empathy is necessary for appropriate moral socialization, we might expect to observe difficulties in moral socialization in children with psychopathic tendencies. Such difficulties have been shown (Wootton *et al.* 1997; Oxford *et al.* 2003). Individuals with psychopathy are more difficult to socialize through standard parenting techniques (Wootton *et al.* 1997; Oxford *et al.* 2003).

In line with this, psychopathy should also be associated with specific difficulties in moral reasoning. Children with psychopathic tendencies and adult individuals with psychopathy have considerable difficulty with the moral–conventional distinction task (Blair 1995, 1997; Blair *et al.* 1995, 2001b). In addition, similar difficulties have been observed with more general populations of children presenting with antisocial behaviour (Nucci and Herman 1982; Arsenio and Fleiss 1996; Hughes and Dunn 2000; Dunn and Hughes 2001). Children with psychopathic tendencies and adult individuals with psychopathy and other antisocial populations do generally regard moral transgressions as more serious than conventional transgressions. However, such populations are far less likely than comparison individuals to make reference to the victim of the transgression when justifying why moral transgressions are bad (Blair 1995; Arsenio and Fleiss 1996; Hughes and Dunn 2000; Blair *et al.* 2001b; Dunn and Hughes 2001). In addition, when the rules prohibiting the transgressions are removed, such populations are far less likely to make the distinction between moral and conventional transgressions that is seen in healthy individuals (Nucci and Herman 1982; Blair 1995; Blair *et al.* 2001b).

7.5 The aetiology of psychopathy

7.5.1 Genetic factors

A comprehensive meta-analysis of behaviour genetic studies on antisocial behaviour concluded that antisocial behaviour is moderately heritable (Rhee and Waldman 2002) or more accurately, since there are no genes coding for antisocial behaviours, the risk factors for antisocial behaviour are moderately heritable. Work on psychopathy, using self-report measures in adult and adolescent populations, has revealed moderate heritability of CU-related traits, no shared environmental influence, and moderate non-shared environmental influence (Blonigen *et al.* 2003, 2005). However, the sizes of these adult samples were small. In recent work, with around 3500 twin pairs, we have shown that CU traits are strongly heritable (67 per cent group heritability) at both 7 and 9 years (Viding *et al.* 2005). Moreover, antisocial behaviour in the presence of elevated levels of CU traits is strongly heritable (81 per cent). However, heritability of antisocial behaviour without CU traits was only moderate (30 per cent) (Viding *et al.* 2005). Importantly, in addition, the high heritability of antisocial behaviour in children with CU traits has been shown to be independent of co-occurring ADHD pathology (Viding *et al.* 2006).

Currently, while behavioural genetics data suggest heritability of CU traits, a molecular level account of psychopathy remains in its infancy. Suggestions have been made that psychopathy might be related to anomalies in noradrenergic neurotransmission (Blair *et al.* 2005b). However, this area is in urgent need of investigation (see section 7.7).

7.5.2 Environmental factors

Many environmental causes have been suggested for an increased risk for aggression and, at least in the lay population, psychopathy. We will consider three sets of potential causes: Exposure to extreme threats (e.g. in the context of childhood abuse/chronic exposure to violence), incompetent parenting, and environmental motivators (e.g. a lack of money).

Exposure to extreme threats increases the risk for aggression This is seen as a result of physical and sexual abuse (Dodge et al. 1995; Farrington and Loeber 2000) as well as a result of exposure to violence in the home/neighbourhood (Miller et al. 1999; Schwab-Stone et al. 1999). However, this does not imply that these environmental factors are risks for the development of psychopathy. Considerable work with animals has revealed the neurobiological impact of acute and prolonged threat/stress on the neural systems that respond to threat (Heim et al. 1997; King 1999; Bremner and Vermetten 2001; Charney 2003; Sanchez et al. 2005). In brief, prolonged threat or stress lead to a long-term potentiation of the neural and neurochemical systems that respond to threat; i.e. the individual becomes more responsive to aversive stimuli. In human clinical work, traumatic exposure, including exposure to violence in the home/neighbourhood, increases the risk for mood and anxiety disorders in general, although not all exposed to trauma will go on to develop these disorders (Gorman-Smith and Tolan 1998; Schwab-Stone et al. 1999). However, a defining feature of psychopathy is a reduction, not elevation, in the individual's responsiveness to threat (Hare 1970; Cleckley 1976; Patrick 1994; Lykken 1995). In short, while prolonged threat/stress leads to psychiatric pathology, it does not lead to the pathology seen in psychopathy.

Incompetent parenting There are also considerable data that exposure to poor parenting increases the risk for aggression/being diagnosed with conduct disorder (Snyder and Stoolmiller 2002; see also Chapter 6, this volume). However, again, this does not imply that poor parenting is a risk factor for the development of *psychopathy*. Work with animals has revealed the neurobiological impact of poor parenting. As with exposure to extreme threats, poor parenting is associated with increased responsiveness to aversive stimuli (Rilling et al. 2001; Rosenblum et al. 2001; Sanchez et al. 2005) and is considered a risk factor for the development of anxiety disorders. Again, while poor parenting may lead to psychiatric pathology, it does not lead to the pathology seen in psychopathy.

But why should exposure to extreme threats and incompetent parenting be associated with an increased risk for aggression/diagnosis of conduct disorder? It is likely that the answer lies with some of those systems that are potentiated by exposure to extreme threats/incompetent parenting. The mammalian response to threat is gradated. At low levels of danger, from a distant threat, animals freeze. At higher levels, from a closer threat, they attempt to escape. At higher levels still, when the threat is very close and escape is impossible, the animal initiates reactive aggression (Blanchard et al. 1977). This response to threat is importantly mediated by the amygdala, hypothalamus, and periaqueductal grey matter (Panksepp 1998; Gregg and Siegel 2001), systems potentiated by exposure to extreme threat/incompetent parenting

(King 1999; Bremner and Vermetten 2001; Charney 2003). Thus, threat exposure to extreme threat/incompetent parenting, by increasing the individual's responsiveness to threat, will increase the likelihood that the individual will display reactive aggression to a lower-level threat than an individual who has not been so exposed. We believe that this is the origin of the association between physical and sexual abuse and increased risk of aggression (Widom 1992; Dodge *et al.* 1995; Miller *et al.* 1999; Schwab-Stone *et al.* 1999; Farrington and Loeber 2000): reactive aggression is elicited in abused individuals by lower-level threats than in individuals who have not been abused.

Environmental motivation. Lower socio-economic status (SES) and lower IQ are both associated with an increased risk for antisocial behaviour, including the antisocial behaviour component of psychopathy (Frick *et al.* 1994; Hare 2003). These data, particularly the SES data, suggest a social contribution to at least the behavioural manifestation of psyhopathy. Importantly, antisocial behaviour shown by individuals with psychopathy is instrumental in nature; it has the goal of gaining another's money, sexual favours, or 'respect' (Williamson *et al.* 1987; Cornell *et al.* 1996). Individuals can attempt to achieve these goals through a variety of means. Having a higher SES (or for that matter intelligence) enables a wider choice of available routes for achieving these goals than having a lower SES (or intelligence). Lower SES/IQ limits the behavioural options available so that antisocial behaviour appears a useful route to the goal. A healthy individual of limited SES/IQ may also have a narrow range of behavioural options but will exclude antisocial behaviour because of aversion to this behaviour formed during socialization (see below). In contrast, individuals with psychopathy may entertain the antisocial option because they do not find the required antisocial behaviour aversive. SES is also likely to impact on the probability of displaying instrumental aggressions by determining relative reward levels for particular actions. If the individual already has £100 000, the subjective value of the £50 that could be gained if the individual mugged another person on the street is low. In contrast, if the individual has only 50 pence, the subjective value of the $50 will be very high indeed (for a discussion of subjective value, see Tversky and Kahneman (1981)).

7.6 Clinical implications

In the short term, the primary clinical implication of the work presented above is for assessment. As indexed by DSM-IV, the main psychiatric disorders associated with elevated levels of antisocial behaviour are conduct disorder in childhood and antisocial personality disorder in adulthood. The problem with the DSM-IV diagnoses is that because they focus on the behavioural feature of antisocial behaviour, they do not differentiate between potential causes for its development.

Psychopathy extends the DSM-IV diagnoses of CD and ASPD by considering emotion (Blair *et al.* 2005b). This is important because the empathic dysfunction seen in the disorder has causal significance for the emergence of the disorder. The diagnosis of CD groups individuals together because they engage in antisocial behaviour. However, it does not consider causality. Thus you can find children with CD whose antisocial behaviour is associated with the specific form of reduced emotional responsiveness associated with the classification of psychopathy as well as children whose antisocial behaviour is associated with heightened emotional responsiveness or dysregulated emotional responding. In short, the DSM-IV diagnosis identifies a highly heterogeneous population who do not share a common aetiology. In contrast, individuals with psychopathic tendencies share a common aetiology—a specific dysfunction in emotional processing.

Identifying the empathy deficit seen in psychopathy allows greater precision with respect to treatment. Empathy-based treatments do lead to reductions in conduct problems. However, such treatments are unlikely to work with individuals with psychopathy. Indeed, as noted above, Hawes and Dadds (2005) found that amongst boys referred for conduct problems to a 10-week behavioural parent-training intervention, CU traits uniquely predicted clinical outcomes when analysed in relation to the severity of the conduct problem, other predictors of antisocial behaviour, and parents' implementation of treatment. Specifically, they found that boys with high CU traits were less responsive to discipline with time-out than boys with low CU traits (Hawes and Dadds 2005).

Unfortunately, however, the above data are not very helpful with respect to the current treatment of individuals with the disorder. This is because it is not clear how to treat individuals with psychopathy given their pronounced emotional deficits. It is quite possible that the basic problem in emotional responding will need to be addressed pharmacologically. It is only then that cognitive therapies based around their problems in empathic responding could be addressed through empathy induction.

7.7 Expected future directions of research

There are three crucial directions for future research. The first is an understanding of psychopathy/empathic dysfunction at the molecular level. To be complete, an account of a psychiatric disorder needs to consider the genetic/social, molecular, neural, cognitive, and behavioural levels. Considerable progress with respect to psychopathy has been made on all of these levels except for the molecular. For example, we know that there is a genetic basis for psychopathy (Viding et al. 2005). However, we know nothing about how that genetic information is expressed at the molecular level. An understanding at the molecular level is particularly important as it is only by following an understanding of a disorder at the molecular level that it is possible to design potential pharmacological treatments on a scientific basis. There are two potential routes in which we might make progress at the molecular level.

The first route is through animal research. As noted above, rats and monkeys will learn to make instrumental responses (press levers/pull chains) which terminate unpleasant occurrences to conspecifics (Church 1959; Rice and Gainer 1962; Masserman et al. 1964; Rice 1965). In short, there is an animal model of psychopathy available—the 'unempathic' rat, the rat that is less likely to make instrumental responses to terminate the unpleasant occurrences to conspecifics. Unfortunately, however, to the author's knowledge there are no groups in the world addressing the molecular basis of psychopathy through animal research.

The second route is through molecular genetic studies. Recently, there has been a flurry of molecular genetic studies where the neurocognitive implications of particular polymorphisms of genes potentially relevant to mental health have been examined. For example, genes regulating serotonergic neurotransmission, in particular monoamine oxidase A (MAOA), have been associated with impulsive antisocial, aggressive, and violent behaviour (Lesch 2003). More recently, research has suggested that experience of environmental maltreatment may be necessary for the low-activity polymorphism of MAOA (MAOA-L) to increase the risk for aggression (Caspi et al. 2002). Recent imaging work has indicated that MAOA-L carriers show increased amygdala responses to emotional stimuli relative to MAOA-H carriers (Meyer-Lindenberg et al. 2006). This relates MAOA-L carriers to threat/frustration-based outbursts of reactive aggression, exactly the aggression seen in clinical populations linked to this gene (Lesch and Merschdorf 2000). However, it is unlikely to be relevant to psychopathy, where decreased rather than increased amygdala responses to emotional stimuli are seen (Kiehl et al. 2001; Birbaumer et al. 2005). In contrast, the 5-HTTLPR allele may have relevance. ll homozygotes of the long (l) 5-HTTLPR allele show decreased amygdala activity relative to carriers of the short 5-HTTLPR allele in response to fear expressions (Hariri et al. 2002, 2005). By understanding the implications for empathic responding of specific polymorphisms of specific genes, we may gain a molecular understanding of the problems seen in psychopathy.

The second major area for future research is to increase an understanding of psychopathy/empathic dysfunction at the neural level. Considerable work has identified the neural systems involved in empathic responding (reviewed by Blair 2005). However, only one study has examined this issue in psychopathy using neuroimaging technology and that was with a subclinical sample (Gordon et al. 2004). There has been no work with children with psychopathic tendencies.

Finally, a third focus of future research should be on the potential treatments for psychopathy/empathic dysfunction. Currently, psychopathy is regarded as untreatable (Hare 2003). This is a highly undesirable situation. Unfortunately, of course, a significant barrier to successful treatment is the profound emotional deficit. It is unlikely that treatment will be efficacious in this population unless the emotional deficit can be addressed pharmacologically. It is only going to be possible to scientifically suggest pharmacological treatments once we have some understanding of the molecular basis of psychopathy.

7.8 Conclusions

Psychopathy is a disorder with a pathology that involves a specific form of emotional dysfunction and a core social cognitive deficit in specific forms of empathy. This deficit leads to pronounced problems in care-based (moral) socialization.

There is a genetic contribution to the disorder. This contribution may interact with environmental variables and these variables certainly have a clear impact with respect to how the underlying pathophysiology manifests. However, environmental variables that have been classically reported to increase the risk for aggression (e.g. trauma and parental neglect) almost certainly do this through effects that are independent of psychopathy. The effects of these variables are to increase emotional responsiveness rather than to decrease it, as is seen in psychopathy.

While considerable progress is being made with respect to the neurocognitive basis of the empathy/emotional deficits seen in psychopathy, an understanding of the molecular basis of this disorder remains in its infancy. Reflecting the parlous state of the molecular understanding of psychopathy, there are no adequate treatment options for this disorder. This should be an area of urgent area for future research interest.

References

Adolphs, R. (2002). Neural systems for recognizing emotion. *Current Opinions in Neurobiology*, **12**, 169–77.

Aniskiewicz, A.S. (1979). Autonomic components of vicarious conditioning and psychopathy. *Journal of Clinical Psychology*, **35**, 60–7.

Armony, J.L., Servan-Schreiber, D., Romanski, L.M., Cohen, J.D., and LeDoux, J.E. (1997). Stimulus generalization of fear responses: effects of auditory cortex lesions in a computational model and in rats. *Cerebral Cortex*, **7**, 157–65.

Arsenio, W.F. and Fleiss, K. (1996). Typical and behaviourally disruptive children's understanding of the emotion consequences of socio-moral events. *British Journal of Developmental Psychology*, **14**, 173–86.

Asendorpf, J.B. and Nunner-Winkler, G. (1992). Children's moral motive strength and temperamental inhibition reduce their immoral behaviour in real moral conflicts. *Child Development*, **63**, 1223–35.

Bandura, A. and Rosenthal, T.L. (1966). Viacarous classical conditioning as a function of arousal level. *Journal of Personality and Social Psychology*, **3**, 54–62.

Baumrind, D. (1971). Current patterns of parental authority. *Developmental Psychology Monographs*, **4**, 1–103.

Baumrind, D. (1983). Rejoinder to Lewis's interpretation of parental firm control effects: are authoritative families really harmonious? *Psychological Bulletin*, **94**, 132–42.

Baxter, M.G. and Murray, E.A. (2002). The amygdala and reward. *Nature Reviews Neuroscience*, **3**, 563–73.

Birbaumer, N., Veit, R., Lotze, M., *et al.* (2005). Deficient fear conditioning in psychopathy: a functional magnetic resonance imaging study. *Archives of General Psychiatry*, **62**, 799–805.

Blair, R.J.R. (1995). A cognitive developmental approach to morality: investigating the psychopath. *Cognition*, **57**, 1–29.

Blair, R.J.R. (1997). Moral reasoning in the child with psychopathic tendencies. *Personality and Individual Differences*, **22**, 731–9.

Blair, R.J.R. (1999). Responsiveness to distress cues in the child with psychopathic tendencies. *Personality and Individual Differences*, **27**, 135–45.

Blair, R.J.R. (2003a). Facial expressions, their communicatory functions and neuro-cognitive substrates. *Philosophical Transactions of the Royal Society of London, Series B: Biological Sciences*, **358**, 561–72.

Blair, R.J.R. (2003b). Neurobiological basis of psychopathy. *British Journal of Psychiatry*, **182**, 5–7.

Blair, R.J.R. (2004). The roles of orbital frontal cortex in the modulation of antisocial behavior. *Brain and Cognition*, **55**, 198–208.

Blair, R.J.R. (2005). Responding to the emotions of others: dissociating forms of empathy through the study of typical and psychiatric populations. *Consciousness and Cognition*, **14**, 698–718.

Blair, R.J.R. and Coles, M. (2000). Expression recognition and behavioural problems in early adolescence. *Cognitive Development*, **15**, 421–34.

Blair, R.J.R., Jones, L., Clark, F., and Smith, M. (1995). Is the psychopath 'morally insane'? *Personality and Individual Differences*, **19**, 741–52.

Blair, R.J.R., Sellars, C, Strickland, I., *et al.* (1996). Theory of mind in the psychopath. *Journal of Forensic Psychiatry*, **7**, 15–25.

Blair, R.J.R., Jones, L., Clark, F., and Smith, M. (1997). The psychopathic individual: a lack of responsiveness to distress cues? *Psychophysiology*, **34**, 192–8.

Blair, R.J.R., Morris, J.S., Frith, C.D., Perrett, D.I., and Dolan, R. (1999). Dissociable neural responses to facial expressions of sadness and anger. *Brain*, **122**, 883–93.

Blair, R.J.R., Colledge, E., Murray, L., and Mitchell, D.G. (2001a). A selective impairment in the processing of sad and fearful expressions in children with psychopathic tendencies. *Journal of Abnormal Child Psychology*, **29**, 491–8.

Blair, R.J.R., Monson, J., and Frederickson, N. (2001b). Moral reasoning and conduct problems in children with emotional and behavioural difficulties. *Personality and Individual Differences*, **31**, 799–811.

Blair, R.J., Mitchell, D.G., Richell, R.A., *et al.* (2002). Turning a deaf ear to fear: impaired recognition of vocal affect in psychopathic individuals. *Journal of Abnormal Psychology*, **111**, 682–6.

Blair, R.J.R., Budhani, S., Colledge, E., and Scott, S. (2005a). Deafness to fear in boys with psychopathic tendencies. *Journal of Child Psychology and Psychiatry*, **46**, 327–36.

Blair, R.J.R., Mitchell, D.G.V., and Blair, K.S. (2005b). *The psychopath: emotion and the brain*. Oxford: Blackwell.

Blair, R.J.R., Peschardt, K.S., Budhani, S., Mitchell, D.G., and Pine, D.S. (2006). The development of psychopathy. *Journal of Child Psychology and Psychiatry*, **47**, 262–76.

Blanchard, R.J., Blanchard, D.C., and Takahashi, L.K. (1977). Attack and defensive behaviour in the albino rat. *Animal Behavior*, **25**, 197–224.

Blonigen, D.M., Carlson, S.R., Krueger, R.F., and Patrick, C.J. (2003). A twin study of self-reported psychopathic personality traits. *Personality and Individual Differences*, **35**, 179–97.

Blonigen, D.M., Hicks, B.M., Krueger, R.F., Patrick, C.J., and Iacono, W.G. (2005). Psychopathic personality traits: heritability and genetic overlap with internalizing and externalizing psychopathology. *Psychological Medicine*, **35**, 637–48.

Bremner, J.D. and Vermetten, E. (2001). Stress and development: behavioral and biological consequences. *Development and Psychopathology*, **13**, 473–489.

Calder, A.J., Keane, J., Manes, F., Antoun, N., and Young, A.W. (2000). Impaired recognition and experience of disgust following brain injury. *Nature Neuroscience*, **3**, 1077–8.

Cale, E.M. and Lilienfeld, S.O. (2002). Sex differences in psychopathy and antisocial personality disorder: a review and integration. *Clinical Psychology Review*, **22**, 1179–1207.

Camras, L.A. (1977). Facial expressions used by children in a conflict situation. *Child Development*, **48**, 1431–5.

Carr, L., Iacoboni, M., Dubeau, M.C., Mazziotta, J.C., and Lenzi, G.L. (2003). Neural mechanisms of empathy in humans: a relay from neural systems for imitation to limbic areas. *Proceedings of the National Academy of Sciences of the USA*, **100**, 5497–502.

Caspi, A., McClay, J., Moffitt, T.E., *et al.* (2002). Role of genotype in the cycle of violence in maltreated children. *Science*, **297**, 851–4.

Chaplin, T.C., Rice, M.E., and Harris, G.T. (1995). Salient victim suffering and the sexual responses of child molesters. *Journal of Consulting and Clinical Psychology*, **63**, 249–55.

Charney, D.S. (2003). Neuroanatomical circuits modulating fear and anxiety behaviors. *Acta Psychiatrica Scandinavica, Supplementum*, **417**, 38–50.

Church, R.M. (1959). Emotional reactions of rats to the pain of others. *Journal of Comparative and Physiological Psychology*, **52**, 132–4.

Cleckley, H. (1941). *The mask of sanity*. Fifth ed. St Louis, MO: Mosby.

Cleckley, H.M. (1976). *The mask of sanity*. Fifth ed. St Louis, MO: Mosby.

Cooke, D.J. and Michie, C. (2001). Refining the construct of psychopathy: towards a hierarchical model. *Psychological Assessment*, **13**, 171–88.

Cornell, D.G., Warren, J., Hawk, G., Stafford, E., Oram, G., and Pine, D. (1996). Psychopathy in instrumental and reactive violent offenders. *Journal of Consulting and Clinical Psychology*, **64**, 783–90.

Cubero, I., Thiele, T.E., and Bernstein, I.L. (1999). Insular cortex lesions and taste aversion learning: Effects of conditioning method and timing of lesion. *Brain Research*, **839**, 323–30.

Decety, J. and Jackson, P.L. (2004). The functional architecture of human empathy. *Behavioral and Cognitive Neuroscience Review*, **3**, 71–100.

de Gelder, B., Vroomen, J., Pourtois, G., and Weiskrantz, L. (1999). Non-conscious recognition of affect in the absence of striate cortex. *Neuroreport*, **10**, 3759–63.

de Haan, M. (2001). The neuropsychology of face processing during infancy and childhood. In *Handbook of developmental cognitive neuroscience* (ed. CA Nelson and M Luciana). Cambridge, MA: MIT Press.

Dodge, K.A., Pettit, G.S., Bates, J.E., and Valente, E. (1995). Social information-processing patterns partially mediate the effect of early physical abuse on later conduct problems. *Journal of Abnormal Psychology*, **104**, 632–43.

Drevets, W.C., Lowry, T., Gautier, C., Perrett, D.I., and Knupfer, D.J. (2000). Amygdalar blood flow responses to facially expressed sadness. *Biological Psychiatry*, **47**, 160S.

Dunn, J. and Hughes, C. (2001). 'I got some swords and you're dead!': Violent fantasy, antisocial behavior, friendship, and moral sensibility in young children. *Child Development*, **72**, 491–505.

Everitt, B.J., Cardinal, R.N., Parkinson, J.A., and Robbins, T.W. (2003). Appetitive behavior: impact of amygdala-dependent mechanisms of emotional learning. *Annals of the New York Academy of Sciences*, **985**, 233–50.

Farrington, D.P. and Loeber, R. (2000). Epidemiology of juvenile violence. *Child and Adolescent Psychiatry Clinics of North America*, **9**, 733–48.

Field, T.M., Woodson, R., Greenberg, R., and Cohen, D. (1982). Discrimination and imitation of facial expression by neonates. *Science*, **218**, 179–81.

Fitzgerald, D.A., Angstadt, M., Jelsone, L.M., Nathan, P.J., and Phan, K.L. (2006). Beyond threat: amygdala reactivity across multiple expressions of facial affect. *NeuroImage*, **30**, 1441–8.

Forth, A.E., Kosson, D.S., and Hare, R.D. (2007). *The Psychopathy Checklist: Youth Version*. Toronto: Multi-Health Systems.

Fowles, D.C. and Kochanska, G. (2000). Temperament as a moderator of pathways to conscience in children: the contribution of electrodermal activity. *Psychophysiology*, **37**, 788–95.

Frick, P.J. (1995). Callous–unemotional traits and conduct problems: a two-factor model of psychopathy in children. *Issues in Criminological and Legal Psychology*, **24**, 47–51.

Frick, P.J. and Hare, R.D. (2001). *The Antisocial Process Screening Device*. Toronto, Multi-Health Systems.

Frick, P.J., O'Brien, B.S., Wootton, J.M., and McBurnett, K. (1994). Psychopathy and conduct problems in children. *Journal of Abnormal Psychology*, **103**, 700–7.

Frith, U. and Frith, C.D. (2003). Development and neurophysiology of mentalizing. *Philosophical Transactioins of the Royal Society, Series B: Biological Sciences*, **358**, 459–73.

Gordon, H.L., Baird, A.A., and End, A. (2004). Functional differences among those high and low on a trait measure of psychopathy. *Biological Psychiatry*, **56**, 516–21.

Gorman-Smith, D. and Tolan, P. (1998). The role of exposure to community violence and developmental problems among inner-city youth. *Development and Psychopathology*, **10**, 101–16.

Gregg, T.R. and Siegel, A. (2001). Brain structures and neurotransmitters regulating aggression in cats: implications for human aggression. *Progress in Neuropsychopharmacology and Biological Psychiatry*, **25**, 91–140.

Happé, F.G.E. and Frith, U. (1996). Theory of mind and social impairment in children with conduct disorder. *British Journal of Developmental Psychology*, **14**, 385–98.

Hare, R.D. (1970). *Psychopathy: theory and research*. New York: John Wiley.

Hare, R.D. (1980). A research scale for the assessment of psychopathy in criminal populations. *Personality and Individual Differences*, **1**, 111–19.

Hare, R.D. (1991). *The Hare Psychopathy Checklist—Revised*. Toronto: Multi-Health Systems.

Hare, R.D. (2003). *The Hare Psychopathy Checklist—Revised (PCL-R)* (2nd edn). Toronto: Multi-Health Systems.

Hare, R.D., Clark, D., Grann, M., and Thornton, D. (2000). Psychopathy and the predictive validity of the PCL-R: an international perspective. *Behavioral Sciences and the Law*, **18**, 623–45.

Hariri, A.R., Mattay, V.S., Tessitore, A., *et al.* (2002). Serotonin transporter genetic variation and the response of the human amygdala. *Science*, **297**, 400–403.

Hariri, A.R., Drabant, E.M, Munoz, K.E., *et al.* (2005). A susceptibility gene for affective disorders and the response of the human amygdala. *Archives of General Psychiatry*, **62**, 146–152.

Harpur, T.J., Hakstian, A.R., and Hare, R.D. (1988). The factor structure of the Psychopathy Checklist. *Journal of Consulting and Clinical Psychology*, **56**, 741–7.

Hart, S., Kropp, P.R., and Hare, R.D. (1988). Performance of male psychopaths following conditional release from prison. *Journal of Consulting and Clinical Psychology*, **56**, 227–32.

Hart, S.D., Forth, A.E., and Hare, R.D. (1990). Performance of criminal psychopaths on selected neuropsychological tests. *Journal of Abnormal Psychology*, **99**, 374–9.

Hawes, D.J. and Dadds, M.R. (2005). The treatment of conduct problems in children with callous–unemotional traits. *Journal of Consulting Clinical Psychology*, **73**, 737–41.

Heim, C., Owens, M.J., Plotsky, P.M., and Nemeroff, C.B. (1997). Persistent changes in corticotropin-releasing factor systems due to early life stress: relationship to the pathophysiology of major depression and post-traumatic stress disorder. *Psychopharmacology Bulletin*, **33**, 185–92.

Hemphill, J.F., Hare, R.D., and Wong, S. (1998). Psychopathy and recidivism: a review. *Legal and Criminological Psychology*, **3**, 139–70.

Herba, A.R. and Phillips, M. (2004). Annotation: development of facial expression recognition from childhood to adolescence: behavioural and neurological perspectives. *Journal of Child Psychology and Psychiatry*, **45**, 1185–1198.

Hobson, J. and Shine, J. (1998). Measurement of psychopathy in a UK prison population referred for long-term psychotherapy. *British Journal of Criminology*, **38**, 504–15.

Hoffman, M.L. (1984). Empathy, its limitations, and its role in a comprehensive moral theory. In *Morality, moral development, and moral behavior*(ed. J. Gewirtz and W. Kurtines), pp. 283–302. New York: John Wiley.

Hoffman, M.L. and Saltzstein, H.D. (1967). Parent discipline and the child's moral development. *Journal of Personality and Social Psychology*, **5**, 45–57.

House, TH. and Milligan, W.L. (1976). Autonomic responses to modeled distress in prison psychopaths. *Journal of Personality and Social Psychology*, **34**, 556–60.

Hughes, C. and Dunn, J. (2000). Hedonism or empathy? Hard-to-manage children's moral awareness and links with cognitive and maternal characteristics. *British Journal of Developmental Psychology*, **18**, 227–45.

Hughes, C. and Ensor, R. (2006). Behavioural problems in 2-year-olds: links with individual differences in theory of mind, executive function and harsh parenting. *Journal of Child Psychology and Psychiatry*, **47**, 488–97.

Hughes, C., Dunn, J., and White, A. (1998). Trick or treat? Uneven understanding of mind and emotion and executive dysfunction in 'hard-to-manage' preschoolers. *Journal of Child Psychology and Psychiatry*, **39**, 981–94.

Johnson, M.H. and Morton, J. (1991). *Biology and cognitive development: the case of face recognition*. Oxford: Blackwell.

Kawasaki, H., Kaufman, O., Damasio, H., et al. (2001). Single-neuron responses to emotional visual stimuli recorded in human ventral prefrontal cortex. *Nature Neuroscience*, **4**, 15–16.

Kiehl, K.A., Smith, A.M., Hare, R.D., et al. (2001). Limbic abnormalities in affective processing by criminal psychopaths as revealed by functional magnetic resonance imaging. *Biological Psychiatry*, **50**, 677–84.

King, S.M. (1999). Escape-related behaviours in an unstable, elevated and exposed environment. II: Long-term sensitization after repetitive electrical stimulation of the rodent midbrain defence system. *Behavioral Brain Research*, **98**, 127–42.

Kochanska, G. (1993). Toward a synthesis of parental socialization and child temperament in early development of conscience. *Child Development*, **64**, 325–47.

Kochanska, G. (1997). Multiple pathways to conscience for children with different temperaments: from toddlerhood to age 5. *Developmental Psychology*, **33**, 228–40.

Kosson, D.S., Cyterski, T.D., Steuerwald, B.L., Neumann, C.S., and Walker-Matthews, S. (2002a). The reliability and validity of the Psychopathy Checklist: Youth Version (PCL:YV) in nonincarcerated adolescent males. *Psychological Assessment*, **14**, 97–109.

Kosson, D.S., Suchy, Y., Mayer, A.R., and Libby, J. (2002b). Facial affect recognition in criminal psychopaths. *Emotion*, **2**, 398–411.

Kotsoni, E., de Haan, M., and Johnson, M.H. (2001). Categorical perception of facial expressions by 7-month-old infants. *Perception*, **30**, 1115–25.

Krebs, D.L. (1975). Empathy and altruism. *Journal of Personality and Social Psychology*, **32**, 1134–46.

LeDoux, J. (1998). *The emotional brain.* New York: Weidenfeld and Nicolson

LeDoux, JE. (2000). Emotion circuits in the brain. *Annual Review of Neuroscience,* **23**, 155–84.

Lesch, K.P. and Merschdorf, U. (2000). Impulsivity, aggression, and serotonin: a molecular psychobiological perspective. *Behavioral Science and the Law,* **18**, 281–604.

Leslie, A.M. (1987). Pretense and representation: the origins of 'theory of mind.' *Psychological Review,* **94**, 412–26.

Luo, Q., Holroyd, T., Jones, M., Hendler, T., and Blair, J. (2007). Neural dynamics for facial threat processing as revealed by gamma band synchronization using MEG. *NeuroImage,* **34**, 839–47.

Lykken, D.T. (1995). *The antisocial personalities.* Hillsdale, NJ: Lawrence Erlbaum.

Marsh, A.A. and Ambady, N. (2007). The influence of the fear facial expression on prosocial responding. *Cognition and Emotion,* **21**, 225–47.

Marsh, A.A. and Ambady, N. Accurate identification of fear facial expressions and the prediction of prosocial behavior. *Emotion,* in press.

Marsh, A.A. and Blair, R.J.R. (2008). Deficits in facial affect recognition among antisocial populations: a meta-analysis. *Neuroscience and Biobehavioral Review,* **32**(3), 454–465.

Masserman, J.H., Wechkin, S., and Terris, W. (1964). 'Altruistic' behavior in rhesus monkeys. *American Journal of Psychiatry,* **121**, 584–85.

Matthews, G. and Wells, A. (1999). The cognitive science of attention and emotion. In *Handbook of cognition and emotion* (ed. T. Dalgleish and M.J. Power), pp. 171–92. New York: John Wiley.

Meyer-Lindenberg, A., Buckholtz, J.W., Kolachana, B., *et al.* (2006). Neural mechanisms of genetic risk for impulsivity and violence in humans. *Proceedings of the National Academy of Sciences of the USA,* **103**, 6269–74.

Miller, L.S., Wasserman, G.A., Neugebauer, R., Gorman-Smith, D., and Kamboukos, D. (1999). Witnessed community violence and antisocial behavior in high-risk, urban boys. *Journal of Clinical Child Psychology,* **28**, 2–11.

Mineka, S. and Cook, M. (1993). Mechanisms involved in the observational conditioning of fear. *Journal of Experimental Psychology: General,* **122**, 23–38.

Morris, J.S., Frith, C.D., Perrett, D.I., *et al.* (1996). A differential response in the human amygdala to fearful and happy facial expressions. *Nature,* **383**, 812–15.

Morris, J.S., Ohman, A., and Dolan, R. (1999). A subcortical pathway to the right amygdala mediating 'unseen' fear. *Proceedings of the National Academy of Sciences of the USA,* **96**, 1680–5.

Morton, J. and Johnson, M.H. (1991). CONSPEC and CONLERN: a two-process theory of infant face recognition. *Psychological Review,* **98**, 164–81.

Nucci, L.P. and Herman, S. (1982). Behavioral disordered children's conceptions of moral, conventional, and personal issues. *Journal of Abnormal Child Psychology,* **10**, 411–25.

Ochsner, K.N. (2004). Current directions in social cognitive neuroscience. *Current Opinions in Neurobiology,* **14**, 254–8.

Oxford, M., Cavell, T.A., and Hughes, J.N. (2003). Callous–unemotional traits moderate the relation between ineffective parenting and child externalizing problems: a partial replication and extension. *Journal of Clinical Child and Adolescent Psychology,* **32**, 577–85.

Panksepp, J. (1998). *Affective neuroscience: the foundations of human and animal emotions*. New York: Oxford University Press.

Patrick, C.J. (1994). Emotion and psychopathy: startling new insights. *Psychophysiology*, 31, 319–30.

Perry, D.G. and Perry, L.C. (1974). Denial of suffering in the victim as a stimulus to violence in aggressive boys. *Child Development*, 45, 55–62.

Phillips, M.L., Young, A.W., Scott, S.K., et al. (1998). Neural responses to facial and vocal expressions of fear and disgust. *Proceedings of the Royal Society of London, Series B: Biological Sciences*, 265, 1809–17.

Preston, S.D. and de Waal, F.B. (2002). Empathy: its ultimate and proximate bases. *Behavioral and Brain Sciences*, 25, 1–20.

Rhee, S.H. and Waldman, I.D. (2002). Genetic and environmental influences on antisocial behaviour: a meta-analysis of twin and adoption studies. *Psychological Bulletin*, 128, 490–529.

Rice, G.E. (1965). Aiding responses in rats: not in guinea pigs. In *Proceedings of the Annual Convention of the American Psychological Association*, pp. 105–106. Washington, DC: American Psychological Association.

Rice, G.E. and Gainer, P. (1962). 'Altruism' in the albino rat. *Journal of Comparative and Physiological Psychology*, 55, 123–5.

Richell, R.A., Mitchell, D.G., Newman, C., Leonard, A., Baron-Cohen, S., and Blair, R.J. (2003). Theory of mind and psychopathy Can psychopathic individuals read the 'language of the eyes'? *Neuropsychologia*, 41, 523–6.

Rilling, J.K., Winslow, J.T., O'Brien, D., Gutman, D.A., Hoffman, J.M., and Kilts, C.D. (2001). Neural correlates of maternal separation in rhesus monkeys. *Biological Psychiatry*, 49, 146–57.

Rizzolatti, G., Fogassi, L., and Gallese, V. (2001). Neurophysiological mechanisms underlying the understanding and imitation of action. *Nature Reviews Neuroscience*, 2, 661–70.

Rosenblum, L.A., Forger, C., Noland, S., Trost, R.C., and Coplan, J.D. (2001). Response of adolescent bonnet macaques to an acute fear stimulus as a function of early rearing conditions. *Developmental Psychobiology*, 39, 40–5.

Rothbart, M., Ahadi, S., and Hershey, K.L. (1994). Temperament and social behaviour in children. *Merrill-Palmer Quarterly*, 40, 21–39.

Rozin, P., Haidt, J., and McCauley, C.R. (1993). Disgust. In *Handbook of emotions* (ed. M. Lewis and J.M. Haviland), pp. 575–94. New York: Guilford Press.

Sanchez, M.M., Noble, P.M., Lyon, C.K., et al. (2005). Alterations in diurnal cortisol rhythm and acoustic startle response in nonhuman primates with adverse rearing. *Biological Psychiatry*, 57, 373–81.

Schwab-Stone, M., Chen, C., Greenberger, E., Silver, D., Lichtman, J., and Voyce, C. (1999). No safe haven. II: The effects of violence exposure on urban youth. *Journal of the American Academy of Child and Adolescent Psychiatry*, 38, 359–67.

Sharp, C. and Kine, S. (2008). The assessment of juvenile psychopathy: strengths and weaknesses of currently used questionnaire measures. *Child and Adolescent Mental Health*, 13(2), 85–95.

Smetana, J.G. (1993). Understanding of social rules. In *The child as psychologist: an introduction to the development of social cognition* (ed. M. Bennett, pp. 111–41. New York: Harvester–Wheatsheaf.

Sprengelmeyer, R., Young, A.W., Calder, A.J., Karnat, A., Lange, H.W., and Homberg, V. (1996). Loss of disgust: perception of faces and emotions in Huntington's disease. *Brain*, **119**, 1647–65.

Stevens, D., Charman, T., and Blair, R.J.R. (2001). Recognition of emotion in facial expressions and vocal tones in children with psychopathic tendencies. *Journal of Genetic Psychology*, **162**, 201–11.

Sutker, P.B. (1970). Vicarious conditioning and sociopathy. *Journal of Abnormal Psychology*, **76**, 380–6.

Sutton, J., Smith, P.K., and Swettenham, J. (1999). Social cognition and bullying: social inadequacy or skilled manipulation? *British Journal of Developmental Psychology*, **17**, 435–50.

Sutton J., Reeves, M., and Keogh, E. (2000). Disruptive behaviour, avoidance of responsibility and theory of mind. *British Journal of Developmental Psychology*, **18**, 1–11.

Turiel, E, Killen M., and Helwig, C.C. (1987). Morality: its structure, functions, and vagaries. In *The emergence of morality in young children* (ed. J. Kagan and S. Lamb), pp. 155–245. University of Chicago Press.

Tversky, A. and Kahneman, D. (1981). The framing of decisions and the psychology of choice. *Science*, **211**, 453–8.

Viding, E., Blair, R.J.R., Moffitt, T.E., and Plomin, R. (2005). Evidence for substantial genetic risk for psychopathy in 7-year-olds. *Journal of Child Psychology and Psychiatry*, **46**, 592–7.

Vuilleumier, P., Armony, J.L., Driver, J., and Dolan, R.J. (2003). Distinct spatial frequency sensitivities for processing faces and emotional expressions. *Nature Neuroscience*, **6**, 624–31.

Whalen, P.J., Shin, L.M., McInerney, S.C., Fischer, H., Wright, C.I., and Rauch, S.L. (2001). A functional MRI study of human amygdala responses to facial expressions of fear versus anger. *Emotion*, **1**, 70–83.

Wicker, B., Keysers, C., Plailly, J., Royet, J.P., Gallese, V., and Rizzolatti, G. (2003). Both of us disgusted in my insula: the common neuron basis of seeing and feeling disgust. *Neuron*, **40**, 655–664.

Widom, C.S. (1978). An empirical classification of female offenders. *Criminal Justice and Behavior*, **5**, 35–52.

Widom, C.S. (1992). *The cycle of violence*. US Department of Justice, Office of Justice Programs, National Institute of Justice.

Williamson, S., Hare, R.D., andWong, S. (1987). Violence: criminal psychopaths and their victims. *Canadian Journal of Behavioral Science*, **19**, 454–62.

Winston, J.S., O'Doherty, J., and Dolan, R.J. (2003). Common and distinct neural responses during direct and incidental processing of multiple facial emotions. *NeuroImage*, **20**, 84–97.

Wootton, J.M., Frick, P.J., Shelton, K.K., and Silverthorn, P. (1997). Ineffective parenting and childhood conduct problems: the moderating role of callous–unemotional traits. *Journal of Consulting and Clinical Psychology*, **65**, 292–300.

Part III
Internalizing disorders

8

Social cognition in depressed children and adolescents

Zoë Kyte and Ian Goodyer

The aim of this chapter is to review current knowledge of the relationship between social cognition and major depressive disorder (MDD) in children and adolescents. Discussion centres on the idea that MDD is regarded as a disorder of both emotion regulation and social cognition. The range of social cognitive deficits characteristic of MDD include distorted mental representations, biased attention, memory, and information processing, poor decision-making, and maladaptive social coping. A profile containing such deficits not only supports some of the most influential cognitive theories of depression, but also the increasingly compelling argument that social cognition plays a vital role in both normal and abnormal development.

This chapter will present both theoretical and experimental evidence ranging from the traditional and well established through to more recently applied neurobiological techniques. It will outline some of the clinical implications of these arguments and make suggestions as to where future research should be directed in order to expand our understanding and appreciation of the social cognitive mechanisms involved in MDD.

8.1 Depression in children and adolescents

MDD is considered to be a serious mental disorder associated with significant risk for recurrence, psychosocial impairment, and suicide. A classic feature of depression is a shift in mood from pleasant to unpleasant (dysphoric) that is experienced as relatively pervasive, persisting over time and place, and sufficiently severe to interrupt everyday functioning. When dysphoric, individuals are likely to experience accompanying social cognitive symptoms such as distorted cognitions about the self, one's environment, and one's experiences, biases in attention and memory, and poor decision-making, in addition to adverse physical alterations including disrupted eating and sleeping patterns, and lack of energy and activity. In order to make a clinical diagnosis of MDD (according to DSM-IV (American Psychiatric Association 1994)), it must be possible to establish firstly the mandatory presence of lowered mood (dysphoria, or irritability if in children) or loss of interest/pleasure (anhedonia) together with four of seven other possible non-mandatory symptoms from the two broad domains of disordered cognition and physical changes. These are shown in Table 8.1.

It is essential that the five symptoms occur concurrently over a minimum 2-week period, and to establish that symptoms are not accounted for by the direct effects of substance misuse, a general medical condition, or recent bereavement. However, it is worth noting that these caveats are not implying that such individuals cannot become clinically depressed as a consequence of these experiences, but rather that symptoms essential to the diagnosis may be acute or transient and therefore increase the liability of a false-positive diagnosis at the time of presentation.

Within this diagnostic framework, there are no requirements for a particular pattern of cognitions and/or physical symptoms, and indeed no distinction is made regarding duration of disorder, provided that symptoms have been present for at least 2 weeks. Consequently, episodes may vary in length from a number of weeks up to a number of years. The disorder may also differ in severity or degree of personal psychosocial impairment ranging from mild, indicating only a modest deviation from normal behavioural functioning, to being unable to care for oneself and requiring 24-hour intensive psychiatric care. Finally, in both community and clinical studies, 50–80 per cent of MDD cases present with concurrent non-depressive comorbid disorders involving symptoms of antisocial behaviour, obsessionality, general anxiety, or substance misuse. The precise temporal relationship between depressive and non-depressive symptoms remains an important component of developmental research. It is likely that a proportion of MDD cases are preceded by the

Table 8.1 Symptoms of MDD in childhood and adolescence

Mood*	Cognitive	Physical
Dysphoria or irritability in children	Anhedonia* Feelings of worthlessness Inappropriate guilt Diminished ability to think or concentrate Recurrent thoughts of death or suicidal ideation	Weight changes (includes a failure to make expected weight gains) Fatigue or loss of energy Psychomotor agitation or retardation

*The diagnosis can only be made when five or more symptoms are present over a 2-week period. Dysphoric mood (or irritability in children) or anhedonia must be present.

existence of non-depressive difficulties, whereas for others the emergence of the depression increases the liability for other comorbid disorders.

It is widely recognized that meeting inclusion criteria for MDD still allows for considerable variation in clinical presentation, including high levels of non-depressive symptoms, giving rise to marked individual differences in the descriptive psychopathology of disorder. With the main research emphasis on the quantity of symptoms as predictors of subsequent onset, little attention has been paid as yet to the relative importance of different types of symptoms or their salience to the subject for evolving a disorder. In addition, many individuals present with a range of symptoms that fall below inclusion threshold for a diagnosis (too few or of insufficient duration) but are of sufficient severity to cause personal impairment (Costello *et al.* 1996). Rutter *et al.* (1976) showed that although only 2 per cent of 14–15-year-olds met criteria for a diagnosis of MDD, 40 per cent reported experiences of significant depressive symptomatology, with 8 per cent reporting suicidal thoughts. Similarly, although prevalence rates of depression in adolescents range between 0.4 and 8.3 per cent (Fleming and Offord 1990; Lewinsohn *et al.* 1993), presence of depressive symptomatology (at least one symptom) has been reported in 60 per cent of adolescents (Harrington and Clark 1998).

One diagnostic assumption is that the phenotype of MDD remains largely constant throughout the lifespan. Certainly in terms of symptom presentation, psychiatric comorbidity, and recurrence rate, there appears to be very little developmental variation in the clinical expression of the disorder (Kovacs 1996). Furthermore, the lifetime prevalence of depression in adolescents ranges between 15 and 20 per cent, which is comparable with that of adults and supports findings of depression onsets during adolescence (Lewinsohn *et al.* 1986; Kovacs 1996). However, some subtle differences have been reported, including the response of patients at different ages to treatment, with depressed children failing to respond to tricyclic antidepressants in the same manner as seen in older age groups (Hazell *et al.* 1995; Keller *et al.* 2001) and the elderly being more responsive to interpersonal therapies than previously supposed (Reynolds *et al.* 1999). Similarly, differences have also been reported in the neurobiological correlates of the disorder across development, with depressed children failing to show evidence of hypercortisolaemia as seen in adolescent and adult populations (Kaufman and Ryan 1999; Lupien *et al.* 1999). Psychosocially, differences have been reported between juvenile-onset (before aged 16) and adult-onset depression with juvenile depression being characterized by an increased family history of antisocial behaviour, indices of family instability such as loss of a parent (through death, separation, or divorce), other mental health problems in childhood, poorer motor skills, and greater temperamental inhibition (Jaffee *et al.* 2002). Discontinuities between pre- and post-pubertal depression have also been reported. Thapar and McGuffin (1996) reported a stronger link to environmental factors in pre-pubertal depression compared with the interaction between genetics and environment implicated in post-pubertal depression. Harrington *et al.* (1996) have also described a strong, but non-specific, risk for adult adjustment problems associated with pre-pubertal depression, compared with a link between post-pubertal depression and recurrent depressive episodes in adulthood. Thus it would seem there are both developmental similarities and differences in MDD across the lifespan, although the extent to which these changes correlate with sociocognitive and affective processes embedded in the liability for and outcome of MDD remains to be established.

8.2 Normal development of social cognition

The study of social cognition is concerned with developing a better knowledge of the mental representations and processes underlying how humans perceive, understand, and interpret themselves and others within their social world. In particular, it is concerned with the ability to select, interpret, perceive, commit to memory, and represent information extracted from social situations. Establishing how individuals accomplish these tasks forms the basis for understanding how they interact with their social environment, and how and why their experiences manifest in the behavioural responses they exhibit. Theoretical and experimental concepts from both social and cognitive psychology have resulted in the formulation of social information processing (SIP) theory (Dodge 1986; Crick and Dodge 1994) aimed at recognizing and explaining the sequence of mental processes (including both cognitive and emotional, conscious and unconscious) underpinning social behaviour. The SIP approach was discussed in detail in Chapter 6. However, for the purposes of the current chapter we summarize the approach again here.

The sequence is proposed to begin with the encoding of relevant aspects of the social situation via sensory input, selectively attending to socially relevant cues, and encoding information in short-term memory. Once encoded, cues are then subjected to mental representation and interpretation, which calls upon the individual's internal attributions and attitudes. Behavioural responses can only be elicited from these mental representations through the process of 'response accessing', which involves retrieval of possible behavioural responses from memory. In order to select and initiate the most appropriate behavioural response in a given situation, the individual must also engage in response evaluation—the decision-making process involving evaluation of the moral acceptability and/or anticipated consequences of a given behavioural response.

Results of this evaluation process allow the individual to settle on an (ideally) optimal behavioural response. The final stage in this sequence involves the transformation of these mental processes into the corresponding verbal and motor behaviours (enactment). Underpinning this entire process and organizing processing at each of these individual stages are 'knowledge structures'. These knowledge structures consist of constructs formulated to explain mnemonic representations of past events that are likely to influence how an individual perceives and responds to future social situations (i.e. frames of reference, schemas, attitudes, stereotypes).

SIP theory acknowledges the interplay between cognitions and emotions. In any social context, our ability to set goals, generate strategic behavioural responses, and evaluate outcomes of our behaviour is likely to influence, and be influenced by, our emotional development. Understanding and regulating our emotions is thought to involve an array of cognitive abilities ('emotional intelligence'), constituting a transition in early childhood from data (biologically) driven emotional behaviour to knowledge-driven behaviour (Meerum Terwogt and Stegge 2001). Hence, gradual gains in cognitive capacity and concurrent insights into determinants of emotional behaviour allow for the use of one's own subjective cognitive representation of events within the context of their emotions. This increased understanding of the subjective nature of emotions helps children to understand not only their own emotions, but also those of others (i.e. to develop a 'theory of mind'). With this comes the skill to regulate one's emotions through an understanding that the emotional impact of a given situation depends on one's interpretation or appraisal of it. As we will show, nowhere is this delicate yet complex relationship between cognition and emotion more apparent than in the case of MDD.

8.3 Maladaptive social information processing in depressed youth

SIP theory proposes that, despite repeatedly engaging in the same sequence of processes across social circumstances, individuals are likely to develop characteristic patterns of processing at each stage of the model in particular situations. It is thought that these characteristic patterns may form the basis for development of psychopathology. Using this theory as a framework, what follows is an account of the empirical (and additional theoretical) evidence supporting the role of social cognitive deficits in the development and maintenance of childhood MDD. Although the focus is on children and adolescents, discussion will adopt a developmental perspective, with relevant literature on adult patients cited where appropriate.

8.3.1 Knowledge structures

The presence of knowledge structures is a prominent feature of one of the most influential theories of depression. According to Beck (1967, 1976), a salient characteristic underpinning the presence of MDD is a negative view about the self and one's experiences. Such a 'negative cognitive schema' is proposed to precede the experience of depression and therefore contribute to an individual's vulnerability for the disorder. Such structures are also thought to influence subsequent cognitions that are important for sequential stages of the SIP model. 'Schemas' are defined as underlying cognitive structures that are implemented in the screening, coding, and evaluation of stimuli to ultimately allow an individual to categorize and interpret experiences in a meaningful way. They are thought to form in childhood and remain relatively stable throughout the lifespan. However, they persist in a latent state, only becoming activated when the individual is exposed to negative circumstances. Once activated, these schemas are thought to bias information processing so as to select and encode negative at the expense of positive stimuli, even if this involves distorting the balance of information being perceived or altering the perception of a situation so as to match the affective tone of the bias.

Knowledge structures of a similar kind underlie Bower's associative network theory of mood and memory (Bower 1981). In this theory, concepts, events, and meaning are all reportedly represented in memory by nodes within a network. Activation within this network depends on a number of factors including the proximity of nodes to each other, the strength of the initial activation, and the time lapse since activation. The theory makes the broad prediction that each emotion has a specific node within the network that becomes associated with a range of perceptual, attentional, and mnemonic biases via the interaction of the emotion node with other nodes. In this sense, a reciprocal relationship is postulated to exist between negative thinking and depressed mood that becomes activated and results in dysphoria in vulnerable individuals experiencing social adversity. This interdependence causes the individual to experience a recursive and potentiating cycle in which depressed mood increases access to negative thoughts, leading to an increase in negative bias for the interpretation of current events and difficulties.

The 'differential activation hypothesis' (Teasdale 1983; Clark and Teasdale 1985; Teasdale and Dent 1987) suggests that vulnerability to intense and persistent depression may be determined by individual differences in the patterns of negative thinking (knowledge structures) that become activated during a state of mild depression or dysphoria. During this time, vulnerable individuals are hypothesized to access qualitatively different types of negative cognitions compared with non-vulnerable individuals, thereby discriminating between individuals who experience moderate to severe compared with mild depression, and those who experience persistent (in which negative self-cognition and dysphoria act upon each other, thus intensifying and maintaining disorder) versus transient depression. According to this hypothesis, the source of the original depression may be less important than the pattern of thinking that is present once an individual is already experiencing mild depression—a pattern characterized by a vicious cycle of negative memories, sad emotion, and negativistic interpretations of current events. Furthermore, the aversiveness of the depressive symptoms themselves may also activate these negative thinking patterns, thus prolonging the depression as the individual becomes 'depressed about their depression' (Teasdale 1985).

Despite some minor technical variations, a common theme in all these theories is the presence of a negative self-concept in which patterns of negative thinking result in distorted processing of information. This in turn biases the individual towards self-deprecating statements and an underestimation of their performance (low self-esteem), negatively biased explanations and interpretations of experiences, and negative expectations of future outcomes (the 'cognitive triad'). Such cognitions may lead the individual into a vicious negative affective–cognitive cycle in which increased negative thinking lowers mood, which in turn increases activation of negative schemas, further increasing negative thinking. This cycle is hypothesized to be important in the aetiology of MDD as part of a pattern of interacting mechanisms which include biological, psychological, and social factors (Teasdale and Barnard 1993).

Attempts to demonstrate evidence of enduring negative self-schemas in well individuals have generally been unsuccessful, leading to an emphasis on the need for the individual to be in lowered (natural or induced) mood before their activation becomes possible (Teasdale and Cox 2001). Working to this specification, empirical evidence has supported the presence of negative self-schema in well children, adolescents, and adults induced into a depressed mood (Zupan *et al.* 1987; Sutton *et al.* 1988; Kelvin *et al.* 1999), formerly depressed adults (Hedlund and Rude 1995), and non-depressed women (Evans *et al.* 2005). In the last of these studies, stable negative self-schemas predicted onset of depression more than 3 years later, suggesting that their presence represents a long-lasting vulnerability to depression rather than being part of the prodrome of a depressive episode (Evans *et al.* 2005). However, the issues of whether depression is associated with a distinct information-processing bias compared with other forms of psychopathology, whether the content of information-processing biases in depression is specific to themes of loss and sadness, or whether biases are consistent across both attention and memory tasks continue to warrant further attention (Gotlib *et al.* 2004a). Also, although social context may play a role in the ontogeny of these schemas (e.g. child maltreatment), or may form the focus of the negative schemas (e.g. 'I will never be loved'), the negative schemas associated with depression are not exclusively social in nature.

8.3.2 Encoding

Critical to encoding is the ability to selectively focus attention on the relevant cues within a social situation in an unbiased manner. Empirical studies support the idea that individuals with depression are not only impaired in their ability to attend to relevant aspects of a situation but also display mood-congruent biases towards the negative. Empirical evidence for this comes largely from studies using either colour-naming or emotional Stroop tasks, or dot-probe tasks (Williams and Nulty 1986; Gotlib and Cane 1987; MacLeod and Rutherford 1992; Mogg *et al.* 1995; Matthews *et al.* 1996; Gallardo Perez *et al.* 1999; Den Hartog *et al.* 2003; Kerr *et al.* 2005; Paelecke-Habermann *et al.* 2005). However, results have not been consistent (MacLeod *et al.* 1986; Mogg *et al.* 1993; Bradley *et al.* 1995, McCabe and Gotlib 1995). Bradley *et al.* (1997) reported a negative attentional bias on a dot-probe task in both induced and naturally occurring dysphoria in adults but only when presentation of stimuli exceeded 500 or 1000 ms. The authors interpret this finding as a lack of negative biases in attention in early automatic aspects of attentional processing; an interpretation supported by recent studies using both faces (Gotlib *et al.* 2004b) and words (Koster *et al.* 2005) as stimuli.

Studies of similar attentional impairments and biases in children are less common. However, depressed children have been shown to attend to and recall negative self-referent words over and above positive words, whereas non-depressed children display the opposite (Hammen and Zupan 1984; Zupan *et al.* 1987). Using an emotional go–no-go task, Kyte *et al.* (2005) also showed an affective bias for negative stimuli in recently depressed adolescents, which was confirmed using the same task with both medicated (Murphy *et al.* 1999) and unmedicated (Erickson *et al.* 2005) depressed adults. However, as with the literature in adults, data for attentional biases in depressed adolescence are inconsistent (Neshat-Doost *et al.* 2000).

8.3.3 Mental representations

Mental representation of encoded cues relies on a number of cognitive features including attributions of causality, inferences about self-worth, and expectations of future outcomes. Much of the work on mental representations in relation to MDD focuses on how efficiently the individual believes they can react to their circumstances and what they believe the causes of their circumstances to be. The 'learned helplessness' theory put forward by Seligman (1975) views depression as the result of the expectation of future helplessness (i.e. expecting bad events to occur and believing that nothing can be done to prevent them). Expectation of a lack of control leads to deficits within three domains: motivational (not initiating subsequent escape responses in the presence of stress), cognitive (slower to learn that responses could control future stress as a result of acquiring a cognitive set in which responses are irrelevant to outcome), and emotional (transient emotional effects as a result of inescapable trauma). Collectively, these are referred to as 'helplessness deficits'.

Although helplessness is thought to arise from the perception of uncontrollability, equally significant determinants include both the type and importance of the event experienced in conjunction with the explanation that the individual attributes to the cause of the event. Based on this, the 'reformulated learned helplessness' theory (Abramson *et al.* 1978) argues for the existence of a 'depressogenic attributional style' which interacts with the experience of a negative life event resulting in the presentation of 'hopelessness depression' (a theoretical subtype of depression that has considerable overlaps with depression as defined by DSM-IV but is characterized by a distinct cluster of symptoms including passivity, cognitive deficits, sadness, lowered self-esteem, and lowered assertiveness and competitiveness). Specifically, a negative life event attributed to causes that are stable (not likely to change) as opposed to unstable (transient), internal (due to something about the individual) as opposed to external (due to something about other people or circumstances), and global (likely to affect many outcomes) as opposed to specific (cause will produce failure only in similar circumstances) may trigger feelings of generalized hopelessness and in turn provoke symptoms of hopelessness depression. A similar consequence is thought to come about if an individual attributes a positive life event to causes that are unstable–external–specific. In this context, hopelessness is defined as '... the expectation that highly desirable outcomes will not occur, and that one is powerless to change the situation' (Needles and Abramson 1990, p.156). Furthermore, an interaction is proposed to exist in which more severe depressogenic attributional styles require less severe negative life events to bring about generalized hopelessness, and less severe attributional styles require more severe life events. This implies that there are varying degrees of depressogenic attributional styles across individuals.

In an extension of the original framework of this theory, Needles and Abramson (1990) state in their model of recovery that an increase in hopefulness (i.e. a decrease in hopelessness) would lead to a reduction in depressive symptoms and thus remission of disorder. They propose that this is brought about by the occurrence of positive life events interacting with an enhancing (rather than depressogenic) attributional style which includes attributing the cause of positive (rather than negative) events as stable–internal–global. There is both theoretical and experimental evidence to suggest that such enhancing attributional styles can coexist alongside depressogenic attributional styles as a consequence of representing separate constructs (reviewed by Sweeney et al. 1986). Indeed, Needles and Abramson (1990) report that '... even among those at risk for hopelessness depression, there may be a subset who have the hypothesized enhancing style for positive events and who thereby may be better able to recover'. If this is true, the restoration of hopefulness may come about as a consequence of the enhancing attributional style being 'greater than' the depressogenic attributional style, assuming equal rates of both positive and negative life events (Voelz et al. 2003). Alternatively, if an individual displays equivalent levels of both enhancing and depressogenic attributional styles, one might expect a more moderate recovery as the two styles work to offset each other, with the experience of either positive or negative life events influencing the rate and degree of recovery from depression (Voelz et al. 2003).

Generally speaking, experimental studies based on both clinical and non-clinical adult (Needles and Abramson 1990; Edelman et al. 1994; Johnson et al. 1996, 1998; Fernandez Prieto et al. 2004), and child/adolescent populations (Seligman et al. 1984; Lewinsohn et al. 1994; Joiner and Wagner 1995; Gladstone and Kaslow 1995; Gladstone et al. 1997; Joiner 2000; Muris et al. 2001; Voelz et al. 2003) have supported these theories. In addition to correlating with concurrent depression, maladaptive attributional style has been shown to predict later depression in children independently from being considered a symptom of the depression or from the influence of earlier depression on attributional style (Nolen-Hoeksema et al. 1986; Spence et al. 2002). In adults, negative attributional style has been shown to persist in remitted depressed patients (Tracy et al. 1992; Gotlib et al. 1993) and remain relatively stable throughout the lifespan for periods of a number of months to a number of years (Fincham et al. 1987; Tiggemann et al. 1991). Presence of negative attributional style has also been documented in children at risk (because of maternal affective disorder), alongside a more negative self-concept and less positive self-schemas compared with children of medically ill or normal mothers (Jaenicke et al. 1987). When considered in the context of interpersonal events (rather than achievement-related events), the presence of a negative attributional style has also been prospectively related to increases in self-reported suicidality (Joiner and Rudd 1995). There is some evidence to suggest that depressogenic attributional style may be mediated by other social cognitive characteristics such as negative coping styles (e.g. as the cause of a negative event is stable there is nothing that can be done about it) and a low sense of self-efficacy and self-esteem (e.g. as the cause of a negative event is both global and stable, there is little belief in one's ability to manipulate the outcome to become favourable) (Tennen *et al.* 1987; Bruder-Mattson and Hovanitz 1990; Muris *et al.* 2001). In turn, such characteristics may exacerbate the effect of negative attributional style on the presence of depressive symptoms (Herman-Stahl *et al.* 1995; Bandura *et al.* 1999).

MDD has been characterized by several other patterns of distorted mental representations. Depressed children have been shown to interpret their (social) performance as more negative compared with well children, as well as setting more stringent criteria for success and failure and being more apt at choosing punishment than reward (Kaslow *et al.* 1984). They have also been shown to have a lower global self-worth (value of oneself as a person) (King *et al.* 1993) and lower social self-confidence (Marton *et al.* 1993). Cognitive errors, as described in Beck's theory (i.e. over-generalization and catastrophizing), have also been reported in depressed children (Leitenberg *et al.* 1986). Dysphoric children have been shown to endorse a greater number of global negative trait adjectives when describing themselves (Hammen and Zupan 1984; Kelvin *et al.* 1999). This has been associated with a slower rate of recovery when compared with equally depressed individuals who do not endorse such self-devaluative adjectives (Dent and Teasdale 1987).

8.3.4 Response accessing

The next stage of the social information processing sequence is to retrieve potential behavioural responses from long-term memory. Nolen-Hoeksema's 'response style' theory (Nolen-Hoeksema 1987, 1991) states that an individual's response to their situation may be connected to their mood. In particular, duration of depressed mood may influence this relationship. The theory states that engaging in rumination (behaviour and/or thoughts focused on mood and presence of depressive symptoms, their causes, and their consequences) maintains an individual's depressed state, leading to prolonged depressive episodes. Several studies have supported the proposition that rumination predicts onset of depressive episodes as well as greater depressive symptoms and longer periods of depressed mood in children and adults (Just and Alloy 1997; Nolan *et al.* 1998; Nolen-Hoeksema *et al.* 1993, 1994, 1999; Lyubomirsky *et al.* 1998; Nolen-Hoeksema 2000; Park *et al.* 2004). Examples of rumination include isolating oneself to think about one's symptoms (i.e. how tired and unmotivated one feels) and worrying about the consequences of one's depression (i.e. how low mood is affecting work and family life). Distraction, on the other hand, involves active and purposeful attempts to turn attention away from one's depressive symptoms and instead engage in neutral or pleasant actions and thoughts. Examples include leisure activities, or concentrating on hobbies or work. Several studies have shown that many individuals engage in self-focused ruminative behaviour and thinking when in a depressed mood, but a large proportion are able to distract themselves after a short period of time by participating in pleasurable activities (Wood et al. 1990; Nolen-Hoeksema et al. 1993).

Engaging in rumination has been shown to influence other aspects of cognition which may contribute to the ability to access suitable responses. In particular, individuals who ruminate have been shown to be poor problem-solvers (Lyubomirsky and Nolen-Hoeksema 1995), generating half as many solutions to a problem compared with individuals who distract (J. Morrow 1990, unpublished). When engaged in problem-solving they are reportedly more likely to participate in maladaptive or risky behaviours (Nolen-Hoeksema and Morrow 1991). The influence on response accessing may also come about indirectly through the relationship between depression, rumination, and memory. Early studies showed that individuals induced into a negative mood found it easier to retrieve negatively toned memories (Teasdale and Fogarty 1979; Teasdale et al. 1980). More recently, when depressed individuals were asked to recall memories of specific autobiographical events, they were more likely than well controls to recall categorical over-general memories (i.e. a summary of repeated memories) as opposed to specific or extended events (taking place over a period of longer than a day) (Williams and Scott 1988; Williams and Dritschel 1992; Goddard et al. 1996; Williams 1996; Park et al. 2002, 2004). This pattern of memory retrieval is thought to remain relatively stable over time, despite clinical improvement (Brittlebank et al. 1993; Peeters et al. 2002), and has been demonstrated in first-episode adolescent as well as recurrent adult depression (Nandrino et al. 2002; Park et al. 2002). In this context, autobiographical memories are defined as episodic, personally salient event memories that are not part of generic script or semantic memory for personal facts, but do form part of an individual's autobiography (Tulving 1983). Increased recall of over-general autobiographical memories appears to be unique to both depression and post-traumatic stress disorder (McNally et al. 1994, 1995). Furthermore, retrieval of a greater proportion of over-general memories may have significant clinical relevance in that depressed individuals who display this kind of memory retrieval take longer to recover (Brittlebank et al. 1993), display a greater degree of hopelessness (Williams and Broadbent 1986), demonstrate more deficits in interpersonal problem-solving (Goddard et al. 1996), and face more of a challenge imagining the future in a specific way (Williams *et al.* 1996). The link between rumination during dysphoria and the recall of categorical over-general autobiographical memories can be extended to include a link with an increased recall of generally negative autobiographical memories (Lyubomirsky *et al.* 1998). The social nature of autobiographical memory stems from several sources, including the expression of theory of mind skills (i.e. understanding the origin of knowledge that contributes to memory, and the ability to consider two conflicting representations simultaneously) and its role in social interactions (i.e. the relationship between reminiscing and the maintenance of social and emotional bonds in the form of attachment) (see Reese 2002).

Rather than being representative of a general failure in the memory system, there are several lines of evidence to suggest that this pattern of memory recollection occurs as a consequence of a specific relationship between over-general autobiographical memory and rumination. Watkins *et al.* (2000) showed that use of a particular distraction technique (Nolen-Hoeksema and Morrow 1993) reduced the degree of categorical over-general memory. Similarly, techniques included in mindfulness-based cognitive therapy, which involves switching out of the analytical self-focused ruminative way of thinking, have been successful in reducing over-general memory in formerly depressed adults (Williams *et al.* 2000; Watkins and Teasdale 2001). This suggests that the elevated retrieval of categorical autobiographical memories associated with MDD may be more modifiable than previously believed (Watkins *et al.* 2000).

More recently, experimental studies have led to the distinction between two subcategories of rumination: reflection ('purposeful turning inward to engage in cognitive problem solving to alleviate one's depressive symptoms') and brooding ('passive comparison of one's current situation with some unachieved standard') (Treynor *et al.* 2003). Reflection has been associated with less depression over time, although with more depression concurrently (Treynor *et al.* 2003). This supports the idea that reflection may be instigated by negative affect or may result in negative affect in the short term, but in fact may be adaptive and effective in reducing negative affect in the longer term because of its efficiency as a problem-solving strategy. In contrast, brooding has been associated both longitudinally and concurrently with greater depression and hence may not contain any adaptive qualities (Treynor *et al.* 2003).

Engaging in distraction may also have implications on response accessing. There are several reasons why deliberately redirecting attention away from depressive thoughts and feelings may be thought of as adaptive as it provides immediate escape from the negative situation or emotions elicited by a given situation. However, it is questionable whether this is an optimal strategy for addressing longer-term, persistent, and recurrent depressions. Such doubt comes from the idea that encouragement to suppress negative thoughts may preclude an individual from knowing and being in touch with their thoughts and feelings, developing alternative interpretations and representations of their thoughts, feelings, and experiences (something which is central to the treatment programmes born out of cognitive theories of depression). This may lead individuals to engage in behavioural and emotional avoidance associated with recurrence rather than remediation of MDD in the wider coping literature (Compas *et al.* 1988; McNaughton *et al.* 1992; Perrez and Reicherts 1992; Saklofske 1993; Zeidner 1994; Kyte 2003). Alternatively, engaging in problem-focused or active coping, which requires an external focus, skill in identifying and defining problem situations, and access to a range of appropriate strategies that manage both the actual stressor and the emotional reaction elicited by the experience (Zeidner and Saklofske 1996), has been associated with fewer psychological problems, including depression (Ayers *et al.* 1990; Sandler *et al.* 1994). However, Nolen-Hoeksema and colleagues (Nolen-Hoeksema and Morrow 1991; Nolen-Hoeksema *et al.* 1994) have provided some evidence for the idea that people who use pleasant events to manage their moods (i.e. distraction techniques) are more likely to progress into active problem-solvers in the long term as a strategy for coping. They argue that this may come about as a consequence of a lift in mood, allowing such individuals to see themselves as capable problem-solvers (Nolen-Hoeksema and Morrow 1991; Nolen-Hoeksema *et al.* 1994). Watkins and Teasdale (2004) argue that this more active approach to negative experiences may come about from an alternative form of rumination which they refer to as 'mindful self-awareness' (rather than analytical rumination which is considered maladaptive). This alternative refocuses attention on the self, relying on strategies that are not considered classic examples of rumination. This supports the idea that rumination should be considered an umbrella term for a number of possible means of self-focus, each with their own distinct functional properties (McFarland and Buehler 1998; Trapnell and Campbell 1999; Watkins and Teasdale 2001; Treynor *et al.* 2003).

Consistent with persistent ruminating in MDD are findings within the neuropsychological literature of a diminished ability to shift attention and response from one affective category to another (Murphy *et al.* 1999) and to shift cognitive set (Franke *et al.* 1993; Beats *et al.* 1996), resulting in perseverative behaviour patterns and consistent use of inappropriate behavioural responses. However, similar results have not been reported in depressed adolescents (Kyte *et al.* 2005), suggesting that this may be a deficit sensitive to either development or stage of illness (i.e. first episode versus recurrent). Murphy *et al.* (1999) interpreted their findings in the context of an abnormal response to negative feedback in depression (Beats *et al.* 1996; Elliott *et al.* 1996, 1997), as it appeared that depressed adults displayed elevated response times on an affective go–no-go task as a strategy for avoiding making a greater number of errors.

8.3.5 Response evaluation

Response evaluation is thought to be dependent on a number of judgements, including self-efficacy, moral acceptability of behaviour, future consequences, and ability to enact a response. According to Dodge (1993), an individual may display impaired response evaluation for a number of reasons: (a) failure to engage in response evaluation altogether due to impulsivity, (b) evaluating outcomes of behaviour in overly positive (or negative) ways, or (c) lacking confidence that engaging in a positive behavioural response would result in a positive outcome. Evidently, a critical skill for response evaluation is the ability to make efficient decisions in order to ensure that the most appropriate and adaptive behavioural response is ultimately enacted. Such skills have been examined in the context of MDD (as well as other psychiatric conditions) by using a computerized task (Rogers *et al.* 1999a) which assesses several key components of decision-making pertinent to response evaluation: (a) decision-making behaviour across a range of contingencies (tested by manipulating the probability of making a correct/adaptive decision), (b) individual efficiency (allowing the individual to place a self-selected bet on their decision being correct), and (c) impulsivity versus genuine risk-taking behaviour (offering a sequence of possible bets in two conditions, ascending or descending). In adults with MDD, administration of this task has resulted in reports of suboptimal decision-making characterized by protracted deliberation times and the employment of less responsive betting strategies (allocation of an inappropriate number of points to a given decision) (Rahman *et al.* 1999; Rubinsztein *et al.* 2000; Murphy *et al.* 2001). However, ability to make decisions that are likely to produce the desired outcome appears to be less impaired (Murphy *et al.* 2001), indicating that adults with MDD remain able to encode information about the likelihood of a reward response effectively and to make decisions accordingly. Using the same task, adolescents experiencing first episode MDD have also displayed a preserved ability to make decisions that are likely to produce the desired outcome (Kyte *et al.* 2005). These adolescents also display suboptimal decision-making in the form of an inappropriate allocation of resources (i.e. betting a large proportion of points on a decision with an unfavourable outcome), although to a greater extent than seen in previous adult populations (Corwin *et al.* 1990; Beats *et al.* 1996; Elliott *et al.* 1996, 1997). This particular pattern of decision-making is indicative of a tendency to be impulsive (i.e. a failure to consider, analyse and reflect prior to engaging in a response). Although this study did not make use of exclusively social situations as stimuli, it points to a general cognitive impairment associated with depression in adolescents which may affect social information-processing. It should also be noted that, although impulsivity is a feature of normal development, it can be both functional and dysfunctional (Dickman 1990) and has been reported as an important dimension of clinical depression (Corruble et al. 1999).

Although increased impulsivity may provide some explanation of the patterns of suboptimal decision-making profiles reported in MDD, studies in adults have suggested that a number of other neuropsychological processes are implicated. These include hyposensitivity to reward (the prospect of a large immediate gain outweighing any prospect of future loss), insensitivity to punishment (prospect of a large loss not overriding any prospect of gain), or insensitivity to future consequences (behaviour always guided by immediate prospects) (Bechara et al. 2000a). Additionally, depressed individuals may display compromised decision-making as a result of an inability to resolve effectively between two competing response options (Rogers et al. 1999b), a loss of ability to ponder over different courses of action (Tranel et al. 2000), or a degree of cognitive (rather than behavioural) impulsivity (Bechara et al. 2000b).

Response evaluations of depressed individuals have also been closely linked with the degree to which specific desired outcomes are under the control of the individual concerned. Within the coping literature, an important distinction exists between events perceived as controllable or uncontrollable (Altshuler and Ruble 1989; Compas et al. 1991). The argument follows that each type of situation is dealt with using very different means of coping, ranging from monitoring or approach strategies for controllable situations to avoidance strategies in uncontrollable situations (Miller et al. 1985). That said, the greater use of avoidance strategies reported in depressed adolescents (e.g. Kyte 2003) may be explained by their perceiving a greater proportion of situations as uncontrollable. Indeed, depressed children and adults apparently display a general tendency towards an external locus of control (Lefkowitz et al. 1980; McCauley et al. 1988), and depressed children perceive themselves as lacking control of their own desired outcomes (Weisz et al. 1987).

8.3.6 Enactment

The final stage of the sequence involves translating decisions regarding behavioural response into verbal and motor behaviours within the context of a specific social interaction. There are no studies that have directly examined this skill in relation to MDD, although it is unlikely that the cognitive profiles described at each of the previous stages of the sequence are exclusive and do not, in any way, impinge on the behavioural manifestations. This is likely to be true not only for enactment, but also across all previous stages of this sequence of social information processing. For example, feelings of hopelessness, discussed within the context of 'mental representations', are also likely to influence a depressed individual's beliefs about the probable outcomes of any behaviour they display and hence will influence cognitions equally pertinent to 'response evaluation'. Similarly, distorted cognitions may impact on overall self-esteem and confidence, which may in turn influence the degree to which a depressed individual is able to execute their chosen behaviour. Therefore the sequence of events involved in the execution of behaviour in a social situation cannot be considered as comprising discrete components, but rather should be viewed as an interacting overlapping collection of cognitions which, in depression, are characterized by distortions and dysfunctions that are likely to underlie the maladaptive behavioural responses that are often manifest.

8.4 Aetiological considerations of social cognitive deficits in child and adolescent major depressive disorder

8.4.1 Gene–environment interactions

Many of the theories discussed in this chapter converge on the opinion that the presence of knowledge structures and the affective–cognitive cycle which ensues exist prior to the experience of depression and hence constitute an important vulnerability factor in the aetiology of MDD. According to Beck (1967, 1976), the content and affective tone of these knowledge structures is likely to be influenced by early life experiences, particularly the experience of adversity. Many have studied the effects of negative life events in the context of depression (Paykel *et al.* 1969; Brown and Harris 1978; Paykel 1978; Goodyer *et al.* 2000), generating support for a relationship to exist between them. In the context of SIP theory, early experience of adversity (i.e. interpersonal loss, threat, disappointment, maltreatment) is thought to influence knowledge structures so that they become characterized by negative self-schema and low self-esteem. Once these knowledge structures become negatively toned as a consequence of early adversity, negative-schema-driven processing influences subsequent cognitions in social situations (i.e. encoding, mental representations, response accessing, and response evaluation), in turn producing the kinds of biases and impairments described in the context of MDD. Such cognitive distortions are likely to encourage the individual to access and select depressive behavioural responses from memory, in turn manifesting in the characteristic symptoms of depression (i.e. sad affect, anhedonia, diminished ability to concentrate, feelings of worthlessness, lack of energy). Dodge (1993) argues that depression may become chronic when the presence of such negative schema and depressogenic processing and behaviour prevents external forces from mitigating these depressive symptoms.

Environmental factors other than direct experience of adversity may also impact on the form and tone of knowledge structures. These may include presence of familial depression (which in turn impacts on parenting style and provides a depressogenic model of thinking/coping), attachment history (development of emotional regulation), and family interactions (i.e. warmth, hostility, conflict). Similarly, individual characteristics such as temperament, aspects of personality (i.e. self-criticism), and relationships with peers have all been implicated in the aetiology of depression and may exert their influence via their effects on the structure and content of self-schema and subsequent cognitive processing (see McCauley et al. 2001).

Identification of a set of affective–cognitive processes which may carry particular risk for subsequent disorder has formed the focus of much of the work conducted within the field of behavioural genetics over the past two decades. Alongside an increasing recognition of the significant contribution of genes to the aetiology of MDD (Corcico and McGuffin 2001; see Goodyer 2003 for a full discussion), attention has focused on the use of quantitative trait markers of behaviour associated with MDD which may be expected to enhance prospects for establishing links between genes and disorder. Examples of such candidate traits include measures of social cognition (Scourfield et al. 1999) and temperament (Eley and Plomin 1997) which provide further support for the involvement of a set of affective–cognitive processes. A second potential set of genetic effects are those which increase liability for environments that are associated with provoking psychopathology (Kendler et al. 1995). Given that much work has already established a link between certain life events and depression (i.e. assault, serious marital problems, divorce/break-up, job loss, serious illness, major financial problems, trouble getting on with friends/family), and that genetic influences on the occurrence of such life events has been documented across the lifespan, the current challenge lies in determining the exact interaction between gene and environment in order to understand this process more clearly (Kendler and Karkowski-Shuman 1997; Silberg et al. 1999).

8.4.2 Neurobiological basis of social cognition

In addition to environmental and genetic origins, there is also likely to be a strong biological (neural) basis to the presence of knowledge structures and associated cognitive processes. Developing our understanding of social cognition beyond established cognitive theory and practice has been aided by recent advances in techniques aimed at characterizing sociocognitive profiles at a neurobiological level. Current focus is on offering a possible reconciliation between biological and psychological approaches to social behaviour by investigating the underlying neural mechanisms of processes collectively involved in social cognition, including decision-making, attention, memory, and emotion (Adolphs 2001).

Studying the neurobiology of social cognition within a developmental context requires consideration of issues surrounding neurodevelopment. In normal development, it is accepted that the brain myelinates from back (caudal) to front (rostral), and from bottom (inferior) to top (superior). Consequently, subcortical structures such as the amygdala, basal ganglia, and thalamus are all thought to have reached both structural and functional maturity by adolescence, unlike the prefrontal cortex which continues to undergo substantial structural and functional development into early adulthood (Casey 1999; Sowell *et al.* 2000; Blumberg *et al.* 2004; Giedd 2004). Potential abnormalities in subcortical structures which may be implicated in emotional disorders may be evident by early adolescence, compared with structural and functional differences in frontal regions which may not become apparent until later adolescence/early adulthood when maturation in these regions is complete (Blumberg *et al.* 2004). Thus complex mood–cognitive differences between healthy individuals and those with mood disorders are unlikely to be evident until the latter part of adolescence or early adulthood. Nevertheless, pre-pubertal children have demonstrated capabilities in complex cognitive processing (i.e. decision-making, memory, and problem-solving) (Luciana and Nelson 1998; Luciana *et al.* 1999; Hughes 2005). Thus, while neural maturation is clearly an ongoing process, it appears that there is sufficient brain development in the pre-pubertal child for the formation of thoughts that may become 'abnormal' in relation to dysphoric mood.

As a consequence of this recent interest in establishing the neurobiological basis of social cognition, Grady and Keightley (2002) outline 10 regions of the brain believed to be associated with various critical components of social cognition.

+ Regions of the anterior cingulate: the *subgenual cingulate* (autonomic responses (Damasio *et al.* 1990) and reward mechanisms (Price 1999)), the *rostral cingulate* (processing of emotional stimuli (Taylor *et al.* 1998; Whalen *et al.* 1998)), and the *dorsal cingulate* (error monitoring and selecting among competing responses (Pardo *et al.* 1990; Paus *et al.* 1993; Bush *et al.* 1998)).

- Regions thought to be involved in face perception: the *fusiform gyrus* (face discrimination (Haxby *et al.* 1994)), the *superior temporal sulcus* (gaze direction and motion of body parts (Puce *et al.* 1998; Decety and Grezes 1999; Hoffman and Haxby 2000)) and the *amygdala* (emotional processing (Le Doux 2000)).

- Regions within the prefrontal cortex (PFC): the *orbitofrontal cortex* (OFC) (decision-making in the context of emotional situations (Rogers *et al.* 1999a; Bechara *et al.* 2000a), the *ventrolateral PFC* (VLPFC) (responding to reward-contingencies (Rogers *et al.* 1999b), the *dorsolateral PFC* (DLPFC) (executive functions and working memory (D'Esposito *et al.* 1999)), and the *dorsomedial PFC* (DMPFC) (self-reference, internal versus external focus (Craik *et al.* 1999; Gusnard *et al.* 2001)).

Thus, social cognition apparently arises from a coordinated neural network which gives rise to a pattern of processes that modulate action responses. The psychological outputs of these processes include memory, decision-making, attention, and motivation. Interestingly, the majority of brain structures subserving social cognition are also implicated in the processing of emotions. This demonstrates a putatively critical set of relations between feeling and thought and, perhaps not surprisingly, implicates the basis of disorders of emotion as occurring in the same neural systems (Grady and Keightley 2002).

In the context of MDD, positron emission tomography (PET) studies conducted on adult patients have demonstrated changes in regional cerebral blood flow (rCBF) and glucose metabolism in areas including the amygdala, the anterior cingulate, the OFC, and the DLPFC (Bench *et al.* 1992; Dolan *et al.* 1994; Elliott *et al.* 1997; Mayberg *et al.* 1999; Drevets 2001). Brain areas reportedly involved in higher cognitive function (i.e. the DLPFC) appear deactivated, while structures mediating emotional and stress responses (i.e. the amygdala) display increased activation. Reports of increased activity in the amygdala, in particular, have been interpreted as possibly reflecting stimulation of cortical structures involved in declarative memory, thus accounting for the tendency of individuals with depression to ruminate about memories that are emotionally negative (Drevets 2000). In addition, increased metabolic activity in the ventromedial PFC (VMPFC) has been associated with severity of depression (Drevets *et al.* 1997), and there is existing evidence that greater activity in the rostral cingulate may be critical in recovery from depression (Mayberg *et al.* 1997).

Of all these abnormalities, those located in regions where cerebral blood flow increases during normal and other pathological emotional states appear to depend on mood state, increasing or decreasing in response to the emotional and cognitive manifestations of the disorder. On the other hand, abnormalities found in orbital and medial PFC areas appear to persist following remission of symptoms, and in this case have been linked more often to the presence of anatomical differences between depressed and non-depressed individuals. These abnormalities are thought to be involved in the pathogenesis of depressive symptoms (Drevets 2000). More specifically, post-mortem studies of patients with MDD have reported reductions in cortical thickness, neuronal size, and neuronal and glial densities (Rajkowska *et al.* 1999), raising the possibility that these neuropathological changes bring about impairment in orbital function which then predispose an individual to disorder.

Both mood-state-dependent and anatomically based abnormalities are consistent not only with abnormalities shown during a state of clinical depression, but also with experimentally induced sad mood. Mayberg *et al.* (1999) demonstrated that provoked sadness was associated with increases in rCBF in ventral limbic and paralimbic regions (including the subgenual cingulate and insula), and also with decreases in rCBF in dorsal cortical regions (namely, right dorsal prefrontal, inferior parietal, dorsal anterior cingulate, and posterior cingulate). When compared with depressed individuals in remission, changes were reported in the same brain regions as in healthy individuals experiencing transient sadness, but in the reverse direction (namely, increases in dorsal cortical regions and decreases in ventral limbic and paralimbic regions). This was interpreted as an association between sad mood and a specific pattern of change in the limbic and cortical areas which are altered in depression, whereby resolution of negative mood symptoms in depressive illness would result in a normalization of this pattern. Similarly, an earlier study reported results from a mood induction procedure comparing individuals in remission with acutely depressed individuals and controls wherein mood-related changes were similar with the exception of the rostral cingulate (Mayberg *et al.* 1998). Decreased activity in this region within the remitted group, increased activity in the acutely ill patients, and no change in the control group suggested that this region may play a unique role in regulating emotional health (Mayberg *et al.* 1998).

Given that MDD appears to be associated with abnormal functioning in both higher cognitive and limbic domains, consensus is now emerging to explain the phenomenology of depression on the basis of a malfunction in the regulation of an entire network of brain regions involved in both emotional behaviour and social cognition (Mayberg *et al.* 1997). Supported by comparative anatomical studies, reciprocal pathways linking limbic structures (amygdala, cingulate, hypothalamus, and hippocampus) with widely distributed brainstem, striatal, paralimbic, and neocortical sites have been defined in rhesus monkeys (Pandya and Yeterian 1996) and associated with specific motivational and emotional behaviours in marmosets (Dias *et al.* 1996). Extrapolating from non-human primates to humans, we can perhaps assume that these same neural structures are responsible for the culmination of sensory, cognitive, and autonomic processing which exists at the core of both normal and abnormal emotional experience (Mayberg *et al.* 1999). These neural structures are now considered within two critical circuits: a limbic–thalamic–cortical (LTC) circuit, involving the amygdala, medial thalamus, and orbital and medial prefrontal cortices, and a limbic–cortical–striatal–pallidal–thalamic (LCSPT) circuit, involving components of the previous circuit with the addition of related parts of the striatum and pallidum (Drevets *et al.* 1992). The presence of these circuits supports a neural model of MDD in which dysfunction involving regions which modulate or inhibit emotional behaviour may, either directly or indirectly, result in the social cognitive deficits and emotional and behavioural manifestations of depression (Figure 8.1).

8.5 Clinical implications

MDD is one of the most disabling illnesses not only amongst mental disorders but also in comparison with the cost and consequences to public health of diseases such as cancer and cardiovascular disease. Studying the social cognition of individuals suffering from MDD has allowed a valuable insight into possible means of identification and treatment of those individuals in need, with many of the influential theories discussed in this chapter contributing significantly to currently available therapeutic approaches (i.e. cognitive behavioural therapy and mindfulness-based cognitive therapy). For this reason, it is clear that the social cognitive profile of a patient requires attention on the part of the clinician not only when it comes to interpreting reports of an individual's circumstances and symptoms, but also when assessing them in terms of suitability for a particular therapeutic approach. Equally valuable is the potential to use the relatively distinct social cognitive profiles described in this chapter to identify individuals either early on in the course of illness or even prior to onset in at-risk individuals; the ultimate goal being to develop a battery of assessments that combine traditional social cognitive tasks, such as those that tap into negative schema, processing biases, and response styles, with contemporary neuropsychological assessments of decision-making and the like to identify individuals who are at risk, but not yet ill, in order to intervene with psychological therapy before onset of illness.

8.6 Future directions of research

Although it is now generally accepted that MDD occurs throughout the lifespan from early childhood through to old age, with slight variations in the nature,

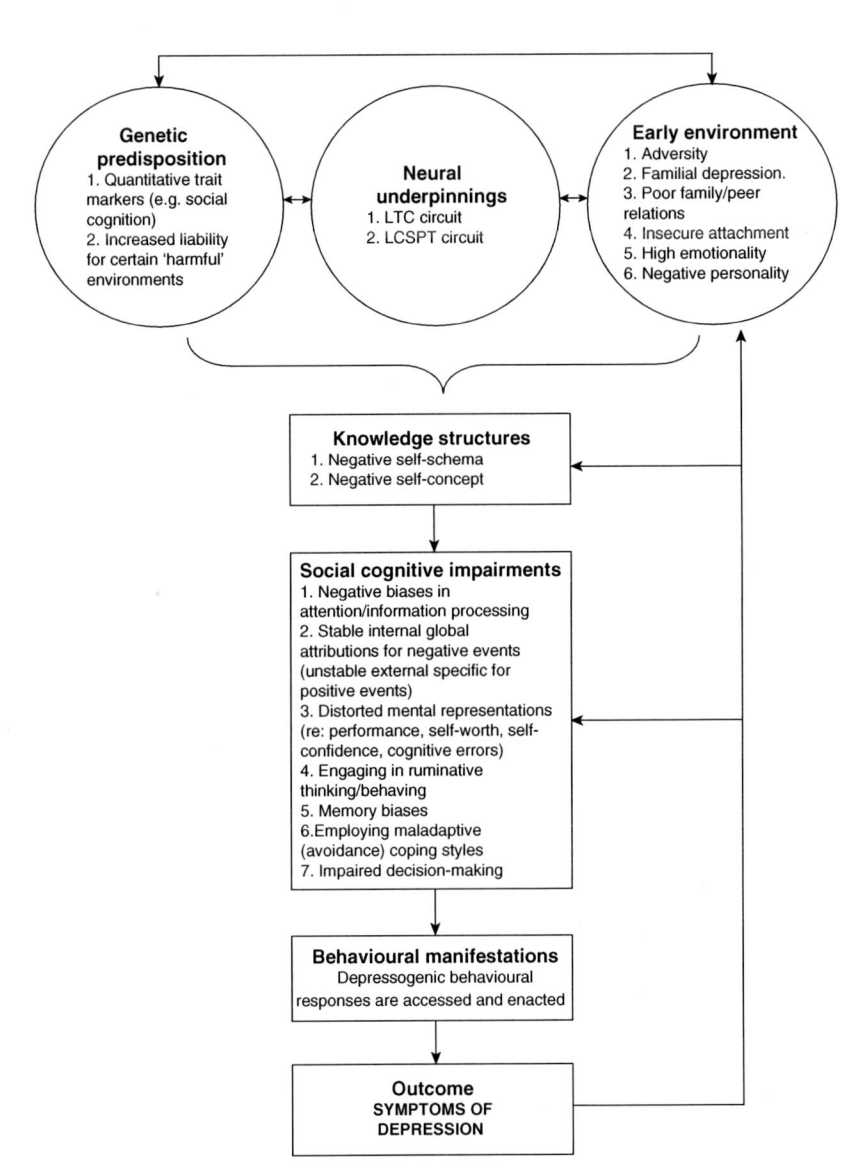

Figure 8.1 Schematic of the aetiology of depression and its associated social cognitive deficits.

characteristics, and outcomes of the condition with age (Kovacs 1996; Goodyer 2003), it remains to be firmly established whether children, adolescents, adults, and the elderly are suffering from the same disorder with a common aetiology and underlying mechanisms, and a similar response to treatment. We are currently not in a position to assume that social cognitive impairments, for example, are the same in first episode versus recurrent disorders, in younger versus older individuals, or in those at high versus low risk for psychopathology. Although studies of the development of neuropsychological processes have begun (Luciana and Nelson 1998; Kyte *et al.* 2005), we currently know little about the individual variations in social cognitive processing in the population at large, or how these critical mental processes evolve with development. Therefore it is important that future research includes a strategy that is focused on determining the similarities and differences in the nature and characteristics of MDD that occur across the lifespan (Goodyer 2003). We have also yet to characterize which social cognitive processing abnormalities predict the onset of an episode and distinguish between sporadic and recurrent or familial and non-familial disorders.

Although a considerable amount of research has already been dedicated to producing solid cognitive theories supported by experimentally sound research studies, one strategy which may assist in documenting the developmental progression, and indeed aetiology, of MDD will be to focus on the continued refinement of the affective–cognitive tasks and scientific approaches used in functional neuroimaging studies. This would allow us to determine the neural correlates that underpin mental processes in normal children, adolescents, adults, and the elderly, as well as in those at high risk for and suffering from serious mental illnesses such as MDD (Elliott *et al.* 2002). It is also hoped that the application of such future thinking will be equally extended to include examination of the wider range of internalizing disorders, including bipolar disorder and other mood disorder subtypes (i.e. dysthmia and cyclothymia), so as to increase specificity in both the formulation and treatment of internalizing disorders.

8.7 Conclusions

This chapter has discussed current knowledge regarding the social cognitive characterizations of child and adolescent MDD. Theoretical accounts and experimental findings converge in their support for a key role of social cognitive processes in the onset and persistence of MDD throughout the lifespan. Exactly how these processes interact with the neural systems thought to be responsible for the disorder remains a challenge for future research to address. Whilst we continue to advance our understanding of these delicate relationships, we remain relatively ignorant of the precise psychological processes which, if not functioning, result in depressive disorders. It seems highly likely that fully integrated social and performance functions are needed for mental competence and that it is the breakdown in one or more components involved in processing environmental stimuli that may result in MDD. Furthermore, it seems possible, even probable, that social cognitive impairments will vary according to the precise nature of the depression. Thus it remains an important objective to understand the phenotype of MDD on a number of psychological levels, in conjunction with developing our knowledge of the neural profiles that underpin these processes.

Acknowledgements

Zoë Kyte was supported by the Isaac Newton and Peterhouse Trusts. Ian Goodyer is supported by the Wellcome Trust and the MRC, UK.

References

Abramson, L.Y., Seligman, M.E.P., and Teasdale, J.D. (1978). Learned helplessness in humans: critique and reformulation. *Journal of Abnormal Psychology*, **87**, 49–74.

Adolphs, R. (2001). The neurobiology of social cognition. *Current Opinion in Neurobiology*, **11**, 231–9.

Altshuler, J.L. and Ruble, D.N. (1989). Developmental changes in children's awareness of strategies for coping with uncontrollable stress. *Child Development*, **60**, 1337–49.

American Psychiatric Association (1994). *Diagnostic and statistical manual for mental and behavioural disorders*, Vol. 4 (DSM-IV). Washington, DC: American Psychiatric Association.

Ayers, TS., Sandler, I.N., West, S.G., and Roosa, M.W. (1990). Assessment of children's coping behaviours: testing alternative models of children's coping. Presented at the American Psychological Association, Boston, MA.

Bandura, A., Pastorelli, C., Barbaranelli, C., and Caprara, G.V. (1999). Self-efficacy pathways to childhood depression. *Journal of Personality and Social Psychology*, **76**, 258–69.

Beats, B.C., Sahakian, B.J., and Levy, R. (1996). Cognitive performance in tests sensitive to frontal lobe dysfunction in the elderly depressed. *Psychological Medicine*, **26**, 591–603.

Bechara, A., Damasio, A., and Damasio, A.R. (2000a). Emotion, decision making and the orbitofrontal cortex. *Psychological Medicine*, **10**, 295–307.

Bechara, A., Tranel, D., and Damasio, H. (2000b). Characterisation of the decision-making deficit of patients with ventromedial prefrontal cortex lesions. *Brain*, **123**, 2189–202.

Beck, A.T. (1967). *Depression: clinical, experimental and theoretical aspects*. New York: Harper & Row.

Beck, A.T. (1976). *Cognitive therapy and the emotional disorders*. New York International Universities Press.

Bench, C.J., Friston, K.L., Brown, R.G., and Scott, L.C. (1992). The anatomy of melancholia: focal abnormalities of cerebral blood flow in unipolar depression. *Psychological Medicine*, **22**, 607–15.

Blumberg, H.P., Kaufman, J., Martin, A., Charney, D.S., Krystal, J.H., and Peterson, B.S. (2004). Significance of adolescent neurodevelopment for the neural circuitry of bipolar disorder. *Annals of the New York Academy of Science*, **1021**, 376–83.

Bower, G.H. (1981). Mood and memory. *American Psychologist*, **36**, 129–48.

Bradley, B.P., Mogg, K., and Williams, R. (1995). Implicit and explicit memory for emotion-congruent information in clinical depression and anxiety. *Behaviour Research and Therapy*, **33**, 755–70.

Bradley, B.P., Moog, K., and Lee, S.C. (1997). Attentional biases for negative information in induced and naturally occurring dysphoria. *Behaviour Research and Therapy*, **35**, 911–27.

Brown, G.W. and Harris, T. (1978). *Social origins of depression: a study of psychiatric disorder in women*. London: Tavistock Publications.

Brittlebank, A.D., Scott, J., Williams, J.M.G., and Ferrier, I.N. (1993). Autobiographical memory in depression: state or trait marker? *British Journal of Psychiatry*, **162**, 118–21.

Bruder-Mattson, S.F. and Hovanitz, C.A. (1990). Coping and attributional styles as predictors of depression. *Journal of Clinical Psychology*, **46**, 557–65.

Bush, G., Whalen, P.J., Rosen, B.R., McInerney, S.C., and Jenike, M.A. (1998). The emotional counting Stroop paradigm: an interference task specialised for functional neuroimaging validation study with functional MRI. *Human Brain Mapping*, **6**, 270–82.

Casey, B.J. (1999). Images in neuroscience. Brain development. XII: Maturation in brain activation. *American Journal of Psychiatry*, **156**, 504.

Clark, D.M. and Teasdale, J.D. (1985). Constraints on the effect of mood on memory. *Journal of Personality and Social Psychology*, **48**, 1595–1608.

Compas, B.E., Malcarne, V., and Fondacaro, K.M. (1988). Coping with stressful events in older children and adolescents. *Journal of Consulting and Clinical Psychology*, **56**, 405–11.

Compas, B.E., Banez, G.A., Malcarne, V., and Worsham, N. (1991). Perceived control and coping with stress: a developmental perspective. *Journal of Social Issues*, **47**, 23–34.

Corcico, A. and McGuffin, P. (2001). Psychiatric genetics: recent advances and clinical implications. *Epidemioligica Psychiatrica*, **10**, 253–9.

Corruble, E., Damy, C., and Guelfi, J.D. (1999). Impulsivity: a relevant dimension in depression regarding suicide attempts? *Journal of Affective Disorders*, **53**, 211–15.

Corwin, J., Peselow, E., Feenan, K., Rotrosen, J., and Fieve, R. (1990). Disorders of decision in affective disease: an effect of β-adrenergic dysfunction? *Biological Psychiatry*, **27**, 813–33.

Costello, E.J., Angold, A., Burns, B.J., *et al*. (1996). The Great Smoky Mountains Study of Youth. Goals, design, methods, and the prevalence of DSM-III-R disorders. *Archives of General Psychiatry*, **53**, 1129–36.

Craik, F.I.M., Moroz, T.M., Moscovitch, M., Stuss, D.T., Winocur, G., and Tulving, E. (1999). In search of the self: a positron emission tomography investigation. *Psychological Science*, **10**, 26–34.

Crick, N.R. and Dodge, K.A. (1994). A review and reformulation of social-information processing mechanisms in children's development. *Psychological Bulletin*, **115**, 74–101.

Damasio, A.R., Tranel, D., and Damasio, H. (1990). Individuals with sociopathic behaviour caused by frontal damage fail to respond automatically to social stimuli. *Behavioural Brain Research*, **4**, 81–94.

Decety, J. and Grezes, J. (1999). Neural mechanisms subserving the perception of human actions. *Trends in Cognitive Science*, **3**, 172–8.

Den Hartog, H.M., Derix, M.M., Van Bemmel, A.L., Kremer, B., and Jolles, J. (2003). Cognitive functioning in young and middle-aged unmedicated out-patients with major depression: testing the effort and cognitive speed hypotheses. *Psychological Medicine*, **33**, 1443–51.

Dent, J. and Teasdale, J.D. (1987). Negative cognitions and the persistence of depression. *Journal of Abnormal Psychology*, **97**, 29–34.

D'Esposito, M., Postle, B.R., Ballard, D., and Lease, J. (1999). Maintenance versus manipulation of information held in working memory: an event-related fMRI study. *Brain and Cognition*, **41**, 66–86.

Dias, R., Roberts, A.C., and Robbins, T.W. (1996). Dissociation in prefrontal cortex of affective and attentional shifts. *Nature*, **380**, 69–72.

Dickman, S.J. (1990). Functional and dysfunctional impulsivity: personality and cognitive correlates. *Journal of Personality and Social Psychology*, **58**, 95–102.

Dodge, K.A. (1986). A social information processing model of social competence in children. In *Minnesota Symposium in Child Psychology*, Vol 18 (ed. M. Perlmutter), pp. 77–125. Hillsdale, NJ: Lawrence Erlbaum.

Dodge, K.A. (1993). Social-cognitive mechanisms in the development of conduct disorder and depression. *Annual Reviews of Psychology*, **44**, 559–84.

Dolan, R.J., Bench, C.J., Brown, R.G., Scott., L.C., and Frackowiak, R.S.J. (1994). Neuropsychological dysfunction in depression: the relationship to regional cerebral blood flow. *Psychological Medicine*, **24**, 849–57.

Drevets, W.C. (2000). Neuroimaging studies of mood disorders. *Biological Psychiatry*, **48**, 813–29.

Drevets, W.C. (2001). Neuroimaging and neuropathological studies of depression: implications for the cognitive-emotional features of mood disorders. *Current Opinion in Neurobiology*, **11**, 240–9.

Drevets, W.C., Videen, T.O., Price, J.L., Preskorn, S.H., Carmichael, S.T., and Raichle, M.E. (1992). A functional anatomical study of unipolar depression. Journal of Neuroscience, **12**, 3628–3641.

Drevets, W.C., Price, J.L., Simpson, J.R., Todd, R.D., Reich, T., and Vannier, M. (1997). Subgenual prefrontal cortex abnormalities in mood disorders. *Nature*, **386**, 824–7.

Edelman, R.E., Ahrens, A.H., and Haaga, D.A.F. (1994). Inferences about the self, attributions, and overgeneralisation as predictors of recovery from dysphoria. *Cognitive Therapy and Research*, **18**, 551–66.

Eley, T.C. and Plomin, R. (1997). Genetic analyses of emotionality. *Cognitive Therapy and Research*, **7**, 279–84.

Elliott, R., Sahakian, B.J., McKay, A.P., Herrod, J.J., Robbins, T.W., and Paykel E.S. (1996). Neuropsychological impairment in unipolar depression: the influence of perceived failure on subsequent performance. *Psychological Medicine*, **26**, 975–89.

Elliott, R., Baker, S.C., Rogers, R.D., *et al.* (1997). Prefrontal dysfunction in depressed patients performing a complex planning task: a study using positron emission tomography. *Psychological Medicine*, **27**, 931–42.

Elliott, R., Rubinsztein, J.S., Sahakian, B.J., and Dolan, R.J. (2002). The neural basis of mood-congruent processing biases in depression. *Archives of General Psychiatry*, **59**, 597–604.

Erickson, K., Drevets, W.C., Clark, L., *et al.* (2005). Mood-congruent bias in affective go, no-go performance of unmedicated patients with Major Depressive Disorder. *American Journal of Psychiatry*, **162**, 2171–2173.

Evans, J., Heron, J., Lewis, G., Araya, R., and Wolke, D. (2005). Negative self-schemas and the onset of depression in women: longitudinal study. *British Journal of Psychiatry*, **186**, 302–7.

Fernandez Prieto, M., Goncalves, O.F., Buela-Casal, G., and Machado, P.P. (2004). Comparative analysis of attributional style and self-esteem in a sample of depressed patients and normal control subjects. *Actas Españolas de Psiquiatría*, 32, 259–63.

Fincham, F.D., Diener, C.I., and Hokoda, A. (1987). Attributional style and learned helplessness: relationship to the use of causal schemata and depressive symptoms in children. *British Journal of Social Psychology*, 26, 1–7.

Fleming, J.E. and Offord, D.R. (1990). Epidemiology of childhood depressive disorders: a critical review. *Journal of the American Academy of Child and Adolescent Psychiatry*, 29, 571–80.

Franke, P., Maier, W., Hardt, J., Frieboes, R., Lichtermann, D., and Hain, C. (1993). Assessment of frontal lobe functioning in schizophrenia and unipolar depression. *Psychopathology*, 26, 76–84.

Gallardo Perez, M., Banos Rivera, R.M., Belloch Fuster, A., and Ruiperez Rodriguez, M.A. (1999). Attentional biases and vulnerability to depression. *Spanish Journal of Psychology*, 2, 11–19.

Giedd, J.N. (2004). Structural magnetic resonance imaging of the adolescent brain. *Annals of the New York Academy of Science*, 1021, 77–85.

Gladstone, T.R.G. and Kaslow, N.J. (1995). Depression and attributions in children and adolescents: a meta-analytic review. *Journal of Abnormal Child Psychology*, 23, 597–606.

Gladstone, T.R.G., Kaslow, N.J., Seeley, J.R., and Lewinsohn, P.M. (1997). Sex differences, attributional style, and depressive symptoms among adolescents. *Journal of Abnormal Child Psychology*, 25, 297–305.

Goddard, L., Dritschel, B., and Burton, A. (1996). Role of autobiographical memory in social problem solving and depression. *Journal of Abnormal Psychology*, 105, 609–16.

Goodyer, I.M. (2003). Unipolar depression across the lifespan: issues and prospects. In *Unipolar depression: a lifespan perspective* (ed. I.M. Goodyer), pp. 180–203. Oxford University Press.

Goodyer, I.M., Herbert, J., Tamplin, A., and Altham, P.M. (2000). Recent life events, cortisol, dehydroepiandrosterone and the onset of major depression in high-risk adolescents. *British Journal of Psychiatry*, 177, 499–504.

Gotlib, I.H. and Cane, D.B. (1987). Construct accessibility and clinical depression: a longitudinal investigation. *Journal of Abnormal Psychology*, 96, 199–204.

Gotlib, I.H., Lewinsohn, P.M., Seeley, J.R., Rohde, P., and Redner, J.E. (1993). Negative cognitions and attributional style in depressed adolescents: an examination of stability and specificity. *Journal of Abnormal Psychology*, 102, 607–15.

Gotlib, I.H., Kasch, K.L., Traill, S., Joorman, J., and Arnow, B.A. (2004a). Coherence and specificity of information-processing biases in depression and social phobia. *Journal of Abnormal Psychology*, 111, 386–98.

Gotlib, I.H., Krasnoperova, E., Yue, D.N., and Joorman, J. (2004b). Attentional biases for negative interpersonal stimuli in clinical depression. *Journal of Abnormal Psychology*, 113, 121–35.

Grady, C.L. and Keightley, M.L. (2002). Studies of altered social cognition in neuropsychiatric disorders using functional neuroimaging. *Canadian Journal of Psychiatry*, 47, 327–36.

Gusnard, D.A., Akbudak, E., Shulman, G.L., and Raichle, M.E. (2001). Medial prefrontal cortex and self-referential mental activity: relation to a default mode of brain function. *Proceedings of the National Academy of Sciences of the USA*, **98**, 4259–4264.

Hammen, C. and Zupan, B.A. (1984). Self-schema, depression, and the processing of personal information in children. *Journal of Experimental Child Psychology*, **37**, 598–608.

Harrington, R. and Clark, A. (1998). Prevention and early intervention for depression in adolescence and early adult life. *Archives of Psychiatry and Clinical Neuroscience*, **248**, 32–45

Harrington, R., Rutter, M., and Fombonne, E. (1996). Developmental pathways in depression: multiple meanings, antecedents, and endpoints. *Development and Psychopathology*, **8**, 601–16.

Haxby, J.V., Horwitz, B., Ungerleider, L.G., Maisog, J.M., Pietrini, P., and Grady, C.L. (1994). The functional organisation of human extrastriate cortex: a PET-rCBF study of selective attention to faces and locations. *Journal of Neuroscience*, **14**, 6336–53.

Hazell, P., O'Connell, D., Heathcote, D., Robertson, J., and Henry, D. (1995). Efficacy of tricyclic drugs in treating child and adolescent depression. *British Medical Journal*, **310**, 897–901.

Hedlund, S. and Rude, S.S. (1995). Evidence of latent depressive schemas in formerly depressed individuals. *Journal of Abnormal Psychology*, **104**, 517–25.

Herman-Stahl, M.A., Stemmler, M., and Petersen, A.C. (1995). Approach and avoidant coping: implications for adolescent mental health. *Journal of Youth and Adolescence*, **24**, 649–65.

Hoffman, E.A. and Haxby, J.V. (2000). Distinct representations of eye gaze and identity in the distributed human neural system for face perception. *Nature Neuroscience*, **3**, 80–4.

Hughes, C. (2005). Executive functions. In *Cambridge Encyclopedia of Child Development* (ed. B. Hopkins), pp. 313–16. Cambridge University Press.

Jaenicke, C., Hammen, C., Zupan, B., Hiroto, D., Gordon, D., Adrian, C., and Burge, D. (1987). Cognitive vulnerability in children at risk for depression. *Journal of Abnormal Child Psychology*, **15**, 559–72.

Jaffee, S.R., Moffitt, T.E., Caspi, A., Fombonne, E., Poulton, R., and Martin, J. (2002). Differences in early childhood risk factors for juvenile-onset and adult-onset depression. *Archives of General Psychiatry*, **59**, 215–22.

Johnson, J.G., Crofton, A., and Feinstein, S.B. (1996). Enhancing attributional style and positive life events predict increased hopefulness among depressed psychiatric inpatients. *Motivation and Emotion*, **20**, 285–97.

Johnson, J.G., Han, Y.S., Douglas, C.J., Johannet, C.M., and Russell, T. (1998). Attributions for positive life events predict recovery from depression among psychiatric inpatients: an investigation of the Needles and Abramson model of recovery from depression. *Journal of Consulting and Clinical Psychology*, **66**, 369–76.

Joiner, T.E., Jr (2000). A test of the hoplessness theory of depression in youth psychiatric inpatients. *Journal of Clinical Child Psychology*, **29**, 167–76.

Joiner, T.E., Jr and Rudd, M.D. (1995). Negative attributional style for interpersonal events and the occurrence of severe interpersonal disruptions as predictors of self-reported suicidal ideation. *Suicide and Life Threatening Behaviour*, **25**, 297–304.

Joiner, T.E., Jr and Wagner, K.D. (1995). Parental, child-centered attributions and outcome: a meta-analytic review with conceptual and methodological implications. *Journal of Abnormal Child Psychology*, **24**, 37–52.

Just, N. and Alloy, L.B. (1997). The Response Styles theory of depression: tests and an extension of the theory. *Journal of Abnormal Psychology*, **106**, 221–9.

Kaslow, N.J., Rehm, L.P., and Siegel, A.W. (1984). Social-cognitive and cognitive correlates of depression in children. *Journal of Abnormal Child Psychology*, **12**, 605–20.

Kaufman, J. and Ryan, N. (1999). The neurobiology of child and adolescent depression. In *The neurobiological foundation of mental illness* (ed. D. Charney, E. Nestler, and B. Bunny), pp. 810–22. New York: Oxford University Press.

Keller, M.B., Ryan, N.D., Strober, M., *et al.* (2001). Efficacy of paroxetine in the treatment of adolescent major depression: a randomised, controlled trial. *Journal of the American Academy of Child and Adolescent Psychiatry*, **40**, 762–72.

Kelvin, R.G., Goodyer, I.M., Teasdale, J.D., and Brechin, D. (1999). Latent negative self-schema and high emotionality in well adolescents at risk for psychopathology. *Journal of Child Psychology and Psychiatry*, **40**, 959–68.

Kendler, K.S. and Karkowski-Shuman, L. (1997). Stressful life events and genetic liability to major depression: genetic control of exposure to the environment? *Psychological Medicine*, **27**, 539–47.

Kendler, K.S., Kessler, R.C., Walters, E.E., *et al.* (1995). Stressful life events, genetic liability, and onset of an episode of major depression in women. *American Journal of Psychiatry*, **152**, 833–42.

Kerr, N., Scott, J., and Philips M.L. (2005). Patterns of attentional deficits and emotional bias in bipolar and major depressive disorder. *British Journal of Clinical Psychology*, **44**, 343–56.

King, C.A., Naylor, M.W., Segal, H.G., Evans, T., and Shain B.N. (1993). Global self-worth, specific self-perceptions of competence, and depression in adolescents. *Journal of the American Academy of Child and Adolescent Psychiatry*, **32**, 745–52.

Koster, E.H., De Raedt, R., Goeleven, E., Franck, E., and Crombez, G. (2005). Mood-congruent attentional bias in dysphoria: maintained attention to and impaired disengagement from negative information. *Emotion*, **5**, 446–55.

Kovacs, M. (1996). Presentation and course of major depressive disorder during childhood and later years of the life span. *Journal of the American Academy of Child and Adolescent Psychiatry*, **35**, 705–15.

Kyte, Z.A. (2003). Executive abilities and social coping in adolescents with and without first episode unipolar depression. PhD thesis, Department of Psychiatry, University of Cambridge.

Kyte, Z.A., Goodyer, I.M., and Sahakian, B.J. (2005). Selected executive skills in adolescents with recent first episode major depression. *Journal of Child Psychology and Psychiatry*, **46**, 995–1005.

Le Doux, J.E. (2000). The amygdala and emotion: a view through fear. In *The amygdala. A functional analysis* (ed. J. P. Aggleton), pp. 289–310. Oxford University Press.

Lefkowitz, M.M., Tesiny, E.P., and Gordon, N.H. (1980). Childhood depression, family income and locus of control. *Journal of Nervous and Mental Diseases*, **168**, 732–5.

Leitenberg, H., Yost, L.W., and Carroll-Wilson, M. (1986). Negative cognitive errors in children: questionnaire development, normative data, and comparisons between children with and without self-reported symptoms of depression, low self-esteem, and evaluation anxiety. *Journal of Consulting Clinical Psychology*, **54**, 528–36.

Lewinsohn, P.M., Duncan, E.M., Stanton, A.K., and Hautziner, M. (1986). Age at onset for first unipolar depression. *Journal of Abnormal Psychology*, **95**, 378–83.

Lewinsohn, P.M., Hops, H., Roberts, R.E., Seeley, J.R., and Andrews, J.A. (1993). Adolescent psychopathology. I: Prevalence and incidence of depression and other DSM-III-R disorders in high school students. *Journal of Abnormal Psychology*, **102**, 133–44.

Lewinsohn, P.M., Roberts, R.E., Seeley, J.R., Rohde, R., Gotlib, I.H., and Hops, H. (1994). Adolescent psychopathology. II: Psychosocial risk factors for depression. *Journal of Abnormal Psychology*, **103**, 302–15.

Luciana, M. and Nelson, C.A. (1998). The functional emergence of prefrontally-guided working memory systems in four-to-eight-year-old children. *Neuropsychologia*, **36**, 273–93.

Luciana, M., Lindeke, L., Georgieff, M., Mills, M., and Nelson, C.A. (1999). Neurobehavioural evidence for working memory deficits in school-aged children with histories of prematurity. *Developmental Medicine and Child Neurology*, **41**, 521–33.

Lupien, S.J., Nair, N.P., Brier, S., *et al.* (1999). Increased cortisol levels and impaired cognition in human ageing: Implication for depression and dementia in later life. *Review of Neuroscience*, **10**, 117–39.

Lyubomirsky, S. and Nolen-Hoeksema, S. (1995). Effects of self-focused rumination on negative thinking and interpersonal problem solving. *Journal of Personality and Social Psychology*, **69**, 176–90.

Lyubomirsky, S., Caldwell, N.D., and Nolen-Hoeksema, S. (1998). Effects of rumination and distracting responses to depressed mood on retrieval of autobiographical memories. *Journal of Personality and Social Psychology*, **75**, 166–77.

McCabe, S.B. and Gotlib, I.H. (1995). Selective attention and clinical depression: performance on a deployment-of-attention task. *Journal of Abnormal Psychology*, **104**, 241–5.

McCauley, E., Mitchell, J.R., Burke, P., and Moss, S. (1988). Cognitive attributes of depression in children and adolescents. *Journal of Consulting Clinical Psychology*, **56**, 903–8.

McCauley, E., Pavlidis, K., and Kendall, K. (2001). Developmental precursors of depression: the child and the social environment. In *The depressed child and adolescent* (ed. I.M. Goodyer), pp. 46–78. Cambridge University Press.

McFarland, C. and Buehler, R. (1998). The impact of negative affect on autobiographical memory: the role of self-focused attention to moods. *Journal of Personality and Social Psychology*, **75**, 1424–40.

MacLeod, C., Matthews, A., and Tata, P. (1986). Attentional bias in emotional disorders. *Journal of Abnormal Psychology*, **95**, 15–20.

MacLeod, C. and Rutherford, E.M. (1992). Anxiety and selective processing of emotional information: mediating roles of awareness, trait and state variables, and personal relevance of stimulus materials. *Behaviour Research Therapy*, **30**, 479–91.

McNally, R.J., Litz, B.T., Prassas, A., Shin, L.M., and Weathers, F.W. (1994). Emotional priming of autobiographical memory in post-traumatic stress disorder. *Cognition and Emotion*, **8**, 351–67.

McNally, R.J., Lasko, N.B., Macklin, M.L., and Pitman, R.K. (1995). Autobiographical memory disturbance in combat-related post-traumatic stress disorder. *Behaviour Research and Therapy*, **33**, 619–30.

McNaughton, M.E., Patterson, T.L., Irwin, M.R., and Grant, I. (1992). The relationship of life adversity, social support and coping to hospitalization with unipolar depression. *Journal of Nervous and Mental Disease*, **180**, 491–7.

Marton, P., Connolly, J., Kutcher, S., and Korenblum, M. (1993). Cognitive social skills and social self-appraisal in depressed adolescents. *Journal of the American Academy of Child and Adolescent Psychiatry*, **32**, 739–44.

Matthews, A., Ridgeway, V., and Williamson, D.A. (1996). Evidence for attention to threatening stimuli in depression. *Behaviour Research and Therapy*, **34**, 695–705.

Mayberg, H.S., Brannan, S.K., Mahurin, R.K., Jerabek, P.A., Brickman, J.S., and Tekell, J.L. (1997). Cingulate function in depression: a potential predictor of treatment response. *Neuroreport*, **8**, 1057–61.

Mayberg, H.S., Liotti, M., Brannan, S.K., McGinnis, S., Mahurin, R.K., and Jerabek, P.A. (1998). Disease and state-specific effects of mood challenge on rCBF. *NeuroImage*, **7**, S901.

Mayberg, H.S., Liotti, M., Brannan, S.K., *et al.* (1999). Reciprocal limbic-cortical function and negative mood: converging PET findings in depression and normal sadness. *American Journal of Psychiatry*, **156**, 675–82.

Meerum Terwogt, M. and Stegge, H. (2001). The development of emotional intelligence. In *The depressed child and adolescent* (ed. I.M Goodyer), pp. 24–45. Cambridge University Press.

Miller, P., Surtees, P.G., Kreitman, N.B., Ingham, J.G., and Sashidharan, S.P. (1985). Maladaptive coping reactions to stress. *Journal of Nervous and Mental Disease*, **172**, 707–16.

Mogg, K., Bradley, B.P., Williams, R., and Matthews, A. (1993). Subliminal processing of emotional information in anxiety and depression. *Journal of Abnormal Psychology*, **102**, 304–11.

Mogg, K., Bradley, B.P., and Williams, R. (1995). Attentional bias in anxiety and depression: the role of awareness. *British Journal of Clinical Psychology*, **34**, 17–36.

Muris, P., Schmidt, H., Lambrichs, R., and Meesters, C. (2001). Protective and vulnerability factors of depression in normal adolescents. *Behaviour Research and Therapy*, **39**, 555–65.

Murphy, F.C., Sahakian, B.J., Rubinsztein, J.S., *et al.* (1999). Emotional bias and inhibitory control processes in mania and depression. *Psychological Medicine*, **29**, 1307–21.

Murphy, F.C., Rubinsztein, J.S., Michael, A., *et al.* (2001). Decision-making cognition in mania and depression. *Psychological Medicine*, **31**, 679–93.

Nandrino, J.L., Pezard, L., Poste, A., Reveillere, C., and Beaune, D. (2002). Autobiographical memory in major depression: a comparison between first-episode and recurrent patients. *Psychopathology*, **35**, 335–40.

Needles, D.J. and Abramson, L.Y. (1990). Positive life events, attributional style and hopefulness: testing a model of recovery from depression. *Journal of Abnormal Psychology*, **99**, 156–65.

Neshat-Doost, H.T., Moradi, A.R., Taghavi, M.R., Yule, W., and Dalgleish, T. (2000). Lack of attentional bias for emotional information in clinically depressed children and adolescents on the dot probe task. *Journal of Child Psychology and Psychiatry*, **41**, 363–8.

Nolan, S.A., Roberts, J.E., and Gotlib, I.H. (1998). Neuroticism and ruminative response style as predictors of change in depressive symptomatology. *Cognitive Therapy and Research*, **22**, 445–55.

Nolen-Hoeksema, S. (1987). Sex differences in unipolar depression: evidence and theory. *Psychological Bulletin*, **101**, 259–82.

Nolen-Hoeksema, S. (1991). Responses to depression and their effects on the duration of depressive episodes. *Journal of Abnormal Psychology*, **100**, 569–582.

Nolen-Hoeksema, S. (2000). The role of rumination in depressive disorders and mixed anxiety/depressive symptoms. *Journal of Abnormal Psychology*, **109**, 504–11.

Nolen-Hoeksema, S. and Morrow, J. (1991). A prospective study of depression and post-traumatic stress symptoms after a natural disaster: the 1989 Loma Prieta earthquake. *Journal of Personality and Social Psychology*, **61**, 115–21.

Nolen-Hoeksema, S. and Morrow, J. (1993). Effects of rumination and distraction on naturally occurring depressed mood. *Cognition and Emotion*, **7**, 561–70.

Nolen-Hoeksema, S., Girgus, J.S., and Seligman, M.E.P. (1986). Learned helplessness in children: a longitudinal study of depression, achievement, and exploratory style. *Journal of Personality and Social Psychology*, **51**, 435–42.

Nolen-Hoeksema, S., Morrow, J., and Fredrickson, B.L. (1993). Response styles and the duration of episodes of depressed mood. *Journal of Abnormal Psychology*, **102**, 20–8.

Nolen-Hoeksema, S., Parker, L.E., and Larson, J. (1994). Ruminative coping with depressed mood following loss. *Journal of Personality and Social Psychology*, **67**, 92–104.

Nolen-Hoeksema, S., Larson, J., and Grayson, C. (1999). Explaining the gender difference in depressive symptoms. *Journal of Personality and Social Psychology*, **77**, 1061–72.

Paelecke-Habermann, Y., Pohl, J., and Leplow, B. (2005). Attention and executive functions in remitted major depression patients. *Journal of Affective Disorders*, **89**, 125–35.

Pandya, D.N. and Yeterian, E.H. (1996). Comparison of prefrontal architecture and connections. *Philosophical Transactions of the Royal Society, London B, Biological Science*, **29**, 1423–32.

Pardo, J.V., Pardo, P.J., Janer, K.W., and Raichle, M.E. (1990). The anterior cingulated cortex mediates processing selection in the Stroop attentional conflict paradigm. *Proceedings of the National Academy of Sciences of the USA*, **87**, 256–9.

Park, R.J., Goodyer, I.M., and Teasdale, J.D. (2002). Categoric overgeneral autobiographical memory in adolescents with major depressive disorder. *Psychological Medicine*, **32**, 267–76.

Park, R.J., Goodyer, I.M., and Teasdale, J.D. (2004). Effects of induced rumination and distraction on mood and overgeneral autobiographical memory in adolescent major depressive disorder and controls. *Journal of Child Psychology and Psychiatry*, **45**, 996–1006.

Paus, T., Petrides, M., Evans, A.C., and Meyer, E. (1993). Role of the human anterior cingulated cortex in the control of oculomotor, manual, and speech responses: a positron emission tomography study. *Journal of Neurophysiology*, **70**, 453–69.

Paykel, E.S. (1978). The contribution of life events to the causation of psychiatric illness. *Psychological Medicine*, **8**, 245–53.

Paykel, E.S., Myers, J.K., and Dienelt, M.N. (1969). Life events and depression: a controlled inquiry. *Archives of General Psychiatry*, **32**, 327–33.

Peeters, F., Wessel, I., Merckelbach, H., and Boon-Vermeeren, M. (2002). Autobiographical memory specificity and the course of major depressive disorder. *Comparative Psychiatry*, **43**, 344–50.

Perrez, M. and Reicherts, M. (1992). Depressed people coping with aversive situations. In *Stress, coping and health: a situation-behaviour approach. Theory, methods and applications* (ed. M. Perrez and Meinrad), pp 103–11. Seattle, WA: Hogrefe and Huber.

Price, J.L. (1999). Prefrontal cortical networks related to visceral function and mood. *Annals of the New York Academy of Science,* **877,** 383–96.

Puce, A., Allison, T., Bentin, S., Gore, J.C., and McCarthy, G. (1998). Temporal cortex activation in humans viewing eye and mouth movements. *Journal of Neuroscience,* **18,** 2188–99.

Rahman, S., Robbins, T.W., and Sahakian, B.J. (1999). Comparative cognitive neuropsychological studies of frontal lobe function: implications for therapeutic strategies in frontal variant frontotemporal dementia. *Dementia and Geriatric Cognitive Disorders,* **10**(Suppl. 1), 15–28.

Rajkowska, G., Miguel-Hidalgo, J.J., Wei, J., *et al.* (1999). Morphometric evidence for neuronal and glial prefrontal cell pathology in major depression. *Biological Psychiatry,* **45,** 1085–98.

Reese, E. (2002). Social factors in the development of autobiographical memory: the state of the art. *Social Development,* **11,** 125–42.

Reynolds, C.F., Frank, E., and Perel, J.M. (1999). Nortryptiline and interpersonal psychotherapy as maintenance therapies for recurrent major depression: a randomised controlled trial in patients older than 59 years. *Journal of the American Medical Association,* **281,** 39–45.

Rogers, R.D., Everitt, B.J., Baldacchino, A., *et al.*(1999a). Dissociable deficits in the decision-making cognition of chronic amphetamine abusers, opiate abusers, patients with focal damage to prefrontal cortex, and tryptophan-depleted normal volunteers: evidence for monoaminergic mechanisms. *Neuropsychopharmacology,* **20,** 322–39.

Rogers, R.D., Owen, A.M., Middleton, H.C., *et al.* (1999b). Choosing between small, likely rewards and large, unlikely rewards activates inferior and orbital prefrontal cortex. *Journal of Neuroscience,* **20,** 9029–2038.

Rubinsztein, J.S., Michael, A., Paykel, E.S., and Sahakian, B.J. (2000). Cognitive impairment in remission in bipolar affective disorder. *Psychological Medicine,* **30,** 1025–36.

Rutter, M., Graham, P., Chadwick, O., and Yule, W. (1976). Adolescent turmoil: fact or fiction? *Journal of Child Psychology and Psychiatry,* **17,** 35–56

Saklofske, D.H. (1993). The position of N with non-clinical groups. *Proceedings of the 6th Meeting of the International Society for the Study of Individual Differences,* Baltimore, MD, p. 32.

Sandler, I.N., Tein, J.Y., and West, S.G. (1994). Coping, stress and the psychological symptoms of children of divorce: a cross-sectional and longitudinal study. *Child Development,* **65,** 1744–63.

Scourfield, J., Martin, N., Lewis, G., and McGuffin, P. (1999). Heritability of social cognitive skills in children and adolescents. *British Journal of Psychiatry,* **175,** 559–64.

Seligman, M.E.P. (1975). *Helplessness.* San Francisco, CA: W.H. Freeman.

Seligman, M.E.P., Peterson, C., Kaslow, N.J., Tanenbaum, R.L., Alloy, L.B., and Abramson, L.Y. (1984). Attributional style and depressive symptoms among children. *Journal of Abnormal Psychology,* **93,** 235–8.

Silberg, J., Pickles, A., Rutter, M., et al. (1999). The influence of genetic factors and life stress on depression among adolescent girls. *Archives of General Psychiatry*, **56**, 225–32.

Sowell, E.R., Thompson, P.M., Holmes, C.J., Jernigan, T.L., and Toga, A.W. (2000). In vivo evidence for post-adolescent brain maturation in frontal and striatal regions. *Nature Neuroscience*, **2**, 859–61.

Spence, S.H., Sheffield, J., and Donovan, C. (2002). Problem-solving orientation and attributional style: moderators of the impact of negative life events on the development of depressive symptoms in adolescence? *Journal of Clinical Child and Adolescent Psychology*, **31**, 219–29.

Sutton, L.J., Teasdale, J.D., and Broadbent, D.E. (1988). Negative self-schema: the effects of induced depressed mood. *British Journal of Clinical Psychology*, **27**, 188–90.

Sweeney, P.D., Anderson, K., and Bailey, S. (1986). Attributional style in depression: a meta-analytic review. *Journal of Personality and Social Psychology*, **50**, 974–91.

Taylor, S.F., Liberson, I., Fig, L.M., Decker, L.R., Minoshima, S., and Koeppe, R.A. (1998). The effect of emotional content on visual recognition memory: a PET activation study. *NeuroImage*, **8**, 188–97.

Teasdale, J.D. (1983). Negative thinking in depression: cause, effect or reciprocal relationship? *Advances in Behaviour Research and Therapy*, **5**, 3–26.

Teasdale, J.D. (1985). Psychological treatments for depression: how do they work? *Behaviour Research and Therapy*, **23**, 157–65.

Teasdale, J.D. and Barnard, P.J. (1993). *Affect, cognition and change: remodelling depressive thought*. Hillsdale, NJ: Lawrence Erlbaum.

Teasdale, J.D. and Cox, S.G. (2001). Dysphoria: self-devaluative and affective components in recovered depressed patients and never depressed controls. *Psychological Medicine*, **31**, 1311–16.

Teasdale, J.D. and Dent, J. (1987). Cognitive vulnerability to depression: an investigation of two hypotheses. *British Journal of Clinical Psychology*, **26**, 113–26.

Teasdale, J.D. and Fogarty, S.J. (1979). Differential effects of induced mood on retrieval of pleasant and unpleasant events from episodic memory. *Journal of Abnormal Psychology*, **88**, 248–57.

Teasdale, J.D., Taylor, M.J., and Fogarty, S.J. (1980). Effects of induced elation-depression on the accessibility of memories of happy and unhappy experiences. *Behaviour Research and Therapy*, **18**, 339–46.

Tennen, H., Herzberger, S., and Nelson, H.F. (1987). Depressive attributional style: the role of self-esteem. *Journal of Personality*, **55**, 631–60.

Thapar, A. and McGuffin, P. (1996). The genetic etiology of depressive symptoms: a developmental perspective. *Development and Psychopathology*, **8**, 751–60.

Tiggemann, M., Winefield, A.H., Winefield, H.R., and Goldney, R.D. (1991). The stability of attributional style and its relation to psychological distress. *British Journal of Clinical Psychology*, **30**, 247–55.

Tracy, A., Bauwens, F., Martin, F., Pardoen, D., and Mendlewicz, J. (1992). Attributional style and depression: a controlled comparison of remitted unipolar and bipolar patients. *British Journal of Clinical Psychology*, **31**, 83–4.

Tranel, D., Bechara, A., and Damasio, A.R. (2000). Decision making and the somatic marker hypothesis. In *The cognitive neurosciences* (2nd edn) (ed. M.S. Gazzaniga), pp. 1047–1106. Cambridge, MA: MIT Press.

Trapnell, P.D. and Campbell, J.D. (1999). Private self-consciousness and the five-factor model of personality: distinguishing rumination from reflection. *Journal of Personality and Social Psychology*, **76**, 284–304.

Treynor, W., Gonzalez, R., and Nolen-Hoeksema, S. (2003). Rumination reconsidered: a psychometric analysis. *Cognitive Therapy and Research*, **27**, 247–59.

Tulving, E. (1983). *Elements of episodic memory*. Oxford University Press.

Voelz, Z.R., Haeffel, G.J., Joiner, T.E., and Wagner, K.D. (2003). Reducing hopelessness: the iteration of enhancing and depressogenic attributional styles for positive and negative life events among youth psychiatric inpatients. *Behaviour Research and Therapy*, **41**, 1183–98.

Watkins, E. and Teasdale, J.D. (2001). Rumination and overgeneral memory in depression: effects of self-focus and analytic thinking. *Journal of Abnormal Psychology*, **110**, 353–7.

Watkins, E. and Teasdale, J.D. (2004). Adaptive and maladaptive self-focus in depression. *Journal of Affective Disorders*, **82**, 1–8.

Watkins, E., Teasdale, J.D., and Williams, R.M. (2000). Decentring and distraction reduce overgeneral autobiographical memory in depression. *Psychological Medicine*, **30**, 911–20.

Weisz, J.R., Weiss, B., Wasserman, A.A., and Rintoul, B. (1987). Control related beliefs and depression among clinic-referred children and adolescents. *Journal of Abnormal Psychology*, **96**, 58–63.

Whalen, P.J., Rauch, S.L., Etcoff, N.L., McInerney, S.C., Lee, M.B., and Jenike, M.A. (1998). Masked presentations of emotional facial expressions modulate amygdala activity without explicit knowledge. *Journal of Neuroscience*, **18**, 411–18.

Williams, J.M.G. (1996). Depression and the specificity of autobiographical memory. In *Remembering our past: studies in autobiographical memory* (ed. D. Rubin), pp. 244–67. Cambridge University Press.

Williams, J.M.G. and Broadbent, K. (1986). Autobiographical memory in suicide attempters. *Journal of Abnormal Psychology*, **95**, 144–9.

Williams, J.M.G. and Dritschel, B.H. (1992). Categoric and extended autobiographical memories. In *Theoretical perspectives on autobiographical memory* (ed. M.A. Conway, D.C. Rubin, H. Spinnler, and W.A. Wagenaar), pp. 391–412. Dordrecht: Kluwer Academic.

Williams, J.M.G. and Nulty, D.D. (1986). Construct accessibility, depression and the emotional Stroop task: transient mood or stable structure? *Personality and Individual Differences*, **7**, 485–91.

Williams, J.M. and Scott, J. (1988). Autobiographical memory in depression. *Psychological Medicine*, **18**, 689–95.

Williams, J.M.G., Ellis, N.C., Tyers, C., Healy, H., Rose, G., and MacLeod, A.K. (1996). The specificity of autobiographical memory and imageability of the future. *Memory and Cognition*, **24**, 116–25.

Williams, J.M.G., Teasdale, J.D., Segal, Z.S., and Soulsby, J. (2000). Mindfulness-based cognitive therapy reduces overgeneral autobiographical memory in formerly depressed patients. *Journal of Abnormal Psychology*, **109**, 150–5.

Wood, J.V., Saltzberg, J.A., Neale, J.M., Stone, A.A., and Rachmiel, T.A. (1990). Self-focused attention, coping responses, and distressed mood in everyday life. *Journal of Personality and Social Psychology*, **58**, 1027–36.

Zeidner, M. (1994). Personal and contextual determinants of coping and anxiety in an evaluative situation: a prospective study. *Personality and Individual Differences*, **16**, 899–918.

Zeidner, M. and Saklofske, D. (1996). Adaptive and maladaptive coping. In *Handbook of coping* (ed. M. Zeidner, and N.S. Endler), pp. 505–31. New York: John Wiley.

Zupan, B.A., Hammen, C., and Jaenicke, C. (1987). The effects of current mood and prior depressive history on self-schematic processing in children. *Journal of Experimental Child Psychology*, **43**, 149–58.

9
Social cognition and anxiety in children
Robin Banerjee

Social cognitive factors associated with anxiety in children and adolescents are addressed in this chapter. First, we examine the nature and prevalence of clinical anxiety disorders in youths, identify common diagnosis and assessment tools, and introduce the thorny issues surrounding comorbidity of anxiety and depression. Then, we turn to the links likely to exist between anxiety and patterns of social cognition. A substantial literature has conceptualized anxiety disorders in terms of cognitive information-processing biases that appear before, during, and after focal events. This research is extended by a smaller, but growing, body of work which concerns socially anxious children's reasoning about mental states and their understanding of social situations. The empirical work conducted on these topics will help to clarify our current state of knowledge regarding the social cognitive profile of anxious children. Next, we review possible factors in the aetiology of the social cognitive characteristics, before turning to the clinical implications of the research and possible directions for further work in this area.

9.1 Anxiety in children and adolescents

9.1.1 Description and assessment

Anxiety disorders are among the most prevalent of psychiatric diagnoses in childhood and adolescence. Taking into account variations in the diagnostic procedures for assessing children, we can expect 6–10 per cent of children to be suffering from an anxiety disorder, with prevalence tending to be higher among girls than among boys (Verhulst 2001). The DSM-IV (American Psychiatric Association 2000) identifies one anxiety disorder–separation anxiety disorder–that is diagnosed solely in children, along with numerous other disorders which can be applied as appropriate to both adults and children. The essential commonality underlying all these disorders is an unusually high level of anxiety or fear, associated with a range of possible internal or external cues which cause significant distress or impairment to everyday functioning. Table 9.1 lists the major forms of anxiety disorder (excluding those whose symptoms follow from medical conditions or substance use), together with the focus of anxiety for each disorder. In general, evidence on age of onset tends to point to specific phobias (especially animal phobias) and separation anxiety disorder as appearing earlier in childhood, with other disorders such as social phobia, agoraphobia, and obsessive–compulsive disorder tending to appear later in adolescence (Öst 1987; Öst and Treffers 2001). However, recent factor analyses of parent ratings of various anxious symptoms exhibited by preschoolers aged 2.5–6.5 years confirm that, even at this age, there is good evidence for differentiation among various subtypes of anxiety, such as social anxiety, fears of physical injury, and obsessive–compulsive disorder (Spence et al. 2001).

Clinical diagnoses of anxiety disorders are made using structured interview schedules, such as the Anxiety Disorders Interview Schedule for DSM-IV (Silverman and Albano 1996), but research on the topic of anxiety often identifies children who score relatively high on parent/teacher rating scales and/or self-report measures. Some such measures may be part of a broader assessment tool (e.g. the anxious–depressed scales within the Youth Self-Report

Table 9.1 Major DSM-IV anxiety disorders

Disorder	Focus of anxiety
Separation anxiety disorder	Separation from home or from attachment figures (e.g. parents)
Generalized anxiety disorder	Various events, activities, settings
Social phobia (social anxiety disorder)	Exposure to social or performance situations
Specific phobia	Exposure to a specific class of objects or situations (e.g. heights, spiders)
Agoraphobia	Open spaces or settings where escape is difficult or help is not accessible
Panic disorder	Sudden and acute physiological symptoms and accompanying fear
Obsessive–compulsive disorder	Persistent or repetitive thoughts or behaviours
Post-traumatic stress disorder	Re-experience of past traumatic event in thoughts, dreams, and responses to cues that symbolize the trauma, lasting more than a month
Acute stress disorder	Re-experience of past traumatic event, lasting no more than 4 weeks

and Child Behaviour Checklist instruments (Achenbach 1991a,b)). However, a number of measurement instruments specifically targeting anxiety and fears are now commonly used by researchers. Among the most established of these are the Fear Survey Schedule for Children–Revised (FSSC-R) (Ollendick 1983), the Revised Children's Manifest Anxiety Scale (RCMAS) (Reynolds and Richmond 1978), and the State-Trait Anxiety Inventory for Children (STAIC) (Spielberger 1973), all of which cover a range of fears and anxieties.

More recently, several scales have been constructed that are intended to fall more closely in line with dominant theoretical and clinical conceptualizations of anxiety, including the DSM classification categories: the Multidimensional Anxiety Scale for Children (MASC) (March et al. 1997), the Screen for Child Anxiety Related Emotional Disorders (SCARED) (Birmaher et al. 1997), and the Spence Children's Anxiety Scale (SCAS) (Spence 1998). A recent study by Muris et al. (2002) evaluated all six scales listed above in a sample of 521 adolescents and reported reasonable internal consistency for all of them as well as good convergent validity (i.e. substantial intercorrelations among the general anxiety scores and between subscale measures of specific forms of anxiety). It should be noted that additional scales have been designed to tap specific anxiety disorders. For example, self-report scales specifically designed to tap social anxiety include the Social Anxiety Scale for Children–Revised (SASC-R) (La Greca and Stone 1993) and the Social Phobia and Anxiety Inventory for Children (SPAI-C) (Beidel et al. 1995), both of which were found to have robust profiles of psychometric properties.

The existence of these types of scale, suitable for completion by children themselves from as young as 7 years of age, has facilitated the collection of data on both the prevalence of anxious symptomatology in large samples of children and the associations that anxious symptoms have with other emotional disorders, behavioural indicators, and cognitive characteristics. In many cases, the opportunity to identify correlates of anxious symptoms in unselected samples of young children serves to highlight factors which could play a role in the later emergence of clinically diagnosed disorders. For example, as discussed in more detail below, typically developing children's scores of self-reported anxiety have been associated with the same kinds of cognitive biases thought to be central to the maintenance of diagnosed anxiety disorders among older adolescents and adults.

9.1.2 Comorbidity with depression

Epidemiological studies as well as research studies into the correlates of anxiety show that anxious symptoms very often co-occur with depressive symptoms, for children as well as for adults. Indeed, Brady and Kendall's (1992) review of studies of children or adolescents, using DSM-III or DSM-IIIR criteria, showed that 15.9–61.9 per cent of samples identified as anxious or depressed met criteria for both conditions. Similarly, within the typically developing sample of children in Muris *et al.*'s (2002) study of six anxiety questionnaires, referred to above, the correlations of the total score on each questionnaire with the Children's Depression Inventory (CDI) score (Kovacs 1981) were high, with 0.50 as the smallest coefficient and four of the six greater than 0.70.

This high rate of co-occurrence of depressive and anxious symptoms raises significant theoretical questions about the conceptualization of the two types of disorder. A prominent framework for making sense of the major commonalities and differences between anxiety and depression is the tripartite model developed by Clark and Watson (1991). This model points to a general 'negative affectivity' factor as underlying the high concordance of anxious and depressed symptoms, but identifies low 'positive affectivity' as differentiating depression from anxiety and high physiological arousal as differentiating anxiety from depression.

In support of the tripartite model, Clark *et al.*'s (1994) study of psychiatric outpatients and undergraduate students provided empirical confirmation that factors specific to depression and anxiety could indeed be identified after controlling for the large negative affectivity factor. Turning to measurement of these factors in children, Chorpita *et al.* (2000) identified a combination of selected items from the CDI and RCMAS to constitute a 'negative affectivity' factor, selected items from the CDI to constitute a 'positive affectivity' factor, and selected items from the RCMAS to constitute a 'physiological hyper-arousal' factor. In a subsequent investigation by Turner and Barrett (2003), confirmatory factor analyses of data from 7-, 10-, and 13-year-olds supported the tripartite model as the most parsimonious and best-fitting model for all age groups. Similar evidence from second-order factor analysis of childhood anxiety and depression inventories is presented by Eley and Stevenson (1999). Thus, even among children, there is good reason to suppose that anxiety and depression share a generalized distress or negative affect factor, but have unique components as well.

A further direction of research focuses on the temporal sequence of anxious and depressed symptoms. Brady and Kendall (1992), for example, suggest that anxious symptoms tend to appear prior to depressed symptoms, explaining why children with comorbid anxiety and depression tend to be older than children with just one disorder. Indeed, Cole *et al.* (1998) conducted a longitudinal investigation of anxious (RCMAS) symptoms and depressed (CDI) symptoms among several hundred third- and sixth-graders over 3 years, and concluded that anxiety predicted increases in depression over time but that the reverse was not true. This is consistent with the proposition that anxiety predates depression, and matches evidence that, for example, age of onset for social phobia is often in mid-adolescence (e.g. Öst (1987) puts the mean at 16 years), while later and more variable ages of onset are typically given for depression (Ingram *et al.* 2001).

Notwithstanding the value of describing the temporal sequence in which anxious and depressive symptoms emerge, the tripartite model described above reminds us that there are likely to be significantly different proximal determinants of anxiety and depression. In particular, the arousal associated with anxiety is likely to be connected to a distinct profile of social cognitive characteristics. The following sections show that research has yielded important evidence pointing to social cognitive factors that are likely to provoke anxious symptoms. The more established literature on broad information-processing biases in anxious children's reasoning is examined first, before turning to recent work on social understanding and mental state reasoning.

9.2 Social information-processing characteristics

In this section we explore theory and empirical findings regarding information-processing characteristics associated with anxiety. It is important to note that, while distinctive patterns of information processing regarding *social* events and encounters are especially significant in the case of social anxiety disorder (as opposed to animal phobias, for example), the underlying theoretical constructs thought to be responsible for these patterns are often common to many or all anxiety disorders. In other words, understanding the social cognitive profile of socially anxious children requires an examination of broad information-processing biases that may operate across multiple domains. Therefore the discussion below introduces broad theoretical frameworks of information processing in relation to anxiety, before turning to specific empirical evidence regarding anxious children's reasoning about the world, and about themselves in relation to the world.

9.2.1 Cognitive theories of anxiety

A dominant approach to understanding anxiety focuses on the cognitive processes associated with perceptions of threat and subsequent processing of both external information (e.g. the threat stimulus) and internal information (e.g. one's coping responses). This emphasis on threat clearly maps onto the suggestion from the tripartite model that anxiety is specifically connected to hyper-arousal (Clark and Watson 1991).

A significant account of the information-processing characteristics related to anxiety was presented by Beck and Clark (1997), drawing on an earlier cognitive framework set out over a decade earlier (Beck *et al.* 1985).

In that paper, the authors pointed to three stages of processing connected to anxiety, involving various automatic and strategic thought processes. In the first stage, the theorists argue, rapid and automatic registration of the threat stimulus takes place. As discussed in the next section, empirical research appears to demonstrate that anxious children, like their adult counterparts, are particularly vigilant with respect to possible negative or threat stimuli. In the second stage of information processing, preparation of a response to the threat stimuli—to ensure safety and avoidance of danger—is considered to involve a range of both automatic and strategic processes. For example, controlled processes are thought to be responsible for constructing an appraisal of the threat stimulus, but automatic processes are engaged in the activation of cognitive (e.g. automatic thoughts), behavioural (e.g. escape), affective (e.g. fear), and physiological (e.g. autonomic arousal) responses. Most significantly for the topic of this chapter, Beck and Clark (1997, p. 53) argue that this stage involves 'a constriction or narrowing of *cognitive processing* that leads to certain biases and inaccuracies', such as hypersensitivity to negative cues at the expense of positive ones, overestimation of the threat, and cognitive elaboration of threat and danger themes. In the final stage, labelled secondary elaboration, a strategic processing of the connection between the perceived threat and one's own coping resources takes place. This reflection on the 'self in relation to the world' can lead to reductions or escalations in anxiety depending on one's appraisal of the current level of threat or of the coping resources available.

How does this framework for understanding anxiety disorders map onto developmental models of social cognition? In fact, the focus on encoding and appraisal of threat cues along with self-evaluation biases is entirely consistent with the social information-processing model constructed by Dodge (1986) and reformulated by Crick and Dodge (1994). Daleiden and Vasey (1997) successfully combined the insights from Kendall's (1985) cognitive-behavioural theory of psychopathology with Crick and Dodge's (1994) model. First, consistent with Beck and Clark's (1997) information-processing model, Kendall (1985) pointed to overactivity of schemas concerned with threat and danger as particularly important in anxiety. Daleiden and Vasey then turned to Crick and Dodge's six-stage model of social information processing to make sense of anxious symptoms. In that model, which can be applied to understanding diverse atypical patterns of responding including aggression as well as anxiety, children are said to (1) encode information in the environment, (2) interpret the encoded information, (3) clarify a goal to meet situational demands, (4) retrieve or construct possible responses, (5) evaluate those responses and make a selection, and (6) enact the selected response.

Crick and Dodge (1994) themselves explicitly highlighted the role of emotional states, including anxiety, in this model. They noted, for example, that anxiety may lead to more negative interpretations of social partners (step 2) and may lead to the construction of avoidant goals (step 3). Daleiden and Vasey's (1997) use of the social information-processing model as a framework for understanding anxiety elaborates on these connections. They argue that encoding biases can be found in terms of selective attention to threat-related information, that interpretation biases can lead to overly negative evaluations of ambiguous stimuli and more negative anticipated outcomes, and that these biases can encourage the adoption of avoidant or escape goals. In a similar vein, Daleiden and Vasey point out that even if knowledge of proactive problem-focused strategies is present, anxiety may be associated with a bias towards the selection of avoidant strategies and with difficulties in the enactment of positive social skills.

Overall, then, cognitive theories of anxiety point to characteristics of children's reasoning about the world around them—and about themselves in relation to that world—as central to their experience of anxiety. Putting together Beck and Clark's (1997) model with the social information-processing steps discussed by Daleiden and Vasey (1997), one can reasonably predict that the social cognition of children with anxiety disorders is likely to be characterized by hypervigilance regarding possible threat, threatening interpretation of social events, and negative appraisal of past encounters. The next section identifies empirical work supporting the existence of such biased social information processing before, during, and after encounters with the focal anxiety-eliciting object/setting.

9.2.2 Encoding of threat and negative cognition

The most prominent source of the 'physiological hyper-arousal' involved in anxiety is the perception of threat. Consistent with the cognitive theories identified above, there is good evidence that anxious children, like anxious adults, are more likely to encode negative/threat cues and more likely to interpret ambiguous stimuli as threatening. These biases are accompanied by other negative cognitions involving anticipation of outcomes and appraisal of the self.

Turning first to evidence regarding attentional biases, Vasey and colleagues have demonstrated that children with anxiety disorders or high levels of test anxiety exhibit a bias to attend to threatening words in comparison with neutral words (Vasey *et al.* 1995, 1996). Intriguingly, there is also some evidence of *avoidance* of negative stimuli. Eley *et al.* (2002), for example, showed with a sample of 79 children aged 8–10 years that increasing anxiety (and in particular social anxiety) was associated with greater avoidance of negative faces, in comparison with neutral faces, on a dot-probe task. Mansell *et al.* (1999) have demonstrated similar findings among socially anxious adults under conditions of social-evaluative threat. However, these two apparently contradictory sets of findings—one pointing to hypervigilance towards threatening stimuli and one suggesting avoidance of threatening stimuli—can be reconciled if one returns to the stage-based information-processing accounts discussed earlier. Specifically, there is increasing evidence that socially anxious adults display an initial rapid automatic orienting towards threat stimuli, but then a pattern of avoidant response to such stimuli. Vassilopoulos (2005) has demonstrated this empirically, showing that an attentional bias towards threatening words on a dot-probe task is present in socially anxious individuals when the probe appears for just 200 ms, but is reversed when the probe appears for 500 ms. Further research is needed to provide support for this hypervigilance–avoidance pattern in children.

The above discussion suggests that, at least in terms of initial orienting responses, there is likely to be a bias to encode threatening information among anxious individuals. Evidence from developmental studies also suggests that children's reasoning about social events is characterized by more negative interpretations of stimuli, expectations of outcomes, and evaluations of self. First, Hadwin *et al.* (1997) showed with a non-clinical sample of children aged 7–9 years that higher levels of trait anxiety were associated with a greater tendency to interpret homophones as threatening rather than neutral (e.g. interpreting 'cross' as angry rather than the symbol). Extending these findings, Muris *et al.* (2003) investigated children's interpretations of threat in response to five-sentence stories with themes relating to social anxiety (e.g. giving an oral report to the class), separation anxiety (e.g. staying with a friend while parents are away), or generalized anxiety (e.g. riding a bike on a very busy street). Children were asked to guess as quickly as possible whether each story they hear is a scary story which will have a bad ending or a non-scary story which will end well. Children also provided threat ratings and open-ended interpretations regarding what would happen in the story situations. Findings showed that both trait anxiety and state anxiety predicted increased perceptions of threat and a lower threat threshold (i.e. faster identification of stories as threatening), but also that trait anxiety continued to predict such threat perception abnormalities after controlling for state anxiety.

Importantly, evidence suggests that this greater perception of threat appears to be domain-general. First, a study using the story paradigm discussed above demonstrated that perception of threat on particular types of stories was not especially connected to corresponding anxiety subtypes (e.g. social anxiety did not have a particular relation to threat perception in the social anxiety stories) (Muris, Kindt, *et al.* 2000). Another study found greater threat perceptions among anxious children even in clearly non-threatening stories, leading the researchers to conclude that anxious children demonstrate a general view of the world as one where 'danger is lurking everywhere' (Muris, Luermans *et al.* 2000).

This notion of domain-generality in perceptions of threat has important implications for our understanding of the links between social cognition and anxiety disorders. If, as these authors suggested, threat perceptions are dependent on the general level of anxiety, rather than on specific anxiety symptoms, biases in *social* cognition should not be attributed only to those with *social* anxiety. Rather, a tendency to view the world in general—including social events and interactants—as threatening could underlie biased social cognition among children with different anxiety disorder subtypes. This proposition needs further examination in work with clinical samples of children with various anxiety disorders.

Notwithstanding this evidence of domain-generality in threat perceptions, it is certainly the case that perception and interpretation of *social* threat has been studied mainly in the context of socially anxious children's reasoning about their own social interactions. In one study of diagnosed social phobic children aged 7–14 years (Spence *et al.* 1999), participants' behaviour and social cognition were measured in the context of a social role-play task. In comparison with non-clinical controls, the social phobic children anticipated significantly poorer performance on the role-play task, in terms of how they thought they would perform compared with others and how they would be seen by others. Furthermore, they reported experiencing more negative cognitions during segments of their performance that were played back to the children on videotape. Not surprisingly, the children's state anxiety ratings were higher than those of controls both before and after the task. This evidence fits with the findings of threat perception abnormalities discussed earlier. Specifically, socially anxious children's negative cognition about interactions with other people, before and during those interactions, could be seen as a manifestation of a broader tendency to perceive threat in the world. Similarly, the heightened negative expectations and negative self-talk are consistent with cognitive-behavioural accounts of anxiety disorder that emphasize cognitive distortions that result from the dominance of schemas relating to threat and danger (see Kendall 1993). Moreover, the perception of social threat among social phobic children clearly corresponds to a view of the self as inadequately equipped to respond to the threat, thereby maintaining or escalating the already high level of anxiety.

The evidence discussed so far relates only to negative cognition before and during anxiety-eliciting encounters. However, Beck and Clark's (1997) information-processing model, discussed earlier, covers the notion of elaborative processing that takes place following the encounter. Clearly, negative or threatening interpretations of stimuli are likely to have psychological significance that extends beyond the duration of the encounter with the stimuli.

In particular, two further aspects of negative cognition could follow from the interpretation biases identified above: a tendency to evaluate one's performance in the encounter more negatively, and a tendency for selective recollection of negative memories.

Indeed, there is already some evidence that anxious individuals rate their own performance more negatively, and recall and ruminate on negative memories (e.g. of past failures) which could maintain or escalate the anxiety. In the study by Spence *et al.* (1999), discussed earlier, there was a general tendency for the social phobic group to evaluate their performance in social-evaluative tasks more poorly than the controls. This negative self-evaluation is likely to be part of a 'post-mortem' which characterizes the post-event processing of socially anxious individuals (Clark and Wells 1995; Rachman *et al.* 2000; Clark 2001). In cognitive models of anxiety disorder, this post-event processing is thought to involve reduced memory for external social cues in general (because of narrowed cognitive processing and increased self-focused attention during the encounter), but biased recall of negative threat-relevant information. For example, Mellings and Alden (2000) found that those high on social anxiety had poorer recall of external (partner-related) details of a social encounter which had taken place the day before, but heightened recall of negative self-related details of the event. Moreover, these patterns were found to be related to the degree of self-focused attention during the social interaction. Similar patterns can also be observed in children, although more research evidence is needed. In a preliminary experimental study conducted by Vassilopoulos (2000), high and low socially anxious 10- to 12-year-olds heard about a hypothetical school day involving 16 events that were either positive or negative and either relevant or irrelevant to public self-image. As expected, the high-anxious group had heightened recall of negative events relevant to public self-image. Finally, it seems possible that the post-event processing of anxious children will be characterized by recall of autobiographical memories that elicit anxiety. This pattern is especially likely to emerge following situations involving social-evaluative threat. Morgan and Banerjee (in press) present evidence for recall by high-anxious adults of autobiographical memories that they earlier rated as significantly more anxiety-eliciting, but only when following negative feedback after a social performance.

However, it is important to stress that the picture from studies exploring anxiety effects on memory is not entirely consistent, and developmental research is clearly needed. Hirsch and Clark's (2004) review of the literature on the topic includes some studies finding no evidence for a memory bias in anxious groups (e.g. Rapee *et al.* 1994). However, Hirsch and Clark point to a tendency for memory effects to emerge in studies where the individual is placed in a situation involving social threat. Putting this together with the evidence regarding threat perception, discussed above, one can legitimately expect that anxious children's social cognitive bias to perceive threat in social encounters may be compounded by subsequent recall of negative self-related information and anxiety-eliciting memories.

In general, the findings of automatic and elaborative negative processing related to anxiety appear to illustrate a general tendency for the anxious child to view the world as threatening. Moreover, these findings are consistent with other work pointing to high levels of negative cognition or self-talk (or a relatively low 'state-of-mind' ratio of positive to negative cognition) as being characteristic of anxiety (Prins 2001). However, unresolved questions remain about the extent and clinical significance of these characteristics. Alfano *et al.* (2002) note that findings of negative cognition are not always consistent across studies, and that the significant differences that are reported are sometimes small in size. Furthermore, they emphasize that it is not yet clear how much of the negative expectancies, interpretations, self-talk, and evaluations relate to threat-arousal processes specific to anxiety compared with the general distress common to emotional problems in general.

9.3 Social understanding and theory of mind

Daleiden and Vasey's (1997) application of the social information-processing model to the cognitive features of anxiety introduced the notion that social skills relating to knowledge and/or choice and enactment of response strategies may be different or impaired in anxious children. While processing biases may certainly play a role here—for example, in directing attention to particular response strategies—one must also consider the possibility that differences in social knowledge and understanding are involved. Indeed, Crick and Dodge (1994) explicitly refer to a database of social knowledge and schemas that influence, and are influenced by, the child's information processing. This database, one may argue, provides a bridge to a large research literature concerning children's social cognitive development. Within this body of work, researchers have explored children's understanding of their own and others' mental states ('theory of mind') as well as broader aspects of social understanding, all of which may underpin the socially effective use of behavioural strategies.

9.3.1 Knowledge of social problem-solving strategies

Turning first to the question of whether anxious individuals have different knowledge of strategies regarding, for example, coping with negative or stressful social events, evidence is somewhat inconclusive. On the one hand, studies with both adults and children suggest that basic knowledge of problem-solving strategies is no different among high- and low-anxious groups. In Davey's (1994) study of worrying, trait anxiety, and social problem-solving, neither worrying nor trait anxiety related to problem-solving ability, although both related to lower problem-solving confidence. Similarly, Vasey *et al.* (1992), cited by Daleiden and Vasey (1997), upon presenting anxiety-disordered children and controls with stories about anxiety-provoking situations (e.g. going to a new school), found no significant differences in the generation of avoidant, problem-focused, and social support coping strategies. However, exhibiting knowledge of response strategies in non-threatening laboratory conditions is clearly not equivalent to using or even accessing that knowledge in socially threatening naturalistic settings.

Davey's (1994) finding that anxious individuals displayed lower problem-solving confidence is critical. In children too, lack of confidence in the use of problem-solving strategies may be responsible for the avoidant behaviour that is disproportionately observed among anxious children. For example, in Vasey *et al.*'s (1992) study, alluded to above, children were more likely to select avoidant responses, and less likely to select proactive responses, when asked what they would do to help themselves feel less anxious. But what could underlie this lack of confidence in the use of known problem-focused strategies?

9.3.2 Social anxiety, theory of mind, and self-presentational understanding

One of the most rapidly expanding bodies of work in developmental psychology over the last two decades has been the research on children's 'theory of mind'–broadly speaking, their understanding of how mental states such as beliefs, desires, intentions, and emotions relate to each other and to behaviour. In much of this work, there is an underlying presumption that children's mental state understanding is part of what gives rise to 'socially competent' behaviour. This notion resonates with Piagetian concepts of egocentrism and perspective-taking, later developed in Selman's (1976, 1980) model of social role-taking. If children have difficulties in understanding their own or others' mental states (and thereby the multiple perspectives that can be taken in viewing the world), it seems reasonable to expect that communication and social relationships will be disadvantaged.

This proposition is particularly credible in view of autistic children's difficulties with standard theory of mind tasks, such as the false-belief task, which requires understanding that a person can hold and act on a belief about the world that is factually untrue (Baron-Cohen *et al.* 1985; see also Chapter 2, this volume). Even among high-functioning autistic children who perform well on the simpler theory of mind tasks, deficiencies can be observed on more advanced measures of mental-state understanding, such as the *faux pas* task (which requires insight into unintentional insults; Baron-Cohen *et al.* 1999). Notwithstanding the vast literature devoted to the precise nature and role of the social cognitive difficulties associated with autistic spectrum disorders (e.g. Baron-Cohen *et al.* 2000; Frith 2003), these kinds of deficits in mental state understanding appear to provide a helpful and logical explanation of the interpersonal and communicative impairments exhibited by individuals with these disorders. Crucially, recent work has shown that these kinds of tasks can also be used to predict individual differences in peer relations and social competence within the typically developing population. Banerjee and Watling (2005), for example, have shown that children with high numbers of negative sociometric nominations (peer-rejected children) performed significantly more poorly on the *faux pas* task. Similarly, Sutton *et al.* (1999) demonstrated that performance on social cognition tasks like these was significantly low among peer-victimized children.

Given these observed connections between mentalizing skills and interpersonal functioning, along with established links between negative peer status/victimization and anxiety (e.g. La Greca and Stone 1993; Inderbitzen *et al.* 1997; Graham and Juvonen 1998), it seems logical to investigate the mentalizing skills of socially anxious children. If mental-state understanding is indeed related to social relationships and competence in social interactions, it is likely that it could explain variability in the translation of social problem-solving knowledge into confident practice. Specifically, difficulties in mental-state understanding could undermine the effective use of problem-focused strategies, thereby maintaining and escalating social anxiety. Indeed, both clinical and research work suggests that the social difficulties faced by children at the higher end of the autistic spectrum do relate to significant anxious symptomatology. In explaining this evidence of chronic anxiety and negative affect in the psychiatric profile of individuals with Asperger syndrome, for example, Frith (2004, p. 682) states, 'if intuitive mentalizing failure makes it hard to predict and interpret other people's behaviour, then the social world cannot be the source of pleasure that it can be for ordinary people'. In fact, even within the typically developing population, recent work described below suggests that anxious symptoms are indeed linked with difficulties on certain advanced mental-state reasoning tasks and with difficulties in translating concerns about social evaluation into effective behavioural strategies.

In a preliminary investigation of the social cognitive correlates of social anxiety, Banerjee and Henderson (2001) investigated the extent to which social anxiety in a non-clinical sample was associated with (1) performance on a standard second-order false-belief task, requiring insights into recursive beliefs about physical object identity (Sullivan *et al*. 1994), (2) performance on the *faux pas* task, referred to above (Banerjee 2000; Baron-Cohen *et al*. 1999), (3) the understanding of self-presentational and prosocial display rules which involve masking emotion to manage one's public self-image and to spare others' feelings, respectively (Banerjee and Yuill 1999), and (4) teacher-rated social skills that require or do not require insight into others' mental states (Happé and Frith 1996).

Analyses of the data from this study showed that social anxiety was *not* associated with impaired performance on the standard false-belief task, which concerned only factual beliefs about physical object identity. However, social anxiety–accompanied by high levels of negative affect relating to shyness–was associated with poorer understanding of *faux pas* scenarios, which constitute a more sensitive measure of social understanding in contexts that involve multiple mental states (beliefs, emotions, and intentions). With respect to the display rule task, anxious children had no particular difficulty in appreciating the prosocial motive for concealing emotion (e.g. when receiving a disappointing gift). However, despite the fact that social anxiety involves deeply-felt concerns about impression management (Schlenker and Leary 1982), it was associated with a *poorer* appreciation of how emotion-masking displays could be motivated by those self-presentational concerns. Thus, it appears that social anxiety may be associated with a difficulty in translating concerns about public self-image into effective behavioural strategies. This proposition is confirmed by further evidence that social anxiety was associated with poorer teacher-rated social skills only when those skills required insight into others' mental states (e.g. the ability to respond to hints and indirect cues in conversation, as opposed to the ability to deliver a simple message (Frith *et al*. 1994)). As expected, this association could be explained by the social cognitive difficulties in understanding *faux pas* and self-presentational display rules.

New evidence confirms that social anxiety may indeed be associated with difficulties in the understanding of self-presentational strategies, which are likely to impede children's attempts to present desired images of the self to others. With a sample of 200 children aged 8–9 years, Banerjee and Watling (2004) demonstrated that social anxiety was positively correlated with the endorsement of fairly crude self-presentational strategies (e.g. agreeing with what others say to ingratiate oneself with them, making up excuses before an event where poor performance is expected, etc. (Lee *et al*. 1999)). This high self-reported use of self-presentational strategies is likely to emanate from anxious children's high levels of concern about the way they are evaluated by others; fear of negative evaluation is a dominant theme in models of social anxiety (see Clark and Wells 2001). However, Banerjee and Watling (2004) also showed that social anxiety was associated—*negatively*—with the ability to differentiate between social audiences known to have different preferences when judging what a character should say to them (an ability that typically improves with age between 6 and 11 years (Banerjee 2002)). Thus, anxious children's strong concerns about positive self-presentation may be undermined by low responsiveness to the preferences of their social partners. Ongoing longitudinal analyses of these children suggest that both these characteristics (the endorsement of crude self-presentational strategies to appear favourable to others, and the difficulties in responding to the distinct preferences of social partners) predicted increases in aspects of social anxiety over time. This profile of how socially anxious children approach the social world is entirely consistent with the self-presentational model of social anxiety, which posits that social anxiety results from a high motivation to make desired impressions on others coupled with low perceived efficacy to achieve that goal (see Schlenker and Leary 1982; Leary 1996).

Few other programmes of research have been explicitly designed to tap different forms of mental state understanding in relation to childhood anxiety. Thus a major task for further research is to identify more precisely the aspects of social understanding that are different or impaired in anxious children. It is important to reiterate that the patterns of social understanding identified so far do not appear to involve a *basic* difficulty in understanding mental states, but rather a specific difficulty with understanding and effectively managing social situations involving multiple mental states and potential social-evaluative threat. Consistent with this, a preliminary study by Southam-Gerow and Kendall (2000) showed that a clinical sample of children and adolescents with anxiety disorder tended to have particular difficulty with understanding strategies for *regulating* emotional experiences (e.g. changing feelings through internal processes) and expressions (e.g. hiding feelings). It is as yet unclear how specific these kinds of difficulties might be to anxiety, as opposed to other emotional disorders. Indeed, Southam-Gerow and Kendall (2002) review evidence linking difficulties in understanding emotion regulation strategies to various disordered groups.

Finally, it is worth noting that there may be important areas of overlap between the research on information-processing biases and the recent work on social understanding in anxious children. For example, a number of studies have examined whether anxious adults and children are distinctive in their decoding of emotional facial expressions. Findings in the adult literature are mixed (e.g. Mullins and Duke 2004; Philippot and Douilliez 2005), but Melfsen and Florin's (2002) investigation with a sample of 8- to 12-year-olds, despite not finding any evidence for a negative interpretational bias, did find longer latencies for classifying basic emotional expressions among anxious children. Simonian *et al.* (2001) have also reported some difficulties among social phobic children in classifying some, but not all, basic emotions. Further work is clearly needed, but in view of research suggesting that emotion recognition processes may be linked to theory of mind development in both typical and atypical populations (e.g. Buitelaar and van der Wees 1997), it would be helpful to think of patterns such as these as possible reflections of mentalizing difficulties as well as of attentional or interpretational biases.

9.4 Aetiology of social cognitive characteristics

This section examines possible causal factors that may be involved in the development of the social cognitive characteristics discussed above. One possibility is that the cognitive features discussed in this chapter are all simply a *consequence* of anxiety, or even 'epiphenomena of various disorders' involving negative emotional states (Alfano *et al.* 2002, p. 1217). However, without denying the importance of anxious states in heightening negative cognition, the weight of research and clinical literature points to cognitive processes as causally implicated in generating, maintaining, and escalating anxiety.

In the next section, we first examine the controversy surrounding the extent to which the negative cognitions of anxious children might be reflections of actual deficits in social competence. Then, we evaluate literature on inherited and social influences on anxiety with respect to the possible role of social cognitive characteristics in mediating genetic and environmental risk.

9.4.1 Social information-processing bias or social skills deficit?

A critical question raised by all the evidence regarding the negative cognitions of anxious children and adults is whether we are right to talk of these as 'biased' or 'distorted'. That is to say, when we refer to anxious individuals as exhibiting greater perceptions of threat, poorer expectancies regarding future social encounters, and more negative evaluations of their performance in past social encounters, are those negative cognitions really unwarranted? Alternatively, could it be that anxious children think more negatively because of difficulties in mentalizing, social understanding, and problem-solving that make the estimation of threat and negative evaluation entirely justified?

The literature on this topic is somewhat mixed. Some research suggests that the negative self-evaluations of anxious children may be unwarranted. Cartwright-Hatton *et al.* (2003), for example, found that children's social anxiety regarding a public performance task was associated with objectively recorded nervous behaviour and subjective negative evaluation of performance, but *not* with observer-rated social skills. Thus it seems entirely possible that at least some children with high levels of social anxiety may have negative self-appraisals (and, plausibly, greater perceptions of threat) that are not founded in observable socio-behavioural impairment.

On the other hand, other research points to clear differences in socially competent behaviour between anxious children and controls. For example, the cognitive characteristics relating to negative expectancies and self-evaluations among the social phobic children in the study by Spence *et al.* (1999) were consistent with evidence from independent observers and peers of poorer social skills among these children during role play and in naturalistic settings. Similar evidence of differences in performance during social role-play tasks is also reported by Beidel *et al.* (1999) and Morgan and Banerjee (2006). Indeed, much research contributing to the validation of social anxiety questionnaires for children presents evidence that children and adolescents scoring high on social anxiety are more likely to be rejected by their peers and have fewer close friendships (e.g. La Greca and Stone 1993; Inderbitzen *et al.* 1997; La Greca and Lopez 1998), implying actual deficits in social competence.

If further evidence confirms that socially anxious children do exhibit impairments in socially competent behaviour, this could not only explain the observed tendencies to perceive threat and think negatively, but could also clarify the role of the difficulties in social understanding and mentalizing referred to above. Specifically, if such social cognitive deficits continue to be found among anxious children, they could potentially explain the difficulties experienced by those children in their peer relationships, and, consequently, the constraints on their opportunities to acquire social problem-solving skills (and confidence in using those skills) from the experience of peer interaction. Thus social cognitive deficits could form part of a vicious cycle whereby difficulties in social understanding lead to fewer or qualitatively poorer peer interactions, which in turn lead to further impairment and negative information processing. However, it is important to note that the research so far points to heterogeneity within the anxious population; although some evidence links anxiety with socio-behavioural impairments that could explain problematic patterns of peer relations, these impairments certainly cannot be assumed to apply to all anxious children. Moreover, further research is needed before we can determine whether any behavioural impairments that are apparent stem from underlying deficits in skills and knowledge, or should rather be seen as performance deficits due to the interference of anxiety-related cognition.

9.4.2 Genetic influences

Behavioural genetic research has provided important insights into the contribution of genetic and environmental factors to childhood anxiety, as well as social cognition (as we will see in Chapter 13). As noted in the discussion of the comorbidity of anxiety and depression earlier in this chapter, the two sets of symptoms are often thought to overlap with respect to general negative affectivity. Eley and Stevenson (1999) present strong evidence that this area of overlap is related to a common genetic risk factor: in a study of 395 twin pairs aged between 8 and 16 years, the genetic influence on the depression and anxiety scores was entirely shared, and largely accounted for the correlation between the two measures. However, they also found evidence that this genetic effect was relatively smaller in size for anxiety symptoms than for depressive symptoms, with environmental factors playing a more significant role in the emergence of anxious symptoms. Moreover, the shared environmental factors (i.e. experiences that similarly influence the twins) for anxiety and depression were much more weakly related to each other, while the non-shared environmental factors (e.g. life events unique to the individual child) were not related at all. These results suggest that the genetic contribution to anxiety is likely to represent a general predisposition towards negative affectivity, while particular types of environmental influence play an important role in the emergence of anxiety-specific symptoms. With respect to the social cognitive characteristics discussed in this chapter, it seems plausible that heritable negative affectivity is implicated in the general propensity for negative cognition among anxious children, whereas differences in social understanding and biases towards threat perception (which would seem to relate more to arousal than to general negativity) are more likely to depend on the child's life experiences.

The evidence for genetic contribution to the overlap between anxiety and depression does not preclude the possible influence of other genetic influences on particular anxiety disorder subtypes. Kendler *et al.* (2001) showed that substantial proportions of variance in social fears were related to genetic factors not connected to other fears. One likely area of such genetic influence concerns the temperamental dimension of 'behavioural inhibition' (Kagan *et al.* 1984), which typically manifests itself in a withdrawn and reticent response to new or unfamiliar situations and interactants, and which has been linked in numerous longitudinal studies to the development of childhood social anxiety (see Biederman *et al.* 2001). Importantly, behavioural inhibition could constrain the development of social cognitive and behavioural skills early in the school years by reducing the opportunity to participate in, and learn from, peer interactions.

9.4.3 Environmental influence

Research on environmental influences on the development of anxiety has focused on two main areas: parent–child interactions and specific life experiences. First, retrospective reports from adult phobics have pointed to the possible significance of over-controlling and less warm parenting (Arrindell *et al.* 1983). Similarly, social anxiety has been associated with children's perceptions of overprotective parenting (Bögels *et al.* 2001). Moreover, Hudson and Rapee (2001, 2002) have provided observational evidence that mothers of anxious children are more intrusive and negative. These kinds of characteristics could conceivably contribute to the negative cognitions evident in anxious children, and indeed to negative affectivity in other disorders as well.

More direct connections between family factors and children's information-processing characteristics have also been investigated. Anxious children's tendency to interpret ambiguous situations as threatening has been connected not only to parents' expectations of such interpretations (Cobham *et al.* 1999; Bögels *et al.* 2003), but also to parents' *own* threatening interpretations (Creswell *et al.* 2005). Furthermore, Barrett, Rapee *et al.* (1996) showed that in addition to making threatening interpretations of ambiguous situations, anxious children demonstrated a stronger tendency to select avoidant responses to those situations following family discussion. In addition, deficits in anxious children's emotion understanding may at least partly be explained by a tendency for anxious children's families to be less emotionally expressive. In one recent study, mothers of anxious children discouraged the discussion of negative emotional experiences more, and used positive emotional words less frequently during discussion (Suveg *et al.* 2005).

However, it is not clear whether parental behaviours towards anxious children are antecedents or consequences of the children's characteristics. Rachman's (1977) framework for understanding the acquisition of fear points to the driving role of information as well as observational learning, and parents are obvious candidates for providing such learning opportunities. Indeed, there is good evidence from prospective studies that verbal information can lead to fear-related beliefs about novel animals and social situations, although more work is needed to compare the roles of different socializing agents (Field and Lawson 2003; Field *et al.* 2008; Lawson *et al.* 2007). Moreover, conditioning models of fear (e.g. Davey 1997; Field and Davey 2001) have pointed to such verbally and culturally transmitted information as setting up negative 'outcome expectancies' regarding encounters with the phobic stimulus. This theory is compatible with the notion that parents' behaviour and verbal communications could generate the negative expectations and threat perceptions exhibited by anxious children. However, in contrast with the proposition that parents are responsible for the emergence of anxious symptoms, Rubin *et al.* (1999) demonstrated that child shyness at age 2 predicted parent protectiveness at age 4, but not vice versa, suggesting that parenting could be the outcome rather than the antecedent of child adjustment. Further longitudinal work on parenting characteristics in relation to both anxious symptoms and their social cognitive correlates is clearly needed.

Besides the enduring influence of relatively stable patterns of parenting, specific life experiences may also contribute to the development of anxiety and relevant social cognitive characteristics. Conditioning models of anxiety have long held that specific traumatic experiences can lead to intense fears of particular stimuli (e.g. Watson and Rayner 1920). Retrospective reports by adult phobics often, although not always, include memories of specific experiences relating to the phobic stimuli; for example, Hackmann *et al.* (2000) have shown that adult social phobics report recurrent negative imagery associated with traumatic memories of being publicly criticized and feeling self-conscious. Similarly, anxious children's difficulties in peer relations could include traumatic incidents relating to the development of specific fears (e.g. social fears could be related to peer bullying or ridicule) and, as noted earlier, could also play a role in limiting the opportunity to develop mentalizing and social understanding skills.

Finally, behavioural genetic research suggests that life events relating to anxiety disorders are often likely to be specific to anxiety, rather than common across multiple emotional disorders; as noted earlier, non-shared environmental influences on anxiety and depression are entirely uncorrelated (Eley and Stevenson 1999). In fact, Eley and Stevenson (2000) have provided evidence that life events revolving around themes of threat (e.g. physical danger, stressful psychological challenges, risk of loss of attachment figure) are strongly and uniquely associated with anxiety rather than depression. The threat-relevant nature of these life events strongly suggests that the threat perception biases discussed in this chapter could mediate the effect of these environmental risks on childhood anxiety.

9.5 Clinical implications and directions for further research

The identification of social cognitive characteristics associated with anxiety has important implications for treatment. Cognitive-behavioural therapy (CBT), a dominant approach to clinical interventions for anxiety disorders, already places considerable emphasis on many of the information-processing and social understanding variables discussed in this chapter. For example, Kendall's (1993) review of CBT approaches to various developmental psychopathologies explicitly emphasizes the mediating role of information-processing characteristics. Thus, as well as working on relaxation to manage hyper-arousal and on modelling and role-play activities to develop socio-behavioural skills, CBT approaches to treating anxiety, such as Kendall's (1990) Coping Cat programme, seek to restructure or remediate automatic negative cognitions, interpretation biases, self-evaluations, and problem-solving strategies (Velting et al. 2004). As Kendall (1993, p. 240) puts it, the 'goal of cognitive interventions is to build a new (or elaborate on an existing) coping template' that will aid in managing the anxiety-eliciting situations. Daleiden and Vasey (1997), for example, have identified possible clinical strategies for dealing with the various stages in Crick and Dodge's (1994) social information-processing model: encoding, interpretation, goals, and generation/selection/enactment of response strategies. Moreover, there is good empirical evidence that CBT programmes that address these processes are effective in treating childhood anxiety disorders. Kendall and colleagues have reported on randomized clinical trials of individual CBT therapy (in comparison with wait-list control conditions) that show significant improvement following the therapy, maintained at follow-up one or more years later (Kendall 1994; Kendall and Southam-Gerow 1996; Kendall et al. 1997). These reports record significant proportions of children as no longer meeting diagnostic criteria for anxiety disorders after CBT.

Notwithstanding the strengths of existing CBT approaches, further research that addresses unresolved issues concerning the links between social cognition and anxiety will be of great value in developing effective treatment and intervention programmes. First, a more precise understanding of the social cognitive characteristics associated with anxiety is required. Although there is good evidence that information-processing characteristics relating to encoding, interpretation, and response choice are connected with anxiety, the above discussion has highlighted a number of questions that require further investigation, such as the nature and extent of hypervigilance-avoidance patterns and of memory biases (including both episodic memory of the focal social encounter and autobiographical memories of past anxiety-eliciting memories) in anxious youths. Moreover, as noted earlier, Alfano et al.'s (2002) review of cognitive processes in anxiety identifies numerous instances of divergent findings regarding the nature and extent of cognitive biases in anxious children. Consequently, the authors identify the need for clearer and agreed-upon definitions for the cognitive processes under investigation and for research that explicitly compares various assessment methods. In the course of this work, particular attention must be paid to how the information-processing variables are connected with children's socio-behavioural skills. The extent to which children's negative cognitions, perceptions of threat, and poor self-evaluations are linked to actual social skills deficits and problems in social interactions will be critical to the therapeutic process. For example, Morgan and Banerjee (2006) have shown that video feedback of social performance will improve self-evaluations of anxious children only if observer ratings indicate skilled performance; where actual impairments in performance are evident, video feedback may actually worsen self-evaluations.

In addition to further work to clarify the information-processing characteristics associated with anxiety, researchers need to follow up the preliminary evidence linking social anxiety to specific patterns of social understanding, including difficulties with advanced mental state reasoning tasks, appreciation of self-presentational strategies, and emotion recognition skills. Such work would be an important complement to the growing body of research on the mentalizing skills and social understanding that emerge after the first 5 or 6 years of life in the typically developing population. Existing intervention and treatment work, including both CBT and universal prevention models relating to emotional competence, such as the Promoting Alternative Thinking Strategies curriculum (Greenberg *et al.* 1995), often covers some of these aspects of social cognition, and in fact some researchers have already reported some preliminary success in incorporating 'theory of mind' topics into social skills training programmes for anxious as well as aggressive children (Steerneman *et al.* 1996). However, a more precise account of exactly where anxious children's social cognitive difficulties lie, relative to the normative development of social competence, would clearly be of great value to both assessment and treatment in clinical settings. In turn, research on the effects of treatments that address these characteristics will be essential for the further development of our theoretical frameworks for understanding anxiety in children.

On a related point, it is important to note that deficits related to reasoning about mental states could have significant implications for the success of CBT, which focuses in detail on the link between cognition and emotion. Alfano *et al.* (2002) have pointed out that both assessment and therapeutic methods must be designed to accommodate developmental factors that may constrain children's reasoning about mental states (e.g. understanding links between cognition and emotion, recognizing simultaneous existence of multiple emotions). Given that anxious children's emotional understanding may be further impaired relative to their non-anxious peers, clinicians must be particularly careful not to make assumptions about the awareness and understanding of these children regarding their own mental states.

More generally, an important challenge for researchers exploring the social cognition of anxious children is to understand the commonalities that link different anxiety disorder subtypes with each other and with other emotional symptoms, as well as the distinctive characteristics which differentiate them. Some studies have reported specific types of negative cognition in anxious groups after taking dysphoria/depression into account (e.g. Epkins 1996; Weems *et al.* 2001). On the other hand, it would probably be oversimplifying matters to assume that depression is linked to cognition about loss and anxiety to cognition about threat; Ambrose and Rholes (1993) have demonstrated that the severity of the threat or loss must be taken into account as well. Similarly, although empirical work suggests that a general tendency to overestimate threat may be common across multiple anxiety disorders, we have little evidence to clarify whether the patterns of social understanding observed in socially anxious children might be apparent in children with other anxious symptoms, or indeed in children with depressive symptoms. Furthermore, the degree of overlap between clinically diagnosed groups and non-clinical samples of children scoring high on self-reported anxiety is still unclear. Although a few studies have included two anxious groups selected in these different ways (e.g. Melfsen and Florin 2002), these are the exception rather than the norm. Such research is needed to clarify the extent to which the observed characteristics of undiagnosed children scoring high on anxiety can be related to categorically diagnosed anxiety disorders.

Finally, given the many promising avenues of research discussed above, work on anxiety that explicitly tracks the connections among genetic and environmental risk factors, social cognitive characteristics, and behaviour would be of great value. As noted above, some studies have already connected family discussion with interpretation biases and problem-solving choices which in turn relate to trait anxiety, and progress has been made in linking social cognitive characteristics to both affective symptoms and social interaction patterns. Indeed, in line with the evidence regarding family processes that contribute to child anxiety, several promising research studies have shown that CBT work that involves parents in managing both their own and their children's anxiety can be particularly effective (e.g. Barrett, Dadds, and Rapee 1996; Cobham *et al.* 1998). However, longitudinal research that addresses the role of specific patterns of social cognition in combination with both antecedent risk factors and clinical outcomes would be valuable for informing treatment approaches. There is already good precedence for such longitudinal work. For example, Dodge *et al.* (1995) have shown that social information-processing patterns mediate the effect of early physical abuse on later externalizing behaviour problems. Such investigations of the development of anxiety would allow us to identify the *mechanisms* by which genetic and environmental risks translate into emotional disorder. For example, negative information-processing biases and social cognitive impairments may have reciprocal relations with social interaction difficulties, and this cognitive and interpersonal maladjustment could operate as a mediator of the influence of distal risk factors on subsequent anxiety. Critically, work of this kind would aid the development of intervention and prevention programmes that could serve to treat and protect children at high risk of anxiety disorders.

References

Achenbach, T.M. (1991a). *Manual for the Youth Self-Report and 1991 profile*. Burlington, VT: Department of Psychiatry, University of Vermont.

Achenbach, T.M. (1991b). *Manual for Child Behavior Checklist 14–18 and 1991 profile*. Burlington, VT: Department of Psychiatry, University of Vermont.

Alfano, C.A., Beidel, D.C. and Turner, S.M. (2002). Cognition in childhood anxiety: conceptual, methodological, and developmental issues. *Clinical Psychology Review*, 22, 1209–38.

Ambrose, B. and Rholes, W.S. (1993). Automatic cognitions and the symptoms of depression and anxiety in children and adolescents: an examination of the content-specificity hypothesis. *Cognitive Therapy and Research*, 17, 153–71.

American Psychiatric Association (1994). *Diagnostic and statistical manual for mental and behavioural disorders*, Vol. 4 (DSM-IV). Washington, DC: American Psychiatric Association.

Arrindell, W.A., Emmelkamp, P.M., Monsma, A., and Brilman, E. (1983). The role of perceived parental rearing practices in the aetiology of phobic disorders: a controlled study. *British Journal of Psychiatry*, 143, 183–7.

Banerjee, R. (2000). The development of an understanding of modesty. *British Journal of Developmental Psychology*, 18, 499–517.

Banerjee, R. (2002). Audience effects on self-presentation in childhood. *Social Development*, 11, 487–507.

Banerjee, R. and Henderson, L. (2001). Social-cognitive factors in childhood social anxiety: a preliminary investigation. *Social Development*, 10, 558–72.

Banerjee, R. and Watling, D. (2004). Social anxiety and depressive symptoms in childhood: models of distinctive pathways. Presented at the British Psychological Association Annual Conference, Imperial College, University of London.

Banerjee, R. and Watling, D. (2005). Children's understanding of *faux pas*: associations with peer relations. *Hellenic Journal of Psychology*, 2, 27–45.

Banerjee, R. and Yuill, N. (1999). Children's explanations for self-presentational behaviour. *European Journal of Social Psychology*, 29, 105–11.

Baron-Cohen, S., Leslie, A.M., and Frith, U. (1985). Does the autistic child have a 'theory of mind'? *Cognition*, 21, 37–46.

Baron-Cohen, S., O'Riordan, M., Stone, V., Jones, R., and Plaisted, K. (1999). Recognition of *faux pas* by normally developing children with Asperger syndrome or high-functioning autism. *Journal of Autism and Developmental Disorders*, **29**, 407–18.

Baron-Cohen, S., Tager-Flusberg, H., and Cohen, D.J. (ed.) (2000). *Understanding other minds: perspectives from developmental cognitive neuroscience* (2nd edn). Oxford University Press.

Barrett, P.M., Dadds, M.R., and Rapee, R.M. (1996). Family treatment of childhood anxiety: a controlled trial. *Journal of Consulting and Clinical Psychology*, **64**, 333–42.

Barrett, P.M., Rapee, R.M., Dadds, M.M., and Ryan, S.M. (1996). Family enhancement of cognitive style in anxious and aggressive children. *Journal of Abnormal Child Psychology*, **24**, 187–203.

Beck, A.T. and Clark, D.A. (1997). An information processing model of anxiety: automatic and strategic processes. *Behaviour Research and Therapy*, **35**, 49–58.

Beck, A.T., Emery, G., and Greenberg, R. (1985). *Anxiety disorders and phobias: a cognitive perspective*. New York: Basic Books.

Beidel, D.C., Turner, S.M., and Morris, T.L. (1995). A new inventory to assess childhood social anxiety and phobia: The Social Phobia and Anxiety Inventory for Children. *Psychological Assessment*, **7**, 73–9.

Beidel, D.C., Turner, S.M. and Morris, T.L. (1999). Psychopathology of childhood social phobia. *Journal of the American Academy of Child and Adolescent Psychiatry*, **38**, 643–50.

Biederman, J., Hirshfeld-Becker, D.R., Rosenbaum, J.F., *et al.* (2001). Further evidence of association between behavioral inhibition and social anxiety in children. *American Journal of Psychiatry*, **158**, 1673–9.

Birmaher, B., Khetarpal, S., Brent, D., *et al.* (1997). The Screen for Child Anxiety Related Emotional Disorders (SCARED): scale construction and psychometric characteristics. *Journal of the American Academy of Child and Adolescent Psychiatry*, **36**, 545–53.

Bögels, S.M., van Oosten, A., Muris, P., and Smulders, D (2001). Familial correlates of social anxiety in children and adolescents. *Behaviour Research and Therapy*, **39**, 273–87.

Bögels, S.M., van Dongen, L., and Muris, P. (2003). Family influences on dysfunctional thinking in anxious children. *Infant and Child Development*, **12**, 243–52.

Brady, E.U. and Kendall, P.C. (1992). Comorbidity of anxiety and depression in children and adolescents. *Psychological Bulletin*, **111**, 244–55.

Buitelaar, J.K. and van der Wees, M. (1997). Are deficits in the decoding of affective cues and in mentalizing abilities independent? *Journal of Autism and Developmental Disorders*, **27**, 539–56.

Cartwright-Hatton, S., Hodges, L., and Porter, J. (2003). Social anxiety in childhood: the relationship with self and observer rated social skills. *Journal of Child Psychology and Psychiatry*, **44**, 737–42.

Chorpita, B.F., Plummer, C.M., and Moffitt, C.E. (2000). Relations of tripartite dimensions of emotion to childhood anxiety and mood disorders. *Journal of Abnormal Child Psychology*, **28**, 299–310.

Clark, D.A., Steer, R.A., and Beck, A.T. (1994). Common and specific dimensions of self-reported anxiety and depression: implications for the cognitive and tripartite models. *Journal of Abnormal Psychology*, **103**, 645–54.

Clark, D.M. (2001). A cognitive perspective on social phobia. In *International handbook of social anxiety* (ed. W.R. Crozier and L.E. Alden), pp. 405–30. Chichester: John Wiley.

Clark, D.M. and Wells, A. (2001). A cognitive model of social phobia. In *Social phobia: diagnosis, assessment, and treatment* (ed. R.G. Heimberg, M.R. Liebowitz, D.A. Hope, and F.R. Schneier), pp. 69–93. New York: Guilford Press.

Clark, L.A. and Watson, D. (1991). Tripartite model of anxiety and depression: psychometric evidence and taxonomic implications. *Journal of Abnormal Psychology*, 100, 316–36.

Cobham, V.E., Dadds, M.R., and Spence, S.H. (1998). The role of parental anxiety in the treatment of childhood anxiety. *Journal of Consulting and Clinical Psychology*, 66, 893–905.

Cobham, V.E., Dadds, M.R., and Spence, S.H. (1999). Anxious children and their parents: what do they expect? *Journal of Clinical Child Psychology*, 28, 220–31.

Cole, D.A., Peeke, L.G., Martin, J.M., Truglio, R., and Seroczynski, A.D. (1998). A longitudinal look at the relation between depression and anxiety in children and adolescents. *Journal of Consulting and Clinical Psychology*, 66, 451–60.

Creswell, C., Schniering, C.A., and Rapee, R.M. (2005). Threat interpretation in anxious children and their mothers: comparison with nonclinical children and the effects of treatment. *Behaviour Research and Therapy*, 43, 1375–81.

Crick, N.R. and Dodge, K.A. (1994). A review and reformulation of social information-processing mechanisms in children's social adjustment. *Psychological Bulletin*, 115, 74–101.

Daleiden, E.L. and Vasey, M.W. (1997). An information-processing perspective on childhood anxiety. *Clinical Psychology Review*, 17, 407–29.

Davey, G.C.L. (1994). Worrying, social problem-solving abilities, and social problem-solving confidence. *Behaviour Research and Therapy*, 32, 327–30.

Davey, G.C.L. (1997). A conditioning model of phobias. In *Phobias: a handbook of theory, research and treatment* (ed. G.C.L. Davey), pp. 301–22. Chichester: John Wiley.

Dodge, K.A. (1986). A social information processing model of social competence in children. In *The Minnesota Symposium on Child Psychology*, Vol. 18 (ed. M. Perlmutter), pp. 77–125. Hillsdale, NJ: Lawrence Erlbaum.

Dodge, K.A., Pettit, G.S., Bates, J.E., and Valente, E. (1995). Social information-processing patterns partially mediate the effect of early physical abuse on later conduct problems. *Journal of Abnormal Psychology*, 104, 632–43.

Eley, T.C. and Stevenson, J. (1999). Using genetic analyses to clarify the distinction between depressive and anxious symptoms in children. *Journal of Abnormal Child Psychology*, 27, 105–14.

Eley, T.C. and Stevenson, J. (2000). Specific life events and chronic experiences differentially associated with depression and anxiety in young twins. *Journal of Abnormal Child Psychology*, 28, 383–94.

Eley, T.C., Stirling, L., Ehlers, A., and Clark, D.M. (2002). Attentional biases and childhood anxiety: a pilot study. Presented at the British Psychological Society Developmental Section Annual Conference, University of Sussex.

Epkins, C.C. (1996). Cognitive specificity and affective confounding in social anxiety and dysphoria in children. *Journal of Psychopathology and Behavioral Assessment*, 18, 83–101.

Field, A.P. and Davey, G.C.L. (2001). Conditioning models of childhood anxiety. In *Anxiety disorders in children and adolescents: research, assessment and intervention,* (ed. W.K. Silverman and P.D.A. Treffers), pp. 187–211). Cambridge University Press.

Field, A.P. and Lawson, J. (2003). Fear information and the development of fears during childhood: effects on implicit fear responses and behavioural avoidance. *Behaviour Research and Therapy,* **41,** 1277–93.

Field, A.P., Lawson, J., and Banerjee, R. (2008). The verbal threat information pathway to fear in children: the longitudinal effects on fear congnitions and the immediate effects on avoidance behaviour. *Journal of Abnormal Psychology,* **117,** 214–224.

Frith, U. (2003). *Autism: explaining the enigma* (2nd ed.). Oxford: Blackwell.

Frith, U. (2004). Emanuel Miller lecture. Confusions and controversies about Asperger syndrome. *Journal of Child Psychology and Psychiatry,* **45,** 672–86.

Frith, U., Happé, F., and Siddons, F. (1994). Autism and theory of mind in everyday life. *Social Development,* **3,** 108–24.

Graham, S. and Juvonen, J. (1998). Self-blame and peer victimization in middle school: an attributional analysis. *Developmental Psychology,* **34,** 587–99.

Greenberg, M.T., Kusche, C.A., Cook, E.T., and Quamma, J.P. (1995). Promoting emotional competence in school-aged children: the effects of the PATHS curriculum. *Development and Psychopathology,* **7,** 117–36.

Hackmann, A., Clark, D.M., and McManus, F. (2000). Recurrent images and early memories in social phobia. *Behaviour Research and Therapy,* **38,** 601–10.

Hadwin, J., Frost, S., French, C.C., and Richards, A. (1997). Cognitive processing and trait anxiety in typically developing children: evidence for an interpretation bias. *Journal of Abnormal Psychology,* **106,** 486–90.

Happé, F.G.E. and Frith, U. (1996). Theory of mind and social impairment in children with conduct disorder. *British Journal of Developmental Psychology,* **14,** 385–98.

Hirsch, C.R. and Clark, D.M. (2004). Information-processing bias in social phobia. *Clinical Psychology Review,* **24,** 799–825.

Hudson, J.L. and Rapee, R.M. (2001). Parent–child interactions and anxiety disorders: an observational study. *Behaviour Research and Therapy,* **39,** 1411–27.

Hudson, J.L. and Rapee, R.M. (2002). Parent–child interactions in clinically anxious children and their siblings. *Journal of Clinical Child and Adolescent Psychology,* **31,** 548–55.

Inderbitzen, H.M., Walters, K.S., and Bukowski, A.L. (1997). The role of social anxiety in adolescent peer relations: differences among sociometric status groups and rejected subgroups. *Journal of Clinical Child Psychology,* **26,** 338–48.

Ingram, R.E., Ramel, W., Chavira, D. and Scher, C. (2001). Social anxiety and depression. In *International handbook of social anxiety* (ed. W.R. Crozier and L.E. Alden), pp. 357–80. Chichester: John Wiley.

Kagan, J., Reznick, J.S., Clarke, C., Snidman, N., and Garcia Coll, C.T. (1984). Behavioral inhibition to the unfamiliar. *Child Development,* **55,** 2212–25.

Kendall, P.C. (1985). Toward a cognitive-behavioral model of child psychopathology and a critique of related interventions. *Journal of Abnormal Child Psychology,* **13,** 357–72.

Kendall, P.C. (1990). *Coping Cat workbook.* Ardmore, PA: Workbook Publishing.

Kendall, P.C. (1993). Cognitive-behavioral therapies with youth: guiding theory, current status, and emerging developments. *Journal of Consulting and Clinical Psychology*, **61**, 235–47.

Kendall, P.C. (1994). Treating anxiety disorders in children: results of a randomized clinical trial. *Journal of Consulting and Clinical Psychology*, **62**, 100–10.

Kendall, P.C. and Southam-Gerow, M.A. (1996). Long-term follow-up of a cognitive-behavioral therapy for anxiety-disordered youth. *Journal of Consulting and Clinical Psychology*, **64**, 724–30.

Kendall, P.C., Flannery-Schroeder, E., Panichelli-Mindel, S.M., Southam-Gerow, M., Henin, A., and Warman, M. (1997). Therapy for youths with anxiety disorders: a second randomized clinical trial. *Journal of Consulting and Clinical Psychology*, **65**, 366–80.

Kendler, K.S., Myers, J., Prescott, C.A., and Neale, M.C. (2001). The genetic epidemiology of irrational fears and phobias in men. *Archives of General Psychiatry*, **58**, 257–65.

Kovacs M (1981). Rating scales to assess depression in school-aged children. *Acta Paedopsychiatrica*, **46**, 305–15.

La Greca, A.M. and Lopez, N. (1998). Social anxiety among adolescents: linkages with peer relations and friendships. *Journal of Abnormal Child Psychology*, **26**, 83–94.

La Greca, A.M. and Stone, W.L. (1993). Social Anxiety Scale for Children–Revised: factor structure and concurrent validity. *Journal of Clinical Child Psychology*, **22**, 17–27.

Lawson, J., Banerjee, R., and Field, A.P. (2007). The effects of verbal information on children's fear beliefs about social situations. *Behaviour Research and Therapy*, **45**, 21–37.

Leary, M.R. (1996). *Self-presentation: impression management and interpersonal behaviour.* Boulder, CO: Westview Press.

Lee, S.J., Quigley, B.M., Nesler, M.S., Corbett, A.B., and Tedeschi, J.T. (1999). Development of a self-presentation tactics scale. *Personality and Individual Differences*, **26**, 701–22.

Mansell, W., Clark, D.M., Ehlers, A., and Chen, Y.P. (1999). Social anxiety and attention away from emotional faces. *Cognition and Emotion*, **13**, 673–90.

March, J.S., Parker, J.D., Sullivan, K., Stallings, P., and Conners, C.K. (1997). The Multidimensional Anxiety Scale for Children (MASC): factor structure, reliability, and validity. *Journal of the American Academy of Child and Adolescent Psychiatry*, **36**, 554–65.

Melfsen, S. and Florin, I. (2002). Do socially anxious children show deficits in classifying facial expressions of emotions? *Journal of Nonverbal Behavior*, **26**, 109–26.

Mellings, T.M.B. and Alden, L.E. (2000). Cognitive processes in social anxiety: the effects of self-focus, rumination and anticipatory processing. *Behaviour Research and Therapy*, **38**, 243–57.

Morgan, J. and Banerjee, R. (2006). Social anxiety and self-evaluation of social performance in a nonclinical sample of children. *Journal of Clinical Child and Adolescent Psychology*, **35**, 292–301.

Morgan, J. and Banerjee, R. (in press). Post-event processing and autobiographical memory in social anxiety: the influence of negative feedback and rumination. *Journal of Anxiety Disorders*.

Mullins, D.T. and Duke, M.P. (2004). Effects of social anxiety on nonverbal accuracy and response time. I: Facial expressions. *Journal of Nonverbal Behavior*, **28**, 3–33.

Muris, P., Kindt, M., Bögels, S., Merckelbach, H., Gadet, B., and Moulaert, V. (2000). Anxiety and threat perception abnormalities in normal children. *Journal of Psychopathology and Behavioral Assessment*, **22**, 183–99.

Muris, P., Luermans, J., Merckelbach, H., and Mayer, B. (2000). 'Danger is lurking everywhere': the relation between anxiety and threat perception abnormalities in normal children. *Journal of Behavior Therapy and Experimental Psychiatry*, **31**, 123–36.

Muris, P., Merckelbach, H., Ollendick, T., King, N., and Bogie, N. (2002). Three traditional and three new childhood anxiety questionnaires: their reliability and validity in a normal adolescent sample. *Behaviour Research and Therapy*, **40**, 753–72.

Muris, P., Rapee, R., Meesters, C., Shouten, E., and Geers, M. (2003). Threat perception abnormalities in children: the role of anxiety disorders symptoms, chronic anxiety, and state anxiety. *Journal of Anxiety Disorders*, **17**, 271–87.

Ollendick, T.H. (1983). Reliability and validity of the Revised Fear Survey Schedule for Children (FSSC-R). *Behaviour Research and Therapy*, **21**, 685–92.

Öst, L.G. (1987). Age of onset in different phobias. *Journal of Abnormal Psychology*, **96**, 223–9.

Öst, L.G. and Treffers, P.D.A. (2001). Onset, course, and outcome for anxiety disorders in children. In *Anxiety disorders in children and adolescents: research, assessment and intervention* (ed. W.K. Silverman and P.D.A. Treffers), pp. 293–312. Cambridge University Press.

Philippot, P. and Douilliez, C. (2005). Social phobics do not misinterpret facial expression of emotion. *Behaviour Research and Therapy*, **43**, 639–52.

Prins, P.J.M. (2001). Affective and cognitive processes and the development and maintenance of anxiety and its disorders. In *Anxiety disorders in children and adolescents: research, assessment and intervention* (ed. W.K. Silverman and P.D.A. Treffers), pp. 23–44. Cambridge University Press.

Rachman, S. (1977). The conditioning theory of fear acquisition: a critical examination. *Behaviour Research and Therapy*, **15**, 375–87.

Rachman, S., Grüter-Andrew, J., and Shafran, R. (2000). Post-event processing in social anxiety. *Behaviour Research and Therapy*, **38**, 611–17.

Rapee, R.M., McCallum, S.L., Melville, L.F., Ravenscroft, H., and Rodney, J.M. (1994). Memory bias in social phobia. *Behaviour Research and Therapy*, **32**, 89–99.

Reynolds, C.R. and Richmond, B.O. (1978). What I think and feel: a revised measure of children's manifest anxiety. *Journal of Abnormal Child Psychology*, **6**, 271–80.

Rubin, K.H., Nelson, L.J., Hastings, P., and Asendorpf, J. (1999). The transaction between parents' perceptions of their children's shyness and their parenting styles. *International Journal of Behavioral Development*, **23**, 937–58.

Schlenker, B.R. and Leary, M.R. (1982). Social anxiety and self-presentation: a conceptualization and model. *Psychological Bulletin*, **92**, 641–69.

Selman, R.L. (1976). Social-cognitive understanding: a guide to educational and clinical practice. In *Moral development and behaviour: theory, research, and social issues* (ed. T. Lickona). New York: Holt.

Selman, R.L. (1980). *The growth of interpersonal understanding*. New York: Academic Press.

Silverman, W.K. and Albano, A.M. (1996). *Anxiety disorders interview schedule for DSM-IV: child interview schedule*. San Antonio, TX: Psychological Corporation.

Simonian, S.J., Beidel, D.C., Turner, S.M., Berkes, J.L., and Long, J.H. (2001). Recognition of facial affect by children and adolescents diagnosed with social phobia. *Child Psychiatry and Human Development*, **32**, 137–45.

Southam-Gerow, M.A. and Kendall, P.C. (2000). A preliminary study of the emotion understanding of youths referred for treatment of anxiety disorders. *Journal of Clinical Child Psychology*, **29**, 319–27.

Southam-Gerow, M.A. and Kendall, P.C. (2002). Emotion regulation and understanding: implications for child psychopathology and therapy. *Clinical Psychology Review*, **22**, 189–222.

Spence, S.H. (1998). A measure of anxiety symptoms among children. *Behaviour Research and Therapy*, **36**, 545–66.

Spence, S.H., Donovan, C., and Brechman-Toussaint, M. (1999). Social skills, social outcomes, and cognitive features of childhood social phobia. *Journal of Abnormal Psychology*, **108**, 211–21.

Spence, S.H., Rapee, R., McDonald, C., and Ingram, M. (2001). The structure of anxiety symptoms among preschoolers. *Behaviour Research and Therapy*, **39**, 1293–1316.

Spielberger, C.D. (1973). *Manual for the State–Trait Anxiety Inventory for Children*. Palo Alto, CA: Consulting Psychologists Press.

Steerneman, P., Jackson, S., Pelzer, H., and Muris, P. (1996). Children with social handicaps: an intervention programme using a theory of mind approach. *Clinical Child Psychology and Psychiatry*, **1**, 251–63.

Sullivan, K., Zaitchik, D., and Tager-Flusberg, H. (1994). Preschoolers can attribute second-order beliefs. *Developmental Psychology*, **30**, 395–402.

Sutton, J., Smith, P.K., and Swettenham, J. (1999). Social cognition and bullying: social inadequacy or skilled manipulation. *British Journal of Developmental Psychology*, **17**, 435–50.

Suveg, C., Zeman, J., Flannery-Schroeder, E., and Cassano, M. (2005). Emotion socialization in families of children with anxiety disorder. *Journal of Abnormal Child Psychology*, **33**, 145–55.

Turner, C.M. and Barrett, P.M. (2003). Does age play a role in structure of anxiety and depression in children and youths? An investigation of the tripartite model in three age cohorts. *Journal of Consulting and Clinical Psychology*, **71**, 826–33.

Vasey, M.W., Daleiden, E.L., Williams, L.L., and Brown, L.M. (1995). Biased attention in childhood anxiety disorders: a preliminary study. *Journal of Abnormal Child Psychology*, **23**, 267–279.

Vasey, M.W., El-Hag, N., and Daleiden, E.L. (1996). Anxiety and the processing of emotionally threatening stimuli: distinctive patterns of selective attention among high- and low-test-anxious children. *Child Development*, **67**, 1173–85.

Vassilopoulos, S.P. (2000). Social anxiety, public self-image and recall of interpersonal information in middle childhood. Unpublished Masters Dissertation, University of Sussex.

Vassilopoulos, S.P. (2005). Social anxiety and the vigilance–avoidance pattern of attentional processing. *Behavioural and Cognitive Psychotherapy*, **33**, 13–24.

Velting, O.N., Setzer, N.J., and Albano, A.M. (2004). Update on and advances in assessment and cognitive-behavioral treatment of anxiety disorders in children and adolescents. *Professional Psychology: Research and Practice*, **35**, 42–54.

Verhulst, F.C. (2001). Community and epidemiological aspects of anxiety disorders in children. In *Anxiety disorders in children and adolescents: research, assessment and intervention* (ed. W.K. Silverman and P.D.A. Treffers), pp. 273–92. Cambridge University Press.

Watson, J.B. and Rayner, R. (1920). Conditioned emotional reactions. *Journal of Experimental Psychology*, **3**, 1–14.

Weems, C.F., Berman, S.L., Silverman, W.K., and Saavedra, L.M. (2001). Cognitive errors in youth with anxiety disorders: the linkages between negative cognitive errors and anxious symptoms. *Cognitive Therapy and Research*, **25**, 559–75.

10

Social cognition and attachment-related disorders

Carla Sharp and Peter Fonagy

10.1 Introduction

One of the most influential psychological theories of the twentieth century has been John Bowlby's attachment theory (Bowlby 1969). Anyone who has observed the immediate and engaged response of a mother to her distressed baby would agree with Bowlby that there is something innate in the preparedness of the infant to seek the protection of attachment figures coupled with the natural disposition of the attachment figures to provide caretaking. The reciprocity between caregiver and infant, which includes behaviours such as touching, holding, and soothing on the parent's side and smiling, clinging, and crying on the infant's side, creates an enduring bond between caregiver and infant. Bowlby referred to this enduring bond as 'attachment', and saw it as the foundation for the infant to develop internal working models of self and other which can then function as templates for future relationships.

Although the above process occurs quite naturally for most, there is a subgroup of people who do not establish secure attachment relationships with primary caregivers. Mary Ainsworth (Ainsworth *et al.*1978) was the first to develop a classification system of infants' responses to their mother's absence and return. She described three types of response to the reunification of mother and infant during the Strange Situation Test: secure, avoidant, and ambivalent. Whilst this system proved useful for classifying infants in general, Main and Solomon (1990) found the system inadequate for classifying children with severe psychiatric problems. Therefore they delineated a fourth attachment category labelled disorganized/disoriented.

Because disorganized/disoriented attachment is often associated with the most severe psychiatric symptoms, our discussion of social cognition and attachment-related disorders will focus on this class of insecure attachment. This will naturally lead to a further focus on borderline personality disorder (BPD). Since the disorganized/disoriented attachments of borderline patients are so central both to their presenting problems and to theories about the pathogenesis of BPD (Agrawal *et al.* 2004), attachment theory is a natural framework for understanding and empirically investigating this devastating diagnosis. This chapter will aim to demonstrate that social cognition provides the essential key to link attachment with borderline symptomatology. First, we discuss the construct of BPD, specifically as it pertains to children and adolescents.

10.2 Definition of juvenile borderline personality disorder

BPD is a complex psychiatric problem typically characterized by numerous deficits in cognitive, emotional, and behavioural functioning. Commonly these include: emotional instability; feelings of emptiness; impulsivity; suicidal ideation and gestures; enmeshed, dysfunctional, and volatile relationships; irrational anxieties about being abandoned by those one cares about; and paranoid thoughts (Lieb *et al.* 2004). Even more than most other personality disorders, BPD has a powerful negative impact on quality of life (Cramer *et al.* 2006). Moreover, patients with BPD use more mental health services than those with major depressive disorder (e.g. Bender *et al.* 2006), and represent a staggering burden to society (Sharp and Bleiberg 2007) in terms of both personal distress and the burden placed on mental health services and families. Such data point to the need for both early identification of those with fledgling BPD features and intervention during childhood and adolescence to prevent youngsters from developing the enduring traits associated with adult BPD.

Therefore it is not surprising that there has been a renewed surge of interest in juvenile BPD, as reflected in several recent reviews (Bondurant *et al.* 2004; Sharp and Bleiberg 2007; Sharp and Romero 2007) and the fact that a special issue of *Development and Psychopathology* was recently devoted to the topic (Lenzenweger and Cicchetti 2005). Sharp and Romero (2007) searched PubMed and PsycInfo from 1940 (the first clinical descriptions of BPD in childhood) to 2006 to review all empirical work with the following keywords: 'personality disorder', 'Cluster B', 'borderline personality disorder', and 'borderline', as well as 'children', 'adolescent', and 'adolescence'. Only studies that included child and adolescent samples were considered (for reviews of retrospective studies investigating childhood precursors of adult BPD see Paris (2003) and Zanarini (2000)). A total of 58 studies were included to compare research findings on diagnostic-related phenomena in child and adolescent samples with those in adult samples to establish the utility of the BPD construct in childhood and adolescence. The review concluded with a suggestion that juvenile BPD overlaps with adult BPD in important ways. For instance, similarities between juvenile BPD and adult BPD have been demonstrated in its diagnostic criteria. More specifically, the childhood markers of this vulnerability have been argued to be: (1) hostile paranoid world view, (2) intense unstable inappropriate emotion, (3) overly close relationships, (4) impulsivity, and (5) lack of a sense of self (Crick et al. 2005). Similar interview-based measures have been used successfully to identify BPD in children and adults. Additional overlap has been observed regarding comorbidity with antisocial behaviour, the stability of the diagnosis, and environmental risk factors.

Empirical research into the diagnostic validity of the construct of juvenile BPD is still in its infancy, and significant research must be conducted before the diagnostic category of juvenile BPD can be included in the psychiatric nomenclature. However, early signs are promising. Moreover, as we hope will become evident in this chapter, we believe that neglecting the developmental social cognitive origins of BPD in children and adolescents leads to an impoverished understanding and treatment of adult BPD.

10.3 Normal development of social cognition: a view from attachment

10.3.1 Attachment and mentalizing

Bretherton et al. (1979) were the first to demonstrate a relation between infant attachment and early social understanding. They found that children who were securely attached at 12 months used more protodeclarative pointing at 11 months than other infants. In addition, a number of studies have reported associations between the quality of children's primary attachment relationships and the passing of standard theory of mind (ToM) tasks (e.g. Fonagy and Target 1997; Fonagy et al. 1997b; Meins et al. 1998; Harris 1999; Steele et al. 1999; Thompson 2000; de Rosnay and Harris 2002; Ontai and Thompson 2002; Symons 2004; Raikes and Thompson 2006). For example, the Separation Anxiety Test, a projective test of attachment security, predicted belief–desire reasoning capacity in 3 1/2–6-year-old children when age, verbal ability, and social maturity were all controlled for (Fonagy et al. 1997a). In this task the child is asked what a character would feel, based on his or her knowledge of the character's belief. Quality of belief–desire reasoning was predicted from attachment security in infancy: 82 per cent of babies classified as secure with mother at 12 months passed the belief–desire reasoning task at 5 1/2 years

(Fonagy *et al.* 1997a), and 46 per cent of those who had been classified as insecure failed. Infant–father attachment (at 18 months) also predicted the child's performance. Underlying this relation between attachment and social cognition is what Bowlby (1969) clearly recognized as a significant developmental step entailed in the emergence of 'the child's capacity both to conceive of his mother as having her own goals and interests separate from his own and to take them into account' (Bowlby 1969 p.368).

It should be noted that not all studies have found a relationship between attachment classification and ToM tasks. The association is somewhat more likely to be observed for emotion understanding than for ToM (Meins *et al.* 2002; Oppenheim *et al.* 2005; Raikes and Thompson 2006). Given the weak and unreliable association between attachment and measures of mentalization, it is most likely that the pathway connecting the two is indirect. For instance, secure attachment and mentalization may both be facilitated by aspects of parenting. The strongest evidence for this comes from observations that the inclination of mothers to take a psychological perspective in relation to their own actions or in relation to their child as they interact with or describe their infants, including maternal 'mind-mindedness' and 'reflective function', is associated with both secure attachment and the child's mentalizing capacity (Fonagy and Target 1997; Meins *et al.* 2002, 2003; Peterson and Slaughter 2003; Slade 2005; Sharp *et al.* 2006). Of course, this raises the question of which qualities of parenting, if not attachment *per se*, appear to facilitate the establishment of robust mentalization?

10.3.2 Parenting and mentalization: the parent's capacity to treat the child as a psychological agent

Precocious understanding of false beliefs has been associated with more reflective parenting practices (Ruffman *et al.* 1999), the quality of parental control (Dunn *et al.* 1991a; Astington 1996; Cutting and Dunn 1999; Ruffman *et al.* 1999; Vinden 2001), parental discourse about emotions (Denham *et al.* 1994; Meins *et al.* 2002), the depth of parental discussion involving affect (Dunn *et al.* 1991b), and parents' beliefs about parenting (Baumrind 1991; Ruffman *et al.* 1999; Vinden 2001). Parenting of this kind is likely to be strongly associated with the child's acquisition of a coherent conceptual apparatus for understanding behaviour in mentalistic terms. It is not hard to understand why parents whose disciplinary strategies focus on mental states (e.g. a victim's feelings or the non-intentional nature of transgressions) should have children who succeed in understanding the importance of mental states better and at an earlier stage, as this capacity is reflected in ToM tasks (Charman *et al.* 2002; Sabbagh and Callanan 1998). In contrast, one might well expect power-assertive parenting (including spanking and yelling) to delay the understanding of false beliefs (Pears and Moses 2003). However, in line with the transactional model we advocate (see section 10.5), we should consider the possibility that less mentalizing children are more likely to elicit controlling parenting behaviour, as well as the parent-to-child causation model positing that more mindful or reflective parenting facilitates both attachment security and the development of mentalization.

The capacity to tolerate negative affect could be a shared characteristic of secure attachment and a family environment facilitating mentalizing. For example, family-wide talk about negative emotions, often precipitated by the child's own emotions, has been shown to predict later success on tests of emotion understanding (Dunn and Brown 2001), and reflecting on intense emotion without being overwhelmed is a marker of secure attachment (Sroufe 1996). The number of references to thoughts and beliefs, and the relationship specificity of children's real-life accounts of negative emotions, correlate with early ToM acquisition (false-belief performance) (Hughes and Dunn 2002). Of course, there are many other characteristics of family function that could link a 'secure base' with mentalization. Considering these may be relevant for both prevention and identifying potentially helpful therapeutic attitudes.

Work by Elizabeth Meins (Meins *et al.* 2001), David Oppenheim (Koren-Karie *et al.* 2002; Oppenheim and Koren-Karie 2002), and Arietta Slade (Grienenberger *et al.* 2005; Schechter *et al.* 2005; Slade 2005; Slade *et al.* 2005), and their respective groups has sought to link parental mentalization to the development of affect regulation and secure attachment by examining interactional narratives between parents and children (for a more comprehensive account of these and other investigations of the impact of the parent's capacity to treat the child as a psychological agent on emotional development, see the review by Sharp and Fonagy (2008)). These studies demonstrate that (1) mind-related mentalizing comments to and about the young child increase the chance of secure attachment, and (2) non-mentalizing descriptions of the child reduce the frequency of maternal behaviours that might undermine the infant's natural progression towards security of attachment.

The findings suggest that a mother's secure attachment history permits and enhances her capacity to explore her own mind and promotes a similar enquiring stance towards the mental state of the infant. This stance is one of open respectful enquiry, in which the mother's awareness of her own mental state helps her to understand her infant without obscuring a genuine awareness of her child as a separate person. The depth of her awareness of the infant in turn reduces the frequency of behaviours that might undermine the infant's natural evolution towards its own sense of mental self, an evolution that occurs through the dialectic of the child's interactions with the mother. Indeed, the work of Goldberg and colleagues (Goldberg *et al.* 2003) shows that atypical maternal behaviour, as coded on the AMBIANCE system, relates not only to infant disorganization of attachment but also to unresolved (disorganized) attachment status on the mother's Adult Attachment Interview (AAI). Thus, while secure mother–infant attachment may not directly facilitate the development of mentalization, it is an indicator of an approach the caregiver takes to the child that may have a direct facilitative effect. Perhaps more crucially, the existence of secure infant attachment suggests that those aspects of parental behaviour that might have undermined mentalization are not present. Preliminary evidence that the capacity for change in attachment organization decreases over development underlines the danger that persistent trauma will lead to long-term disorganization of attachment, with attendant poor development of social cognition and substantially raised risks of psychopathology (Kobak *et al.* 2006).

However, we are not suggesting that parental mind-mindedness is inevitably helpful for the children's emotional development. Mind-mindedness is likely to be one of those parental attributes that is most adaptive in moderation. While evidence on this issue is still lacking, on the basis of our clinical observations we have proposed that maladaptive aspects of parental mentalizing of a child can be either deficient (concrete and stimulus-bound) or excessive or hypermentalizing (necessarily going beyond the data, often quite distorted and sometimes paranoid or intrusive) (Fearon *et al.* 2006; Williams *et al.* 2006). In the research considered above, the measure of mind-mindedness was confounded with the accuracy in the scoring: low scorers could be either deficient or excessive mentalizers because both would be rated as failing to reflect the child's mental state with what we may refer to as 'grounded imagination' (Allen 2006). Indeed, Sharp, Croudace, and Goodyer (2007) showed that the children of mothers who are super-mentalizers (mothers who are outstanding in their accuracy of mentalizing the contents of their children's minds) show similar pathology ratings as children of average mentalizers. However, regardless of the confounding of accuracy and concreteness in assessments of parenting, the literature suggests that it is not attachment *per se*, but correlated features of parenting, particularly an adult's taking an interest in a child's mental state, which may be critical in the robust establishment of mentalization.

Next, we explore how the above links between attachment and mentalizing via the parent's capacity to treat the child as a psychological agent map onto the symptoms of BPD.

10.4 Social cognitive deficits associated with borderline personality disorder

10.4.1 Mentalizing problems associated with adult BPD

Evidence in support of mentalization problems in adult patients with BPD has been documented more fully elsewhere (Bateman and Fonagy 2004). Here, we will only briefly point to some pertinent data. Disturbed interpersonal relatedness has been identified as a key aspect of BPD pathology differentiating it from other personality disorders (e.g. Nurnberg *et al.* 1991; Livesley and Jackson 1992; Blais *et al.* 1997; Skodol *et al.* 2002; Stevenson *et al.* 2003). Social experience triggers key problem behaviours. Environmental triggers of suicide attempts are more likely to be interpersonal stressors in BPD than in other disorders associated with depression (Brodsky *et al.* 2006). Observational studies consistently suggest that individuals with BPD exhibit abnormalities in interpersonal emotional perception, experience, and expression. Specifically, they show that individuals with BPD exhibit emotional hyper-responsiveness (summarized in Herpertz 2003; Leichsenring and Sachsse 2002) and deficits in emotion recognition and the capacity for empathy (Wagner and Ambrosini 2001; Guttman and Laporte 2002; Soloff *et al.* 2003; Bland *et al.* 2004).

However, it is not clear how best to understand the connection between BPD and various social cognitive deficits. The connection is situation and context dependent. For example, in relation to their deficit in facial emotion processing, while patients with BPD show a normal ability to recognize isolated facial or prosodic emotions, they appear to have impaired recognition of emotions with integrated facial/prosodic stimuli, as well as impaired discrimination of non-emotional facial features (e.g Minzenberg *et al.* 2006). However, the deficit clearly relates to functioning: impaired recognition of integrated emotional stimuli has been shown to be associated with interpersonal antagonism, particularly suspiciousness and assaultiveness (Minzenberg *et al.* 2006). As this chapter aims to illustrate, when mentalization is less precariously established, its loss will be more apparent in the emergence of unusual alternative strategies rather than in the loss of the capacity as such. For example, mentalization underpins normal self-regulation via self-talk and other processes that involve thinking about internal states (e.g. Dennett 2001). A limited capacity for self-regulation is also part of the clinical picture of BPD patients (see below). This may also be manifest as self-punishing negative vocalization as a self-regulation strategy (e.g. Rosenthal *et al.* 2006).

In social contexts where mentalization is impaired, a number of indications of a failure of self-organization become apparent. Mentalization (a psychological self-narrative) normally maintains an agentive sense of self (Fonagy and Target 1997). Self here is not considered as a representation but rather as a process with specific qualities that are closely related to the notion of autonomy, a consciously accessible sense of regulating one's own behaviour (Ryan 2005). There are many other constructs which cover more or less the same ground as mentalization, such as reflectiveness (Bleiberg 2001), mindfulness (Brown and Ryan 2003), or coherence of 'self-narrative' (Westen and Cohen 1993). The failure of self-narrativization creates characteristic gaps or discontinuities in self-experience. While our emphasis is on the *process* of self rather than its representation, changes in the phenomenology of the self are invariably associated with the temporary failure of mentalization. In the face of negative affect, patients may feel unable to experience themselves as authors of their actions, leading not only to a sense of temporally diffused identity (Kernberg 1983), but also to experiences of inauthenticity or painful incoherence, a feeling of emptiness, an inability to make commitment, gender dysphoria, and disturbances of body image (Akhtar 1992), all borne out by factor-analytical studies of data from clinically experienced informants for adult patients (Wilkinson-Ryan and Westen 2000) and adolescent patients (Betan and Westen 2005, unpublished data).

Ultimately, failure of mentalization in borderline patients is marked by an inclination to misread minds, both their own and those of others, resulting in 'distorted mentalizing' (Sharp *et al.* 2006). They consequently perform dramatically badly in social contexts, not only upsetting people whom they wish to recruit but also frequently exhibiting deficits in social problem-solving. This tendency may be considered a general marker of psychopathology, but certain features of temporary social cognitive deficit appear not to characterize other clinical groups (e.g. producing less specific solutions during means–end problem-solving, and reporting higher levels of negative problem orientation and a more impulsive/careless style towards solving social problems (Bray *et al.* 2007). Work from Drew Westen's productive laboratory has consistently demonstrated that patients with BPD represent others' internal states with less complexity and differentiation than patients with other disorders, such as major depression (Baker *et al.* 1992; Westen *et al.* 1990a). When emotionally aroused, and as their relationship with another person moves into the sphere of attachment, the intensification of that relationship means that their ability to think about the mental state of the other person can rapidly disappear. When this happens, prementalistic modes of organizing subjectivity emerge, which have the power to disorganize these relationships and destroy the coherence of self-experience that the narrative provided by normal mentalization generates (see below).

Taken together, we believe that the clinical and experimental data show that patients with BPD have vulnerabilities in the higher-order integration of social information, and ways of coping with this vulnerability which may be related to some of the more serious symptoms of the disorder. Although interpersonal problems can refer to a whole constellation of difficulties, including dramatic shifts from idealization of to disillusionment with others, frantic efforts to avoid perceived abandonment, and inappropriate interpersonal aggression (e.g. Raine 1993), an emerging literature suggests that all of these may share common mechanisms to do with the unstable perception of the other, where the stability of that social perspective—its depth—is normally guaranteed by a relatively clear perception of intentionality behind behaviour.

In conclusion, the 'mentalization' account of BPD is based on clinical evidence (Allen 2000, 2004; Allen and Fonagy 2002; Bateman and Fonagy 2004) and some empirical evidence (Fonagy *et al.* 1996; Bateman and Fonagy 2001; Vermote *et al.* 2003; Bateman and Tyrer 2004; Levy *et al.* 2006), and points to a specific difficulty that individuals with BPD appear to have in accurately differentiating and representing the mental states of people who are significant to them, as well as in having a clear grasp of their own subjective experience (Fonagy *et al.* 2000; Gunderson 2001; Holmes 2003). The diagnosis of BPD may be associated with low scores on Baron-Cohen's Reading the Mind in the Eyes Test (Fonagy *et al.* 2003a) and Happé's Strange Stories Test (Stokes *et al.*, submitted). However, we do not believe that a simple deficit model provides an adequate dynamic developmental account of this complex and multifaceted condition. Taking into account the links between attachment and BPD on the one hand (section 10.1), and attachment and mentalizing on the other hand (section 10.3), we present a model of the developmental origins of maladaptive social cognition in BPD.

10.4.2 The developmental origins of maladaptive social cognition in BPD: insecure attachment

There is limited but suggestive evidence that those suffering from BPD have a history of insecure disorganized attachment. Two longitudinal studies following children from infancy to early adulthood have found associations between insecure attachment in early childhood and BPD symptoms on follow-up (Lyons-Ruth *et al.* 2005; Sroufe *et al.* 2005). Summarizing across several longitudinal studies over 18+ years, it appears that early insecurity is a relatively stable characteristic of the individual, particularly in conjunction with subsequent negative life events (stability 94 per cent) (Hamilton 2000; Waters *et al.* 2000; Weinfield *et al.* 2000). Given evidence of the continuity of (insecure) attachment from early childhood, at least in adverse environments, the extent to which attachment is observed to be disorganized in adulthood may be relevant to our developmental model.

This growing literature was recently reviewed by Levy (2005). To date, nine studies have examined attachment patterns with patients diagnosed with BPD. Most of these studies used the best available assessment tool for adult attachment, the AAI; two further studies used rating scales; and over a dozen used self-report measures. While the relationship between BPD diagnosis and specific attachment category is not obvious, there is little doubt that BPD is strongly associated with insecure attachment (only 6–8 per cent of interviews are secure), most notably disorganization (unresolved attachment and cannot classify category of attachment) in interview-based studies and fearful, avoidant, and preoccupied attachment in questionnaire-based studies (Levy 2005).

Earlier (sections 10.3.1 and 10.3.2), we discussed the data demonstrating a link between attachment and the development of optimal mentalizing capacity in children. We suggested that it is not attachment *per se* that facilitates the development of mentalizing, but a particular property of the secure attachment relationship, namely parental mind-mindedness or reflective function. If these findings are to form the basis of our developmental model of dysfunctional social cognition in BPD, then we need to demonstrate that borderline individuals have not benefited from parental experience that could be regarded as mind-minded, reflective, or mentalizing. Below, we review the evidence in support of this claim.

10.4.3 'Mindless' parenting

While far from confirming the assumptions that all borderline patients have a borderline parent, there is consistent evidence of problematic parenting and parental bonding in individuals with BPD (Soloff and Millward 1983; Frank and Hoffman 1986; Paris and Frank 1989; Young and Gunderson 1995; Johnson *et al.* 2001; Paris 2003; Russ *et al.* 2003). Most of these studies are retrospective in design. Perhaps the most relevant observations come from the longitudinal study by Johnson *et al.* (2006). This was a community-based investigation of a sample of 593 families interviewed during the index offspring's childhood (mean age, 6 years), adolescence (mean ages, 14 and 16 years), emerging adulthood (mean age, 22 years), and adulthood (mean age, 33 years). The Structured Clinical Interview for DSM-IV Personality Disorders was used to assess personality disorders in the index offspring, and these were related to parenting behaviours observed during the child-rearing years. In addition to its longitudinal design, a further strength of the study was the rigorous control for childhood behavioural or emotional problems and parental psychiatric disorders. The number of different types of problematic parental behaviours observed in the home during the child-rearing years was associated with increasing offspring risk for personality disorders at the ages of 22 and 33 years. In particular, low parental affection or nurturing was associated with elevated risk for offspring borderline, antisocial, paranoid, and schizotypal personality disorders. Aversive parental behaviours, such as harsh punishments, also increased the risk for offspring borderline and paranoid personality disorders. These findings suggest that problematic parental behaviour towards the child increases the risk of BPD, while BPD is not predictable from childhood behavioural problems or parental Axis I disorder. While the former reduces (if not precludes) the possibility of a child-to-parent effect, the latter argues against genetic rather than environmental mediation.

The strength of the association between parenting and personality disorders does not decrease between emerging and full adulthood, indicating that long-term vulnerability has been created by these experiences. It seems from this study that both neglect and physical abuse additively increase the likelihood of personality problems, and, as we shall try to demonstrate, both types of experience may undermine the full development of mentalization. First, we discuss other evidence supporting the notion that social cognitive development may be impeded by 'mindblindness' in parenting.

In general, low family cohesion and high instability have been shown to characterize families of BPD patients (Feldman *et al.* 1995). In some older cross-sectional studies, the disrupted communication of mothers of BPD adolescents was assessed in less sophisticated ways, but mothers tended to rate themselves or be rated as less empathic, more egocentric, and less differentiated (Golomb *et al.* 1994; Guttman and Laporte 2000). Parents of high BPD scoring college students rated themselves retrospectively as over-involved and/or inconsistent (Bezirganian *et al.* 1993; Brennan and Shaver 1998).

A fascinating study from Lyons-Ruth's laboratory gives an indication of the level of detail that might be necessary. She showed, in a small sample, that disrupted maternal communications in infancy correlated significantly ($r = 0.31$) with borderline symptoms as assessed at age 18 (Lyons-Ruth *et al.* 2005). Such disruptions typically included frightening behaviour, grossly misattuned emotional responding, and role reversals involving seeking comfort from the infant—precisely the behaviours that may suggest a significant parental failure in mentalizing the child. Forty per cent of the infants of mothers with disrupted affective communication displayed BPD features compared with only 12 per cent of the infants of non-disrupted mothers. We should note, in relation to the separate effects of neglect and aversive treatment, that abuse in adolescence did not mediate the relationship. The strongest correlation reported was between inappropriate maternal withdrawal from her infant and borderline symptoms in her child 17 years later. Predictors of BPD status in young adulthood included both the mother's referral for documented maltreatment when the child was an infant and total abuse reported in adolescence, in addition to mother–infant disrupted communication. The specificity is considerable. Half of the high-risk clinically referred infants displayed BPD features compared with only 9 per cent of matched socio-economic status (SES) controls.

It seems, then, that behind broad descriptors such as low cohesion and high instability may lie quite subtle behaviours that create a vulnerability to BPD through compromising the process of parental mentalizing to a point where, at least at certain moments, the young child might feel that the process of trying to locate their experience in the other is likely to generate aversive experience and is therefore avoided.

In the absence of an adequate number of longitudinal studies, there is a further indirect way in which the early experiences of BPD patients can be investigated. Given the general consensus on the transgenerational transmission of attachment behaviours, we might learn something about the mothering received by BPD patients through direct observations of mothering by women with this diagnosis (Fraiberg *et al.* 1975; Lebovici 1988; van Ijzendoorn 1992, 1995; Fonagy *et al.* 1995; van Ijzendoorn and Bakermans-Kranenburg 1997; Smith and Farrington 2004).

Indeed, studies of caregiving by BPD mothers suggest significant anomalies in child care practices for this group. Borderline mothers show an incapacity to modulate their emotional expression in laboratory interaction with their infants, heightening non-contingency at the 'reunion phase' of the 'still face' paradigm (Danon and Graignic 2003). A more carefully controlled experimental study, also using the still face paradigm, revealed that BPD mothers show more intrusiveness and insensitivity towards 2-month-olds (Crandell *et al.* 2003). The same group of researchers also report more intrusive mothering with 12-month-olds who are more likely to be disorganized in their attachment (Hobson *et al.* 2005).

A severe class of anomaly in child care practices is, of course, maltreatment. Along with de Rosnay, Harris, and Pons (Chapter 12, this volume), our review of the literature suggests that maltreatment of children is associated with a delay in development of emotion understanding. Maltreated children are, by definition, deprived of expectable attuned social input, which could be argued to cause the distortion and deficit in mentalization in such children. There is reasonable evidence linking the maltreatment of young children with problems of mentalization.

1. Maltreated children engage in less symbolic and dyadic play (Alessandri 1991).
2. They may fail to show typical empathic responses to distress in other children (Howes and Espinosa 1985; Main and George 1985; Klimes-Dougan and Kistner 1990).
3. They make fewer references to internal states, and maltreating mother–child dyads discuss emotions less frequently than non-maltreating dyads (Beeghly and Cicchetti 1994; Shipman and Zeman 1999).
4. Maltreated children also manifest a range of problems indicative of difficulties in processing emotional expressions.

Preschool children who were maltreated have poorer understanding of universal adult (During and McMahon 1991) and child (Camras et al. 1983) facial expressions of emotion, even when controlled for verbal IQ (Camras et al. 1990). There is little evidence for affect-specific deviation (Camras et al. 1988; Smith and Walden 1999), except for the tendency by maltreated children to misattribute anger (Camras et al. 1996) and for maltreated 6–12-year-olds to show elevated event-related potential (ERP) to angry faces (Pollak et al. 2001; Pollak and Sinha 2003).

The question then is whether evidence exists to suggest that the extent of the delay in emotion-focused mentalization observed in maltreated children (Frodi and Smetana 1984; Rogosch et al. 1995; Smith and Walden 1999; Pears and Fisher 2005) is of developmental significance relevant to BPD. There is some suggestive evidence that this might be the case. For example, the quality of understanding of the possible situational determinants of sad and angry emotions at approximately 6 years of age was found to predict social competence at 8 years of age (Rogosch et al. 1995). Further, the experience of physical abuse was found to predict social isolation at 8 years of age to the extent that it had impacted on emotion understanding (controlling for verbal ability) (Rogosch et al. 1995). We have noted that emotion dysregulation and social competence problems are among the early precursors of BPD (see above, and Crick et al. 2005).

Beyond problems of affect processing and affect regulation, is there evidence that maltreatment predisposes to a non-mentalizing style of cognition? There is evidence, for example, of delayed ToM understanding in maltreated children (Cicchetti et al. 2003; Pears and Fisher 2005). This could be a function of the broader intellectual delays experienced by many maltreated children. A persuasive study from the Rochester Mount Hope Family Center (Cicchetti et al. 2003) tested 203 maltreated low-SES children and 104 non-maltreated controls using the unexpected content false-belief task.

Children's language was assessed, and verbal mental age (VMA) was estimated based on the Peabody Picture Vocabulary Test. There was a highly significant effect of maltreatment on ToM ($p < 0.001$). Controlling for chronological age and SES reduced the effect, but it remained statistically significant (Cicchetti *et al.* 2003).

In addition to the above, in a study of 80 maltreated preschoolers Macfie *et al.* (1999) showed clear limitations in the representation of social cognition in a story stem completion task where the story stem called for the relief of distress. In a further study of narratives (Macfie *et al.* 2001), maltreated children, especially physically or sexually abused children, were shown to manifest more dissociation, disruptions of identity, and incoherence of parental representations. We would see all of this as indicating the potential failure of mentalizing capacities (Fonagy *et al.* 2002).

Observed developmental trends support this argument. In maltreated children, the capacity for social cognition, particularly the complexity of the representation of the parent in conflict-imbued settings, decreases with development, while the children's representations of themselves become increasingly simplified and exaggerated (Toth *et al.* 2000). Arguably, these simplified and exaggerated representations are the precursors of the extreme problems of achieving complex representations that may be a hallmark of borderline functioning (Westen *et al.* 1990b).

Given the strong relation between maltreatment and delayed or disrupted development of mentalizing, it is noteworthy that 40–71 per cent of inpatients with BPD retrospectively report having been sexually abused as children (e.g. Herman *et al.* 1989; Zanarini *et al.* 1989, 1997; Shearer *et al.* 1990; Westen *et al.* 1990b; Paris 1994). Moreover, in a recent study, we found that of three groups of patients matched for gender, age, education, and Axis I diagnoses, the group who also met criteria for BPD scored lower in Baron-Cohen's Reading the Mind in the Eyes test (Baron-Cohen and Cross 1992; Baron-Cohen *et al.* 1997) than a group without Axis II diagnoses or a group with Axis II but not cluster B diagnoses (Fonagy *et al.*, submitted). Structural equation modelling revealed that those with a history of adversity who had low scores on the Eyes task were also more likely to have BPD diagnoses. When low mentalizing scores were placed in the structural equation model as an outcome of BPD diagnosis, the model fitted more poorly, suggesting that low mentalizing is consequent on maltreatment history, whilst not all those with low mentalizing associated with maltreatment acquire a BPD diagnosis.

Taken together, the subtle anomalies in parenting described earlier, or the more severe instances of maltreatment, create a mechanism by which the child's subjective experience is invalidated, thereby increasing the risk of developing BPD. In particular, these environmental influences lead to a systematic undermining of a person's experience of their own mind, either through direct disconfirmations and the minimizing of difficulties, or by failing to teach children to discriminate effectively between what they feel and what the caregiver feels. A pervasive history of invalidating, or more specifically, non-mentalizing responses from attachment figures is considered to generate skills deficits primarily in emotionally charged interpersonal situations where social cognitive capacities are essential. The failure of interpersonal understanding further exaggerates the social stress, leading to major difficulties of emotion regulation, problem-solving, and social and interpersonal dysregulation.

10.5 An aetiological model of borderline personality disorder

In keeping with the developmental psychopathology approach taken in this volume, we aim to take a dynamic developmental view (e.g. Crick *et al.* 2005; see also Chapter 5, this volume) in considering the role of social cognition, or more specifically a dysfunction of mentalization in BPD. This entails the following assumptions.

1. Symptoms of the disorder will manifest differently at different developmental periods (heterotypic continuity).
2. A specific influence may be critical at a certain stage of development but matter less at others.
3. The impact of a specific deficit will relate to the child's stage of development.
4. A complex function such as mentalization will have multiple components (developmental precursors, alternative mediating mechanisms, and strategies for compensating for a deficit).
5. Contextual determinants will moderate the relationship of risk factors and pathogenic outcomes. Thus atypical personality development can only be identified by considering the difficulties in negotiating developmentally appropriate, normative tasks that have relevance for BPD.
6. Given what we know about the natural course, particularly the reversible character of the disorder, the dynamic model must explain not just the emergence of the disease but also the process of often spontaneous and sometimes dramatic recovery.

The ideal developmental model from our standpoint describes the emergence of both the capacity to mentalize and the characteristic failure of this function in BPD. Such a developmental model will always be transactional, even if data are rarely available that speak to models of that degree of complexity. In other words, individual difference models based on genetic and biological parameters, or environmental models that focus on stressful or traumatic experience, or interaction models (e.g. the diathesis stress model) which identify individual vulnerabilities to particular types of environmental challenges will all be inadequate to the task of depicting the likely unfolding of BPD and its volatile course and sometimes rapid resolution. Transactional models have the potential for change built into them in that they take into consideration the impact that individuals have on their environment, which can change the characteristics of both the person and the environment in ways that could alter the nature of future interactions between the two (Steinberg and Avenevoli 2000; Cicchetti and Rogosch 2002).

The transactional nature of development is probably key to understanding the emergence of most complex mental health problems, not just BPD. However, BPD may be a particularly strong example. The disorganization of the attachment system may, for instance, cause a child to be increasingly manipulative and controlling towards their environment, but such controlling actions may undermine the caregiver's capacity to provide a normative playful environment for their young child. A similar idea is reflected in the description of BPD symptoms as '... the manifestations and consequences of complex interactions among cognitive-affective units that are triggered by specific situational contingencies and through synergistic and recursive activation, lead to characteristic patters of action, thought and feelings' (Meyer and Pilkonis 2005, p. 240).

We have discussed our developmental model of BPD in detail elsewhere (Fonagy *et al.* 2002; Fonagy *et al.* 2003b; Bateman and Fonagy 2004). Essentially, our account focuses on the development of the social affiliative system that we consider to drive many higher-order social cognitive functions. These in turn underpin interpersonal interaction, specifically in an attachment context. Four of these are of primary importance in understanding BPD: affect representation and, related to this, affect regulation; attentional control, also with strong links to the regulation of affect; the dual arousal system involved in maintaining an appropriate balance between mental functions undertaken by the anterior and posterior portions of the brain; finally, mentalization, a system for interpersonal understanding within the attachment context. Since these capacities evolve in the context of the child's relationship with the primary caregiver(s), in addition to the child's constitutional vulnerabilities, they are vulnerable to extremes of environmental deficiency as exemplified by severe neglect, psychological or physical abuse, childhood molestation, or other forms of maltreatment.

As individual difference in normal personality has a large genetic component, it would be surprising if extremes of personality types such as BPD did not also have major genetic components. Current evidence suggests that genes may have both main effects (Torgersen *et al.* 2000; White *et al.* 2003) and interactive effects with anomalous environmental influences (Caspi *et al.* 2002, 2003). Longitudinal and genetically sophisticated studies of early environment are essential, as we know that children who go on to develop BPD are vulnerable not least because they are likely to bring hard-to-manage temperaments to the parent–child relationship (Depue and Lenzenweger 2001). A child who is high in novelty-seeking and need for stimulation, and high in reactivity and anxiety proneness (Cloninger *et al.* 1993), will be relatively hard to interact with in a manner which optimally supports his or her autonomy.

As for the genetic underpinnings of social cognition, behaviour genetic data have traditionally been considered key to the assessment of social influences (see also Chapter 13, this volume). At the extreme of low mentalizing, there has for some time been compelling evidence of genetic influences (e.g. Dorris *et al.* 2004). Despite initial reports that revealed little if any shared environmental variance in ToM performance in preschool-aged twins (Hughes and Cutting 1999), a larger study with a longitudinal twin sample of 1116 60-month-old twin pairs, who completed a comprehensive battery of ToM tasks, showed that environmental factors explained the largest part (48 per cent) of the variance in ToM performance (Hughes *et al.* 2005).

The genetic evidence above, coupled with the arguments put forward in favour of environmental influences (section 10.4), supports the notion of an interaction between nature and nurture in the development of BPD and associated social cognition. A genetic predisposition for social cognitive capacity may prepare the infant either positively or negatively to make use of her social environment through the innate capacity for social cognition. In turn, nurture may modify nature. Thus, although some biological preparedness exists that allows the infant to utilize her social environment, the environment may negatively impact this preparedness in the form of, for instance, an abusive parent.

10.6 Mentalization-based treatment

Whilst most people, since they live without major psychological problems, are in a relatively strong position to utilize the alternative perspective presented by the psychological therapist, individuals who have a very poor appreciation of their own and others' perception of mind are unlikely to benefit from traditional (particularly insight-oriented) psychological therapies. Earlier we have discussed evidence to suggest that individuals with BPD have an impoverished model of their own and others' mental function. They have schematic, rigid, and sometimes extreme views, which make them vulnerable to powerful emotional storms and apparently impulsive actions, and which create profound problems of behavioural regulation, including affect regulation. The weaker an individual's sense of their own subjectivity, the more difficult it is for them to compare the validity of their own perceptions regarding the way their mind works with those presented by a 'mind expert'. When presented with a coherent and perhaps even accurate view of mental function in the context of psychotherapy, they are not able to compare the picture offered to them with a self-generated model and may all too often accept alternative perspectives uncritically or reject them wholesale. Even focusing on how the patient feels can have its dangers. A person who has little capacity to discern the subjective state associated with anger cannot benefit from being told both that they are feeling angry and the underlying cause of that anger. This assertion addresses nothing that is known or can be integrated. It can only be accepted as true or rejected outright, but in neither case is it helpful. The dissonance between the patient's inner experience and the perspective given by the therapist, in the context of feelings of attachment to the therapist, leads to bewilderment, which in turn leads to instability as the patient attempts to integrate the different views and experiences. Unsurprisingly, this results in more, rather than less, mental and behavioural disturbance.

It follows from the data we discussed in the preceding sections of this chapter that the recovery of mentalizing capacity in the context of attachment relationships must be a primary objective of all psychosocial treatments for BPD. Treatments likely to be effective with BPD should contain certain common features.

1. They should be well-structured.
2. They should devote considerable effort to enhancing compliance.
3. They should be clearly focused, whether that focus is a problem behaviour, such as self-harm, or an aspect of interpersonal relationship patterns.
4. They should be theoretically highly coherent to both therapist and patient, sometimes deliberately omitting information incompatible with the theory.
5. They should be relatively long term.
6. They should encourage a powerful attachment relationship between therapist and patient, enabling the therapist to adopt a relatively active rather than a passive stance.
7. They should be well integrated with other services available to the patient.

To this end, Bateman and Fonagy (1999, 2001) developed mentalization-based treatment (MBT). MBT aims to develop a therapeutic process in which the *mind* of the patient becomes the focus of treatment. The objective is for the patient to find out more about how he/she thinks and feels about him/herself and others, how that dictates his/her responses, and how 'errors' in understanding him/herself and others lead to actions born of the attempt to retain stability and to make sense of incomprehensible feelings. It is not for the therapist to 'tell' the patient about how he/she feels, what he/she thinks, how he/she should behave, or what the underlying reasons are, conscious or unconscious, for his/her difficulties. We believe that any therapy approach which moves towards 'knowing' how a patient 'is', how he/she should behave and think, and 'why he/she is like he/she is', is likely to be harmful. The therapist has to ensure that a focus on the mind of the patient is retained so that both his/her mind and awareness of the independent minds of others can be experienced at any given moment.

In an attempt to capture the therapeutic stance that gives the best chance of achieving mentalizing goals, we have defined a mentalizing, inquisitive, or not-knowing stance. The mentalizing or not-knowing stance is not synonymous with having no knowledge. The term is an attempt to capture a sense that mental states are opaque and that the therapist can have no more of an idea of what is in the patient's mind than the patient him/herself. When the therapist takes a different perspective to the patient, this should be verbalized and explored in relation to the patient's alternative perspective with no assumption being made about whose viewpoint has greater validity. The task is to determine the mental processes which have led to alternative viewpoints and to consider each perspective in relation to the other, acknowledging that diverse outlooks may be acceptable.

A randomized control trial for MBT with BPD patients in a partial hospital programme showed significant and enduring changes in mood states and interpersonal functioning associated with an 18-month programme (Bateman and Fonagy 2001). The benefits, relative to treatment as usual, were large (numbers needed to treat (NNTs) around 2) and were observed to increase during the follow-up period of 18 months, rather than staying level as with dialectical behaviour therapy (DBT).

These promising results led to the development of a mentalization-based treatment protocol for use with children and their families called Short-term Mentalizing and Relational Therapy (SMART). A more detailed description of SMART is provided elsewhere (Fearon *et al.* 2006). Here, we present only the philosophy and core components of SMART.

Fearon *et al.* (2006) described the philosophy of SMART as based on the view that, to promote longer-term resilience in a family—particularly in the context of multiple psychological and social problems—directly relieving symptoms may be a less critical therapeutic goal than promoting means of coping, particularly in relation to the quality and supportiveness of family attachment relationships. By the end of treatment, the aim is not only to offer solutions in relation to the problems identified but also for the family to feel that they are in a position to solve problems themselves and to be better equipped in the future to tackle new ones. Although there is scope for longer-term versions of SMART, the manual in its current incarnation assumes a period of treatment ranging from six to 12 sessions.

Although there are a large (and growing) number of possible ways of intervening to promote mentalizing, seven core interventions have been described as being central to SMART (Fearon *et al.* 2006).

1. **Identifying, highlighting, and praising examples of skilful mentalizing** Families more or less frequently demonstrate mentalizing in sessions. When they do, particularly if the example is relevant to the way the therapist understands mentalizing to be problematic in the family, the therapist communicates to the family how interested she is in this, how impressive and significant she thinks it is, and why. The therapist may, for example, intervene, and pause a conversation, and then draw the family's attention to the mentalizing that was observed. The therapist may say, 'Sorry, I just want to come back to something here, because I think it might be really important. Joanna, I noticed a moment ago you said to Johnny X and it seemed like he really noticed and liked how interested you were in his point of view ...'.

2. **Sharing and provoking curiosity** As noted above, the most important feature of a mentalizing stance is respect for and curiosity about the minds of others and an attitude/belief that learning about how others are thinking and feeling will be enlightening. Thus the therapist models this attitude as frequently as possible, by asking about how others are feeling or what they might be thinking—and by not making assumptions about either of these. Thus the therapist may say, 'This is interesting. I wonder, Sally, what it feels like for you when your dad does X?' 'Let me see if I got this right: are you saying that when your dad does X, that makes you feel Y, and you think to yourself z?' If the therapist wants to share a hypothesis about what someone might be feeling, he/she qualifies this by saying 'I'm not sure I've got this right, so please tell me, but I was wondering whether Sally might feel X. Is that right Sally?'

3. **Pausing and searching** During a non-mentalizing interaction, the therapist stops the interaction and deliberately slows it down, noting that he/she is very interested in exactly what each person is feeling as this interaction unfolds.

The therapist then lets the interaction slowly move forward, checking with each person exactly what the action of the other person makes them feel and what it makes them think. In other words, the therapist stops a non-mentalizing interaction and tries to help the family piece together the sequence of mental states, emotions, and behaviours that occurred during that interaction. Having done so, the therapist sometimes follows up by asking the relevant parties to try to empathize with one person's feelings, perhaps by asking them to recall a time when they felt similarly, or by asking them to role-play with the other person. All attempts by family members to add typical non-mentalizing narratives (as considered next) are actively limited by the therapist.

4. **Identifying preferred nonmentalizing narratives** When non-mentalizing occurs, a person often has a characteristic style of non-mentalistic thinking and speaking that they use to try to explain another person's (or their own) behaviour. If this process appears to be blocking a shift to a more mentalizing perspective, the therapist highlights that, for example, the family seems to get in quite similar repetitive conversations that don't appear to get anywhere. This observation may form the basis for a move to a mentalizing intervention, and provides a shared reference, so that later on the therapist is able to say, 'It feels a bit like we're getting into one of those round-in-circles conversations again' (or whatever label is most fitting). When done with gentle humour, this approach can be a very effective way of drawing attention to, and hopefully changing, non-mentalizing interactions.

5. **Identifying and labeling hidden feeling states** During family discussions of a problem-relevant situation, the therapist actively elicits a feeling state or, if one is mentioned but not dwelt on, the therapist highlights the importance of this feeling. The therapist actively encourages family members to label their feelings and, when they have done so, to reflect on what labelling of their feeling must be like for them. In addition, the therapist strives to search for subtleties in emotional experience that are not routinely expressed. For example, the therapist might say, 'You say you were feeling angry. Were there any other feelings you had at that time?' Often, simple probes like this will elicit a richer, and less hostile or hurtful, picture of someone's thinking. Ultimately, the therapist aims to learn from the person in question what would need to happen to allow them to not feel this way and, more specifically, how this person would need other members of the family to think about them such that they would help them feel differently.

6. **Using hypotheticals and counterfactuals** The therapist aims to activate the family's capacity to think about states of mind. This is tantamount to

increasing the level of abstraction at which the family functions, particularly at times of stress. A relatively easy way of achieving this goal is using hypotheticals, or 'What if?' questions, often building on the client's implicit assumptions. An extension of this technique is asking clients to conceive of states of mind diametrically opposed to the assertion they have made. For example, the therapist might say 'You said that you expect David would leave if you said X. What if he did not leave? What do you think might have been going on in his mind if he decided not to leave?'

7. **Therapist's making use of self** Therapists ask families to focus on and express feelings that have triggered non-mentalizing responses. Therapists encourage family members to be direct, honest, and vulnerable with each other. Therapists use their own experience of current interactions to communicate openly, clearly, and honestly about their own mental states and the way these are affected by the behaviour and interactions of others. This requires tremendous trust and courage from all participants. The therapist's willingness to enter intense personal conversations with honesty, conviction, commitment, and vulnerability greatly affects the outcome by modelling the integrity that the therapist attempts to promote in all family members.

10.7 Conclusions

Three questions should remain the focus of future research if we are to arrive at an understanding of maladaptive social cognition associated with juvenile BPD that is adequate to inform treatment.

1. What biobehavioural developmental processes create the cognitive vulnerabilities we encounter clinically?
2. What factors control the presence or absence of this dysfunction at any one time, and in the course of the patient's progress with the disorder?
3. What secondary difficulties are created for the patient by the dysfunction, and what are the developmentally expectable attempts at coping with the dysfunction of a key aspect of social cognition?

In this chapter, we have reviewed an approach to answering the above questions, but clearly we have only begun to scratch the surface. Given the devastating consequences of BPD—for individuals, their families, and society—a better understanding of the early precursors of BPD, with associated opportunities for intervention, is of crucial importance. As we have shown in this chapter, social cognition provides the key to identifying and understanding the developmental origins of BPD, and with its associated treatment may provide essential opportunities for early intervention.

References

Agrawal, H.R., Gunderson, J., Holmes, B.M., and Lyons-Ruth, K. (2004). Attachment studies with borderline patients: a review. *Harvard Review of Psychiatry*, **12**, 94–104.

Ainsworth, M.D.S., Blehar, M.C., Waters, E., and Wall, S. (1978). *Patterns of attachment: a psychological study of the Strange Situation*. Hillsdale, NJ: Lawrence Erlbaum.

Akhtar, S. (1992). Broken structures: severe personality disorders and their treatment. Northvale, NJ: Jason Aronson.

Alessandri, S.M. (1991). Play and social behaviours in maltreated preschoolers. *Development and Psychopathology*, **3**, 191–206.

Allen, J.G. (2000). *Traumatic attachments*. New York: John Wiley.

Allen, J.G. (2004). *Coping with trauma: a guide to self-understanding* (2nd edn). Washington, DC: American Psychiatric Press.

Allen, J.G. (2006). Mentalizing in practice. In *Handbook of mentalization-based treatment* (ed. J.G. Allen and P.Fonagy). New York: John Wiley.

Allen, J.G. and Fonagy, P. (2002). *The development of mentalizing and its role in psychopathology and psychotherapy*. Technical Report 02–0048), Research Department, Menninger Clinic, Topeka, KS.

Astington, J. (1996). What is theoretical about the child's theory of mind? A Vygotskian view of its development. In *Theories of theories of mind* (ed. P. Carruthers and P.K. Smith), pp. 184–99). Cambridge University Press.

Baker, L., Silk, K.R., Westen, D., Nigg, J.T., and Lohr, N.E. (1992). Malevolence, splitting, and parental ratings by borderlines. *Journal of Nervous Mental Disorders*, **180**, 258–64.

Baron-Cohen, S. and Cross, P. (1992). Reading the eyes: evidence for the role of perception in the development of a theory of mind. *Mind and Language*, **6**, 173–86.

Baron-Cohen, S., Jolliffe, T., Mortimore, C., and Robertson, M. (1997). Another advanced test of theory of mind: evidence from very high functioning adults with autisms or Asperger syndrome. *Journal of Child Psychology and Psychiatry*, **38**, 813–22.

Bateman, A.W. and Fonagy, P. (1999). The effectiveness of partial hospitalization in the treatment of borderline personality disorder: a randomised controlled trial. *American Journal of Psychiatry*, **156**, 1563–9.

Bateman, A.W. and Fonagy, P. (2001). Treatment of borderline personality disorder with psychoanalytically oriented partial hospitalization: an 18-month follow-up. *American Journal of Psychiatry*, **158**, 36–42.

Bateman, A.W. and Fonagy, P. (2004). *Psychotherapy for borderline personality disorder: mentalization-based treatment*. Oxford University Press.

Bateman, A.W. and Tyrer, P. (2004). Psychological treatment for personality disorders. *Advances in Psychiatric Treatment*, **10**, 378–88.

Baumrind, D. (1991). Parenting styles and adolescent development. In *The encyclopedia on adolescence* ((ed. J. Brooks-Gunn, R. Lerner, and A.C. Petersen), pp. 746–58. New York: Garland.

Beeghly, M. and Cicchetti, D. (1994). Child maltreatment, attachment, and the self system: emergence of an internal state lexicon in toddlers at high social risk. *Development and Psychopathology*, **6**, 5–30.

Bender, D.S., Skodol, A.E., Pagano, M.E., *et al.* (2006). Prospective assessment of treatment use by patients with personality disorders. *Psychiatric Services*, **57**, 254–7.

Bezirganian, S., Cohen, P., and Brook, J.S. (1993). The impact of mother–child interaction on the development of borderline personality disorder. *American Journal of Psychiatry*, 150, 1836–42.

Blais, M.A., Hilsenroth, M.J., and Castlebury, F.D. (1997). Content validity of the DSM-IV borderline and narcissistic personality disorder criteria sets. *Comprehensive Psychiatry*, 38, 31–7.

Bland, A.R., Williams, C.A., Scharer, K., and Manning, S. (2004). Emotion processing in borderline personality disorders. *Issues in Mental Health Nursing*, 25, 655–72.

Bleiberg, E. (2001). *Treating personality disorders in children and adolescents: a relational approach*. New York: Guilford Press.

Bondurant, H., Greenfield, B., and Tse, S.M. (2004). Construct validity. of adolescent BPD. *Canadian Journal of Child and Adolescent Psychiatry Review*, 13, 53–7.

Bowlby, J (1969). *Attachment and loss*. Vol. 1: *Attachment*. London: Hogarth Press–Institute of Psycho-Analysis.

Bray,S. Barrowclough,C., and Lobban, F. (2007). The social problem-solving abilities of people with borderline personality disorder. *Behavioral Research and Therapy*, 45, 1409–17.

Brennan, K.A. and Shaver, P.R. (1998). Attachment styles and personality disorders: their connections to each other and to parental divorce, parental death, and perceptions of parental caregiving. *Journal of Personality*, 66, 835–78.

Bretherton, I., Bates, E., Benigni, L., Camaioni, L., and Volterra, V. (1979). Relationships between cognition, communication, and quality of attachment. In *The emergence of symbols: cognition and communication in infancy* (ed. E. Bates, L. Benigni, I. Bretherton, L. Camaioni, and V. Volterra), pp. 223–69. New York: Academic Press.

Brodsky, B.S,, Groves, S.A., Oquendo, M.A., Mann, J.J., and Stanley, B. (2006). Interpersonal precipitants and suicide attempts in borderline personality disorder. *Suicide and Life Threatening Behaviors*, 36, 313–22.

Brown, K.W. and Ryan, R.M. (2003). The benefits of being present: mindfulness and its role in psychological well-being. *Journal of Personality and Social Psychology*, 84, 822–48.

Camras, L.A., Grow, G., and Ribordy, S. (1983). Recognition of emotional expressions by abused children. *Journal of Consulting and Clinical Psychology*, 12, 325–8.

Camras, L.A., Ribordy, S., Hill, J., Martino, S., Spaccarelli, S., and Stefani, R. (1988). Recognition and posing of emotional expressions by abused children and their mothers. *Developmental Psychology*, 24, 776–81.

Camras, L.A., Ribordy, S., Hill, J., et al. (1990). Maternal facial behavior and the recognition and production of emotional expression by maltreated and nonmaltreated children. *Developmental Psychology*, 26, 304–12.

Camras, L.A., Sachs-Alter, E., and Ribordy, S.C (1996). Emotion understanding in maltreated children: Recognition of facial expressions and integration with other emotion cues. In *Emotional development in atypical children* (ed. M.D. Lewis and M. Sullivan), pp. 203–25). Mahwah, NJ: Lawrence Erlbaum.

Caspi, A., McClay, J., Moffitt, T.E., et al. (2002). Role of genotype in the cycle of violence in maltreated children. *Science*, 297, 851–4.

Caspi, A., Sugden, K., Moffitt, T.E., et al. (2003). Influence of life stress on depression: moderation by a polymorphism in the 5-HTT gene. *Science*, 301, 386–9.

Charman, T., Ruffman, T., and Clements, W. (2002). Is there a gender difference in false belief development? *Social Development*, **11**, 1–10.

Cicchetti, D. and Rogosch, F.A. (2002). A developmental psychopathology perspective on adolescence. *Journal of Consulting and Clinical Psychology*, **70**, 6–20.

Cicchetti, D., Rogosch, F.A. Maughan, A., Toth, S.L., and Bruce, J. (2003). False belief understanding in maltreated children. *Development and Psychopathology*, **15**, 1067–91.

Cloninger, C.R., Svrakic, D.M., and Przybeck, T.R. (1993). A psychobiological model of temperament and character. *Archives of General Psychiatry*, **50**, 975–90.

Cramer, V., Torgersen, S., and Kringlen, E. (2006). Personality disorders and quality of life. A population study. *Comprehensive Psychiatry*, **47**, 178–84.

Crandell, L.E., Patrick, M.P.H., and Hobson, R.P. (2003). 'Still-face' interactions between mothers with borderline personality disored and their 2-month-old infants. *British Journal of Psychiatry*, **183**, 239–47.

Crick, N.R., Murray-Close, D., and Woods, K. (2005). Borderline personality features in childhood: a short-term longitudinal study. *Development and Psychopathology*, **17**, 1051–70.

Cutting, A.L. and Dunn, J. (1999). Theory of mind, emotion understanding, language, and family background: individual differences and interrelations. *Child Development*, **70**, 853–65.

Danon, G. and Graignic, R. (2003). Borderline personality disorder and mother–infant interaction. Presented at the Society for Child Development, Atlanta, GA.

Denham, S.A., Zoller, D., and Couchoud, E.A. (1994). Socialization of preschoolers emotion understanding. *Developmental Psychology*, **30**, 928–36.

Dennett, D. (2001). Are we explaining consciousness yet? *Cognition*, **79**, 221–37.

Depue, R.A. and Lenzenweger, M.F. (2001). A neurobehavioral dimensional model of personality disorders. In *The handbook of personality disorders* (ed. W.J. Livesley), pp. 136–76. New York: Guilford Press.

de Rosnay, M. and Harris, P.L. (2002). Individual differences in children's understanding of emotion: the roles of attachment and language. *Attachment and Human Development*, **4**, 39–54.

Dorris, L., Espie, C.A., Knott, F., and Salt, J. (2004). Mind-reading difficulties in the siblings of people with Asperger's syndrome: evidence for a genetic influence in the abnormal development of a specific cognitive domain. *Journal of Child Psychology and Psychiatry*, **45**, 412–18.

Dunn, J. and Brown, J. (2001). Relationship, talk about feelings, and the development of affect regulation in early childhood. In J. Garber and K. Dodge (Eds.). *Affect Regulation and Dysregulation in Childhood* pp. 89–108. Cambridge: Cambridge University Press.

Dunn, J., Brown, J., and Beardsall, L. (1991a). Family talk abut feeling states and children's later understanding of others' emotions. *Developmental Psychology*, **27**, 448–55.

Dunn, J., Brown, J., Somkowski, C., Telsa, C., and Youngblade, L. (1991b). Young children's understanding of other people's feelings and beliefs: individual differences and their antecedents. *Child Development*, **62**, 1352–66.

During, S. and McMahon, R. (1991). Recognition of emotional facial expressions by abusive mothers and their children. *Journal of Consulting and Clinical Psychology*, **20**, 132–9.

Fearon, P, Target, M., Fonagy, P., et al. (2006). Short-Term Mentalization and Relational Therapy (SMART): an integrative family therapy for children and adolescents. In *Handbook of mentalisaiton based treatments* (ed. J. Allen and P. Fonagy), Chichester: John Wiley.

Feldman, R.B., Zelkowitz, P., Weiss, M., Vogel, J., Heyman, M., and Paris, J. (1995). A comparison of the families of mothers with borderline and nonborderline personality disorders. *Comprehensive Psychiatry*, **36**, 157–63.

Fonagy, P. and Target, M. (1997). Attachment and reflective function: their role in self-organization. *Development and Psychopathology*, **9**, 679–700.

Fonagy, P., Steele, M., Steele, H., et al. (1995). The predictive validity of Mary Main's Adult Attachment Interview: a psychoanalytic and developmental perspective on the transgenerational transmission of attachment and borderline states. In *Attachment theory: social, developmental and clinical perspectives* (ed. S Goldberg, R. Muir, and J. Kerr), pp. 233–78. Hillsdale, NJ: Analytic Press.

Fonagy, P., Leigh, T., Steele, M., et al. (1996). The relation of attachment status, psychiatric classification, and response to psychotherapy. *Journal of Consulting and Clinical Psychology*, **64**, 22–31.

Fonagy, P., Redfern, S., and Charman, T. (1997a). The relationship between belief–desire reasoning and a projective measure of attachment security (SAT). *British Journal of Developmental Psychology*, **15**, 51–61.

Fonagy, P., Steele, H., Steele, M., and Holder, J. (1997b). Attachment and theory of mind: Overlapping constructs? *Association for Child Psychology and Psychiatry Occasional Papers*, **14**, 31–40.

Fonagy, P., Target, M., and Gergely, G. (2000). Attachment and borderline personality disorder: a theory and some evidence. *Psychiatric Clinics of North America*, **23**, 103–22.

Fonagy, P., Gergely, G., Jurist, E., and Target, M. (2002). *Affect regulation, mentalization and the development of the self*. New York: Other Press.

Fonagy, P., Stein, H., Allen, J., and Fultz, J. (2003a). The relationship of mentalization and childhood and adolescent adversity to adult functioning. Presented at the Biennial Meeting of the Society for Research in Child Development, Tampa, FL.

Fonagy, P., Target, M., Gergely, G., Allen, J.G., and Bateman, A (2003b). The developmental roots of borderline personality disorder in early attachment relationships: a theory and some evidence. *Psychoanalytic Inquiry*, **23**, 412–59.

Fonagy, P., Stein, H., Allen, D., Chen, C.F., Allen, J.G., and Vrouva, I. The relationship of childhood and adolescent adversity to impairment of mentalizing capacity and psychological disorder. *Development and Psychopathology*, submitted for publication.

Fraiberg, S.H., Adelson, E., and Shapiro, V. (1975). Ghosts in the nursery: a psychoanalytic approach to the problem of impaired infant-mother relationships. *Journal of the American Academy Child Psychiatry*, **14**, 387–422.

Frank, H. and Hoffman, N. (1986). Borderline empathy: an empirical investigation. *Comprehensive Psychiatry*, **27**, 387–95.

Frodi, A. and Smetana, J. (1984). Abused, neglected, and nonmaltreated preschoolers' ability to discriminate emotions in others: the effects of IQ. *Child Abuse and Neglect*, **8**, 459–65.

Goldberg, S., Benoit, D., Blokland, K., and Madigan, S. (2003). Atypical maternal behavior, maternal representations, and infant disorganized attachment. *Development and Psychopathology*, **15**, 239–57.

Golomb, A., Ludolph, P., Westen, D., Block, M.J., Maurer, P., and Wiss, F.C. (1994). Maternal empathy, family chaos, and the etiology of borderline personality disorder. *Journal of the American Psychoanalytic Association*, **42**, 525–48.

Grienenberger, J., Kelly, K., and Slade, A. (2005). Maternal reflective functioning, mother–infant affective communication, and infant attachment: exploring the link between mental states and observed caregiving behaviour in the intergenerational transmission of attachment. *Attachment and Human Development*, **7**, 299–311.

Gunderson, J.G. (2001). *Borderline personality disorder: a clinical guide*. Washington, DC: American Psychiatric Publishing.

Guttman, H.A. and Laporte, L. (2000). Empathy in families of women with borderline personality disorder, anorexia nervosa, and a control group. *Family Process*, **39**, 345–58.

Guttman, H.A. and Laporte, L. (2002). Alexithymia, empathy, and psychological symptoms in a family context. *Comprehensive Psychiatry*, **43**, 448–55.

Hamilton, C.E. (2000). Continuity and discontinuity of attachment from infancy through adolescence. *Child Development*, **71**, 690–4.

Harris, P.L. (1999). Individual differences in understanding emotions: the role of attachment status and emotional discourse. *Attachment and Human Development*, **1**, 307–24.

Herman, J.L., Perry, C., and van der Kolk, B.A. (1989). Childhood trauma in borderline personality disorder. *American Journal of Psychiatry*, **146**, 490–5.

Herpertz, S.C. (2003). Emotional processing in personality disorder. *Current Psychiatry Reports*, **5**, 23–7.

Hobson, P., Patrick, M., Crandell, L.E., Garcia-Perez, R., and Lee, A. (2005). Personal relatedness and attachment in infants of mothers with borderline personality disorder. *Development and Psychopathology*, **17**, 329–47.

Holmes, J. (2003). Borderline personality disorder and the search for meaning: an attachment perspective. *Australian and New Zealand Journal of Psychiatry*, **37**, 524–31.

Howes, C. and Espinosa, M.P. (1985). The consequences of child abuse for the formation of relationships with peers. *International Journal of Child Abuse and Neglect*, **9**, 397–404.

Hughes, C. and Cutting, A. (1999). Nature, nurture and individual differences in early understanding of mind. *Psychological Science*, **10**, 429–32.

Hughes, C. and Dunn, J. (2002). 'When I say a naughty word.' Children's accounts of anger and sadness in self, mother and friend: longitudinal findings from ages four to seven. *British Journal of Developmental Psychology*, **20**, 515–35.

Hughes, C., Jaffee, S.R., Happè, F., Taylor, A., Caspi, A., and Moffitt TE (2005). Origins of individual differences in theory of mind: from nature to nurture? *Child Developoment*, **76**, 356–70.

Johnson, JG, Cohen, P., Smailes, E., Skodol, A., Brown, J., and Oldham, J. (2001). Childhood verbal abuse and risk for personality disorders during adolescence and early adulthood. *Comprehensive Psychiatry*, **42**, 16–23.

Johnson, J.G., Cohen, P., Kasen, S., Ehrensaft, M.K., and Crawford, T.N. (2006). Associations of parental personality disorders and axis I disorders with childrearing behavior. *Psychiatry*, **69**, 336–350.

Kernberg, O.F. (1983). Object relations theory and character analysis. *Journal of the American Psychoanalytic Association*, **31**, 247–71.

Klimes-Dougan, B. and Kistner, J. (1990). Physically abused preschoolers' responses to peers' distress. *Developmental Psychology*, **25**, 516–24.

Kobak, R., Cassidy, J., Lyons-Ruth, K., and Ziv, Y. (2006). Attachment, stress and psychopathology: a developmental pathways model. In *Development and psychopathology. Vol. 1: Theory and method* (2nd edn) (ed. D. Cicchetti and D.J. Cohen), pp. 334–69. New York: John Wiley.

Koren-Karie, N., Oppenheim, D., Dolev, S., Sher, S., and Etzion-Carasso, A. (2002). Mother's insightfulness regarding their infants' internal experience: relations with maternal sensitivity and infant attachment. *Developmental Psychology*, **38**, 534–42.

Lebovici, S. (1988). Fantasmatic interactions and intergenerational transmission. *Infant Mental Health Journal*, **9**, 10–19.

Leichsenring, F. and Sachsse, U. (2002). Emotions as wishes and beliefs. *Journal of Personality Assessment*, **79**, 257–73.

Lenzenweger, M.F. and Cicchetti, D. (2005). Toward a developmental psychopathology approach to borderline personality disorder. *Development and Psychopathology*, **17**, 893–8.

Levy, K.N. (2005). The implications of attachment theory and research for understanding borderline personality disorder. *Development and Psychopathology*, **17**, 959–86.

Levy, K.N., Meehan, K.B., Kelly, K.M., *et al.* (2006). Change in attachment patterns and reflective function in a randomized control trial of transference-focused psychotherapy for borderline personality disorder. *Journal of Consulting and Clinical Psychology*, **74**, 1027–40.

Lieb, K., Zanarini, M.C., Schmahl, C., Linehan, M.M., and Bohus, M. (2004). Borderline personality disorder. *Lancet*, **364**, 453–61.

Livesley, W.J. and Jackson, D.N. (1992). Guidelines for developing, evaluating and revising the classification of personality disorders. *Journal of Nervous and Mental Disease*, **180**, 609–18.

Lyons-Ruth, K., Yellin, C., Melnick, S., and Atwood, G. (2005). Expanding the concept of unresolved mental states: hostile/helpless states of mind on the Adult Attachment Interview are associated with disrupted mother–infant communication and infant disorganization. *Development and Psychopathology*, **17**, 1–23.

Macfie, J., Toth, S.L., Rogosch, F.A., Robinson, J., Emde, R.N., and Cicchetti, D. (1999). Effect of maltreatment on preschoolers' narrative representations of responses to relieve distress and of role reversal. *Developmental Psychology*, **35**, 460–5.

Macfie, J., Cicchetti, D., and Toth, S.L. (2001). The development of dissociation in maltreated preschool-aged children. *Development and Psychopathology*, **13**, 233–54.

Main, M. and George, C. (1985). Responses of abused and disadvantaged toddlers to distress in agemates: a study in the daycare setting. *Developmental Psychology*, **21**, 407–12.

Main, M. and Solomon, J. (1990). Procedures for identifying infants as disorganized/ disoriented during the Ainsworth Strange Situation. In *Attachment during the preschool years: theory, research and intervention* (ed. M Greenberg, D. Cicchetti and E.M. Cummings, pp. 121–60. University of Chicago Press.

Meins, E., Fernyhough, C., Russel, J., and Clark-Carter, D. (1998). Security of attachment as a predictor of symbolic and mentalising abilities: a longitudinal study. *Social Development*, 7, 1–24.

Meins, E., Fernyhough, C., Fradley, E., and Tuckey, M. (2001). Rethinking maternal sensitivity: mothers' comments on infants mental processes predict security of attachment at 12 months. *Journal of Child Psychology and Psychiatry*, 42, 637–48.

Meins, E., Fernyhough, C., Wainwright, R., Das Gupta, M., Fradley, E., and Tuckey, M. (2002). Maternal mind-mindedness and attachment security as predictors of theory of mind understanding. *Child Development*, 73, 1715–26.

Meins, E., Fernyhough, C., Wainwright, R., *et al.* (2003). Pathways to understanding mind: construct validity and predictive validity of maternal mind-mindedness. *Child Development*, 74(4), 1194–1211.

Meyer, B. and Pilkonis, P.A. (2005). An attachment model of personality disorder. In *Major theories of personality disorder* (ed. M.F. Lenzenweger and J.F. Clark). New York: Guilford Press.

Minzenberg, M.J., Poole, J.H., and Vinogradov, S. (2006). Social-emotion recognition in borderline personality disorder. *Comprehensive Psychiatry*, 47, 468–74.

Nurnberg, H.G., Raskin, M., Levine, P.E., and Pollack, S. (1991). Hierarchy of DSM-III-R criteria efficiency for the diagnosis of borderline personality disorder. *Journal of Persoanlity Disorders*, 5, 211–24.

Ontai, L.L. and Thompson, R.A. (2002). Patterns of attachment and maternal discourse effects on children's emotion understanding from 3 to 5 years of age. *Social Development*, 11, 433–50.

Oppenheim, D. and Koren-Karie, N. (2002). Mothers' insightfulness regarding their children's internal worlds: the capacity underlying secure child-mother relationships. *Infant Mental Health Journal*, 23, 593–605.

Oppenheim, D., Koren-Karie, N., Etzion-Carasso, A., and Sagi-Schwartz, A. (2005). Maternal insightfulness but not infant attachment predicts 4 year olds' theory of mind. Presented at the Biennial meeting of the Society for Research in Child Development, Atlanta, GA.

Paris, J. (1994). The etiology of borderline personality disorder: a biopsychosocial approach. *Psychiatry*, 57, 316–25.

Paris, J. (2003). *Personality disorders over time: precursors, course, and outcome*. Washington, DC: American Psychiatric Association.

Paris, J. and Frank, H. (1989). Perceptions of parental bonding in borderline patients. *American Journal of Psychiatry*, 146, 1498–9.

Pears, K.C. and Fisher, P.A. (2005). Emotion understanding and theory of mind among maltreated children in foster care. *Development and Psychopathology*, 17, 47–65.

Pears, K.C. and Moses, L.J. (2003). Demographics, parenting, and theory of mind in preschool children. *Social Development*, 12, 1–20.

Peterson, C. and Slaughter, V. (2003). Opening widows into the mind: mothers' preference for mental state explanations and children's theory of mind. *Cognitive Development*, 18, 399–429.

Pollak, S.D. and Sinha, P. (2003). Effects of early experience on children's recognition of facial displays of emotion. *Developmental Psychology*, **38**, 784–91.

Pollak, S.D., Klorman, R., Thatcher, J.E., and Cicchetti, D. (2001). P3b reflects maltreated children's reactions to facial displays of emotion. *Psychophysiology*, **38**, 267–74.

Raikes, H.A. and Thompson, R.A. (2006). Family emotional climate, attachment security, and young children's emotion knowledge in a high-risk sample. *British Journal of Developmental Psychology*, **24**, 89–104.

Raine, A. (1993). Features of borderline personality and violence. *Journal of Clinical Psychology*, **49**, 277–81.

Rogosch, F.A., Cicchetti, D., and Aber, J.L. (1995). The role of child maltreatment in early deviations in cognitive and affective processing abilities and later peer relationship problems. *Development and Psychopathology*, **7**, 591–609.

Rosenthal, M.Z., Cukrowicz, K.C., Cheavens, J.S., and Lynch, T.R. (2006). Self-punishment as a regulation strategy in borderline personality disorder. *Journal of Personality Disorders*, **20**, 232–46.

Ruffman, T., Perner, J., and Parkin, L. (1999). How parenting style affects false belief understanding. *Social Development*, **8**, 395–411.

Russ, E., Heim, A., and Westen, D. (2003). Parental bonding and personality pathology assessed by clinician report. *Journal of Personality Disorders*, **17**, 522–36.

Ryan, R.M. (2005). The developmental line of autonomy in the etiology, dynamics, and treatment of borderline personality disorders. *Development and Psychopathology*, **17**, 987–1006.

Sabbagh, M.A. and Callanan, M.A. (1998). Metarepresentation in action: 3-, 4-, and 5-year-olds developing theories of mind in parent-child conversations. *Developmental Psychology*, **34**, 491–502.

Schechter, D.S., Coots, T., Zeanah, C.H., *et al.* (2005). Maternal mental representations of the child in an inner-city clinical sample: violence-related posttraumatic stress and reflective functioning. *Attachment and Human Development*, **7**, 313–31.

Sharp, C. and Bleiberg, E. (2007). Borderline personality disorder in children and adolescents. In *Lewis' Child and adolescent psychiatry* (4th edn) (ed. A. Martin and F Volkmar), pp. 680–691. Baltimore, MD: Lippincott–Williams and Wilkins.

Sharp, C. and Fonagy, P. The parent's capacity to treat the child as a psychological agent: Constructs, measures and implications for developmental psychopathology. *Social Development*, in press.

Sharp, C. and Romero, C. (2007). Borderline personality disorder: a comparison between children and adults. *Bulletin of the Menninger Clinic*, **71**, 121–50.

Sharp, C., Fonagy, P., and Goodyer, I. (2006). Imagining your child's mind: psychosocial adjustment and mothers' ability to predict their children's attributional response styles. *British Journal of Developmental Psychology*, **24**, 197–214.

Sharp, C., Croudace T.J. and Goodyer, I. (2007) Biased mentalising in children aged 7–11: Latent class confirmation of response styles to social scenarios and associations with psychopathology. *Social Development*, **16**(1), 181–202.

Shearer, S.L., Peters, C.P., Quaytman, M.S., and Ogden, R.L. (1990). Frequency and correlates of childhood sexual and physical abuse histories in adult female borderline inpatients. *American Journal of Psychiatry*, **147**, 214–16.

Shipman, K.L. and Zeman, J. (1999). Emotional understanding: a comparison of physically maltreating and nonmaltreating mother–child dyads. *Journal of Clinical Child Psychology*, **28**, 407–17.

Skodol, A.E., Gunderson, J.G., McGlashan, T.H., *et al.* (2002). Functional impairment in patients with schizotypal, borderline, avoidant, or obsessive–compulsive personality disorder. *American Journal of Psychiatry*, **159**, 276–83.

Slade, A. (2005). Parental reflective functioning: an introduction. *Attachment and Human Development*, **7**, 269–81.

Slade, A., Grienenberger, J., Bernbach, E., Levy, D., and Locker, A. (2005). Maternal reflective functioning, attachment and the transmission gap: a preliminary study. *Attachment and Human Development*, **7**, 283–98.

Smith, C.A. and Farrington, D.P. (2004). Continuities in antisocial behavior and parenting across three generations. *Journal of Child Psychology and Psychiatry*, **45**, 230–47.

Smith, M. and Walden, T. (1999). Understanding feelings and coping with emotional situations: a comparison of maltreated and nonmaltreated preschoolers. *Social Development*, **8**, 93–116.

Soloff, P. and Millward, J. (1983). Developmental histories of borderline patients. *Comprehensive Psychiatry*, **24**, 574–88.

Soloff, P.H., Kelly, T.M., Strotmeyer, S.J., Malone, K.M., and Mann, J.J. (2003). Impulsivity, gender, and response to fenfluramine challenge in borderline personality disorder. *Psychiatry Research*, **119**, 11–24.

Sroufe, L.A. (1996). *Emotional development: the organization of emotional life in the early years*. New York: Cambridge University Press.

Sroufe, L.A., Egeland, B., Carlson, E., and Collins, W.A. (2005). *The development of the person: the Minnesota study of risk and adaptation from birth to adulthood*. New York: Guilford Press.

Steele, M., Steele, H., Croft, C., and Fonagy, P. (1999). Infant mother attachment at one year predicts children's understanding of mixed emotions at 6 years. *Social Development*, **8**, 161–78.

Steinberg, L. and Avenevoli, S. (2000). The role of context in the development of psychopathology: a conceptual framework and some speculative propositions. *Child Development*, **71**, 66–74.

Stevenson, J., Meares, R., and Comerford, A. (2003). Diminished impulsivity in older patients with borderline personality disorder. *American Journal of Psychiatry*, **160**, 165–6.

Stokes, N.A., Feigenbaum, J.D., Fonagy, P., and Channon, S. Theory of mind in borderline personality disorder, submitted for publication.

Symons, D.K. (2004). Mental state discourse, theory of mind, and the internalization of self-other understanding. *Developmental Review*, **24**, 159–88.

Thompson, R.A. (2000). The legacy of early attachments. *Child Development*, **71**, 145–52.

Torgersen, S., Lygren, S., Oien, P.A., *et al.* (2000). A twin study of personality disorders. *Comprehensive Psychiatry*, **41**, 416–25.

Toth, S.L., Cicchetti, D., Macfie, J., Maughan, A., and Vanmeenen, K. (2000). Narrative representations of caregivers and seld in maltreated pre-schoolers. *Attachment and Human Development*, **2**, 271–305.

van Ijzendoorn, M.H. (1992). Intergenerational transmission of parenting: a review of studies in non-clinical populations. *Developmental Review*, **12**, 76–99.

van Ijzendoorn, M.H. (1995). Adult attachment representations, parental responsiveness, and infant attachment: a meta-analysis on the predictive validity of the Adult Attachment Interview. *Psychological Bulletin*, **117**, 387–403.

van Ijzendoorn, M.H. and Bakermans-Kranenburg, M.J. (1997). Intergenerational transmission of attachment: a move to the contextual level. In *Attachment and psychopathology* (ed. L. Atkinson and K.J. Zucker), pp. 135–70. New York: Guilford Press.

Vermote, R., Vertommen, H., Corveleyn, J., Verhaest, Y., Franssen, M., and Peuskens, J. (2003). The Kortenberg–Louvain process-outcome study. Presented at the IPA Congress, Toronto.

Vinden, P.G. (2001). Parenting attitudes and children's understanding of mind: a comparison of Korean American and Anglo-American families. *Cognitive Development*, **16**, 793–809.

Wagner, K.D. and Ambrosini, P.J. (2001). Childhood depression: pharmacological therapy/treatment (pharmacotherapy of childhood depression). *Journal of Clinical Child Psychology*, **30**, 88–97.

Waters, E., Merrick, S.K., Treboux, D., Crowell, J., and Albersheim, L. (2000). Attachment security from infancy to early adulthood: a 20 year longitudinal study. *Child Development*, **71**, 684–9.

Weinfield N, Sroufe LA and Egeland B (2000). Attachment from infancy to early adulthood in a high risk sample: Continuity, discontinuity and their correlates. *Child Development*, **71**(3), 695–702.

Westen, D. and Cohen, R.P. (1993). The self in borderline personality disorder: a psychodynamic perspective. In *The self in emotional distress: cognitive and psychodynamic perspectives* (ed. Z.V. Segal and S.J. Blatt, pp. 334–60. New York: Guilford Press.

Westen, D., Lohr, N., Silk, K., Gold, L., and Kerber, K. (1990a). Object relations and social cognition in borderlines, major depressives, and normals: a TAT analysis. *Psychological Assessment*, **2**, 355–64.

Westen, D., Ludolph, P., Misle, B., Ruffins, S., and Block, J. (1990b). Physical and sexual abuse in adolescent girls with borderline personality disorder. *American Journal of Orthopsychiatry*, **60**, 55–66.

White, C.N., Gunderson, J.G., Zanarini, M.C., and Hudson J.I. (2003). Family studies of borderline personality disorder: a review. *Harvard Review of Psychiatry*, **11**, 8–19.

Wilkinson-Ryan, T. and Westen, D. (2000). Identity disturbance in borderline personality disorder: an empirical investigation. *American Journal of Psychiatry*, **157**, 528–41.

Williams, L., Fonagy, P., Target, M., *et al.* (2006). Training psychiatry residents in mentalization-based therapy. In *Handbook of mentalisation based treatments* (ed. J. Allen and P. Fonagy), London: John Wiley.

Young, D.W. and Gunderson, J.G. (1995). Family images of borderline adolescents. *Psychiatry*, **58**, 164–72.

Zanarini, M.C. (2000). Childhood experiences associated with the development of borderline personality disorder. *Psychiatric Clinics of North America*, **23**, 89–101.

Zanarini, M.C., Gunderson, J.G., Marino, M.F., Schwartz, E.O., and Frankenburg, F.R. (1989). Childhood experiences of borderline patients. *Comprehensive Psychiatry*, **30**, 18–25.

Zanarini, M.C., Williams A.A., Lewis, R.E., *et al.* (1997). Reported pathological childhood experiences associated with the development of borderline personality disorder. *American Journal of Psychiatry*, **154**, 1101–6.

Part IV

Other considerations

11

Attachment, affect-regulation, and mentalization: the developmental origins of the representational affective self

György Gergely and Zsolt Unoka

In this chapter we propose an evolutionary-based social cognitive theory of the early development of the representational affective self in humans and its role in emotional self-regulation and control. We first identify species-unique properties of human caregiver–infant interactions and critically discuss alternative proposals concerning the functional role of the human attachment system in the development of mentalizing on the one hand, and emotional self-awareness and affective self-control on the other. We propose that the human-specific features of early caregiver–infant interactions provide the necessary input conditions for specialized representation-building and attention socialization mechanisms (such as contingency detection, social biofeedback, and natural 'pedagogy'). These mechanisms play a crucial role in establishing primary self–other affective relationship representations that capture the characteristic causal structure of contingent reactivity of early attachment relationships. They also set up cognitively accessible second-order emotion representations with associative links to the self's procedurally represented prewired basic emotions. We then characterize different levels of primary and secondary emotion-control systems and show how the developmentally established affective self–other representations subserve these emotion-regulative mechanisms. Finally, we argue that the socially constructed second-order emotion representations support the ontogenetic extension of the domain of mentalizing to include the self's own causal mental states (apart from those of others) and show how this enables the functional use of mentalization for the purposes of emotional self-regulation and control in affectively charged interactions and relationships in humans.

11.1 Species-unique properties of human attachment interactions and their functions: challenging current views on the development of mentalizing

Humans are just one of the many social animal species with an attachment instinct system where the quality of early caregiving (Harlow 1961; Bowlby 1969; Hofer 1995; Suomi 1995, 1999; Polan and Hofer 1999) has formative effects on the organism's later capacity to function adaptively in affiliative relationships. In contrast, humans may be unique in their ability to rely on a specialized inferential and representational system for mentalizing, or 'theory of mind' (ToM) (Dennett 1978, 1987; Baron-Cohen *et al*. 1985; Wellman 1990; Perner 1991; Fodor 1992; Baron-Cohen 1995; Leslie 2000) that has evolved to predict, interpret, and manipulate others' actions by inferring and attributing causal intentional mind states (such as desires, intentions, and beliefs) to them.

Arguably, attachment and mentalizing are two independent adaptations selected to serve qualitatively different evolutionary functions. This is suggested, for example, by the fact that many social species, such as rodents or rhesus monkeys (Hofer 1995; Polan and Hofer 1999; Suomi 1999), that apparently lack the capacity for mentalizing, nevertheless possess an innate infant–caregiver attachment system. According to Bowlby's (1969) original proposal, the basic evolutionary function of the attachment instinct is to provide a specialized interactive mechanism to ensure predator evasion for the immature offspring through a prewired goal-directed signal system serving proximity seeking and maintenance between caregiver and infant. This function certainly seems independent and qualitatively different from the primary function served by the specialized social cognitive adaptation for mentalizing, which is to predict and interpret the actions of conspecifics during adult competitive or cooperative situations through attributing causal mental states to them.

However, it is noteworthy that the structural organization of early attachment interactions in humans has become qualitatively enriched by species-unique evolved features that are conspicuously absent from mother–infant attachment interactions of other social species (including our closest primate relatives). Thus human mother–infant interactions show a unique 'proto-conversational' turn-taking contingency structure (Brazelton *et al.* 1974; Trevarthen 1979; Brazelton and Tronick 1980; Stern 1985; Sander 1988; Tronick 1989; Tronick and Cohn 1989; Trevarthen and Aitken 2001). Human infants exhibit early sensitivity and preference for highly response-contingent stimulus events characteristic of the interactive style of infant-attuned social partners (Watson 1972, 1985, 1994; Bahrick and Watson 1985; Lewis *et al*. 1990; Rochat and Morgan 1995; Bigelow 1999; Bigelow and

De Coste 2003; Bigelow and Rochat 2006). They also show special sensitivity to so-called ostensive-communicative cues (Csibra and Gergely 2006) such as eye contact (Farroni *et al.* 2002), infant-directed speech or 'motherese' (Fernald 1985, 1992; Cooper and Aslin 1990), and contingent reactivity (Watson 1994, 1995, 2001; Floccia *et al.* 1997; Johnson *et al.* 1998; Movellan and Watson 2002). Young human infants spontaneously attend to and gaze-follow others' referential cues (such as gaze shift), but only if these are preceded by direct eye contact or infant-contingent reactivity (Johnson *et al.* 1998; Farroni *et al.* 2002; Movellan and Watson 2002; reviewed by Csibra and Gergely 2006). Unlike apes, by 12 months humans show a communicative and referential understanding and use of pointing in triadic joint attention interactions (Liszkowski *et al.* 2004; Behne *et al.* 2005; Southgate *et al.* 2007b; Tomasello *et al.* 2007). Human mother–infant interactions also involve frequent exchanges of an increasingly differentiated repertoire of basic emotion expressions (Izard and Malatesta 1987; Cohn and Tronick 1988; Malatesta *et al.* 1989; Tronick 1989; Camras 1992; Gergely and Watson 1996, 1999; Sroufe 1996; Gergely 2002, 2007a; Bennett *et al.* 2004, 2005). This contrasts with the small range and low frequency of emotion displays in non-human infant–caregiver attachment interactions. Even in primates mother-directed affect displays by infants are rare and restricted to expressions of distress and protest triggered by loss of proximity (e.g. De Marco and Visalberghi 2007, Ferrari *et al.* 2006). Empathic affect-mirroring emotion displays by the caregiver seem unique to human mother–infant interactions (Cohn and Tronick 1988; Malatesta *et al.* 1989; Tronick 1989; Uzgiris *et al.* 1989; Gergely and Watson 1996, 1999; Bigelow 1999; Gergely 2004, 2007a; Fonagy *et al.* 2002, 2007). In this chapter we will explore the question of whether these apparently species-unique properties of human attachment interactions are related functionally or developmentally to the emergence of the capacity to mentalize, or whether they serve other basic functions that are independent of, or at least not directly related to, mindreading.

In recent years several attachment theorists and developmental psychologists have put forward different versions of the general hypothesis that, in the case of humans, there is an inherent causal and functional link between the quality of early infant attachment on the one hand, and the development of the ability for mentalizing on the other. In particular, the acquisition of mindreading skills by about 4 years of age, as indicated by passing the standard verbal false-belief attribution tasks (Wimmer and Perner 1983; Wellman *et al.* 2001), has been suggested to be facilitated by the security of early attachment relationships (e.g. Fonagy and Target 1997; Fonagy *et al.* 1997a,b; Meins *et al.* 1998, 2003; Hobson 2002). It has been proposed that secure attachment and early parental interactive behaviours which correlate with infant attachment security at 12 months, such as maternal mind-mindedness at 6 months (Meins *et al.* 2001), play an important causal role in fostering the development of mentalizing as they facilitate the early appearance of explicit mindreading skills in preschoolers (e.g. Fonagy and Target 1997; Fonagy *et al.* 1997a,b; Meins *et al.* 1998, 2002, 2003; Fonagy 2001). The supporting evidence consists mainly of correlational findings showing that secure infant attachment at 1 year (as well as its earlier correlates such as maternal mind-mindedness at 6 months) predict earlier ability to pass the standard verbal false-belief tasks at around 4 years (e.g. Fonagy and Target 1997; Fonagy *et al.* 1997a,b; Meins *et al.* 1998, 2003; de Rosnay and Harris 2002; Ontai and Thompson 2002).

However, there are a number of empirical and theoretical reasons to question the strong form of the hypothesis which postulates a specific evolutionary role and/or a direct ontogenetic causal developmental and functional link between security of infant attachment and its early interactive predictors on the one hand, and the development of explicit mindreading abilities in later childhood on the other. First, one problem lies in the fact that the correlational findings linking infant attachment security during the first year to earlier success in passing the explicit ToM tasks have not been supplemented with specific causal developmental models. Ideally, such models should spell out the particular ways in which the secure quality of preverbal attachment and/or factors such as parental talk involving mental state attributions to the baby at 6 months exert their facilitating effects on the acquisition of the cognitive skills involved in inferring, attributing, representing, and reasoning about the epistemic mind states of others (such as beliefs). Numerous plausible causal linking factors have been suggested in this regard which, however, exert their effect later in development. These include the frequency of perspective taking in caregiver–child linguistic exchanges (e.g. Harris 2005; Lohmann *et al.* 2005; de Rosnay and Hughes 2006), the amount of complementary role play in the family, the degree of family talk about conflicting emotions and differential conflict- and emotion-regulation strategies (Dunn *et al.* 1991; Sabbagh and Callanan 1998; Cutting and Dunn 1999; Ruffman *et al.* 1999; Vinden 2001), and the number of references to thoughts and beliefs and the relationship specificity of children's real-life accounts of negative emotions (Hughes and Dunn 2002). The independent effects of these (and other) factors on the earlier appearance of explicit ToM performance around 4 years are well documented (reviewed by Fonagy *et al.* 2007). Other facilitating factors that are unlikely to be related to infant attachment security include having older siblings (Perner *et al.* 1994; Ruffman *et al.* 1998), the relative frequency and precocity of using complex syntactic complement structures (Astington and Jenkins 1999; de Villiers and de Villiers 2000, de Villiers and Plyers 2002), and the maturational development of executive function, selective attention, and response inhibition capacities (Leslie 2000; Perner and Lang 2000; Leslie *et al.* 2004).

Secondly, the demonstrated facilitating effects of early secure attachment on ToM development are not strong. Moreover, in several studies they only show up in ToM tasks which involve reasoning about both beliefs and emotions (such as belief–desire tasks) in contrast with tasks probing purely epistemic states such as false beliefs (e.g. Fonagy *et al.* 1997a; reviewed by Fonagy *et al.* 2007). Furthermore, there are strong recent arguments and supporting evidence showing that the standard use of explicit verbal false-belief tasks (Wellman *et al.* 2001) to diagnose the developmental achievement of 'full' mindreading skills around age 4 involves several complex linguistic, pragmatic interpretational, and executive function requirements. Thus it is possible that young children have difficulty passing false-belief tasks not because they still lack the capacity to mentalize (or at least some components of ToM), but rather because of deficits with some of the non-ToM-related component skills that these tasks require (Bloom and German 2000; Leslie *et al.* 2004). This may have seriously distorted the validity of the generally accepted developmental timetable for the ontogenetic establishment of mentalizing abilities. For these reasons, some researchers have recently argued explicitly for the abandonment of the standard false-belief tasks as a general diagnostic tool for establishing the attainment of ToM skills (e.g. Bloom and German 2000).

Complementary to these methodologically based doubts, there is converging recent evidence (based on paradigms not plagued with the methodological problems outlined above) demonstrating mentalization much earlier in human ontogeny. For example, Tomasello and his colleagues have shown that infants exhibit a variety of ToM abilities as early as 12 months. These include spontaneously monitoring others' perceptual access to transformations of relevant aspects of reality, inferring and attributing to them the corresponding epistemic mental states of informedness or ignorance, and relying on such mental attributions to modulate one's own goal-directed behaviours in the presence of the other (e.g. Tomasello and Haberl 2003; Tomasello *et al.* 2005). Similarly, there is convergent new evidence based on implicit non-verbal versions of the standard false-belief tasks using violation-of-expectation looking-time paradigms which show that infants as young as 13 months of age monitor others' perceptual access to reality, infer, attribute, and represent their true or false beliefs about the situation accordingly, and predict the other's subsequent behaviour by relying on the representational content of such attributed mental states (Onishi and Baillargeon 2005; Csibra and Southgate 2006; Onishi *et al.* 2007; Southgate *et al.* 2007a; Surian *et al.* 2007).

Finally, recent evidence from comparative animal literature calls into doubt the notion that the basic ability for implicit mindreading is an exclusively human-specific capacity. These studies suggest that some rudimentary and possibly highly domain-restricted forms of mentalizing seem to have also evolved independently and convergently in a number of non-human social species, such as apes, goats, and avian species including crows, ravens, and scrab-jays (Hare et al. 2001; Tomasello et al. 2003; Emery and Clayton 2004; Bugnyar and Heinrich 2005; Kaminski et al. 2006).

Based on this brief review, we argue that the currently popular view endorsed by a number of attachment theorist and infant researchers which assumes a (possibly evolutionary-based and human-specific) direct causal and functional link between early security of infant attachment on the one hand, and the acquisition of explicit mentalizing skills on the other, must be significantly revised. The relevant developmental and comparative evidence of recent years seems more compatible with the alternative view that an implicit and automatic capacity for mentalizing about others is not a developmental achievement, but an innate social cognitive evolutionary adaptation implemented by a specialized and prewired mindreading mechanism which seems to be active and functional at least as early as 12 months in humans. Furthermore, this capacity for implicit mentalizing is unlikely to be a uniquely human competence as, in its basic form, it also seems to have evolved independently and convergently in a number of non-human social species which live in highly competitive niches.

The above does not imply that certain types of early interactive patterns characteristic of specific attachment relationships of human infants would have no developmental effect whatsoever on later ability to use the capacity for mentalizing functionally and efficiently in coping with interpersonal interactions and relationships. There are, in fact, good empirical reasons to believe that certain dysfunctional types of early attachment relations, involving severe neglect, abuse, or dissociative, highly intrusive, or grossly unpredictable patterns of parental reactivity, have significant and long-term detrimental and disruptive effects on later capacity to use the innate competence for on-line mentalization functionally as an adaptive interpersonal coping strategy (e.g. Fonagy et al. 2000, 2002, 2003, 2007; Gergely et al. 2002b).

In this chapter we advance the argument that the specialized capacity for mentalization is likely to be an independent social cognitive adaptation whose primary evolutionary function is separate and unrelated to the basic evolutionary function for which the attachment instinct system has been selected. If so, it would not be surprising if security of early infant attachment in humans did not turn out to play a direct causal functional role in the ontogenetic development of our mentalizing capacity. Nevertheless, we propose that when maladaptive patterns of affective parental reactivity become the dominant features of the recurring interactive structure of the infant's primary attachment relationships, they can and do play a significant causal role in pathologically undermining the developing self's potential to rely on its innate mentalizing capacity as its dominant social cognitive strategy to cope with interpersonal situations and intimate and affiliative relationships during later life. Elsewhere we have argued, and analysed a specific clinical example as illustration (Gergely and Unoka 2007), that the ensuing inhibitory or distorting effects on the self's later capacity to mentalize stem from the continued influence that the self's non-conscious and procedurally represented primary affective self–other relationship representations exert on perceiving, anticipating, and interpreting the behavioural and affective reactions of interactive partners. In the rest of this chapter, we describe an evolutionary-based social developmental model about the structural nature and ontogenetic origins of such primary affective relationship representations. In particular, we shall specify the role of representation-building and attention-socialization mechanisms which result in the early establishment of such affective self–other representations that capture the causal properties of the recurring patterns of specific attachment interactions during early development.

11.2 The social construction of the representational affective self in humans

11.2.1 The 'constitutional self': the evolutionary function of basic emotions, their modular organization, and prewired causal properties

We assume that the infant's innate 'constitutional self' (Gergely and Watson 1996, 1999; Fonagy *et al.* 2002, 2007; Gergely 2007a) has a rich prewired affective structural organization. Apart from genetically based individual temperamental differences (Rothbart 1989; Kagan 1994), we assume, in line with current evolutionary theories of emotions (Ekman *et al.* 1972; Izard and Malatesta 1987; Ekman 1992; Tomkins 1995; see also Darwin 1872), that the constitutional self also contains innate specifications of the core physiological, motor, and functional components that make up the organizational structure of basic emotion programs (such as fear, anger, joy/interest, disgust, and sadness). Current cross-cultural and experimental research has identified about six basic categorical emotions that are characterized by specific and differential patterns of physiological bodily arousal states on the one hand and/or motor programs of emotion expressive facial display patterns on the other.

These are universally recognized and cross-culturally shared by adult humans around the world (Ekman *et al.* 1972; Ekman 1992). The basic emotions are types of adaptations that originate from similar automatic emotional coping systems present in several non-human social animal species such as our primate ancestors (Panksepp 1998; Suomi 1999).

Basic emotion programs are prewired stimulus-driven and procedurally represented behavioural automatisms (Ekman 1992). They have evolved to generate rapid and adequate automatic coping responses (e.g. fight or flight) to deal with the specific types of environmental challenges that their causal triggering conditions represent (e.g. predator threat, territorial conflicts, mating competition, etc.). Such largely invariant, stereotypic, and recurring environmental stimulus conditions became represented through evolution as innately specified causal inputs which automatically activate the basic emotions. These primary emotion programs consist of two major structural components: (a) a specific pattern of physiological bodily arousal state, and (b) prewired emotion-specific motor routines. The latter component consists of two types of fixed behavioural automatisms: (i) stereotypic action tendencies (approach/avoidance, fight/flight, etc.) and (ii) expressive emotion-specific fixed facial–vocal display patterns and body postures. The evolutionary function of both components is to provide specific coping responses with the built-in goal to change (i.e. to eliminate, modify, or maintain) the environmental triggering conditions adaptively so that the challenges represented by these triggers are altered and thereby resolved.

In non-human animal species the activation of basic emotions is largely stimulus-driven and automatic, and under the external control of pre-specified inputs. Furthermore, the range of causal consequences that the execution of their fixed behavioural components (e.g. attack, threat displays, courting behaviour, distress calls) can bring about in the animal's environment is also highly restricted to a small set of stereotypic outcomes. This is so because the scope of their social environmental effects is restricted to the equally small number of innately pre-specified stereotypic reactions that they can induce in other conspecifics (e.g. flight/fight, submission, acceptance/refusal of mating approaches). Therefore the ensuing stereotyped emotional interactions among conspecifics transform the original causal environmental emotion-triggering conditions in a relatively small number of largely invariant ways. The consequent environmental changes then induce either automatic termination of the organism's basic emotional arousal, or inhibition of its behavioural expressions (by modifying its original triggering conditions), or activation of a different basic emotion (by establishing new environmental triggering conditions).

Clearly, this type of innately specified, automatic, and stimulus-controlled modular organization of basic emotions can fulfill its primary function described above only in evolutionary niches that are characterized by stable, recurring, and largely invariant social environmental conditions. Indeed, the specialized and modularly organized behavioural coping systems provided by the basic emotion programs must have evolved under the selective pressure that such invariant and stable conditions of the species' evolutionary environment represented.

11.2.2 The emergence of context-sensitive modifiability of the control mechanisms of basic emotion programs in humans

Such highly stable evolutionary conditions have ceased to characterize the increasingly complex and changing cultural, social, and technological environment of early humans. In human social interactions the same expressions of a basic emotion can evoke largely variable responses from different individuals as a function of their personality traits, social status, current dispositions, informedness about relevant aspects of the situation, and cognitive evaluation of the significance of the emotion-inducing context. During ontogenetic development, individuals can also acquire variably large and flexible repertoires of non-stereotypic emotional response alternatives whose context-sensitive selective activation comes to be, at least partially and some of the time, under their cognitive voluntary control. This results in large variability and significant individual differences in the range and types of reactions that the automatic behavioural expressions of a conspecific's basic emotional arousal can induce in others under different situational and social contexts.

We suggest that the evolutionary emergence of such significantly growing variability and increase in the types of relevant social environmental conditions must have co-evolved with correspondingly significant modifications in the inhibitory and response selective control mechanisms of basic emotion programs in humans to ensure their continued role as functional coping systems. For the basic emotion programs to remain adaptive in the face of such conditions of situational and individually variable social environmental reactivity, their control systems must have evolved to incorporate mechanisms (a) to evaluate, anticipate, and represent the variable causal consequences that specific emotional reactions are likely to result in under different interpersonal and situational contexts, and (b) to selectively inhibit or flexibly modify their automatic emotion-induced behaviours and expressive displays as a function of their anticipated situation-specific causal effects.

11.2.3 Early maternal emotion-regulation of the infant's primary affective states within the human attachment system

In early phases of ontogenetic development the affective behaviour of young infants provides no indication of the availability of such flexible and context-sensitive emotion-control mechanisms. Infants seem largely unable to modulate or inhibit the automatic motor expressions of their basic emotional arousal states. Their affective state regulation is largely under the external control of the attachment figure's adequate reactions (Tronick 1989; Gergely and Watson 1996, 1999; Sroufe 1996; Fonagy *et al.* 2002, 2007; Gergely 2007a). If the caregiver can sensitively monitor and correctly interpret the infant's automatic affective state signals, she can react to them with adequate contingent emotional expressions or instrumental coping responses to regulate the baby's emotional arousal. This can be achieved by at least two different mechanisms: first, through the prewired direct physiological state-modulating effects of certain maternal attachment reactions, for example through the innate soothing effect that gentle bodily contact or the specific intonation pattern of 'motherese' induces in babies (Fernald 1985, 1992; Cooper and Aslin 1990; Hofer 1995; Polan and Hofer 1999); secondly, through instrumental actions transforming the baby's proximal environment, thereby appropriately changing the external conditions that have triggered (or would continue to maintain) the infant's emotional arousal.

By this process the infant's basic emotion programs start to become modified so that the young child is increasingly able to anticipate and cope with the characteristic situational variability of the habitual causal consequences to which his/her specific emotional reactions typically lead. This requires the establishment of experience-based representations of the expected causal consequences that different emotion responses tend to induce from particular attachment figures under specific situational contexts. However, it should be noted that, to enable the construction of such context-sensitive emotion representations during different person- and situation-specific affective interactions, the infant must possess a suitable event-monitoring and representation-building mechanism which can register, analyse, and represent the characteristic causal dependencies between the self's particular emotion responses and the specific reactions they invoke in others.

11.2.4 The causal contingency detection mechanism and its role in building context-specific primary emotion representations

Elsewhere we have proposed that human infants are, indeed, equipped with a specialized innate information-processing and representation-building device, the so-called 'contingency detection mechanism' (Watson 1994; Gergely and Watson 1996, 1999) which, when applied to the domain of emotional interactions, can construct the required type of experience-based and context-sensitive primary emotion representations. This mechanism is specialized for the detection and representation of causal contingency relations between the infant's specific responses and consequent environmental outcomes by registering the degree of causal dependency (in terms of conditional probability of co-occurrence over time) between responses and stimulus outcomes within particular situational contexts; for technical details and reviews of supporting evidence see Watson (1985, 1994, 1995, 2001), Gergely and Watson (1996, 1999), and Gergely (2002, 2004, 2007a). One basic developmental function of the contingency detection device is to identify and represent the degree of the infant's causal control over different responses of the social environment and the specific contextual factors modulating these causal effects (Watson 1995, 2001). The resulting experience-based primary representations of the degree of causal efficacy of the infant's responses form the basis of the young child's developing primary sense of self-efficacy and social self-agency (Gergely and Watson 1996; Gergely 2002; 2007a).

We shall not describe the details of the structural and functional characteristics of this specialized causal representation-building mechanism here; the interested reader is referred to Watson (1985, 1994, 1995; 2001), Gergely and Watson (1996, 1999), or Fonagy et al. (2002). For our present purposes we call attention to only one of its crucial properties: To discover and represent the actual degree of causal control that a specific infant behaviour has over a particular response by the caregiver requires the monitoring, assessment, and representation of two different (and independent) aspects of the causal dependency relation that are obtained between these two target events over time. In other words, the contingency detection mechanism must construct two separate representations. The first must monitor the occurrences of a specific target behaviour of the self and represent the degree of causal likelihood that it is followed by a particular monitored response of the other. The second must monitor the occurrences of the target response of the other and represent the degree of causal likelihood that it was preceded by the self's target behaviour that was monitored. Only the aggregate of these two values can provide a correct estimate and representation of the actual degree of causal relatedness of the two target events monitored (Watson 1994; Gergely and Watson 1996).

Let us clarify this point with an example (cf. Watson 1995). Imagine a frightened boy whose negative emotional arousal automatically activates a fear-expressive facial display towards his mother. Assume that she promptly responds to the infant's emotion-expression by picking him up. By monitoring the causal structure of this specific type of attachment interaction over recurring episodes, the infant's contingency detection mechanism will register that his fear-expressive facial–vocal display results in being picked up by his mother, say, 80 per cent of the time. On this basis alone, it would seem safe to conclude that the degree of causal efficacy of this specific attachment behaviour in inducing the desired maternal response is, in fact, quite high. But would this provide a correct estimate of the actual degree of the infant's causal control over the mother's specific response? Not necessarily. Imagine that this mother is over-controlling, or physically intrusive, or has an anxious, worried, and fearful disposition (projecting these emotions onto her baby), or is emotionally unstable and insecure with a constant need for physical proximity herself. Any of these maternal dispositions can result in highly frequent occurrences of picking her baby up even when this was not preceded (and evoked) by her infant's fear-expression. To take into account such occasions when the maternal response was not brought about by the infant's fear-expressive behaviour, the contingency detection mechanism needs to, and does (see Watson 1985, 1994; Gergely and Watson 1996, 1999), separately monitor the occurrences of the maternal target behaviour, checking the conditional probability with which her reaction was actually preceded (and evoked) by the infant's fear-expressive display. Assume that this second type of assessment indicates that only 20 per cent of the mother's target behaviours were, in fact, preceded by her infant's fear-expression. Clearly, under such circumstances it would be grossly misleading to represent the actual degree of causal control that the infant's fear-expression has over being picked up by his mother as being very high.

In fact, as the evidence indicates (e.g. Watson 1985, 1994), the design structure of the contingency detection mechanism is sensitive to this problem and solves it by separately monitoring and representing the two types of target events and their respective degrees of (prospective and retrospective) causal dependency in relation to each other. This results in setting up two separate representations for the two behavioural events: one representing the monitored target behaviour of the infant and its degree of causal efficacy in bringing about the particular target response of the other (the 'sufficiency index'), and one representing the monitored target response of the other and its degree of causal dependence on the previous occurrence of the specific target behaviour of the infant (the 'necessity index') (Watson 1994; Gergely and Watson 1996).

11.2.5 Two types of primary emotion representation of early affective attachment interactions and their causal properties: self-to-other versus other-to-self emotion schemes

Let us examine what kind of experience-based primary emotion representations are constructed when the contingency detection mechanism is applied to recurring affective infant–caregiver attachment interactions. There are three features of the resulting primary affective self–other representations that we think are of central importance because of the functional role they will play in supporting the infant's emerging capacity for emotional self-regulation and control during affectively charged attachment interactions. First, they will represent crucial information about the characteristic causal properties of the specific emotion responses that are monitored (representing both their causal triggering conditions and their expectable consequences). Secondly, the characteristic profile of these causal conditions will be separately represented for different situational and person-contexts in which the specific target responses tend to occur. Thirdly, separate primary emotion schemes will be established to represent the causal and situational properties of the self's own emotion responses on the one hand, and those of the monitored target responses of different caregivers on the other.

Clearly, it can be highly adaptive for the infant to actively monitor and separately represent the causal and situational conditions under which different caregivers tend to produce specific types of responses. This is particularly relevant when such target behaviours of the other represent significant challenges for the self's physical well-being and emotional state of arousal. Such representations provide vital information for the infant to anticipate emotionally highly charged and potentially self-endangering interactions with particular caregivers in specific attachment situations and therefore can facilitate the generation of adaptive anticipatory coping reactions to deal with them.

Thus we propose that the contingency detection mechanism creates two basic kinds of experience-based primary emotion representations that capture the causal properties of recurring types of affective interactions with particular attachment figures under specific situational contexts.

- **Self-to-Other causal emotion schemes** These represent two types of predictable causal consequences that a specific emotion reaction is likely to lead to when performed in the presence of a particular attachment figure in a given situational context:
  (i) the relative likelihood that the infant's emotion-expression will induce a particular response by the caregiver in the situation;
  (ii) the probable consequences that the infant-induced reaction of the caregiver will give rise to in that situation, i.e. the ways in which it is likely to modify the environmental conditions that had triggered the emotional reaction in the first place.

- **Other-to-Self causal emotion schemes** These represent the characteristic causal properties of specific target behaviours that are likely to be performed by the caregiver under certain attachment contexts. These behaviours of specific caregivers become active targets of monitoring either because they belong to the likely consequences of some of the infant's own monitored emotion-expressive responses (by her Self-to-Other emotion schemes), or because their occurrence is likely to trigger a basic emotional reaction in the infant (thus representing a significant environmental challenge for the self).

Such Other-to-Self emotion schemes will include causal information about the types of environmental triggering conditions that are likely to induce (and therefore can be used to anticipate) the other's monitored target behaviours. Importantly, such causal conditions may also include the infant's representation of his/her own specific emotion-expressive responses as having triggered the caregiver's monitored reactions in the past during particular situations and with differential likelihoods. In such cases the infant can use this represented causal information to control, modify, or pre-empt the occurrence of the other's anticipated target reaction by inhibiting its potential cause, i.e. by suppressing or modifying the behavioural expression of his/her own emotion reactions that are represented as likely to induce the other's, potentially self-endangering, target behaviour whose occurrence the infant is trying to avoid.

11.2.6 Primary response inhibition and substitution mechanisms of automatic emotional self-control

Two basic types of emotion control processes (involving primary automatic versus secondary cognitive control mechanisms) serve affective self-regulation and coping in humans during emotionally charged interactions. We discuss primary automatic response inhibition first.

In our view, the basic developmental function of the infant's experience-based primary emotion schemes is to provide him/her with representational means to anticipate and adaptively influence the course of affective attachment interactions with particular caregivers in the service of emotional self-control and coping. By extracting and representing the context- and person-specific causal patterns of affective interactions, these primary representations equip the infant with a repertoire of specific emotion schemes which can be used to anticipate, and to some degree actively modulate, the emotional consequences that particular types of attachment interactions will bring about.

There are two types of mechanism through which the infant's primary emotion control system can utilize the representational contents of the Self-to-Other and Other-to-Self emotion schemes for these purposes. The first is a primary response inhibitory control mechanism which can automatically suppress the behavioural expression of a basic emotional arousal state. One condition that leads to the triggering of such a response-inhibitory process is when the activation of the self's basic emotion reaction primes a specific Self-to-Other emotion scheme which represents the behavioural expression of the activated emotion state as likely to lead to severe negative consequences for the self in the given attachment context. In such cases, the anticipatory activation of the represented negative consequences exerts a direct and automatic inhibitory effect, blocking the impending motor expression of the activated emotion and thereby avoiding the realization of the negative consequences anticipated. This type of primary response-inhibitory emotion control mechanism is automatic and procedural in nature.

Evidence from attachment research (Cassidy and Shaver 1999) indicates that this primary response-inhibitory coping mechanism becomes operational rather early. An example is the separation-induced response pattern observed in the Strange Situation Test (Ainsworth *et al.* 1978) in a subgroup of 1-year-olds who show avoidant attachment to their caregiver. Unlike other (securely or insecurely attached) infants, avoidantly attached babies typically do not exhibit the behavioural-expressive signs of distress or protest that would indicate negative physiological arousal induced by separation from their caregiver (Ainsworth *et al.* 1978; Goldberg *et al.* 1995; Cassidy and Shaver 1999). Despite this apparent lack of emotion-expressive reactivity to separation, physiological measures (heart rate and cortisol elevation) indicate that, similarly to infants belonging to other attachment categories, separation from the caregiver induces clear bodily indices of high negative emotional arousal and stress in such infants (e.g. Spangler and Grossmann 1993; Cassidy and Shaver 1999).

Importantly, this automatic inhibition of the expression of separation-induced distress is relationship specific; no strong correlation has been found between the types of attachment infants exhibit towards different caregivers (reviewed by Cassidy and Shaver 1999; Fonagy 2001). There is evidence (Ainsworth *et al.* 1978; Cassidy and Shaver 1999) that the establishment in avoidant infants of the primary response-inhibitory coping strategy towards a particular caregiver is related to (and is best explained as an adaptation to cope with) the predictable and systematically negative emotional reactivity habitually exhibited by the caregiver in response to the infant's expressions of negative affect across situations (Watson 2001).

Note that the same automatic response-inhibitory control mechanism can also be triggered by the activation of some of the infant's Other-to-Self emotion schemes which represent the causal properties of those target behaviours of a given caregiver that are likely to induce negative emotional consequences for the infant in the given attachment context. This can happen when the situation triggers in the baby a basic emotional arousal whose behavioural expression is represented in the infant's Other-to-Self scheme as one of the potential causes that are likely to invoke the self-endangering target behaviour of the caregiver. In such cases the infant's emotional arousal activates the Other-to-Self scheme in question, leading to the anticipatory evocation of its representational content: the potential occurrence of the caregiver's target behaviour and its expectable negative consequences. This will trigger the automatic response-inhibition control mechanism to suppress the expression of the infant's basic emotion arousal and thereby avoid the realization of its anticipated negative consequences by blocking their causal triggering event from occurring.

However, it should be pointed out that, when exercised in isolation, this kind of automatic response-inhibitory coping reaction is of rather limited adaptive value for the infant's emotion regulation for two reasons. First, while it automatically suppresses the expression of the activated emotion, it does so without affecting the physiological arousal reaction itself. One of the undesirable consequences is that while the inhibition of the emotion expression removes the source of likely further escalation of the infant's emotional reaction, the negative physiological arousal already activated remains unmodified and unmodulated. Secondly, the inhibition of the emotion expression also leaves unchanged the environmental triggering conditions that led to the activation of the basic emotion reaction in the first place. Therefore the infant's emotional arousal will be maintained as long as its environmental triggering source continues to be present. In short, such an automatic inhibitory 'freezing' of the emotion response system can leave the self helplessly overwhelmed by its uncontrolled and continued state of heightened physiological arousal and stress which, if occurring frequently, can lead to deleterious long-term toxic consequences, resulting in the development of a rigid and dysfunctional organization of the physiological stress-regulation system (Francis and Meaney 1999; Francis et al. 1999; Fonagy et al. 2002; Pruessner et al. 2004; Wismer Fries et al. 2005).

The danger of toxic consequences can be coped with only by applying the second type of primary emotion control mechanism which involves response substitution. This mechanism exploits the possibility provided by the representational contents of primary Self-to-Other and Other-to-Self emotion schemes to automatically activate a suitable substitute behaviour which is represented as having a high likelihood to change the environmental conditions that had activated the infant's original basic emotional arousal in the first place. Clearly, this can be accomplished only if the infant possesses a sufficiently rich and differentiated repertoire of response alternatives suitable to serve as adequate substitute responses in the given situation.

11.2.7 Secondary cognitive appraisal mechanisms and top-down voluntary processes of emotional self-control

We have argued that the automatic primary emotion control mechanisms, when applied over a sufficiently differentiated repertoire of primary emotion representations, allow the infant to exert a certain measure of adaptive behavioural control in the service of emotional self-regulation during early affective interactions. However, this primary emotional coping system is severely limited in both its scope and its flexibility. This is because the Self-to-Other and Other-to-Self emotion schemes are stimulus-driven and procedurally represented emotion representations which are automatically activated whenever the stimulus situation is sufficiently similar to their represented environmental triggering conditions or their associated situational and person-contexts. By necessity, this restricts their scope of adaptive applicability to the narrow domain of the recurring types of affective attachment interactions with caregivers, whose features are represented by the primary emotion schemes in the first place.

However, as children develop, they encounter an increasing variety of new interpersonal contexts of affective interactions, often involving unfamiliar persons and situations. This results in two basic problems of adaptation that the primary emotion representations and their automatic emotion control mechanisms cannot satisfactorily cope with and that necessitate the establishment of an additional type of secondary top-down cognitive mechanism of emotion control (e.g. Lazarus 1991; Lazarus and Lazarus 1994; Thompson 1994; LeDoux 2000; Posner and Rothbart 2000; Ellsworth and Scherer 2003; Ochsner and Gross 2005).

The first problem arises when the new interactive situations encountered represent significant challenges for the self that would call for adaptive emotional coping responses, but which, because of their unfamiliarity and lack of sufficient similarity to the triggering conditions represented in the child's primary emotion schemes, do not automatically trigger a basic emotion reaction. To recognize the realistic nature of the challenge that such situations represent for the self (and consequently to generate appropriate emotional coping reactions to them), the child has to rely on secondary cognitive appraisal mechanisms. By having access to an increasingly large pool of relevant knowledge and being able to derive relevant inferences from situational cues, these top-down cognitive appraisal processes can generate realistic evaluations of the significance that these new types of input condition represent for the self. The interpretation that such secondary cognitive appraisals provide can then be used by top-down executive action control systems to activate relevant emotion responses to cope with the situational challenge thus recognized.

The second type of problem arises when the surface features of the current interactive context automatically trigger the self's primary and procedural emotion representations leading to non-adaptive and inappropriate emotion reactions. This can occur whenever the environmental situation shows sufficient similarity with the triggering conditions or associated situational and person-contexts that are represented by some of the self's primary Self-to-Other or Other-to-Self emotion schemes. Since the input specifications of such primary emotion schemes represent the recurring patterns specific to the self's early attachment interactions, their 'spurious' triggering by a featurally partially overlapping current context is highly unlikely to generate an automatic emotional reaction that is adaptive in the present situation. Therefore, if left cognitively unchecked, such automatic and similarity-driven contextual activation of the procedurally organized primary emotion schemes are likely to result in inappropriate and reality-distorting projective constructions of the emotional significance of the current interpersonal situation. In order to control such dysfunctional automatic activation of primary emotion schemes, the self must again rely on top-down processes of secondary cognitive reappraisal of current situational cues (e.g. Lazarus 1991; Thompson 1994; Ellsworth and Scherer 2003; Ochsner and Gross 2005) to inhibit and override the impending execution of the spuriously activated primary emotions. This ontogenetically developing capacity for top-down control over one's primary emotional automatisms relies on two related aspects of cognitive processes of secondary evaluation. Both result in a reinterpretation of events and the generation of alternative response options.

First, the secondary reappraisal processes can reinterpret the actual significance for the self of the causal evoking conditions that have automatically activated the primary emotional reaction in the first place. Based on stored or situationally inferred relevant information, one can reappraise and revise the interpretation of what the emotion-triggering events signify for the self. This top-down cognitive re-evaluation can override the automatic output of the 'quick-and-dirty' stimulus-driven primary perceptual appraisal processes (LeDoux 1995, 1996, 2000; Ochsner and Gross 2005) which led to the original automatic triggering of one's primary emotion reaction. Secondly, the secondary cognitive evaluative processes can also reappraise the realistic significance of the expectable causal consequences to which the automatic expression of the spuriously activated primary emotional reaction would lead.

However, several developmental, representational, and cognitive preconditions need to be established before such secondary cognitive reappraisal processes can be successfully applied to serve their emotion-regulative function adaptively. First, top-down cognitive processes of emotional self-control need to be 'alerted' when a specific emotional arousal state has been activated. Therefore the cognitive emotion control system must be able to monitor, detect, and introspectively access internal state cues that signal the onset of a basic emotional reaction in the self. Secondly, this introspective emotion recognition must be based on sufficiently differentiated internal state signals to allow for the correct identification and self-attribution of the particular emotion category that has been triggered. Thirdly, the cognitive processes of secondary reappraisal must have access to sufficient and relevant (stored or inferred) information in the light of which adaptive re-evaluation of the realistic significance of the causal conditions of the basic emotion reaction can be successfully performed. Importantly, these processes of representational access and situational reappraisal must be implemented under time pressure to deliver their output before the execution of the stereotypic behavioural components of the activated basic emotion program is automatically implemented.

11.3 The establishment of second-order emotion representations: developmental mechanisms and social environmental preconditions

11.3.1 The development of the subjective sense of a differentiated affective self

Many currently popular developmental and attachment theories consider the human-specific characteristics of early caregiver–infant attachment interactions (see section 11.1) as evidence supporting a 'rich' mentalistic interpretation of such interactions in terms of primary 'intersubjectivity'. These theories assume that during the first months of life human infants already have introspective access to a variety of differential mental states (such as emotions, goals, intentions, or motives), can recognize and attribute such internal states to the other's mind, and experience subjective and mutual awareness of 'being in' and 'sharing' such internal states with the caregiver (Meltzoff and Moore 1977, 1989, 1998; Trevarthen 1979, 1993; Stern 1985; Braten 1988, 1992, 1998; Giannino and Tronick 1988; Meltzoff and Gopnik 1993; Hobson 1993, 2002; Trevarthen and Aitken 2001; Meltzoff 2002). Elsewhere we have criticized this primary intersubjectivist interpretation on a number of grounds, arguing that it attributes to very young infants overly 'rich' mentalizing capacities that are not necessary to explain the characteristics of early mother–infant interactions in humans (for details see Gergely and Watson 1996, 1999; Fonagy et al. 2002, 2007; Gergely 2002, 2007a). We have proposed an alternative model of early socio-emotional self development

(Gergely and Watson 1996, 1999; Fonagy et al. 2002) within the framework of contingency detection and attachment theory (Watson 1985, 2001). We hypothesized that infants' subjective awareness of differentiated emotional self-states has important social interactional origins with an individually variable developmental course of ontogenetic unfolding. In this view, subjective self-awareness and sense of differential affective self-states is viewed as a (relatively hard-won) developmental achievement rather than being a universally given prewired capacity. Similarly, we see the establishment and 'intersubjective' recognition of mutual 'sharing' of affective states with others as an emergent property of the subjective self, rather than an initial and universal starting state of human infants' mental life.

In particular, we have proposed that the subjective sense of discrete emotional self-states (e.g. awareness of being 'angry', rather than just experiencing an undifferentiated negative state of tension) is established as a result of infants' repeated experience with the pattern of contingent parental reactivity and social 'mirroring' feedback reactions that the automatic expressions of these, initially non-conscious, basic emotional arousal states evoke from the attachment environment. Our model is based on two central assumptions.

1. **The introspectively inaccessible constitutional affective self** We assume (together with numerous others) that the infant's innate constitutional self has a richly structured internal organization at birth. While on the one hand the constitutional self is characterized by significant genetically based individual temperamental differences, it also contains a basic set of prewired universal categorical emotion programs that are primary biological adaptations (Ekman et al. 1972; Ekman 1992; Gergely and Watson 1996). As argued earlier, these basic emotions are best understood as prewired stimulus-driven procedural physiological and motor automatisms that are initially not accessible to conscious awareness and over which the baby has no voluntary control at first. Early affect-regulation is carried out mainly by the attachment environment, as the caregiver, reading the infant's automatic emotion expressions, reacts to them with appropriate affect-modulating interactions and emotion displays (Gergely and Watson 1996, 1999; Fonagy et al. 2002; Gergely 2007a). Thus, while infants may be sensitive to the general (positive versus negative) hedonic quality of their affective states, we assume that they have no initial introspective awareness of their discrete basic emotion states as categorically distinct subjective self-states (Gergely and Watson 1996). It is in this sense that we consider the constitutional affective self to be initially introspectively inaccessible; while it contains discrete and categorical basic emotional states, these prewired primary automatisms are at first not subject

to introspective awareness and so they do not present themselves as subjectively experienced differential internal self-states. We further hypothesize, contrary to classical approaches such as Bruner *et al.* (1966) and Mahler *et al.* (1975) (cf. Gergely 2000), that in human infants, because of a prewired directionality bias, the attention system is initially dominantly externally oriented showing a primary sensitivity bias towards exteroceptive stimulation. Therefore it is assumed that very little introspectively directed attentional monitoring of internal self-states takes place in the earliest months of life (for supporting arguments see Gergely and Watson 1996, 1999; Fonagy *et al.* 2002).

2. **The social interactive origins of affective subjectivity: the development of introspectively accessible emotional self-representations** We assume that for the categorical basic emotion states of the constitutional self to become introspectively accessible and subjectively differentially experienced, two basic conditions must be established developmentally. On the one hand, the primary and procedural basic emotion programs need to become associated with second-order representations which, when activated, are cognitively accessible to introspectively oriented attentional self-monitoring processes. In other words, we suggest that the initially non-conscious primary emotion states become introspectively detectable differentiated states of subjective awareness through the activation and cognitive access of their associated second-order representations only. For this to happen, it is also necessary that the primary orientation bias of the young infant's attention system towards external stimulus events should become modified. The infant's attentional system must become partially directed towards the self's internal states to allow the active introspective monitoring and detection of the activation of the self's second-order emotion representations. Introspective emotion recognition then becomes possible whenever the second-order emotion representations are triggered by the stimulus-induced automatic arousal of the self's basic emotions to which they are associatively linked. This leads to the introspective self-perception of 'being in' a particular differentiated emotion state, giving rise to the discrete subjective awareness of that state.

The cognitively accessible and introspectively monitored second-order representations of the primary emotion states can then provide the basis for the establishment of a (continuously updated) representation of the dynamically changing affective states of the self. This makes it possible to generate self-predictions about what kind of emotion-induced behaviour one is about to perform by anticipating the impending execution of the emotion-specific action schemes that the self's activated basic emotional arousal state is about to trigger. To become subjectively aware of one's current dispositional affective states before the automatic activation of the primary emotion-induced action tendencies would take effect is a central precondition for the self's emerging capacity to exercise online affective self-control (Gergely and Watson 1996). The introspective detection of one's emotional arousal state allows the self to foresee and cognitively evaluate the likely consequences to which the anticipated primary emotion reactions would lead in the given interpersonal context. The self can then avoid such non-adaptive outcomes by inhibiting or modifying the anticipated primary emotional reactions in time (i.e. before they are executed) rather than being automatically driven to act them out.

Our developmental proposal is that both of these preconditions for the establishment of the introspectively accessible subjective self are fulfilled as a result of, and to the degree to which, the attachment environment provides systematic contingent feedback reactions to the automatic expressions of the initially non-conscious primary emotional arousal states of the infant. In other words, it is the repeated experience that one's current internal states are externally 'mirrored' or 'reflected' through the infant-attuned contingent reactions of the social environment that leads to the development of a subjective sense and awareness of one's differentiated affective self-states.

Of course, no amount of social 'mirroring' could result in the establishment of these two (representational and attentional) preconditions unless infants were equipped with an adequate mechanism to detect and represent the contingent relatedness between their automatic state-expressive displays on the one hand, and the ensuing environmental mirroring reactions on the other. This mechanism must be able to internalize the representation of the external 'mirroring' feedback signal as a second-order representation of the primary self-state whose automatic expression invokes the contingent 'mirroring' reaction in question.

In previous work on the social biofeedback theory of parental affect-mirroring (Gergely and Watson 1996, 1999) we have proposed that the infant's contingency detection device has the necessary structural properties to establish second-order emotion representations when applied to contingent affect-mirroring interactions. As already discussed, this prewired causal contingency analyser (Watson 1985, 1994) automatically monitors and assesses the degree of contingent relatedness between the infant's responses and subsequent external stimulus events. By monitoring three different aspects of contingent relatedness in parallel (temporal contingency, spatial similarity, and relative intensity) (reviewed by Gergely and Watson 1999), the mechanism can identify those aspects of the social environment that are under (some specific degree of) causal control of the infant's state expressive displays. One important developmental consequence of this causal contingency analysis is that the resulting discovery of the degree of contingent control that the self exercises over aspects of the social environment generates a subjective sense of causal efficacy and self-agency in the infant.

11.3.2 The role of 'markedness' of affect-mirroring expressions in the internalization of second-order representations of affective self-states

One of the human-specific characteristics of infant–caregiver interactions (see section 11.1) is that infant-attuned caregivers are inclined to produce 'marked' affect-mirroring expressions that are induced by their baby's automatic emotion displays. Such 'marked' affect-reflecting expressions are saliently transformed versions of the stereotypic motor displays of categorical emotions which normally express the caregiver's actual affective states (Gergely and Watson 1996, 1999; Fonagy et al. 2002). 'Markedness' involves motor transformations that result in an exaggerated, slowed down, schematic, abbreviated, or only partially executed normative display pattern of basic emotion expressions. Furthermore, marked affect-mirroring is typically accompanied by ostensive-communicative cues (such as direct eye contact, eyebrow raising, and vocal intonation pattern characteristic of 'motherese') that are also among the human-specific features of early caregiver–infant interactions (Csibra and Gergely 2006).

Our original functional interpretation of 'markedness' (Gergely and Watson 1996) emphasized its importance as a cue to signal that the displayed emotion 'is not for real' and should therefore be 'decoupled' from the mother, i.e. its attribution as her actual and real emotion state should be inhibited. Here we further propose that 'marked' affect-mirroring interactions constitute a specific form of 'pedagogical' manifestation of cultural knowledge transfer (Csibra and Gergely 2006) in the domain of emotion socialization. This new theoretical perspective allows us to extend the original functional account of 'marked' affect-mirroring interactions in two ways.

- We shall show why 'marked' affect-mirroring displays become interpreted self-referentially by the infant, leading to their referential 'anchoring' as second-order emotion representations of the constitutional self's primary emotions.

- We shall explicate how the 'markedness' of contingent affect-mirroring expressions contributes to the modification of the primary directional bias of the infant's initially dominantly externally oriented attention system, resulting in its eventual internally directed deployment to introspectively monitor the self's internal affectivef states.

11.3.3 Natural 'pedagogy': the functions of cues of 'ostensive communication' and 'referential knowledge manifestation' in communicative knowledge transfer

Recently, Csibra and Gergely (2006) developed a new evolutionary-based theory of cultural transmission, postulating a human-specific learning system that they call natural 'pedagogy' (Gergely 2007b; Gergely *et al.* 2007). They propose that humans have become adapted to spontaneously manifest relevant cultural knowledge to conspecifics who are naturally inclined to attend to and learn from such knowledge manifestations through a specialized cue-driven social communicative learning mechanism of mutual design. Human pedagogy ensures efficient intergenerational transfer of relevant cultural knowledge in a variety of knowledge domains including words, gestural symbols, artefact functions and novel means actions, valence properties of object kinds, social habits, rituals, etc. (Gergely *et al.* 2002a, 2007; Gergely and Csibra 2005, 2006; Csibra and Gergely 2006; Gergely 2007b).

Here we argue that natural pedagogy is also employed in the domain of emotion socialization to identify those categorical emotions that are culturally universal and shared among humans, to sensitize the infant to them, and to transfer relevant knowledge about them to the infant. In this view, early infant–caregiver affective interactions (involving ostensively cued 'marked' forms of contingent emotion-mirroring) constitute a special case of pedagogical knowledge transfer whereby sensitive caregivers establish second-order representations in infants that identify and encode the categorical emotions that are culturally universal and can be shared with and communicated to other humans.

The built-in mutual design structure of natural pedagogy involves biological preparedness for both providing and receiving relevant cultural information among humans. Knowledgeable caregivers show a natural inclination to express their 'communicative intention' (cf. Sperber and Wilson 1986) to transfer new and relevant knowledge to ignorant juveniles by addressing them through specific 'ostensive' communicative cues (such as eye contact, eyebrow flashing, contingent reactivity, or the prosodic pattern of 'motherese') to which infants show prewired sensitivity and preferential orientation (for a review of the supporting evidence see Csibra and Gergely 2006). Ostensive cues are followed by referential cues (such as gaze-shift) to help the infant identify the referent object about which new and relevant information is going to be demonstrated through the caregiver's 'marked' forms of knowledge manifestations. These ostensive and manifestative pedagogical cues trigger a specially receptive learning attitude in infants which induces fast mapping of the manifested information to their representation of the referent.

Cues of 'referential knowledge manifestations' help the infant to identify and extract the content of the adult's 'referential intention' (cf. Sperber and Wilson 1986), i.e. the new and relevant knowledge manifested about the referent, which the infant then encodes as a property of the referent kind. Such knowledge manifestations are cued by being performed in a specially 'marked' manner which involves a modified and saliently transformed version of the normative and primary form of application of the novel cultural knowledge skill that is being demonstrated for the infant to learn. (Imagine, for example, the difference between the 'marked' manifestative form of demonstrating to a novice 'how to' hammer in a nail versus the standard motor execution of the same routine when it is performed simply to fulfill its primary function of driving in a nail.) The features of 'markedness' which characterize knowledge manifestations serve several pedagogical functions. They cue the infant that the demonstrated content conveys relevant and culturally shared information about some essential property of the referent to be identified and represented. They also help the infant infer what aspect of the manifested knowledge should be encoded by foregrounding and selectively emphasizing the new and relevant information that should be extracted and internalized as part of the referent representation (for details see Gergely 2007b).

11.3.4 The role of cues of 'ostension' and 'markedness' in inducing the self-referential interpretation of 'marked' emotion-mirroring displays

We propose that the cues of 'markedness' of emotion-mirroring parental expressions constitute a special instance of the 'marked' forms of manifestative knowledge displays which characterize communicative acts of pedagogical knowledge transfer. 'Marked' affect-mirroring displays are also accompanied by ostensive cues that signal the adult's communicative intent during pedagogical interactions (such as direct eye contact, raised eyebrows, the vocal pattern of 'motherese', and addressing the infant by name). We argued above (Gergely and Watson 1996, 1999; Fonagy et al. 2002) that as a consequence of these cues the infant inhibits the attribution of the expressed emotion to the caregiver as her 'real' feeling by referentially 'decoupling' the emotion display from her. We can now add that the cues of ostension and 'markedness' of emotion manifestation during affect-mirroring interactions also function to trigger the referential interpretive and receptive learning attitude of the infant's 'pedagogical stance'. In other words, these pedagogical cues induce the infant to search for and identify the intended referent of the caregiver's 'marked' emotion manifestation and to 'anchor' the mirroring display to some referent other than the caregiver's actual emotion state (from which it has been 'decoupled'). In trying to establish the referent of the 'marked' emotion display, the infant will rely on cues of referent identification (such as eye-gaze direction) which accompany the caregiver's affect-mirroring expression. Since the caregiver is looking at the infant while displaying her emotion-reflecting expressions, the infant's attention will be directed towards his/her own face and body as the likely spatial locus of the referent to which the 'marked' (and 'decoupled') emotion-mirroring display should be referentially 'anchored'. Note that the infant's automatic facial–vocal emotion expressions that are being mirrored by the caregiver emanate from the very same locus as well. The infant's contingency detection mechanism identifies these emotion expressive responses of the self (and their proprioceptive bodily correlates) as the source of contingent control that the infant exercises over the caregiver's mirroring response (Gergely and Watson 1996). These two sources of information converge to identify the infant's own internal emotional arousal state and its motor expressions as the referent of the caregiver's 'marked' mirroring display. As a result, the infant will referentially 'anchor' the representation of the 'marked' mirroring display to his/her own primary and procedural emotion program and will internalize it as its second-order representation. In sum, this is how, through activating the infant's pedagogical stance, repeated experience with ostensively cued 'marked' affect-mirroring feedback reactions of infant-attuned caregivers can 'teach' the infant about the self's differential categorical emotion states which become represented as universal and cognitively accessible emotion categories shared by other humans. This is achieved by the referential 'anchoring' and internalization of the caregiver's 'marked' mirroring displays as second-order emotion representations which become associated with the infant's primary and procedural emotional self-states. Through this process the infant's attentional system becomes introspectively sensitized and internally directed to detect and monitor the activation of the self's affective states. This, together with the sensitization effects of the contingency-based social biofeedback mechanism as described by Gergely and Watson (1996), also results in heightened sensitivity to the internal proprioceptive cues that accompany emotional self-expressions. A further consequence is the development of subjective awareness and emergent voluntary induction of the instrumental effects of contingent control that the self exerts through its emotion responses over the infant-attuned reactivity of the social environment.

Through these processes the infant's social mirroring environment contributes significantly to the establishment of the introspectively detectable subjective self by populating it with cognitively accessible second-order representations of internal affective self-states. This provides the representational basis which, together with the infant's introspectively socialized attentional system, make the developmental emergence of top-down cognitive emotional self-monitoring and secondary reappraisal processes possible.

11.4 Mentalizing and its role in secondary cognitive reappraisal processes of emotional self-control

We now turn to the important role that the ability to mentalize can play in enhancing the self's developing competence to achieve top-down cognitive emotional self-regulation and control by increasing the efficiency and scope of the secondary cognitive reappraisal processes involved. We speculate that the proper evolutionary domain (cf. Sperber and Hirschfeld 2004) of the cognitive adaptation for mentalizing may have originally been restricted to infer and represent the causal intentional mental states of other minds only. This was sufficient to confer significant evolutionary benefits on the mindreader by allowing him/her to anticipate the likely actions of other conspecifics in primarily competitive situations. However, we hypothesize that with the human-specific establishment during early social and emotional development of cognitively accessible second-order representations of internal self-states, the proper domain of the mentalizing capacity becomes ontogenetically extended to include in its actual domain the mind of one's own self as well. This is likely to result in significantly better coping strategies in the realm of competitive and cooperative interactions and affective relationships by enabling the self to anticipate its own actions and reactions, as well as those of others, through introspectively detecting, self-attributing, representing, and reflecting about one's own internal mental states that are the causal sources underlying one's actions.

So how is the inferential system for mentalizing applied introspectively in the domain of emotional self-regulation and control to make coping with affectively charged interpersonal interactions more effective? Clearly, one's mindreading abilities can often provide highly useful and relevant information to instruct the self's secondary cognitive emotion reappraisal mechanisms. This would be the case, for example, when these top-down cognitive processes are applied to re-evaluate the realistic significance for the self of the causal input conditions that have induced one's primary and automatic emotional arousal reactions in situations where these triggering conditions involve another person's actions, reactions, or emotion expressions directed towards the self. In such cases mentalizing processes can support secondary cognitive reappraisals by accessing and reasoning about stored knowledge concerning the other person's enduring mental dispositions, self-related attitudes, long-term aspirations, temperamental and personality traits, or recent life events that are relevant for the reconstruction of the mental reasons behind the other's self-directed actions. Similarly, one's mentalizing ability can be recruited to detect and interpret current situational or behavioural cues that are relevant for inferring what particular present desires, intentions, and (possibly false) beliefs about the situation and/or one's own self may have induced the other's responses towards the self that led to the triggering of one's automatic basic emotional arousal response.

Mentalizing can also significantly facilitate the generation of secondary cognitive evaluations of the likely causal consequences that automatically acting out or expressively displaying one's basic emotional arousal reactions would lead to in the given interpersonal context. The validity and scope of the predictions generated by such secondary cognitive evaluations can be qualitatively enriched by mentalistic reasoning about what kind of causal mental states and reactions would be expected to be induced in the other person by the self's automatic emotion-induced responses. Such mentalizing inferences can take into consideration a range of accessible or inferable information about relevant situation- and person-specific motivational factors such as the other's temperamental features, personality traits, childhood history, current dispositional states, his/her quality of relationship with and available relevant knowledge about one's own self, etc. Importantly, in generating predictions about the other's likely reactions to one's potential emotional outburst a good mentalizer may also be able to take into account available knowledge about the quality of the other's mentalizing skills that the latter can be counted on to apply when evaluating the reasons behind one's own emotional reactions towards him/her in the given situation.

11.5 Conclusions

One of the, arguably, species-unique abilities of humans is the exercise of online introspective control over their primary emotional impulses in affectively charged interpersonal situations and relationships. However, individuals differ significantly in the degree to which this remarkable capacity is available to them or can be put to functional use. In this chapter we have outlined a social cognitive developmental theory specifying the early social environmental preconditions and cognitive representation-building and attention socialization mechanisms that underlie the ontogenetic unfolding of the introspectively accessible representational affective self. This approach relates the individual variability in the capacity for introspective access to affective self-states and emotional self-control to the differences in the availability of a contingently reactive infant-attuned attachment environment in which the infant's automatic emotion expressive responses induce contingent external feedback reactions and 'marked' forms of affect-mirroring displays by caregivers. We have argued that these human-specific features of early caregiver–infant interactions constitute necessary environmental input conditions for the infant's representation-building and attention socialization mechanisms to establish second-order cognitively accessible representations for the initially non-conscious, stimulus-controlled, and procedural basic emotional automatisms of the innate constitutional self. Our approach sheds new light on the functional role of the human-specific features of early affective attachment interactions (such as contingent turn-taking reactivity, 'marked' forms of affect-mirroring, or ostensive-communicative cues of 'pedagogical' knowledge manifestations) in early social cognitive development. It interprets ostensively cued 'marked' affect-reflective interactions as a special case of 'pedagogical' knowledge manifestations (Csibra and Gergely 2006) which function to transfer relevant cultural knowledge about universally shared emotion categories by establishing second-order representations for the infant's primary emotion states. We have contrasted this view with currently popular primary 'intersubjectivist' interpretations which consider the species-unique features of caregiver–infant interactions as characteristics of early secure attachment relationships that function as developmental precursors and facilitating conditions fostering the acquisition of mentalizing by early childhood. Finally, we have argued that the developmentally established second-order emotion representations allow the self to extend the original domain of the innate capacity for mentalizing about other minds to include introspective mentalizing about one's own internal affective mental states and anticipated emotion-induced actions as well. As a result the introspectively accessible representational affective self can employ its innate mentalizing ability in the service of emotional self-regulation and control by anticipating and adaptively modifying its own emotion-induced action tendencies to cope more efficiently with affectively charged interpersonal interactions.

References

Ainsworth, M.D.S., Blehar, M.C., Waters, E., and Wall, S. (1978). *Patterns of attachment: a psychological study of the Strange Situation*. Hillsdale, NJ, Lawrence Erlbaum.

Astington, J.W. and Jenkins, J.M. (1999). A longitudinal study of the relation between language and theory-of-mind development. *Developmental Psychology*, 35, 1311–20.

Bahrick, L.R. and Watson, J.S. (1985). Detection of intermodal proprioceptive–visual contingency as a potential basis of self-perception in infancy. *Developmental Psychology*, 21, 963–73.

Baron-Cohen, S. (1995). *Mindblindness:an essay on autism and theory of mind*. Cambridge, MA, Bradford–MIT Press.

Baron-Cohen, S., Leslie, A.M., and Frith, U. (1985). Does the autistic child have a 'theory of mind'? *Cognition*, 21, 37–46.

Behne, T., Carpenter, M., and Tomasello, M. (2005). One-year-olds comprehend the communicative intentions behind gestures in a hiding game. *Developmental Science*, 8, 492–9.

Bennett, D.S., Bendersky, M., and Lewis, M. (2004). On specifying specificity: facial expressions at 4 months. *Infancy*, 6, 425–9.

Bennett, D.S., Bendersky, M., and Lewis, M. (2005). Does the organization of facial expression change over time? Facial expressivity from 4 to 12 months. *Infancy*, 8, 167–87.

Bigelow, A.E. (1999). Infants' sensitivity to imperfect contingency in social interaction. In *Early social cognition* (ed. P Rochat), pp 137–154. Hillsdale, NJ: Lawrence Erlbaum.

Bigelow, A.E. and De Coste, C. (2003). Infants' sensitivity to contingency in social interactions with familiar and unfamiliar partners. *Infancy*, 4, 111–40.

Bigelow, A.E. and Rochat, P. (2006). Two-month-old infants' sensitivity to social contingency in mother–infant and stranger–infant interaction. *Infancy*, 9, 313–25.

Bloom, P. and German, T.P. (2000). Two reasons to abandon the false belief task as a test of theory of mind. *Cognition*, 77, B25–31.

Bowlby, J. (1969). *Attachment and loss*: Vol. 1: *Attachment*. London: Hogarth Press and Institute of Psycho-Analysis.

Braten, S. (1988). Dialogic mind: the infant and the adult in protoconversation. In *Nature, cognition, and system*, Vol. 1 (ed. M Carvallo), pp. 187–205. Dordrecht: Kluwer Academic.

Braten, S. (1992). The virtual other in infants' minds and social feelings. In *The dialogical alternative* (ed. H Wold), pp. 77–97. Oslo: Scandinavian University Press.

Braten, S. (ed.) (1998). *Intersubjective communication and emotion in early ontogeny*. Paris: Cambridge University Press–Editions de la Maison des Science de l'Homme.

Brazelton, T.B. and Tronick, E. (1980). Preverbal communication between mothers and infants. In *The social foundations of language and thought* (ed. D.R. Olson), pp. 299–315. New York: Norton.

Brazelton, T.B., Koslowski, B., and Main, M. (1974). The origins of reciprocity: the early mother–infant interaction. In *The effect of the infant on its caregiver* (ed. M. Lewis and L. Rosenblum), pp. 49–76. New York: John Wiley.

Bruner, J.S., Olver, P.R., and Greenfield, P.M. (1966). *Studies on cognitive growth*. New York: John Wiley.

Bugnyar, T. and Heinrich, B. (2005). Ravens, *Corvus corax*, differentiate between knowledgeable and ignorant competitors. *Proceedings of the Royal Society of London*, 272, 1641–6.

Camras, L.A. (1992). Expressive development and basic emotions. *Cognition and Emotion*, 6, 269–83.

Cassidy, J. and Shaver, P.R. (1999). *Handbook of attachment: theory, research and clinical implications*. New York: Guilford Press.

Cohn, J.F. and Tronick, E.Z (1988). Mother–infant face-to-face interaction: influence is bidirectional and unrelated to periodic cycles in either partner's behavior. *Developmental Psychology*, 24, 386–92.

Cooper, R.P. and Aslin, R.N. (1990). Preference for infant-directed speech in the first month after birth. *Child Development*, 61, 1584–95.

Csibra, G. and Gergely, G. (2006). Social learning and social cognition: the case of pedagogy. In *Processes of change in brain and cognitive development. Attention and Performance XXI*, (ed. M.H. Johnson and Y.M. Munakata), pp. 249–74. Oxford University Press.

Csibra, G. and Southgate, V. (2006). Evidence for infants understanding false beliefs should not be dismissed. *Trends in Cognitive Sciences*, **10**, 4–5.

Cutting, A.L. and Dunn, J. (1999). Theory of mind, emotion understanding, language, and family background: individual differences and interrelations. *Child Development*, **70**, 853–65.

Darwin, C. (1872). *The expression of emotions in man and animals*. New York: Philosophical Library.

De Marco, A. and Visalberghi, E. (2007). Facial displays in young tufted capuchin monkeys (*Cebus apella*): appearance, meaning, context and target, *Folia Primatologica*, **78**, 118–37.

Dennett, D.C. (1978). Beliefs about beliefs. *Behavioral and Brain Sciences*, **4**, 568–70.

Dennett, D.C. (1987). *The intentional stance*. Cambridge, MA: MIT Press.

de Rosnay, M. and Harris, P.L. (2002). Individual differences in children's understanding of emotion: the roles of attachment and language. *Attachment and Human Development*, **4**, 39–54.

de Rosnay, M. and Hughes, C. (2006). Conversation and theory of mind. Do children talk their way to socio-cognitive understanding? *British Journal of Developmental Psychology*, **24**, 7–37.

de Villiers, J.G. and de Villiers, P. (2000). Linguistic determinism and the understanding of false belief. In *Children's reasoning and the mind* (ed. P Mitchell and K Riggs), pp. 191–228. Hove: Psychology Press.

de Villiers, J.G. and Pyers, J.E. (2002). Complements to cognition: a longitudinal study of the relationship between complex syntax and false-belief-understanding. *Cognitive Development*, **17**, 1037–60.

Dunn, J., Brown, J., and Beardsall, L. (1991). Family talk about feeling states and children's later understanding of others' emotions. *Developmental Psychology*, **27**, 448–55.

Ekman, P. (1992). Facial expressions of emotion: new findings, new questions. *Psychological Science*, **3**, 34–8.

Ekman, P., Friesen, W.V., and Ellsworth, P. (1972). *Emotion in the human face*. New York: Pergamon Press.

Ellsworth, P.C. and Scherer, K.R. (2003). Appraisal process in emotion. In *Handbook of affective sciences* (ed. R.J. Davidson, K.R. Scherer, and H.H. Goldsmith), pp. 572–95. Oxford University Press.

Emery, N.J. and Clayton, N.S. (2004). The mentality of crows: convergent evolution of intelligence in corvids and apes. *Science*, **306**, 1903–7.

Farroni, T., Csibra, G., Simion, F., and Johnson, M.H. (2002). Eye contact detection in humans from birth. *Proceedings of the National Academy of Sciences of the USA*, **99**, 9602–5.

Fernald, A. (1985). Four-month-old infants prefer to listen to motherese. *Infant Behavior and Development*, **8**, 181–95.

Fernald, A. (1992). Human maternal vocalizations to infants as biological signals: an evolutionary perspective. In *The adapted mind: evolutionary psychology and the generation of culture* (ed. J.H. Barkow, J. Tooby, and L.C. Cosmides), pp. 391–428. Oxford University Press.

Ferrari, P.F., Visalberghi, E., Paukner, A., Fogassi, L., Ruggiero, A., and Suomi, S.T. (2006). Neonatal limitation in rhesus monkeys. *PLoS Biology*, 4(9), 302.

Floccia, C., Christophe, A., and Bertoncini, J. (1997). High-amplitude sucking and newborns: the quest for underlying mechanisms. *Journal of Experimental Child Psychology*, 64, 175–89.

Fodor, J, (1992). A theory of the child's theory of mind. *Cognition*, 44, 283–96.

Fonagy, P. (2001). *Attachment theory and psychoanalysis*. New York: Other Press.

Fonagy, P. and Target, M. (1997). Attachment and reflective function: their role in self-organization. *Development and Psychopathology*, 9, 679–700.

Fonagy, P., Redfern, S., and Charman, T. (1997a). The relationship between belief–desire reasoning and a projective measure of attachment security (SAT). *British Journal of Developmental Psychology*, 15, 51–61.

Fonagy, P., Steele, H., Steele, M., and Holder, J. (1997b). Attachment and theory of mind: overlapping constructs? *Association for Child Psychology and Psychiatry Occasional Papers*, 14, 31–40.

Fonagy, P., Target, M., and Gergely, G. (2000) Attachment and borderline personality disorder: a theory and some evidence. *Psychiatric Clinics of North America*, 23, 103–23.

Fonagy, P., Gergely, G., Jurist, E. and Target, M. (2002). *Affect-regulation, mentalization and the development of the self*. New York: Other Press.

Fonagy, P., Target, M., Gergely, G., Allen, J.G. and Bateman, A. (2003). The developmental roots of borderline personality disorder in early attachment relationships: a theory and some evidence. *Psychoanalytic Inquiry*, 23, 412–59.

Fonagy, P., Gergely, G. and Target, M. (2007). The parent–infant dyad and the construction of the subjective self. *Journal of Child Psychology and Psychiatry*, 48, 288–328.

Francis, D.D. and Meaney, M.J. (1999) Maternal care and the development of stress responses. *Current Opinions in Neurobiology*, 9,128–34.

Francis, D.D., Diorio, J., Liu, D., and Meaney, M.J. (1999). Variations in maternal care form the basis for a non-genomic mechanism of inter-generational transmission of individual differences in behavioral and endocrine responses to stress. *Science*, 286(5442), 1155–8.

Gergely, G. (2000). Reapproaching Mahler: new perspectives on normal autism,
normal symbiosis, splitting and libidinal object constancy from cognitive developmental theory. *Journal of the American Psychoanalytic Association*, 48(4), 1197–1228.

Gergely, G. (2002). The development of understanding self and agency. In *Blackwell handbook of childhood cognitive development* (ed. U. Goshwami), pp. 26–46. Oxford: Blackwell.

Gergely, G. (2004). The role of contingency detection in early affect-regulative interactions and in the development of different types of infant attachment. *Social Development*, 13, 468–88.

Gergely, G. (2007a). The social construction of the subjective self: the role of affect-mirroring, markedness, and ostensive communication in self development.

In *Developmental science and psychoanalysis* (ed. L. Mayes, P. Fonagy, and M. Target). London: Karnac.

Gergely, G. (2007b). Learning 'about' versus learning 'from' other minds: human pedagogy and its implications. In *Innateness*. Vol. III: *Foundations and mechanisms* (ed. P Carruthers). Oxford University Press.

Gergely, G. and Csibra, G. (2005). The social construction of the cultural mind: imitative learning as a mechanism of human pedagogy. *Interaction Studies*, 6, 463–81.

Gergely, G. and Csibra, G. (2006). Sylvia's recipe: the role of imitation and pedagogy in the transmission of cultural knowledge. In *Roots of human sociality: culture, cognition, and human interaction* (ed. S. Levenson and N. Enfield), pp. 229–255. Oxford: Berg.

Gergely, G. and Unoka, Z. (2007). The development of the unreflective self. In *Mentalization: theoretical considerations, research findings, and clinical implications* (ed. F.N. Bush). Hillsdale, NJ: Analytic Press.

Gergely, G. and Watson, J.S. (1996). The social biofeedback theory of parental affect-mirroring: the development of emotional self-awareness and self-control in infancy. *International Journal of Psycho-Analysis*, 77, 1–31.

Gergely, G. and Watson, J.S. (1999). Early social-emotional development: contingency perception and the social biofeedback model. In *Early social cognition* (ed. P Rochat), pp. 101–37. Hillsdale, NJ: Lawrence Erlbaum.

Gergely, G., Bekkering, H., and Király, I. (2002a). Rational imitation in preverbal infants. *Nature*, 415, 755.

Gergely, G., Fonagy, P., and Target, M. (2002b). Attachment, mentalization, and the etiology of borderline personality disorder. *Self Psychology*, 3, 73–82.

Gergely, G., Király, I., and Egyed, K. (2007). On pedagogy. *Developmental Science*, 10, 139–46.

Giannino, A. and Tronick, E.Z (1988). The mutual regulation model: the infant's self and interactive regulation and coping and defensive capacities. In *Stress and coping across development* (ed. T.M. Field, P.M. McCabe, and N. Schneiderman), pp. 47–68. Hillsdale, NJ: Lawrence Erlbaum.

Goldberg, S., Muir, R., and Kerr, J. (1995). *Attachment theory: social, developmental and clinical perspectives*. Hillsdale, NJ: Analytic Press.

Hare, B., Call, J., and Tomasello, M. (2001). Do chimpanzees know what conspecifics know? *Animal Behavior*, 61, 139–151.

Harlow, H.F. (1961). The development of affectional patterns in infant monkeys. In *Determinants of infant behaviour* (ed. BM Foss), Vol. 1, pp. 75–88. London: Methuen.

Harris, P. (2005). Conversation, pretence and theory of mind. In *Why language matters for theory of mind* (ed. J. Astington and J. Baird), pp. 70–83. New York: Oxford University Press.

Hobson, R.P. (1993). *Autism and the development of mind*. Hove: Lawrence Erlbaum.

Hobson, P (2002). *The cradle of thought: exploring the origins of thinking*. Oxford University Press.

Hofer, M.A. (1995). Hidden regulators: implications for a new understanding of attachment, separation and loss. In *Attachment theory: social, developmental and clinical perspectives* (ed. S. Goldberg, R. Muir, and J. Kerr), pp. 203–30. Hillsdale, NJ: Analytic Press.

Hughes, C. and Dunn, J. (2002). 'When I say a naughty word.' Children's accounts of anger and sadness in self, mother and friend: longitudinal findings from ages four to seven. *British Journal of Developmental Psychology*, **20**, 515–35.

Izard, C.E. and Malatesta, C.Z. (1987). Perspectives on emotional development. I: Differential emotions theory of early emotional development. In *Handbook of Infant Development* (2nd edn) (ed. J.D. Osofsky), pp. 494–554. New York: John Wiley.

Johnson, S.C., Slaughter, V., and Carey, S. (1998). Whose gaze will infants follow? The elicitation of gaze-following in 12-month-olds. *Developmental Science*, **1**, 233–8.

Kagan, J. (1994). *Galen's prophecy: temperament in human nature.* New York: Basic Books.

Kaminski, J., Call, J., and Tomasello, M. (2006). Goat's behaviour in a competitive food paradigm: evidence for perspective taking? *Behaviour*, **143**, 1341–56.

Lazarus, R.S. (1991). *Emotion and adaptation.* New York: Oxford University Press.

Lazarus, R.S. and Lazarus, B.N. (1994). *Passion and reason: making sense of our emotions.* New York: Oxford University Press.

LeDoux, J.E. (1995). Emotion: clues from the brain. *Annual Review of Psychology*, **46**, 209–35.

LeDoux, J.E. (1996). *The emotional brain: the mysterious underpinnings of emotional life.* New York: Simon & Schuster.

LeDoux, J.E. (2000). Emotion circuits in the brain. *Annual Review of Neuroscience*, **23**, 155–84.

Leslie, A.M. (2000). 'Theory of Mind' as a mechanism of selective attention. In *The new cognitive neurosciences* (2nd edn) (ed. M.S. Gazzaniga), pp. 1235–47. Cambridge, MA: MIT Press.

Leslie, A.M., Friedman, O., and German, T.P. (2004). Core mechanisms in 'theory of mind'. *Trends in Cognitive Sciences*, **8**, 528–33.

Lewis, M., Allessandri, S.M., and Sullivan, M.W. (1990). Violation of expectancy, loss of control and anger expressions in young infants. *Developmental Psychology*, **26**, 745–51.

Liszkowski, U., Carpenter, M., Henning, A., Striano, T., and Tomasello, M. (2004). Twelve-month-olds point to share attention and interest. *Developmental Science*, **7**, 297–307.

Lohmann, H., Tomasello, M., and Meyer, S. (2005). Linguistic communication and social understanding. In *Why language matters for theory of mind* (ed. J. Astington and J. Baird), pp. 245–65. Oxford University Press.

Mahler, M., Pine, F., and Bergman, A. (1975). *The psychological birth of the human infant: symbiosis and individuation.* New York: Basic Books.

Malatesta, C.Z., Culver, C., Tesman, R.J., and Shepard, B. (1989). The development of emotion expression during the first two years of life. *Monographs of the Society for Research in Child Development*, **54**, No. 219.

Meins, E., Fernyhough, C., Russel, J., and Clark-Carter, D. (1998). Security of attachment as a predictor of symbolic and mentalising abilities: a longitudinal study. *Social Development*, **7**, 1–24.

Meins, E., Fernyhough, C., Fradley, E., and Tuckey, M. (2001). Rethinking maternal sensitivity: Mothers' comments on infants mental processes predict security of attachment at 12 months. *Journal of Child Psychology and Psychiatry*, **42**, 637–48.

Meins, E., Fernyhough, C., Wainwright, R., Das Gupta, M., Fradley, E., and Tuckey, M. (2002). Maternal mind-mindedness and attachment security as predictors of theory of mind understanding. *Child Development*, **73**, 1715–26.

Meins, E., Fernyhough, C., Wainwright, R., et al. (2003). Pathways to understanding mind: construct validity and predictive validity of maternal mind-mindedness. *Child Development*, **74**, 1194–1211.

Meltzoff, A.N. (2002). Imitation as a mechanism of social cognition: origins of empathy, theory of mind, and the representation of action. In *Blackwell handbook of childhood cognitive development* (ed. U. Goshwami), pp. 6–25. Oxford: Blackwell.

Meltzoff, A.N. and Gopnik, A. (1993). The role of imitation in understanding persons and developing a theory of mind. In *Understanding other minds: perspectives from autism* (ed. S. Baron-Cohen, H. Tager-Flusberg, and D.J. Cohen), pp. 335–65. Oxford University Press.

Meltzoff, A.N. and Moore, M.K. (1977). Imitation of facial and manual gestures by human neonates. *Science*, **198**, 75–8.

Meltzoff, A.N. and Moore, M.K. (1989). Imitation in newborn infants: exploring the range of gestures imitated and the underlying mechanisms. *Developmental Psychology*, **25**, 954–62.

Meltzoff, A.N. and Moore, M.K. (1998). Infant intersubjectivity: broadening the dialogue to include imitation, identity and intention. In *Intersubjective communication and emotion in early ontogeny* (ed. S. Braten), pp. 47–62. Paris: Cambridge University Press–Editions de la Maison des Science de l'Homme.

Movellan, J.R. and Watson, J.S. (2002). The development of gaze following as a Bayesian systems identification problem. *UCSD Machine Perception Laboratory Technical Reports*, 2002(1).

Ochsner, K.N. and Gross, J.J. (2005). The cognitive control of emotion. *Trends in Cognitive Sciences*, **9**, 242–9.

Onishi, K.H. and Baillargeon, R. (2005). 15-month-old infants understand false beliefs. *Science*, **308**, 255–8.

Onishi, K.H., Baillargeon, R., and Leslie, A.M. (2007). 15-month-old infants detect violations in pretend scenarios. *Acta Psychologica*, **124**, 106–28.

Ontai, L.L. and Thompson, R.A. (2002). Patterns of attachment and maternal discourse effects on children's emotion understanding from 3 to 5 years of age. *Social Development*, **11**, 433–50.

Panksepp, J. (1998). *Affective neuroscience: the foundations of human and animal emotions*. Oxford University Press.

Perner, J. (1991). *Understanding the representational mind*, Cambridge, MA: MIT Press.

Perner, J. and Lang, B. (2000). Theory of mind and executive function. Is there a developmental relationship? In *Understanding other minds: perspectives from autism* (ed. S. Baron-Cohen, H. Tager-Flusberg, and D.J. Cohen), pp. 150–81. New York: Oxford University Press.

Perner, J., Ruffman, T., and Leekman, S.R. (1994). Theory of mind is contagious: You catch it from your sibs. *Child Development*, **65**, 1228–38.

Polan, H.J. and Hofer, M.A. (1999). Psychobiological origins of attachment and separation responses. In *Handbook of attachment: theory, research and clinical implications* (ed. J. Cassidy and P.R. Shaver), pp.162–80. New York: Guilford Press.

Posner, M.I. and Rothbart, M.K. (2000). Developing mechanisms of self-regulation. *Development and Psychopathology*, **12**, 427–41.

Pruessner, J.C., Champagne, F., Meaney, M.J., and Dagher, A. (2004). Dopamine release in response to a psychological stress in humans and its relationship to early life maternal care: a positron emission tomographystudy using [^{11}C]raclopride. *Journal of Neuroscience*, **24**, 2825–31.

Rochat, P. and Morgan, R. (1995). Spatial determinants in the perception of self-produced leg movements in 3- and 5-month-old infants. *Developmental Psychology*, **31**, 626–36.

Rothbart, M.K. (1989). Temperament and development. In *Temperament in childhood* (ed. G.A. Kohnstamm, J.E. Bates, and M.K. Rothbart), pp. 187–247. New York: John Wiley.

Ruffman, T., Perner, J., Naito, M., Parkin, L., and Clements, W. (1998). Older (but not younger) siblings facilitate false belief understanding. *Developmental Psychology*, **34**, 161–74.

Ruffman, T., Perner, J., and Parkin, L. (1999). How parenting style affects false belief understanding. *Social Development*, **8**, 395–411.

Sabbagh, M.A. and Callanan, M.A. (1998). Metarepresentation in action: 3-, 4-, and 5-year-olds' developing theories of mind in parent–child conversations. *Developmental Psychology*, **34**, 491–502.

Sander, L. (1988). The event-structure of regulation in the neonate–caregiver system as a biological background for early organisation of psychic structure. In *Frontiers in self psychology* (ed. A. Goldberg), pp. 64–77. Hillsdale, NJ: Analytic Press.

Spangler, G. and Grossmann, K.E. (1993). Bio-behavioral organization in securely and insecurely attached infants. *Child Development*, **64**, 1439–50.

Southgate, V., Senju, A., and Csibra, G. (2007a). Action anticipation through attribution of false beliefs by two-year-olds. *Psychological Science*, **18**, 587–92.

Southgate, V., van Maanen, C., and Csibra, G. (2007b). Infant pointing: communication to cooperate or communication to learn? *Child Development*, **78**, 735–40.

Sperber, D. and Wilson, D. (1986). *Relevance: communication and cognition*. Oxford: Blackwell.

Sperber, D. and Hirschfeld, L. (2004). The cognitive foundations of cultural stability and diversity. *Trends in Cognitive Sciences*, **8**, 40–6.

Sroufe, L.A. (1996). *Emotional development. The organization of emotional life in the early years*. Cambridge University Press.

Stern DN (1985). The Interpersonal Word of the Infant. New York: Basic Books.

Suomi, S.J. (1995). Influence of Bowlby's attachment theory on research on non-human promate biobehavioral development. In *Attachment theory: social, developmental and clinical perspectives* (ed. S. Goldberg, R. Muir, and J. Kerr), pp.185–201. Hillsdale, NJ: Analytic Press.

Suomi, S.J. (1999). Attachment in rhesus monkeys. In *Handbook of attachment: theory, research and clinical implications* (ed. J. Cassidy and P.R. Shaver), pp. 181–97. New York: Guilford Press.

Surian, L., Caldi, S., and Sperber, D. (2007). Attribution of beliefs by 13-month-old infants. *Psychological Science*, **18**, 580–6.

Thompson, R.S. (1994). Emotion regulation: a theme in search of definition. *Monographs of the Society for Research on Child Development*, **59**, 25–52.

Tomasello, M. and Haberl, K. (2003). Understanding attention: 12- and 18-month-olds know what's new for other persons. *Developmental Psychology*, **39**, 906–12.

Tomasello, M., Call, J., and Hare, B. (2003). Chimpanzees understand psychological states—the question is which ones and to what extent. *Trends in Cognitive Sciences*, **7**, 153–6.

Tomasello, M., Carpenter, M., Call, J., Behne, T., and Moll, H. (2005). Understanding and sharing intentions: the origins of cultural cognition. *Behavioral and Brain Sciences*, **28**, 675–91.

Tomasello, M., Carpenter, M., and Liszkowski, U. (2007). A new look at infant pointing. *Child Development*, **78**, 705–22.

Tomkins, S. (1995). *Exploring affect: the selective writings of Silvan Tomkins*. Cambridge University Press.

Trevarthen, C. (1979). Communication and cooperation in early infancy: a description of primary intersubjectivity. In *Before speech: the beginning of interpersonal communication* (ed. M Bullowa), pp. 321–47. New York: Cambridge University Press.

Trevarthen, C. (1993). The self born in intersubjectivity: an infant communicating. In *The perceived self* (ed. U Neisser), pp. 121–73. New York: Cambridge University Press.

Trevarthen, C. and Aitken, K.J. (2001) Infant intersubjectivity: research, theory, and clinical applications. *Journal of Child Psychology and Psychiatry*, **42**, 3–48.

Tronick, E.Z (1989). Emotions and emotional communication in infants. *American Psychologist*, **44**, 112–19.

Tronick, E.Z and Cohn, J.F. (1989). Infant–mother face-to-face interaction: age and gender differences in coordination and the occurrence of miscoordination. *Child Development*, **60**, 85–92.

Uzgiris, I.C., Benson, J.B., Kruper, J.C., and Vasek, M.E. (1989). Contextual influences on imitative interactions between mothers and infants. In *Action in social context: perspectives on early development* (ed. J.J. Lockman and N.L. Hazen), pp. 103–27. New York: Plenum Press.

Vinden, P.G. (2001). Parenting attitudes and children's understanding of mind: a comparison of Korean American and Anglo-American families. *Cognitive Development*, **16**, 793–809.

Watson, J.S. (1972). Smiling, cooing, and 'the game'. *Merrill-Palmer Quarterly*, **18**, 323–39.

Watson, J.S. (1985). Contingency perception in early social development. In *Social perception in infants* (ed. T.M. Field and N.A. Fox), pp.157–76. Norwood, NJ: Ablex.

Watson, J.S. (1994). Detection of self: the perfect algorithm. In *Self-awareness in animals and humans: developmental perspectives* (ed. S.T. Parker, R.W. Mitchell, and M.L. Boccia), pp.131–48. New York: Cambridge University Press.

Watson, J.S. (1995). Mother–infant interaction: dispositional properties and mutual designs. In *Perspectives in ethology*. Vol. 11: *Behavioral design* (ed. N.S. Thompson). New York: Plenum Press.

Watson, J.S. (2001). Contingency perception and misperception in infancy: some potential implications for attachment. *Bulletin of the Menninger Clinic*, **65**, 296–321.

Wellman, H. (1990). *The child's theory of mind*. Cambridge, MA: Bradford Books–MIT Press.

Wellman, H.M., Cross, D., and Watson, J. (2001). Meta-analysis of theory-of-mind development: the truth about false belief. *Child Development*, **72**, 655–84.

Wimmer, H. and Perner, J. (1983). Beliefs about beliefs: representation and constraining function of wrong beliefs in young children's understanding of deception. *Cognition*, **13**, 103–28.

Wismer Fries, A.B., Ziegler, T.E., Kurian, J.R., Jacoris, S., and Pollak, S.D. (2005). Early experience in humans is associated with changes in neuropeptides critical for regulating social behavior. *Proceedings of the National Academy of Sciences of the USA*, **102**, 17237–40.

12
Emotion understanding and developmental psychopathology in young children

Marc de Rosnay, Paul L. Harris, and Francisco Pons

12.1 Introduction

What aspects of their own emotional experiences do children bring to their understanding of others' emotions? Main and George (1985) offer a provocative and somewhat disturbing insight into this question. They were interested to see how abuse and maltreatment might affect children's responses to distress in playmates. Two groups of children from similarly disadvantaged backgrounds were compared: those who suffered abuse and maltreatment and those who did not. Children were between 1 and 3 years of age and were observed in a daycare setting. The children who had no history of abuse or maltreatment showed a range of responses to distress in others. They most commonly looked on or patted the distressed playmate in a mechanical fashion. However, they also engaged in more active empathic strategies to placate the distressed playmate, showing signs of concern and sadness and behaving in a motherly fashion. In contrast, expressions of active concern were absent from the abused and maltreated group. Although abused and neglected children did sometimes look on and pat the distressed playmate in a mechanical fashion, they frequently responded negatively. Negative responses had a varied character; sometimes these children became distressed and fearful themselves, and sometimes they became hostile—even physically hostile—towards the distressed playmate.

Stewart and Marvin (1984) also considered how children differ in their responses to others' distress but they emphasized individual differences in children's perspective-taking abilities. In their study, children between 3 and 5 years of age were left in a waiting room with a younger sibling. Upon the departure of the mother all the younger siblings responded with varying degrees of distress. Approximately half of the older children offered some type of comfort to their younger sibling. Comforting strategies ranged from verbal reassurance to hugs, but by and large they were appropriate given the distress of the sibling. Furthermore, the majority of those children offering comfort to their younger sibling performed better on two perspective-taking tasks. In the first of these tasks they had to take into account the idiosyncratic preferences of a story protagonist engaging in a series of activities. In the second, they had to account for the knowledge of other people when it differed from their own.

Both investigations point to the important role of individual differences for children's empathic responding and both have implications for children's emotional competence. The findings presented by Stewart and Marvin (1984) suggest that advanced socio-cognitive understanding furnishes more flexible and accurate understanding of others' emotions and helps children to respond appropriately to others' distress. Sociocognitive understanding, which encompasses emotion understanding (EU), refers to the insights children have into others' perspectives, including their idiosyncratic desires, motivations, beliefs, and emotions (de Rosnay and Hughes 2006). In contrast, research by Main and George (1985) vividly illustrates that children somehow bring their unique emotional experiences—in the case of abuse and maltreatment at least—to the emotional situations they encounter, and that such experiences colour their subsequent responses to emotional situations. These two investigations also convey a persistent division in the study of children's emotional development between the child as someone who experiences emotion and someone who seeks to understand it. Nevertheless, these two pioneering investigations dramatically illustrate the importance of both aspects for the development of children's emotional competence (Harris 1994; Saarni 1999).

In this chapter, we examine the role of EU and, to a lesser extent, the related construct theory of mind (ToM) in research on developmental psychopathology. Our discussion centres on children who do not have any obvious developmental delays or disorders, such as those affected by Down syndrome or autism, because there is mounting evidence that these groups differ in fundamental ways from other children (Cicchetti and Sroufe 1978; Cicchetti 1990; Dawson *et al.* 2002; Peterson *et al.* 2005). We seek to explicate the normative developmental processes involved in EU, their function in organizing children's behaviour, and the ways in which they can become diverted or derailed. Such an analysis is also timely given recent growth in research on individual differences in children's socio-cognitive understanding (e.g. Repacholi and Slaughter 2003).

Although there is an intuitive connection between mainstream developmental research on EU and developmental psychopathology, a rapid survey of the empirical literature reveals relatively few attempts at integration (e.g. Southam-Gerow and Kendall 2002; Pears and Fisher 2005). This remains true despite the fact that developmental psychopathology is inherently concerned with emotional development, processes, and organization (Sroufe and Rutter 1984; Cicchetti 1990; Izard and Harris 1995; Southam-Gerow and Kendall 2002). In fact, it is not yet possible to set out the relations between children's EU and specific childhood psychopathologies, if indeed such relations exist. In contrast, there is steady growth in research on typical and low-SES children's socio-cognitive understanding, including the factors that promote such understanding and the importance of individual differences for children's subsequent development, social integration, and well-being (e.g. Repacholi and Slaughter 2003; Astington and Baird 2005; de Rosnay and Hughes 2006). Thus normative developmental trajectories in children's emotional development can be described, including distinct developmental benchmarks in EU and the function of such understanding in social and emotional development.

It is instructive, in the first instance, to give a brief outline of the domain of EU. We conceptualize EU in relatively narrow terms and see it as only one aspect of children's emotional development, for which emotion is treated as an object of knowledge. Hence, EU traditionally focuses on the ways in which children identify, predict, and explain emotion in themselves and in others (Harris 1989). EU defined in this way can be contrasted with much more elaborate and clinically grounded accounts of children's emotional competence. For instance, several emotion theorists and researchers have put forward integrated accounts of children's emotional lives within a developmental framework that simultaneously addresses many important dimensions, including the fact that emotion both regulates behaviour and is the object of regulation, the impact of cognitive development on emotional competence, and the processes of emotion socialization (e.g. Denham 1989; Saarni 1999; Halberstadt *et al.* 2001; Cole *et al.* 2004). Despite this bigger picture, we believe that a focused analysis of EU has much to offer, particularly as a framework for studying children's attempts to make sense of and integrate their socio-emotional experiences.

Therefore our main purpose in this chapter is to establish an empirically grounded account of the function of EU in the adaptation of typically developing young children to their social worlds. The relevance of this account for developmental psychopathology will, we hope, become self-evident as we work through the extant literature. The last 20 years have seen extensive and detailed studies in many areas of children's EU that span toddlerhood to late childhood. Because of the nature of EU, researchers have relied heavily on children's abilities to reveal what they know through dialogue or behavioural predictions. However, we begin our discussion with a short overview of the capacities evident in late infancy and toddlerhood that underpin children's expanding EU (section 12.2). A continuous view of the development of EU that stresses stage-relevant capacities and achievements takes on particular relevance within a developmental psychopathology context, for which it is important to be cognisant of the complex nature of developmental processes and the possibility of disturbance or disruption at all stages (Sroufe and Rutter 1984). We then describe the organization and changing nature of children's EU throughout childhood and explore some different approaches to measurement (section 12.3). With this general description in place, we summarize the rapidly expanding literature concerning the individual and social factors influencing the development of children's socio-cognitive understanding (section 12.4). We include in this discussion a survey of the research that makes associations between maltreatment and young children's understanding of mind and emotion. Granted the existence of profound individual differences in children's EU and ToM, we shift our focus to the impact of such individual differences for young children's socio-emotional interactions with their peers (section 12.5). Our discussion includes both positive and negative manifestations of children's adjustment, and we attempt to distil the ways in which EU is likely to influence children's socio-emotional competence. We conclude our discussion with some thoughts on how an EU framework could be used productively in future research (section 12.6). Specifically, we emphasize the significance of EU as an organizing influence on children's experience rather than as a predictor of specific behaviours.

12.2 **Foundations of emotion understanding**

The underlying and apparently universal capacity of normally developing infants to recognize and respond appropriately to emotional facial expressions, albeit in limited terms (Haviland and Lelwica 1987; Termine and Izard 1988; Tronick 1989), is doubtless seminal to children's later EU. Nevertheless, these capacities have generally been viewed as species specific and probably having an innate basis (Harris 1989). However, by the time children can accurately identify and label simple emotional expressions and their representations in their third year, they have undergone an enormous transition in their emotional competence. Emotion is now something that can be identified, articulated, and discussed, and it is also something that can be represented outside the immediate experiential context (Bretherton *et al.* 1981; Dunn *et al.* 1987; Wellman *et al.* 1995). Therefore it is tempting to treat EU as contingent on language development; indeed, there is every indication that linguistic ability promotes the elaboration of EU (e.g. Hughes and Dunn 1998; Cutting and Dunn 1999; Harris *et al.* 2005). In keeping with this view, some assessments of EU begin with children's capacity to recognize and produce the verbal labels for emotional expressions (e.g. Denham 1986; Pons *et al.* 2004). However, it is also apparent that preschool children's emotional insights rest on an appreciation of the emotional experience and agency of persons (Harris 1989). In fact, at least three research domains converge in suggesting that, even in the second year, toddlers have some understanding of their social partners as emotional agents with whom emotional experiences can be shared, communicated, and modified. We pick up this discussion before moving on to more conventional notions of EU as 'conscious knowledge' about emotional processes (Southam-Gerow and Kendall 2002).

Research on social referencing, for example, provides mounting evidence that towards the end of the first year, and certainly in the second year, infants utilize emotional input from social partners to inform their own responses to ambiguous situations, objects, and persons (Baldwin and Moses 1996; Moses *et al.* 2001). Relatedly, within the context of the attachment relationship, it is commonplace to see affective sharing through affiliative gestures, whereby infants actively share pleasurable experiences, such as the discovery of a new toy, with the caregiver (Ainsworth *et al.* 1978; Sroufe 1996). The second year also witnesses rapid developments in children's empathic understanding. Whereas infants do not initially attempt to comfort another person in distress, by 18 months of age many toddlers make simple but appropriate efforts to alleviate such distress. By 24 months many toddlers understand what others are distressed about, provided that it is readily interpretable from current circumstances, and they begin to take more sophisticated interventions to placate—or torment—others (Zahn-Waxler *et al.* 1982, 1992; Dunn and Munn 1985). Thus, by the end of the second year, toddlers tacitly understand that discrete emotional displays have referents (objects, persons, and situations), they understand the motivational salience of these displays, and they engage in social interactions based on such an understanding.

This sketch of EU in the first 2 years is commensurate with the contention of Bretherton *et al.* (1986, p. 534) that the '… toddler's naive "theory of emotions" is a functionalist one', insofar as toddlers grasp the central position of emotion in regulating behaviour through appraisal and interpretation of both their own behaviour and that of others. Admittedly, the behaviours illustrated above are open to alternative interpretations, but when children begin to talk about emotion in the third year they place emotional concepts in a very similar folk psychological explanatory framework to that of adults, although their explanations are less sophisticated. In fact, various studies using different methodologies confirm that young children talk about emotion regularly from the beginning of the third year, and they do so appropriately. They also discuss emotions in non-present situations (past and future) and pretend entities. Although development brings a broader emotional vocabulary and an increasing appreciation of mental life, these essential features of talk about emotion are present in many children from 2 years of age, and they support the interpretation that there is remarkable continuity in young children's appreciation of the subjective nature of emotional experience (Bretherton *et al.* 1981; Bretherton and Beeghly 1982; Dunn *et al.* 1987; Wellman *et al.* 1995).

We stress continuities in EU from infancy, through toddlerhood, and into childhood to emphasize the fact that, even in toddlerhood, young children are not merely regulated by their emotions and the emotional communications of others, but are also emotionally aware. To see the implications of such emotional awareness, it is useful to consider a distinction made by Izard and Harris (1995) between the basic emotion appraisal system and the attributional system. The former, '… allows a person to assess a situation in terms of his or her beliefs and desires, and generates emotions depending on the outcome of that appraisal' (Izard and Harris 1995, p. 494): It is an embodied and automatic process. The latter allows the appraisal sequence and its emotional 'output' to be conceptualized. Conventionally, the area of inquiry captured by EU deals with the attributional system, and it is tempting to make a sharp distinction between the two systems (Harris 1994); after all, treating emotion as an object of knowledge requires reasonable linguistic skill, developing self-awareness, and, arguably, a capacity for imaginative thinking (Harris 1989; Harris *et al.* 2005). However, it is evident from our brief discussion above that the capacity to label and discuss emotions in a contextually appropriate manner probably also rests on a *grasp* of the functional role of emotions in human behaviour and interaction; which is evident in social referencing, affective sharing, and empathic behaviour. These earliest manifestations of EU are not adequately described by either the appraisal or attributional systems. Rather, they occupy the territory between the two.

The majority of our ensuing discussion will focus on EU in the conventional sense, but it would be naive to maintain too sharp a distinction between emotion as understood and emotion as experienced (Harris 1994). The shortcomings of such an approach are nowhere more evident than in the study of developmental psychopathology. The emotional disturbances that are the hallmark features of various psychopathologies have many potential starting points and may assume different significance at distinct developmental periods (Sroufe and Rutter 1984). Izard and Harris (1995, p.496) explain how early emotion socialization can affect infants' emotional organization:

> Socialization, particularly parenting practices during early development, creates an emotional climate that can have long-term effects on emotional development. It can determine whether the child perceives a given context as threatening or rewarding and whether the child expresses negative or positive emotions. Parenting practices can also bring about a wide-ranging recalibration of the appraisal system. Following such alterations, the infant can be more disposed to appraise a variety of contexts as fearful or distressing.

Thus we should expect variation in early emotion socialization, mother–infant emotional co-regulation (including attachment organization), and emotion-based communication (e.g. social referencing) to have an impact on children's later emotional organization; this is a cornerstone assumption within developmental psychopathology (Sroufe and Rutter 1984; Cicchetti and Toth 1995; Sroufe 1996; Rutter 2005). Studying EU to the exclusion of these antecedent factors risks telling only half the story about children's understanding of others as emotional agents (Harris 1994; Hughes and Leekam 2004). That said, the elaboration of EU in preschool and primary school also constitutes a series of developmental-stage-relevant capacities that open a world of communicative and representational possibilities for children, and it is also important to understand the function of these capacities in formulating and organizing behaviour. In the following discussion we provide an overview of what is known about the development of children's EU and discuss some important conceptual distinctions that also have implications for measurement.

12.3 The nature and measurement of emotion understanding

In the previous section, we emphasized that children's abilities to identify, predict, and explain emotions were a natural progression from less explicit and consciously accessible features of EU. We shall return to the importance of this developmental progression at the end of this chapter. In this section, we focus on the developmental-stage-relevant accomplishments in EU through the preschool and primary school years. Our focus in this chapter is on young children, but we also briefly discuss middle childhood to give a fuller developmental view.

12.3.1 The development of emotion understanding

Twenty years of research on EU has helped to isolate some clear milestones in children's capacities, and comprehensive overviews of this literature already exist (Harris 1989; Meerum Terwogt and Harris 1993; Saarni et al. 1998; Pons et al. 2004). One way of describing development from the third year to the end of elementary school is to divide children's understanding into three broad, and imperfect, categories: public and situational, mental, and reflective (Pons et al. 2004). By 4 or 5 years of age, most children have a firm grasp of the public and situational aspects of emotion, including: the outward expression of basic emotions, the situational causes of emotion, and circumstances or objects that can reactivate emotional experiences by serving as a reminder. Thus 4-year-olds can recognize and appropriately label emotional expressions on the basis of expressive cues (Bullock and Russell 1985; Denham 1986), and they can appreciate how certain situations or actions can influence another person's emotions or their own emotions under different circumstances (Yuill 1984; Denham 1986). Also around this period, children have firm ideas about the continuity of personal emotional experience, so whilst they recognize that emotions wane over time, they can also appreciate that a reminder can rekindle positive or negative feelings. In fact, if explicitly asked to explain why a reminder has such an impact, even some 3-year-olds can make reference to mental processes (e.g. memory), but when spontaneously explaining why people's emotions change they rarely make reference to memories and, instead, rely on situational cues. Similarly, if asked how a story protagonist can become less happy or less sad, young children focus on situational rather than cognitive mechanisms (Harris et al. 1985; Harris 1989; Lagattuta and Wellman 2001; Pons et al. 2004).

During this first phase, children can most certainly associate people's desires and preferences with their concomitant emotions (e.g. someone will be happy if they get what they want or like) (Harris et al. 1989; Bartsch and Wellman 1995), but they quickly run into trouble-making emotion attributions when two individuals hold conflicting preferences or desires, or when they are asked to attribute an emotion to story protagonists whose preferences or desires differ markedly from their own (Moore et al. 1995; Rieffe et al. 2001).

From 4 to 7 years of age, children assume an increasingly mentalistic understanding of emotion. During this period they are able to explain different emotional reactions concerning the same situation or elicitor on the basis of conflicting desires or preferences, they develop an appreciation of the relationship between emotion on the one hand and mental states (e.g. beliefs) and processes (e.g. thoughts) on the other, and they come to recognize the distinction between real and expressed emotion. For example, Lagattuta and Wellman (2001) found that by 5 years of age most children from a predominantly middle-class sample could make explicit mental connections between a story protagonist's current emotions and past events (e.g. 'She's sad because the dog makes her think about her lost bunny'). By 6 or 7 years of age, children '… demonstrated a pervasive, extended understanding of mind and emotion—one that did not differ significantly from adults' (Lagattuta and Wellman 2001, p.97). Also between 5 and 7 years of age, children start to understand how (false) beliefs relate to emotions (Harris *et al.* 1989; Hadwin and Perner 1991; Ruffman and Keenan 1996), and so they understand that someone's emotions will turn on their expectations rather than on the true state of the world.

At approximately 7 years of age, children's EU has taken on a distinctively adult character; they are able to explain emotions within a belief–desire framework in which people's emotional response turns on the match between their desires and their beliefs (Harris 1989; Bartsch and Wellman 1995). Notwithstanding these considerable advances, the subsequent years still witness profound changes. The final stage of childhood EU is characterized by an increasing awareness of the ways in which an individual can reflect upon a given situation from various perspectives, and thereby trigger different feelings either concurrently or successively (Pons *et al.* 2004). From approximately 8 years of age, children begin to understand mixed or ambivalent feelings, they become aware of the emotional determinants of pride, shame, and guilt, and they start to realize that someone can change the way they feel by changing what they think (reviewed by Harris 1989).

The public and situational, mental, and reflective aspects of emotion provide a convenient structure within which we can conceptualize the profound changes in children's EU throughout childhood. It is worth emphasizing that these abilities are hard won and represent a tremendous advance in children's capacities for reflexive self-awareness. Development of EU should also be distinguished from the counterpart skills manifest in *online* emotional appraisals. For example, children experience the feeling of surprise before they understand why someone might feel surprised, and they hide their feelings before they understand that emotions can be concealed to mislead others or to protect the self (Izard and Harris 1995). This décalage between the appraisal and attribution systems has received relatively little attention in the study of children's emotion regulation or developmental psychopathology, and we return to this issue in the final section of this chapter.

It is also worth stressing the overlap between emotion and ToM understanding. In fact, many widely used ToM tasks are also EU tasks (cf. Wellman and Liu 2004). That said, the two fields have typically been studied separately or treated as distinct features of children's socio-cognitive development. What does the extant literature reveal about the relationship between these two fields? First, there are impressive correlations between EU and ToM tasks, and both are strongly influenced by children's linguistic abilities (e.g. Hughes and Dunn 1998; Cutting and Dunn 1999). Secondly, they show similar developmental patterns; insofar as children acquire new ToM and emotion insights or *concepts* in a predictable sequence (Pons *et al.* 2004; Wellman and Liu 2004; Peterson *et al.* 2005). Thirdly, children's early insights about emotion (e.g. that emotions result from the satisfaction or frustration of desires) and mind (e.g. that two people can hold different desires) are not discarded as children's psychological understanding of others becomes more sophisticated. Rather, earlier insights in both domains become incorporated into a richer and more nuanced folk psychological framework.

In sum, EU and ToM are both essential aspects of children's burgeoning socio-cognitive understanding, and it would be misleading to treat them as wholly independent domains (de Rosnay and Hughes 2006) or to study one to the exclusion of the other. Whilst EU and ToM (in particular false-belief understanding) may ultimately cleave along certain lines (Cutting and Dunn 1999; de Villiers 2005; Peterson *et al.* 2005), it is manifestly clear that the hallmark insights measured in classic ToM tasks (e.g. deception, conflicting knowledge, the difference between appearance and reality, and false-belief understanding) are essential underpinnings of emotion constructs. Therefore in the following sections, although our investigation centres on EU, we also draw on research that examines children's ToM understanding in the context of socio-emotional development.

12.3.2 Children's 'folk theories of emotion'

We have presented a view of EU that extends naturally from classical developmental research. It is a view which stresses universal and normative accomplishments that are distilled in relatively abstract terms (Harris 1994). From a clinical point of view, in which the emotional lives of children are given very detailed consideration, such an emphasis may seem jarring because it neglects many aspects of children's appraisals and responses to emotional interactions or situations. To bridge this divide, Saarni's (1999) work on children's emotional competence is very instructive. Saarni weaves a subtle tapestry in which children's cognitive development, their socialization within the family, broader cultural influences, contextual constraints, and unique experience combine and together account for an individual's emotional competence. Central to her account of children's emotional lives is the notion of folk theories of emotion. Broadly, these are beliefs about what emotions are and how they function. Saarni explains this as follows:

> Children are exposed to emotion-eliciting circumstances, learn about the emotions involved, and subsequently incorporate that learning into their own emotional 'map' of when to feel, what to feel, how to express feelings, and whom to express them to. (Saarni 1999, pp. 63–4)

Folk theories, in Saarni's terms, are grounded in real experiences, convey cultural, familial, and age- and gender-appropriate values, and are closely linked with coping in emotion-eliciting situations. For example, a 7-year-old girl might have the following folk theories: (i) when someone gives you a present that you don't like, you must act happy to protect their feelings; (ii) when other children are being nasty or teasing you, you must act as though you don't care, so as to protect your feelings. A 7-year-old boy may share (i), but in the circumstances described in (ii) may be less preoccupied with hiding feelings and more focused on retaliation and expressing anger. This gender-biased caricature illustrates that both the girl and the boy grasp a key tenet of EU: emotions can be hidden or masked with another emotional expression to deceive others (Harris et al. 1986). However, it also illustrates that children's responses to emotionally complex situations are determined by multiple factors, not merely their level of EU.

EU and folk theories of emotion are complementary; both are manifestations of children's broader knowledge of emotion, and both can inform their responses to emotional situations synergistically. Nevertheless, children's level of EU puts conceptual limitations or *constraints* on the ways in which they are able to think about emotion-eliciting situations and to reflect on or anticipate those situations. We turn now to the measurement of children's EU.

12.3.3 Measurement

Whilst we have drawn distinctions between children's EU and folk theories of emotion, the measurement of children's knowledge about emotion has sometimes, justifiably, incorporated elements of both and at other times focused on very specific capacities. To facilitate future research with atypical populations, we discuss four approaches to assessing young children's EU and highlight measurement issues that are still in need of clarification.

The first approach is to tap into children's knowledge of the emotional expressions of real people. Facial expressions are commonly used as a stimulus (e.g. Izard 1971; Izard et al. 2001), but it is also possible to assess children's understanding of other expressions (e.g. vocal, postural, or integrated expressions) and some researchers have even considered children's capacities to produce emotional expressions (both automatically and deliberately) (e.g. Walden and Field 1990). For the purpose of illustration, we describe an intriguing procedure used by various authors (e.g. Frodi and Smetana 1984; Dunn et al. 1991a) which required children to identify emotional transitions in audiotaped conversations between a man and a woman. The procedure, developed by Rothenberg (1970), was conceptualized as an index of social sensitivity and required children to identify, using photographs of emotional expressions, emotions expressed in a naturalistic conversational interactions (happiness, sadness, anger, and anxiety). Therefore children actually have to decode the emotional content of the verbal interaction and generate an appropriate cross-modal representation of that content—a demanding and apparently ecologically valid procedure.

The second approach, which has proved very popular with researchers studying young children, is Denham's (1986) affective labelling and perspective-taking tasks which incorporate both expressive emotional cues and developmental-stage-relevant conceptual demands. In the first section of this procedure, affective labelling, children have to make connections between emotion labels (happy, sad, angry, and afraid), representations of those emotions as depicted on felt faces, and the experimenter's corresponding expressive emotional cues. In the second section, vignettes with emotional outcomes are acted out with a faceless doll and children must attach appropriate faces. The initial vignettes depict situations which have predictable emotional outcomes (e.g. being afraid upon having a nightmare), but the latter situations are tailored to individual children and require them to identify protagonists' idiosyncratic responses to situations. For example, if a mother judges that her child will be afraid upon seeing a big dog, the child is presented with a vignette in which the protagonist's actions betray happiness when confronted with the dog. For each vignette in the second section, the experimenter acts out the emotional response on behalf of the protagonist (i.e. the correct response) and children must answer by affixing the matching facial expression. Whereas in the predictable stories children can obtain the correct answer by relying on either situational or expressive cues (from the experimenter), in the idiosyncratic stories they must be able to identify expressive cues to appraise the emotional perspective of the protagonist correctly.

The third approach is reflected in a large body of research which centres on the identification of the various components of EU (i.e. public and situational, mental and reflective). Whilst spanning a very wide developmental period, the methodologies have been surprisingly consistent (Pons et al. 2004). A common approach is to present children with a hypothetical story or situation which taps a developmental-stage-appropriate facet of EU, typically described in terms of conceptual milestones (e.g. the capacity to hide emotions). Such procedures can be acted out with props, depicted in illustrations, or merely described. The choice between each of these possible methods usually turns on children's age and the desire to maximize story comprehension. Critically, this approach has largely avoided genuine emotional expressions in the telling of stories (see de Rosnay and Harris (2002) for an exception). When expressive cues are involved in the telling of such stories or in the faces of the story protagonists, they do not convey the emotional outcome of the story, and so children have to figure out the answer rather than apperceive it. Regarding children's responses, it is usually assumed that they have mastered the linguistic labels for basic emotions and they can identify iconic cartoon facial expressions expressing such emotions. However, with very young children, labelling and identification of basic emotions is sometimes investigated first and regarded as the most rudimentary manifestation of EU.

Finally, there are procedures to assess children's emotional comprehension that draw children into richer emotional narratives. For example, Cassidy *et al.* (1992) devised a procedure in which children's recognition of real emotional facial expressions, their understanding of the causes of emotion, and their responses to such emotions were assessed simultaneously. Children, who were approximately 5 years of age, were shown a picture of a same sex child posing an emotional expression (one each for happiness, sadness, anger, and fear) and asked a series of 15 questions to ascertain the sophistication of their emotional comprehension. Children who scored highly labelled emotions more accurately, acknowledged experiencing the emotions, were able to invoke situations that elicited the emotions, acknowledged having expressed the emotions, and demonstrated an awareness of appropriate responses (both actions and feelings) to other people's experience of the emotions.

We describe these four approaches because they illustrate how diverse the assessment of EU can be. No approach has an obvious and inherent advantage, and we can imagine ways in which they all have a place in exploring children's emotional lives. However, each approach limits the kinds of conclusions that can be drawn. Thus, while the emotional comprehension procedure described by Cassidy *et al.* (1992) provides a rich emotional narrative, it is hard to ascertain, for example, the reasons for poor performance (e.g. there may be genuine conceptual failures or an unfamiliarity with extended discussions of emotion). In contrast, classical EU tasks which hone in on a specific relations or emotion *concepts* (e.g. the dependence of emotion on belief) may tell us little or nothing about children's use of such understanding when making sense of more complex everyday situations (e.g. Pons *et al.*, 2004).

12.3.4 Implications

There are many procedures for assessing children's knowledge about emotion, but insufficient attention is still given to the conclusions that such procedures allow. The task developed by Denham (1986) has proved very popular because it effectively taps into inter-individual variation and is nicely pitched to its young audience. However, the strong dependence on expressive emotional cues means that there is ambiguity surrounding the extent to which it accesses children's knowledge of emotional expressions, their understanding of the situational determinants of emotion, and their emotional perspective-taking abilities. For each emotional vignette it is possible that children correctly appraise the emotion of the protagonist based on expressive cues, without necessarily seeing the implications for the protagonist's desires, preferences, or dispositions. That is to say, depending on a given child's strategy, correct responses on the predictable stories need not reflect an understanding of situation—emotion regularities and correct responses on the idiosyncratic stories need not imply that the child is genuinely able to take the emotional perspective of the story protagonist. Furthermore, such ambiguity is exacerbated by the existence of very similar procedures to Denham's which appear to provide information about the same dimensions of EU but, on closer inspection, have significant procedural variations (Iannotti 1985; Garner *et al.* 1994; Cassidy *et al.* 2003).

It is difficult to make definite distinctions between children's knowledge of emotional expressions and more abstract notions of EU; in real emotional encounters the two are often inseparable. However, this may prove to be an important distinction for young children, who have less reflexive self-awareness about emotion, and atypical groups. It is probably accurate to say that children's knowledge of emotional expressions is developmentally foundational to other manifestations of EU, the latter of which conventionally focus on abstract relations. Even though quite young children agree that certain situations or circumstances will provoke a given emotion (e.g. birthday parties make people happy), the meaning of others' emotional expressions is to some extent at least informed by children's unique experiences, such as the emotion socialization processes within the family (for a discussion, see Izard and Harris 1995) and individual differences in development. Thus the conventions governing the recognition, labelling, and perhaps also production of emotional expressions are important features of children's EU that deserve attention in their own right, even if they have a different character from those aspects usually accessed in cognitive EU tasks (see section 12.3.1).

In conclusion, it is not yet clear how different EU tasks relate to one another. To evaluate connections between EU and developmental psychopathology, it is prudent to keep such limitations in mind. Of particular importance for young children is the distinction between knowledge of emotional expressions and EU as defined in section 12.3.1. Whilst both are important facets of children's EU, there is a meaningful distinction to be made between them, to which we return throughout the remaining sections of this chapter. In the following section, we pick up on the factors that influence the development of children's EU.

12.4 Developmental precursors and correlates of children's emotion understanding

Researchers from many different backgrounds have endeavoured to isolate the factors that influence children's socio-cognitive understanding. Whereas some investigations have focused exclusively on narrow definitions of ToM, others have incorporated EU or studied EU exclusively. Despite these differences in emphasis, such investigations are broadly relevant to the current discussion because they provide a view on the sorts of abilities, interactions, and environments that foster children's psychological understanding of others. Developmental precursors and correlates of children's socio-cognitive understanding that have come to prominence include:

(1) children's linguistic competence (e.g. Astington and Jenkins 1999; Cutting and Dunn 1999; Pons *et al.* 2003; Astington and Baird 2005; Harris *et al.* 2005);

(2) children's conversational interactions (e.g. Dunn *et al.* 1991a; Dunn 1996; Ruffman *et al.* 2002; Harris *et al.* 2005; Nelson 2005; de Rosnay and Hughes 2006);

(3) the inclination of mothers to take the psychological perspective of their child, including maternal mind-mindedness and the reflective function (Fonagy and Target 1997; Meins *et al.* 2002; Peterson and Slaughter 2003);

(4) the quality of children's play (Youngblade and Dunn 1995; Jenkins and Astington 2000; Harris 2005);

(5) the quality of children's primary attachment relationship (e.g. Fonagy and Target 1997; Meins *et al.* 1998; Harris 1999; Steele *et al.* 1999; Thompson 2000; Raikes and Thompson 2006);

(6) children's Internal Working Model (IWM) of the attachment relationship (Fonagy and Target 1997; de Rosnay and Harris 2002);

(7) other features of the emotional climate within the family (e.g. Cassidy *et al.* 1992; Denham *et al.* 1994).

The wide-ranging literature summarized above is unified in that it seeks to isolate specific child or parent factors within a normative spectrum that are causally related to the development of children's understanding of mind and emotion. In this section, we selectively highlight those developmental precursors and correlates of children's socio-cognitive understanding that have come to prominence in the research literature. In contrast with the normative literature, there is a relatively circumscribed literature examining associations between childhood psychopathologies and EU or ToM understanding in young children (Southam-Gerow and Kendall 2002). However, there has been sustained investigation of maltreated children, and whilst this group is not constitutive of any particular psychopathology, they are highly at risk for various psychopathological outcomes (Cicchetti and Toth 1995). Therefore, in this section, we also consider the influence of maltreatment on young children's understanding of mind and emotion.

12.4.1 Children's linguistic abilities and their conversational environments

The importance of children's linguistic abilities for their EU and ToM has been demonstrated repeatedly: children with more advanced linguistic ability are also reliably more advanced in their psychological perspective-taking (for a detailed discussion see Astington and Baird (2005)). Whilst there is some evidence that specific aspects of verbal competence may be associated with false-belief understanding (de Villiers 2005), the overall pattern suggests that the impact of linguistic ability on psychological understanding is very general (e.g. Cutting and Dunn 1999; Ruffman *et al.* 2003). The close link between children's linguistic abilities and their EU is perhaps unsurprising because EU assessments are typically language-based, children's negotiation of social situations is to a large extent mediated by language, and conversational exchange is a 'royal road' to others' viewpoints (e.g. Dunn 1996; Nelson 2005). Therefore it stands to reason that studies investigating EU in atypical populations or exploring the influence of EU on children's socio-emotional competence, for example, should ideally also take into account children's linguistic abilities and explore the relationship between these two factors.

Another factor that has been reliably linked with individual differences in children's EU is the quality of their conversational interactions. Verbal explanations about emotions have long been recognized as an important forum for emotion socialization; sometimes labelled coaching or induction (Lewis and Saarni 1985). More recently, causally coherent mother–child psychological discourse has emerged as an important correlate and causal influence on children's socio-cognitive understanding (reviewed by de Rosnay and Hughes 2006). Very similar patterns have emerged regarding child–child and child–sibling conversations, but it remains less clear how these latter interactions influence development, although a parallel pattern of influence is entirely plausible (Brown *et al.* 1996; Hughes and Dunn 1998; Jenkins *et al.* 2003).

In a similar vein, various authors have emphasized that the mother's regard for her child as an independent psychological being plays a significant role in the development of the child's psychological understanding of others (e.g. Light 1979; Fonagy and Target 1997; Meins 1997). The influence of such a maternal mindset has been vividly illustrated by Meins *et al.* (2002), who showed that the mother's mind-mindedness—appropriate mental-state comments on her infant's behaviours at 6 months—predicted the child's mental-state understanding at 4 years of age independently of the child's concurrent linguistic ability. The exact relationship between mind-mindedness and the quality of mothers' conversational interactions with their children is not yet determined, but it is reasonable to conjecture that a mind-minded mother will also engage in more causally coherent psychological discourse with her children (Harris 1999; de Rosnay and Hughes 2006).

12.4.2 The primary attachment relationship

Recently, there has also been an increasing focus on the quality of mother–infant attachment status as a predictor of children's later socio-cognitive understanding, with many researchers suggesting that a secure attachment relationship promotes children's understanding of mind and emotion (e.g. Fonagy and Target 1997; Meins *et al.* 1998; Thompson 2000; Symons 2004). The role of attachment status can be conceptualized in various ways (Fonagy and Target 1997; Harris 1999) but there is emerging consensus from different research traditions that the quality of the attachment relationship is likely to set the tone for conversational interactions that take place between mother and child, and it is the quality of such conversational interactions, in turn, that exert a direct influence on children's socio-cognitive development (Main *et al.* 1985; Fonagy and Target 1997; Thompson 2000; Reese 2002; Symons 2004). For example, Fonagy and Target, who put forward various possible connections between secure attachment and superior mental state understanding in children, also explicitly proposed that 'Secure attachment may then engender patterns of verbal interaction between child and caregiver which in turn support thinking about feelings and intentions' (Fonagy and Target 1997, p. 688). Within such a framework, a positive association between secure attachment in infancy and higher levels of socio-cognitive understanding in childhood is to be expected, but this relationship should be mediated by qualitative aspects of mother–child conversational interactions. The empirical basis of such an account is still uncertain. Crucially, the evidence linking observational measures of attachment with higher levels of socio-cognitive understanding is very inconsistent, although it is marginally more consistent for EU than for ToM (Laible and Thompson 1998; Steele *et al.* 1999; Meins *et al.* 2002; Ontai and Thompson 2002; de Rosnay and Harris 2005; Oppenheim *et al.* 2005; Raikes and Thompson 2006). Where a link between attachment and socio-cognitive understanding has emerged, the interpretation that it is mediated by the mother's conversational style has to some extent been supported (Meins et al. 1998; Raikes and Thompson 2006).

To summarize, the proposal that secure attachment promotes children's understanding of mind and emotion does not yet rest on a firm empirical base, although it is noteworthy that the findings discussed above all come from normative samples and therefore may underestimate the significance of attachment for children's subsequent socio-cognitive understanding.

12.4.3 Child maltreatment

Maltreated children have been the focus of sustained investigation within a developmental psychopathology context, and it is clear that they encounter many developmental challenges over and above those ordinarily facing typical children: The extent and diversity of these challenges have been described by Cicchetti and his colleagues (e.g. Cicchetti 1990; Cicchetti and Toth 1995). For example, infants and toddlers experiencing maltreatment have aberrant emotional responses to ordinary social situations, such as maternal or stranger approach (Gaensbauer et al. 1980), and their attachment organization with their primary caregiver is likely to be characterized by insecurity and/or disorganization (Carlson et al. 1989). Such severe emotional disturbance in the mother–infant relationship suggests that atypical patterns of emotional appraisal are likely to be deeply entrenched in children who have been subjected to early maltreatment (Izard and Harris 1995). Young maltreated children also engage in less symbolic and dyadic play than non-maltreated children (Alessandri 1991), they often fail to show typical empathic responses to distress in other children (Howes and Espinosa 1985; Main and George 1985; Klimes-Dougan and Kistner 1990), and they have a higher incidence of emotionally dysregulated behaviour (e.g. Maughan and Cicchetti 2002). Regarding their emotional communications, maltreated toddlers make proportionately fewer references to internal states and maltreating mother–child dyads discuss emotions less frequently than non-maltreating dyads (Beeghly and Cicchetti 1994; Shipman and Zeman 1999). Finally, physical abuse and neglect are associated with considerable delays in school assessments of children's intellectual development (Erickson et al. 1989; Eckenrode et al. 1993). In sum, the effects of maltreatment are pervasive (Cicchetti and Toth 1995)

In terms of the developmental precursors and correlates of EU outlined above, it is evident that maltreated children are at risk of disturbance on nearly every front. Therefore it is easy to imagine that a normative developmental framework may be an inappropriate backdrop against which to evaluate the emotional development of maltreated children. However, a close reading of the literature reveals much continuity between the development of

EU in normal and maltreated children. Below, we examine the deficits in EU and ToM that have been associated with maltreatment, and we also ask whether they can be understood within the context of the preceding discussion or whether they need special consideration within the context of maltreatment. For clarity, we divide the child maltreatment literature into studies that focus on children's understanding of emotional expressions and studies that focus on more conventional notions of EU and ToM.

Maltreatment and understanding emotional expressions

In section 12.3 we expressed the view that understanding emotional expressions, whilst different in nature to other aspects of EU, is likely to be an important foundation for later EU abilities. Given the aberrant emotional experience of maltreated children from early on in development, it is plausible that such experience has an enduring influence on their understanding of emotional expressions. To test this possibility, two research groups have measured maltreated and non-maltreated children's recognition of emotional transitions occurring in audiotaped naturalistic conversations between a man and a woman (see section 12.3.2) (Barahal *et al.* 1981; Frodi and Smetana 1984). The findings of Frodi and Smetana for children between 3 and 5 years of age revealed no differences in recognition accuracy between abused, maltreated, matched-control (for verbal ability), and typical control children. However, this young sample may have produced insufficient variability in recognition accuracy to reveal group differences. Indeed, the findings of Barahal *et al.* with children aged from 6 to 8 years showed that maltreated children were significantly poorer at recognizing emotional expressions than their non-maltreated counterparts. But close inspection of these latter data also revealed that differences in recognition accuracy were carried by children's IQ rather than a history of maltreatment.

More reliable differences between maltreated and non-maltreated children have emerged in research focusing exclusively on facial expression recognition. In three separate studies, Camras and colleagues (Camras *et al.* 1983, 1988, 1990) showed that maltreated children between 3 and 7 years of age had poorer understanding of universal facial expressions of emotion and, in the two later studies, poorer understanding of masked negative emotional facial expressions. All facial expressions were posed by a boy or girl model and subjects had to match facial expressions to emotion stories. Importantly, independent confirmation of these findings was obtained by During and McMahon (1991) despite significant procedural variations (including the use of adult and child facial expressions of emotion). Furthermore, Camras *et al.* (1990) examined the possibility that children's verbal abilities related to their recognition of emotional facial expressions and/or explained the observed differences in performance between maltreated and non-maltreated children. In their study, no association between verbal ability and recognition of emotional facial expressions emerged. However, this finding should be treated with some caution because independent research groups have repeatedly documented such associations with similarly aged children (Izard *et al.* 2001; Schultz *et al.* 2001; Mostow *et al.* 2002) and Smith and Walden (1999) showed that, whilst both maltreated and high-risk children matched for verbal ability were poorer at recognizing line drawings of facial expressions when compared with typical control children, all group differences disappeared once differences in verbal ability were accounted for.

The findings of Camras and colleagues, During and McMahon (1991), and Smith and Walden (1999) also suggest that there is a high degree of continuity in the recognition of emotional facial expressions between maltreated and non-maltreated children. Specifically, these studies reported that maltreated children, despite performing at a lower overall level, differentiated between facial expressions in the same way as non-maltreated children (e.g. Camras *et al.* 1988; Smith and Walden 1999). Thus, even though children found some emotion judgement harder than others (e.g. masked negative emotions were harder to identify than simple facial expressions (Camras *et al.* 1988)), response patterns were not affected by maltreatment status. Continuity in patterns of responding between maltreated and non-maltreated children strongly suggests that maltreated children are delayed in their recognition rather than deviant or deficient in any specific manner. Additional support for this conclusion comes from Camras *et al.* (1988), who compared the relationship between children's ability to pose emotional expressions and their recognition of emotional expressions. They found a robust correspondence and a very similar pattern between the two capacities for maltreated and non-maltreated children.

The only qualitative discontinuity to surface between maltreated and non-maltreated children in this literature emerged in the analysis of children's errors (Camras *et al.* 1990): Camras *et al.* (1996) reported that maltreated children were more likely to make anger misattributions (27 per cent) than non-maltreated children (18 per cent). Whilst this trend was non-significant, it resonates with more recent research showing that older maltreated children (6–12 years of age) have significantly different levels of event-related brain potential activation specific to angry faces (Pollak *et al.* 2001) and they are quicker to recognize degraded facial expressions depicting anger than their non-maltreated counterparts (Pollak and Sinha 2002).

In sum, there is ample evidence that maltreated children perform more poorly than non-maltreated children in the recognition of emotional expressions, in particular facial expressions. For the most part, such recognition deficits are consistent with delayed development along a normative trajectory. Where maltreated children may differ qualitatively from their non-maltreated counterparts is in their readiness to perceive or attribute anger; this bias possibly derives from their hyper-vigilance to aggressive stimuli (Rieder and Cicchetti 1989) and may relate to their proclivity to attribute hostile intentions within ambiguous situations (Dodge et al. 1995).

Maltreatment and socio-cognitive understanding

At least four separate research groups have documented delayed EU in maltreated young children (Frodi and Smetana 1984; Rogosch et al. 1995; Smith and Walden 1999; Pears and Fisher 2005). All these studies employed EU tasks in which children had to appreciate the external aspects or situational determinants of emotion (see section 12.3.1). Two studies are notable in that they were conducted on a small scale but provided excellent control groups; including demographically and intellectually matched control children as well as typical children (Frodi and Smetana 1984; Smith and Walden 1999). In both studies, maltreated children performed very similarly on the EU tasks to the intellectually and socially matched controls. Whilst typical control children performed at a higher level on EU tasks, all group differences in performance disappeared once children's verbal abilities were accounted for. In contrast with the findings of these two small-scale studies, the results presented by Pears and Fisher and by Rogosch et al. indicate that maltreatment may have a negative influence on EU even when differences in intellectual ability have been statistically accounted for. These latter studies were conducted with larger samples but did not have intellectually and demographically matched controls, and so it is difficult to ascertain whether the findings reflect the unique influence of maltreatment on EU or whether group differences would disappear if suitable matched control groups were obtained.

Two of the aforementioned studies also analysed whether children's sensitivity to specific emotions differed as a function of maltreatment status (Smith and Walden 1999; Pears and Fisher 2005). Results from both studies revealed that maltreated children did not exhibit any particular pattern of deviance or specific deficits. Therefore, although maltreated children may have lower levels of EU, there is relatively little evidence that the link between maltreatment and EU should be conceptualized in qualitatively different terms to normal children with poor EU, except insofar as it is likely to be only one of many negative ramifications stemming from maltreatment.

Regarding ToM understanding, two studies have recently documented poorer performance by maltreated children (Cicchetti et al. 2003; Pears and Fisher 2005). The study by Cicchetti et al. employed a large and socially diverse sample of children aged between 3 and 8 years, and provides good evidence that maltreated children are at a considerable disadvantage in their understanding of other minds. However, it is unclear whether the deficits experienced by maltreated children result from maltreatment *per se* or whether they are a function of the broader intellectual delays experienced by many maltreated children. Despite the compelling link between linguistic competence and ToM (Peterson and Siegal 2000; Astington and Baird 2005), neither investigation employed a straightforward control for verbal ability, although such a measure was available. Cicchetti *et al.* (2003) used a comprehensive composite index of children's verbal mental age (VMA) to restrict their sample; they only examined the relationship between maltreatment and ToM understanding in children with VMA > 48 months. This decision was based on the analyses of Jenkins and Astington (1996) who showed, using a small sample, that children with a VMA < 49 mo did not have the requisite verbal skills to pass ToM tasks. Notwithstanding the merits of the cautious approach adopted by Cicchetti *et al.*, Jenkins and Astington in fact argued that VMA continues to be relevant for ToM understanding *beyond* a VMA of 48 months. However, Cicchetti *et al.* did not examine whether VMA explained differences in ToM understanding between maltreated and non-maltreated children within their restricted sample despite robust negative correlations between maltreatment status and VMA. Pears and Fisher (2005) measured both verbal and performance IQ but, unfortunately, used a composite measure of general IQ in their analyses. Therefore it is possible that the relation between maltreatment and EU may have been further attenuated (and possibly non-significant) if only the verbal IQ index was employed in the analyses.

To summarize, young maltreated children have poorer EU and ToM understanding than their non-maltreated counterparts but it is far from clear whether these deficits are particular to the experience of maltreatment. When maltreated children are compared with carefully matched control groups, which seems to be a prudent research strategy given the profound range of developmental challenges facing them, there is little evidence of maltreatment-specific EU deficits. Thus the impact of maltreatment on children's socio-cognitive understanding is likely to be mediated by the mechanisms outlined earlier in this section, i.e. linguistic development and restricted access to causally coherent psychological discourse.

12.4.4 Implications

This brief discussion illustrates that children's understanding of mind and emotion is closely linked to their linguistic abilities and conversational environments, and it also alerts us to the possibility that other qualitative aspects of their close relationships may be of significance. When making links between EU and developmental psychopathology, it is important to keep these findings in mind. The co-occurrence of EU deficits and distinctive patterns of emotional or behavioural disturbance, for example, need not imply that the former is in any way conceptually linked with the latter. As we have seen in this section, deficits in EU could arise because of delays in linguistic development or restricted opportunities for social interaction. For example, Cook et al. (1994) identified young primary school children who had high or moderate levels of disruptive behaviour problems and showed that these children also had relatively poor understanding of their own emotional experience and the cues for recognizing basic emotion. However, in a similar vein to the maltreatment literature, when intellectual functioning was statistically controlled for, the association between EU and disruptive behaviour reduced dramatically.

In sum, when studying EU in the context of developmental psychopathology, differences between disordered and non-disordered groups, such as relative delays in reaching normative milestones or distinctive patterns of deviation, should be interpreted with caution. Before specific links are made between a given childhood disorder and EU, more commonplace explanations for children's performance on EU assessments, such as poor linguistic development or social exclusion, deserve attention. Whilst these latter factors may be a direct consequence of the disorder or the factors bringing it about, their influence on EU can probably be understood within a normal developmental framework. However, if distinctive patterns of EU can be reliably linked to a specific childhood disorder, and this association cannot be accounted for within a normal developmental framework, it is plausible that such distinctive patterns of EU will provide an important window on the developmental history of the disorder and, potentially, a basis for ongoing maladaptive child behaviours: A readiness amongst maltreated children to perceive or attribute anger in facial expressions and ambiguous situations may be a case in point. From the child's point of view, of course, the reasons for delayed or deviant EU may be of less importance than the fact that the child's EU differs in significant ways from his/her age-mates; assuming that children rely on their socio-cognitive understanding to make sense of complex social situations, delay or deviance relative to peers is likely to carry a heavy price. Therefore, in the following section, we explore the empirical relations between children's EU and their social integration with peers.

12.5 Children's emotion understanding and their socio-emotional competence

In this section, close attention is directed to links between children's EU and their socio-emotional competence. Although we focus on EU, we also draw on recent research seeking to link individual differences in ToM understanding and children's social competence. By choosing the term 'competence', we are casting a broad net in the hope of establishing normative relations between socio-cognitive understanding and children's socio-emotional functioning along many dimensions (e.g. prosocial behaviour, friendship maintenance, aggressive behaviour, etc). Such normative developmental relations or trajectories are useful on various fronts for research on developmental psychopathology. For example, they illustrate and contextualize critical developmental-stage-relevant skills. They also provide an empirically grounded backdrop against which more searching questions about the development of various psychopathologies can be scrutinized.

Therefore we examine whether EU influences children's socio-emotional competence with peers, whether this relationship is direct or mediated by other factors (e.g. children's verbal abilities), and whether this relationship is specific to EU or is a more general feature of children's psychological understanding of persons. We break up our discussion along thematic lines: first we address positive and then negative manifestations of socio-emotional competence. Because of space limitations, we do not address gender differences in this discussion.

12.5.1 Positive manifestations of socio-emotional competence: prosocial behaviour and likeability

The work of Dunn and her colleagues has repeatedly emphasized links between children's socio-cognitive understanding and the quality of their friendship interactions (Youngblade and Dunn 1995; McGuire and Dunn 1997; Hughes and Dunn 1998; Dunn and Cutting 1999). One study of particular note (Dunn and Cutting 1999) compared the influence of ToM understanding, two indices of EU (Cassidy *et al.* 1992; Denham 1986), and verbal competence on the quality of children's friendship interactions between 3 and 4 years of age. By and large, results showed that better performance in all these domains increased the occurrence of children's cooperative pretend play, but it was not possible to tease apart the relative contribution of each.

Does this same pattern of influence, observed within friendship pairs, hold for young children's prosocial behaviour? Broadly speaking, prosocial behaviour is an index of children's voluntary positive overtures and interactions which benefit others within their social environment (Eisenberg and Mussen 1989) and it is also, implicitly or explicitly, a reflection of their ability to establish harmonious or cooperative peer interactions. Prosocial behaviours typically depend on children's understanding or interpretation of current circumstances, and therefore many authors have reasoned that EU will influence children's ability to act in a prosocial manner (Iannotti 1985; Denham 1986; Denham *et al.* 1990; Garner *et al.* 1994). Investigations of prosocial behaviour have revealed that it is a highly contextually dependent construct, and so generalizations should be made cautiously (e.g. Iannotti 1985; Rose-Krasnor 1997). Nevertheless, evidence has accumulated over many years to suggest that higher levels of EU promote young children's prosocial behaviour and also their acceptance and popularity with peers (Denham 1986; Denham *et al.* 1990, 2002; Cassidy *et al.* 1992; Garner *et al.* 1994; Izard *et al.* 2001).

Two early studies are particularly notable because they allow a comparison of the relationship between children's EU, their perspective-taking abilities in a non-emotional context (which were similar to more contemporary notions of ToM), and prosocial behaviours (Iannotti 1985; Denham 1986). Denham's results (for children aged 2–3 years) and Iannotti's results (for children aged 4–5 years) both indicated that only EU was a reliable correlate of children's prosocial behaviour. A feature of Denham's findings deserves emphasis: there was impressive continuity between children's performance on the EU and cognitive perspective-taking tasks, but only EU was closely linked with children's positive social behaviours. Whilst open to different interpretations, the cross-sectional findings presented by Denham (1986) and Iannotti (1985) indicate that children who are better able to take the emotional perspective of another person are also more likely to initiate and engage in prosocial behaviour in various contexts.

More recently, Denham *et al.* (1992, 2002), Cassidy *et al.* (1992), and Garner *et al.* (1994) have all examined the influence of EU on children's popularity with peers or 'likeability'. Insofar as it is possible to summarize across these four studies, the association between children's EU, their social competence, and their likeability has mostly been upheld: greater EU was associated with increased likeability both concurrently and, to a limited extent, longitudinally (Denham *et al.* 1990). The results presented by Denham *et al.* (2002) deserve mention because they did not find robust concurrent association between EU and children's social competence—a pattern which deviates considerably from the literature reviewed here. Nevertheless, they did show that children's EU between 3 and 4 years of age (time$_1$) predicted their social competence between 4 and 5 years of age (time$_2$), controlling for continuity in children's social competence between time$_1$ and time$_2$.

The findings summarized above highlight the importance of EU for children's prosocial behaviour and their likeability, even when other aspects of their emotional regulation and their parent's emotional expressivity have been accounted for (Denham *et al.* 1990; Cassidy *et al.* 1992). Do such findings also hold when children's verbal abilities are taken into account? Several recent studies speak to this important issue (Izard et al. 2001; Schultz et al. 2001; Mostow et al. 2002; Cassidy et al. 2003). Cassidy et al. replicated the positive association between children's EU and their prosocial behaviours at ages 3–5 years, but found that these associations fell away dramatically once children's verbal abilities were taken into account. The findings of Izard and his colleagues, in contrast, tell a different story. In two longitudinal studies, one started when children were 5 years of age (Izard et al. 2001) and one started when children were 7 years of age (Mostow et al. 2002), they showed that EU was a better longitudinal predictor of children's social skills than their verbal abilities, despite robust correlations between the two domains. Social skills was comprised of three subscales from the Social Skills Rating System (SSRS) (Gresham and Elliott 1990): cooperation, assertion, and self-control. The social skills index resembles other measures of children's prosocial behaviour.

Inconsistencies between research groups regarding the independent influence of EU on children's positive social behaviours may turn, to some extent, on the age group of children examined. The findings of both Dunn and Cutting (1999) and Cassidy et al. (2003), with children aged 3–5 years, speak to the joint influences of linguistic competence and EU on children's positive social behaviours. Contrastingly, in older samples (Izard et al. 2001; Mostow et al. 2002), there is clearer evidence for the specific influence of EU.

Additional evidence for this conclusion comes from research with maltreated children. Recall the findings of Rogosch et al. (1995), who documented an independent and negative association between maltreatment and EU (see section 12.4.3). This study was notable in that the authors explored longitudinal relations between early maltreatment, EU at approximately 6 years of age, and social competence at 8 years of age. Regarding physically abused children, a history of maltreatment predicted social isolation at 8 years of age. However, physical abuse also predicted EU (controlling for verbal ability), and EU, in turn, was a robust predictor of both maltreated and control children's social isolation from peers (controlling for verbal ability). In fact, EU mediated the association between physical maltreatment and isolation from peers. In these analyses, EU indexed children's understanding of the situational determinants of sad and angry emotions. When viewed in conjunction with the findings of Izard et al. (2001) and Schultz et al. (2001) (see above), these results support the wide-ranging conclusion that higher levels of EU between five and six years of age facilitate children's social integration and friendship maintenance.

Finally, recall the findings of Denham (1986) and Iannotti (1985) which placed EU, rather than non-emotional perspective-taking abilities, at the forefront of children's socio-emotional competence. More recently, at least four studies have shown that superior ToM understanding is in fact associated with greater socio-emotional competence. Measures included teacher reports of positive social behaviours involving a mentalistic dimension (e.g. cooperative play or make-believe) among 3-year-olds (Lalonde and Chandler 1995), social preference and popularity amongst 3- to 6-year-olds (Slaughter *et al.* 2002; Cassidy *et al.* 2003), teacher ratings of social skill and popularity among 3- to 6-year-olds (Watson *et al.* 1999; Cassidy *et al.* 2003), and observer ratings of children's positive social overtures, interactions, and sensibilities among 3- to 5-year-olds (Cassidy *et al.* 2003). However, when the effects of verbal ability were taken into account, the strength of the association between ToM understanding and socio-emotional competence diminished (Watson *et al.* 1999), in some cases profoundly (Cassidy *et al.* 2003), or disappeared altogether (Slaughter, Dennis and Pritchard 2002). This overall null finding is supported by research with Spanish children aged 4–6 years (Badenes *et al.* 2000).

Therefore, on current evidence, there is a more compelling association between EU and children's socio-emotional competence between than ToM and their socio-emotional competence, particularly for children between 5 and 6 years of age. However, this conclusion is not unproblematic; there are significant procedural variations that make the extant literature very hard to integrate. We return to this discussion below in section 12.5.3. In the next section, we consider the ways in which children's EU relates to their experience of conflict and aggression, and to hard-to-manage behaviours.

12.5.2 Manifestations of poor socio-emotional competence: conflict, aggression, and hard-to-manage behaviours

We have shown above that there are reasonable grounds to conclude that more advanced EU promotes children's socio-emotional competence. In this section, we first examine the role of children's EU in their management and resolution of conflict, and then ask whether children's EU is likely to exert an influence on negative social behaviours with peers, such as aggression.

Dunn and Herrera (1997) present a rare insight into the antecedents of young children's management and resolution of conflict with friends. Their analysis derives from a sample of 50 second-born children observed and assessed extensively between 33 months and 6 years of age (Dunn *et al.* 1991b, 1995). Drawing on this rich database, Dunn and Herrera explore the influence of relationship-specific patterns of conflict management (child–mother and child–sibling), EU, and ToM understanding on children's naturally occurring conflicts with friends. Summarizing across this impressive investigation, mothers and siblings who at earlier time points were more sensitive to the child's point of view promoted an interpersonal style in the child characterized by avoidance of direct conflict and active attempts to resolve conflicts with friends. The overall picture of familial conflict management and resolution corresponded nicely with the longitudinal influences of children's socio-cognitive understanding; for example, when involved in conflict with a friend at 6 years of age, children who had higher levels of EU at 40 and 67 months were less likely to use threats, whereas those with better ToM performance at 47 months were more likely to seek clarification of the other person's point of view. In sum, children treated as independent psychological agents within the family and children having greater psychological insight were more likely to negotiate conflicts in ways that minimized the opportunity for aggression and maintain amicable friendship relations. Furthermore, it seems that children's socio-cognitive understanding is more closely tied to their management and resolution of conflict than its frequency of occurrence; at least in young and relatively *typical* children's friendship interactions (Dunn and Cutting 1999).

The careful observational work of Dunn and colleagues opens a window on children's management and resolution of conflict, and it tells us a great deal about the ways in which children can maintain their friendships. Given the central position of EU in their findings, we might also expect that children who engage in high levels of aggressive behaviour or meet hard-to-manage criteria might have lower levels of EU. Whilst some findings suggest that deficits in EU might play a role in such maladaptive behaviour patterns, albeit a minor one (Cook *et al.* 1994; Hughes *et al.* 1998; Denham *et al.* 2002), others report no significant influence of EU (MacQuiddy *et al.* 1987; Hughes *et al.* 2000, 2001). Furthermore, factors which have come to prominence in explaining aggressive and hard-to-manage behaviour, such as executive function, effortful control, and linguistic ability (e.g. Hughes *et al.* 2000; Olson *et al.* 2005), were not accounted for in some of those studies suggesting a role for EU (e.g. Denham *et al.* 2002). In sum, the evidence linking EU deficits to young children's aggressive or hard-to-manage behaviour is poor at best. However, there is reasonable evidence that such behavioural patterns are linked to a preoccupation with anger, the attribution of hostile intent, and violent fantasy throughout childhood (e.g. Jenkins and Greenbaum 1999; Dunn and Hughes 2001; van Tijen *et al.* 2004).

12.5.3 Synthesis

One of the most remarkable features of this literature is its heterogeneity. Barely two studies are directly comparable because of methodological and procedural differences. Nevertheless, persistent associations between EU, ToM, and children's socio-emotional competence suggest that this is an important domain of study; particularly because the formation and maintenance of friendships constitute such an important part of children's adaptation to the social world (Gottman 1983; Ladd and Kochenderfer 1996), and in light of the long-term risks facing children who are isolated, rejected, and withdrawn (e.g. Kupersmidt et al. 1990; Rubin 1993; Nangle et al. 2003). How, then, can we put some order on this mixed collection of findings? Below we attempt a synthesis of the literature reviewed above in sections 12.4, 12.5.1, and 12.5.2, and we discuss some outstanding empirical and theoretical issues.

The research presented above gives EU an important role in the development of young children's prosocial behaviour and their likeability. Furthermore, at least two independent studies suggest that EU mediates or accounts for relations between the family emotional climate and positive manifestations of children's socio-emotional competence with their peers (Cassidy et al. 1992; Garner et al. 1994). To a lesser extent, children's ToM understanding has also been associated with prosocial behaviour and likeability, but it is unclear whether the influence of ToM understanding can be differentiated from verbal competence. Thus, in conjunction with the overview presented in section 12.4, a viable and intuitive story about the role of socio-cognitive understanding begins to emerge: Certain socialization practices, such as mothers' causally coherent psychological discourse and children's verbal abilities, support the elaboration of psychological understanding, and this understanding, in turn, equips children to respond increasingly sensitively and appropriately to complex social interactions with peers and cultivate good relationships. This conclusion is reminiscent of the positive association documented by Underwood and Moore (1982), in their major meta-analysis, between children's perspective-taking abilities and altruism. Children's sensitivity to and understanding of emotion may have particular salience for their socio-emotional competence, although the reason for this is not yet clear. Furthermore, antisocial or aggressive behavioural patterns may cut across children's social interactions but they do not appear, on current evidence, to be a function of poor EU. Admittedly, the empirical basis of this story is not watertight, but research from various perspectives suggest that it is plausible. Three aspects of this story also deserve close scrutiny. We take these up below.

First, it is possible that the relationship between socio-cognitive understanding and socio-emotional competence is mediated by some other variable. The most obvious candidate is children's linguistic abilities, which have been linked with both positive and negative manifestations of socio-emotional competence (e.g. Putallaz 1983; Hughes et al. 2000; Cassidy et al. 2003), as well as their socio-cognitive understanding (e.g. Harris et al. 2005). The role played by children's linguistic abilities is still far from clear, but at least two findings with children aged 5–9 years suggest that the longitudinal impact of EU on social skills is more profound than the impact of verbal abilities (Izard et al. 2001; Mostow et al. 2002). Therefore a certain level of verbal competence may be a necessary, but not a sufficient, condition for children to enact their prosocial behaviours and interventions.

Secondly, the possibility that EU, rather than cognitive perspective-taking abilities or ToM understanding, has a unique influence on children's prosocial behaviour and likeability needs clarification. In teasing apart the influences of these closely related domains, various possible explanations present themselves. Regarding measurement, there are typically discrepancies between EU and ToM. With young children, EU assessments tap into substantial variability in performance: ToM assessments are rarely so comprehensive. Regarding validity, EU tasks often ask children to think about situations that have transparent relevance to their own everyday social interactions. However, it is also possible that EU and ToM tasks may access fundamentally different abilities despite the considerable overlap frequently documented between them (see section 12.3.1). For young children in particular, it is possible that better knowledge of emotional expressions makes a unique contribution to their positive social behaviours (Izard 1971). In fact, there exists reasonable evidence that skills in decoding, and to a lesser extent producing, emotional expressions are linked with positive social behaviours and popularity in younger and older children (Edwards et al. 1984; Custrini and Feldman 1989; Walden and Field 1990; Boyatzis and Satyaprasad 1994; Izard et al. 2001). ToM assessments do not generally draw on children's understanding of expressive behaviours and it is plausible that this is one of the lines along which they cleave with EU assessments in explaining socio-emotional competence (Cutting and Dunn 1999).

Finally, the influence of socio-cognitive understanding on children's socio-emotional competence is likely to shift with development. As we have already noted, it is generally assumed that EU allows children to read and respond to complex social situations *in vivo*. Our own reading of the literature is that this account is very plausible for children until about 5 or 6 years of age; even once linguistic competence has been accounted for. For these young children, the data testify to considerable concurrent relations between EU, prosocial behaviour, and likeability (e.g. Denham *et al.* 1990). However, as children become older, their social interactions are likely to be increasingly influenced by their history of previous interactions. The implication is that measurements of likeability in young children will be more sensitive to their current level of prosocial behaviour and EU when compared with older children. However, as children become older, their social 'track-record' probably takes on more significance. Thus their repertoire of social skills will be increasingly dependent on their previous interactions, and peer perceptions of a given child are likely to be more stable. In keeping with this overall analysis, Mostow *et al.* (2002) showed that, between about 7 and 8 years of age, children's social skills were very stable indeed and, furthermore, mediated the relationship between EU and likeability. Nevertheless, even in this older group, EU predicted social skills but the reverse relationship did not hold. Also as children become older, the relative importance of their knowledge about emotional expressions is likely to diminish as their explicit capacity to reason about psychological states and motives blossoms (e.g. Schultz *et al.* 2001; Slaughter *et al.* 2002).

In this section, we have seen that children's EU supports their prosocial behaviour, friendship maintenance, and likeability. Maltreated children, who are often delayed in their understanding of mind and emotion, struggle to maintain friendships in terms of both their management of interpersonal conflict and their tendency to become withdrawn from and avoid peer interactions (reviewed by Cicchetti and Toth 1995). Thus the development of EU has clear relevance for developmental psychopathology.

12.6 **Future directions**

In this chapter we have given an account of young children's EU with a view to thinking about developmental psychopathology and further studying emotional disturbance in childhood. We have tried to emphasize that EU cannot be viewed as an isolated phenomenon (Harris 1994). Although the basic relations underpinning EU are part of a shared folk psychological explanatory framework, EU emerges in the context of children's personal emotional histories and social interactions, and is constrained by their ongoing cognitive development. However, a focus on EU reminds us that children are actively seeking to make sense of their own and others' emotional experiences from a very young age (Bretherton *et al.* 1981). The finding that EU is associated with and predicts children's socio-emotional competence should direct our attention to the fact that task-based indices of EU are a proxy index of children's capacity to appropriately read and respond to complex social situations. Therefore it follows that children who have not reached age-appropriate milestones in their EU or have distorted conceptions of emotion are at risk of being poorly synchronized with their peers. Throughout this chapter, we have attempted to synthesize and draw out the implications of what is a complex literature concerning young children's EU. We have provided conclusions along the way and do not recapitulate them here. Instead, we present two perspectives for future research that extend from our discussion above.

First, we return to the persistent issue of children's knowledge of emotional expressions and its link with more wide-ranging notions of EU. In surveying the literature in sections 12.4 and 12.5 we were struck by the fact that associations between EU and socio-emotional competence may rest, to some extent at least, on children's ability to recognize and label emotional expressions, despite the fact that other aspects of young children's EU are commonly emphasized (e.g. situational determinants) (see sections 12.3.4 and 12.4.3). One possible interpretation of such findings is that children's knowledge of emotional expressions taps into their empathic sensitivity. The problem in likening emotion expression knowledge to empathy is that the empathy construct typically captures both sensitivity to the contextual salience of others' emotional expressions and, crucially, a desire, willingness, or ability to intervene (Hoffman 1982; Zahn-Waxler *et al.*1982, 1992). However, this latter feature of the empathy construct means that it is grounded in social conduct. Therefore in future research it may be productive to examine children's empathic arousal to others' emotions (Hoffman 1982; Zahn-Waxler *et al.* 1995; Strayer and Roberts 2004), rather than their recognition of emotional expressions in isolation, and to ask how the recognition—arousal relation interacts with EU to inform children's actions. In order to discover how children come to enact increasingly sophisticated prosocial behaviours or why they fail to do so, an experimental approach that emphasizes recognition of emotional expressions in conjunction with children's motivation to act and their burgeoning conscious understanding of emotion may prove very powerful.

Secondly, in section 12.3.1 we noted that there is décalage between children's experience of emotion and their EU; for example, children feel surprised before they understand how surprise functions (Izard and Harris 1995). In fact, children's capacities to understand the causes and consequences of emotion and to think about emotion–environment relations undergoes dramatic elaboration throughout childhood. The consequence is that, with development, children stand in a fundamentally different relation to the emotional interactions they encounter. The significance of children's changing mental attitude to their emotional environments has been eloquently described by Vygotsky (1995) in his dramatic case study of three children referred to the clinic because of maltreatment suffered at the hands of their alcoholic and psychologically disturbed mother. Vygotsky explains how the youngest, middle, and oldest child experienced the punitive and disorganizing environment created by her:

> [The youngest] experienced it as an inexplicable, incomprehensible horror which has left him in a state of defencelessness. The second was experiencing it consciously, as a clash between his strong attachment, and his no less strong feeling of fear, hate and hostility. And the third child experienced it, to some extent, as far as it is possible for a 10–11 year old boy, as a misfortune which has befallen the family and which required him [...] to try somehow to mitigate the misfortune [...].' (Vygotsky 1995, p. 341)

In this extract we see that the impact of harsh parenting differs dramatically depending on each child's capacity to understand his/her mother's behaviour. Such clinical insights remind us that children's EU helps to structure their experience of interpersonal interactions. By contrast, in the research presented in section 12.5, EU has been treated as a correlate or predictor of children's social behaviours and integration. Whilst the implication is that different levels of EU exert an influence on children's behavioural organization, it is noteworthy that this possibility has not been examined directly. Treating EU as a predictor of prosocial behaviour, for example, has some inherent problems: there is no guarantee that children's level of understanding will translate into predictable actions or even that children bring their understanding to all the situations they encounter. An alternative organizational approach for future research is to explore how EU moderates children's interactions with the environment and affects their interpretations of the situations they encounter (Sroufe 1996). For example, it may be productive to focus less on whether EU correlates with prosocial behaviour and ask, instead, how EU relates to the sophistication of children's social acts, be they prosocial or antisocial. From a clinical point of view, it may also be productive to explore the extent to which developmentally immature modes of understanding emotion persist in salient interpersonal domains, despite the increasing elaboration of EU manifest in other contexts (see mobility of behavioural functions in Sroufe and Rutter (1984, p.21)). Whilst an organizational approach has not been adopted in EU research to date, there are preliminary findings in the ToM literature to suggest that it will be a productive strategy (e.g. Cutting and Dunn 2002; Cahill *et al.* 2007).

To summarize, EU is a dynamic construct despite the fact that it is often treated in empirical research as a given quantity. Developments in children's EU necessitate and afford opportunities for emotional and behavioural reorganization, and this ongoing process has obvious relevance for the study of emotional disturbance in childhood.

Ackowledgements

We thank Churchill College, Cambridge, for their generous support of this research. We are indebted to Alex Gillespie, Nigel MacKay, and Rosie Ensor for their critical and constructive comments on earlier versions of this manuscript. Thank you also to the Bagnati family for providing such wonderful music while the manuscript was being completed.

References

Ainsworth, M.D.S., Blehar, M.C., Waters, E., and Wall, S. (1978). *Patterns of attachment: a psychological study of the Strange Situation*, Hillsdale, NJ: Lawrence Erlbaum.

Alessandri, S.M. (1991). Play and social behaviors in maltreated preschoolers. *Development and Psychopathology*, **3**, 191–206.

Astington, J.W. and Baird, J.A. (2005). Introduction: Why language matters. In *Why language matters for theory of mind* (ed. J.W. Astington and J.A. Baird), pp. 3–25. Oxford University Press.

Astington, J.W. and Jenkins, J.M. (1999). A longitudinal study of the relation between language and theory-of-mind development. *Developmental Psychology*, **35**, 1311–20.

Badenes, L.V., Clemente Estevan, R.A., and Garcia Bacete, F.J. (2000). Theory of mind and peer rejection at school. *Social Development*, **9**, 271–83.

Baldwin, D.A. and Moses, L.J. (1996). The ontogeny of social information gathering. *Child Development*, **67**, 1915–39.

Barahal, R.M., Waterman, J., and Marin, H.P. (1981). The social cognitive development of abused children. *Journal of Consulting and Clinical Psychology*, **49**, 508–16.

Bartsch, K. and Wellman, H.M. (1995). *Children's talk about the mind*, New York: Oxford University Press.

Beeghly, M. and Cicchetti, D. (1994). Child maltreatment, attachment and the self system: emergence of an internal state lexicon in toddlers at high social risk. *Development and Psychopathology*, **6**, 5–30.

Boyatzis, C. and Satyaprasad, C. (1994). Children's facial and gestural decoding and encoding: relations between skills and with popularity. *Journal of Nonverbal Behavior*, **18**, 37–55.

Bretherton, I. and Beeghly, M. (1982). Talking about internal states: the acquisition of an explicit theory of mind. *Developmental Psychology*, **18**, 906–21.

Bretherton, I., McNew, S., and Beeghly-Smith, M. (1981). Early person knowledge as expressed in gestural and verbal communication. When do infants acquire a 'theory of mind'. In *Infant social cognition* (ed. M.E. Lamb and L.R. Sherrod). Hillsdale, NJ: Lawrence Erlbaum.

Bretherton, I., Fritz, J., Zahn-Waxler, C., and Ridgeway, D. (1986). Learning to talk about emotions: a functionalist perspective. *Child Development*, **57**, 529–48.

Brown, J.R., Donelan-McCall, N., and Dunn, J. (1996). Why talk about mental states? The significance of children's conversations with friends, siblings, and mothers. *Child Development*, **67**, 836–49.

Bullock, M. and Russell, J.A. (1985). Further evidence on preschoolers' interpretation of facial expressions. *International Journal of Behavioral Development*, **8**, 15–38.

Cahill, K.R., Deater-Deckard, K., Pike, A., and Hughes, C. (2007). Theory of mind, self-worth, and the mother–child relationship. *Social Development*, **16**, 45–56.

Camras, L.A., Grow, G., and Ribordy, S. (1983). Recognition of emotional expressions by abused children. *Journal of Clinical and Consulting Psychology*, **12**, 325–8.

Camras, L.A., Ribordy, S., Hill, J., Martino, S., Spaccarelli, S., and Stefani, R., (1988). Recognition and posing of emotional expressions by abused children and their mothers. *Developmental Psychology*, **24**, 776–81.

Camras, L.A., Ribordy, S., Hill, J., *et al*. (1990). Maternal facial behavior and the recognition and production of emotional expression by maltreated and nonmaltreated children. *Developmental Psychology*, **26**, 304–12.

Camras, L.A., Sachs-Alter, E., and Ribordy, S.C. (1996). Emotion understanding in maltreated children: recognition of facial expressions and integration with other emotion cues. In *Emotional development in atypical children* (ed. M. Lewis and M.W. Sullivan), pp. 203–25. Mahwah, NJ: Lawrence Erlbaum.

Carlson, V., Cicchetti, D., Barnett, D., and Braunwald, K. (1989). Disorganized/disoriented attachment relationships in maltreated infants. *Developmental Psychology*, **25**, 525–31.

Cassidy, J., Parke, R.D., Butkovsky, L., and Braungart, J.M. (1992). Family–peer connections: the roles of emotional expressiveness within the family and children's understanding of emotion. *Child Development*, **63**, 603–18.

Cassidy, K.W., Werner, R.S., Rourke, M., and Zubernis, L.S. (2003). The relationship between psychological understanding and positive social behaviors. *Social Development*, **12**, 198–221.

Cicchetti, D. (1990). The organization and coherence of socioemotional, cognitive, and representational development: illustrations through a developmental psychopathology perspective on Down syndrome and child maltreatment. In *Nebraska Symposium on Motivation*. Vol. 36: *Socioemotional development* (ed. R. Thompson), pp. 259–366. Lincoln, NB: University of Nebraska Press.

Cicchetti, D. and Sroufe, L.A. (1978). An organizational view of affect: illustration from the study of Down's syndrome infants. In *The Development of Affect* (ed. M. Lewis and L. Rosenblum), pp. 309–50. New York: Plenum Press.

Cicchetti, D. and Toth, S.L. (1995). A developmental psychopathology perspective on child abuse and neglect. *Journal of the American Academy of Child and Adolescent Psychiatry*, **34**, 541–65.

Cicchetti, D., Rogosch, F.A., Maughan, A., Toth, S.L., and Bruce, J. (2003). False belief understanding in maltreated children. *Development and Psychopathology*, **15**, 1067–91.

Cole, P.M., Martin, S.E., and Dennis, T.A. (2004). Emotion regulation as a scientific construct: Methodological challenges and directions for child development research. *Child Development*, **75**, 317–33.

Cook, E.T., Greenberg, M.T., and Kusche, C.A. (1994). The relations between emotional understanding, intellectual functioning, and disruptive behaviour problems in elementary-school-aged children. *Journal of Abnormal Child Psychology*, **22**, 205–19.

Custrini, R.J. and Feldman, R.S. (1989). Children's social competence and nonverbal encoding and decoding of emotions. *Journal of Clinical Child Psychology*, **18**, 336–42.

Cutting, A.L. and Dunn, J. (1999). Theory of mind, emotion understanding, language, and family background: individual differences and interrelations. *Child Development*, **70**, 853–65.

Cutting, A.L. and Dunn, J. (2002). The cost of understanding other people: social cognition predicts young children's sensitivity to criticism. *Journal of Child Psychology and Psychiatry*, **43**, 849–60.

Dawson, G., Carver, L., Meltzoff, A.N., Panagiotides, H., McPartland, J., and Webb, S.J. (2002). Neural correlates of face and object recognition in young children with autism spectrum disorder, developmental delay, and typical development. *Child Development*, **73**, 700–17.

Denham, S.A. (1986). Social cognition, prosocial behavior, and emotion in preschoolers: contextual validation. *Child Development*, **57**, 194–201.

Denham, S.A. (1989). *Emotional development in young children*. New York: Guilford Press.

Denham, S.A., McKinly, M., Couchoud, E.A., and Holt, R. (1990). Emotional and behavioral predictors of preschool peer ratings. *Child Development*, **61**, 1145–52.

Denham, S.A., Zoller, D., and Couchoud, E.A. (1994). Socialization of preschooler's emotion understanding. *Developmental Psychology*, **30**, 928–36.

Denham, S.A., Caverly, S., Schmidt, M., et al. (2002). Preschool understanding of emotions: contributions to classroom anger and aggression. *Journal of Child Psychology and Psychiatry*, **43**, 901–16.

de Rosnay, M. and Harris, P. (2002). Individual differences in children's understanding of emotion. *Attachment and Human Development*, **4**, 39–54.

de Rosnay, M. and Harris, P.L. (2005). Maternal comments on Strange-Situation videos: natural clusters, and links with child attachment status and emotion understanding. Presented at the Biennial Meeting of the Society for Research in Child Development, Atlanta, GA.

de Rosnay, M. and Hughes, C. (2006). Conversation and theory of mind. Do children talk their way to socio-cognitive understanding? *British Journal of Developmental Psychology*, **24**, 7–37.

de Rosnay, M., Pons, F., Harris, P.L., and Morrell, J.M.B. (2004). A lag between understanding false belief and emotion attribution in young children: relationships with linguistic ability and mothers' mental-state language. *British Journal of Developmental Psychology*, **22**, 197–218.

de Villiers, J. (2005). Can language acquisition give children a point of view? In *Why language matters for theory of mind* (ed. J.W. Astington and J.A. Baird), pp. 186–219. Oxford University Press.

Dodge, K., Pettit, G.S., Bates, J.E., and Valente, E. (1995). Social information-processing patterns partially mediate the effect of early physical abuse on later conduct problems. *Journal of Abnormal Psychology*, **104**, 632–43.

Dunn, J. (1996). The Emannuel Miller Memorial Lecture 1995. Children's relationships: bridging the divide between cognitive and social development. *Journal of Child Psychology and Psychiatry*, **37**, 507–18.

Dunn, J. and Cutting, A.L. (1999). Understanding others, and individual differences in friendship interactions in young children. *Social Development*, **8**, 202–19.

Dunn, J. and Herrera, C. (1997). Conflict resolution with friends, siblings, and mothers: a developmental perspective. *Aggressive Behavior*, **23**, 343–57.

Dunn, J. and Hughes, C. (2001). 'I got some swords and you're dead!' Violent fantasy, antisocial behavior, friendship, and moral sensibility in young children. *Child Development*, **72**, 491–505.

Dunn, J. and Munn, P. (1985). Becoming a family member: family conflict and the development of social understanding in the first year. *Child Development*, **50**, 306–18.

Dunn, J., Bretherton, I., and Munn, P. (1987). Conversations about feeling states between mothers and their young children. *Developmental Psychology*, **23**, 132–9.

Dunn, J., Brown, J., and Beardsall, L. (1991a). Family talk about feeling states and children's later understanding of others' emotions. *Developmental Psychology*, **27**, 448–55.

Dunn, J., Brown, J.R., Slomkowski, C., Tesla, C., and Youngblade, L. (1991b). Young children's understanding of other people's feelings and beliefs: individual differences and their antecedents. *Child Development*, **62**, 1352–66.

Dunn, J., Slomkowski, C., Donelan, N., and Herrera, C. (1995). Conflict, understanding, and relationships: developments and differences in the preschool years. *Early Education and Development*, **6**, 303–16.

During, S., and McMahon, R. (1991). Recognition of emotional facial expressions by abusive mothers and their children. *Journal of Clinical and Consulting Psychology*, **20**, 132–9.

Eckenrode, J., Laird, M., and Doris, J. (1993). School performance and disciplinary problems among abused and neglected children. *Developmental Psychology*, **29**, 53–62

Edwards, R., Manstead, A.S.R., and MacDonald, C.J. (1984). The relationship between children's sociometric status and ability to recognize facial expression of emotion. *European Journal of Social Psychology*, **14**, 235–8.

Eisenberg, N. and Mussen, P.H. (1989). *The roots of prosocial behavior in children*. New York: Cambridge University Press.

Erickson, M., Egeland, B., and Pianta, R. (1989). The effects of maltreatment on the development of young children. In *Child maltreatment: theory and research on the causes and consequences of child abuse and neglect* (ed. D Cicchetti and V. Carlson), pp. 647–84. New York: Cambridge University Press.

Fonagy, P. and Target, M. (1997). Attachment and the reflective function: their role in self-organisation. *Development and Psychopathology*, **9**, 679–700.

Frodi, A. and Smetana, J. (1984). Abused, neglected, and nonmaltreated preschoolers' ability to discriminate emotions in others: the effects of IQ. *Child Abuse and Neglect*, **8**, 459–65.

Gaensbauer, T., Mrazek, D., and Harmon, R. (1980). Emotional expression in abused and/or neglected infants. In *Psychological approaches to child abuse* (ed. N Frude). London, Batsford.

Garner, P.W., Jones, D.C., and Miner, J.L. (1994). Social competence among low-income preschoolers: emotion socialization practices and social cognitive correlates. *Child Development*, **65**, 622–37.

Gottman, J.M. (1983). How children become friends. *Monographs of the Society for Research in Child Development*, **48**(3).

Gresham, F.M. and Elliott, S.N. (1990). *Social Skills Questionnaire: Social Skills Rating System (teacher form)*. Circle Pines, MN: American Guidance Service.

Hadwin, J. and Perner, J. (1991). Pleased and surprised: children's cognitive theory of emotion. *British Journal of Developmental Psychology*, **9**, 215–34.

Halberstadt, A.G., Denham, S.A., and Dunsmore, J.C. (2001). Affective social competence. *Social Development*, **10**, 79–119.

Harris, P.L. (1989). *Children and emotion*. Oxford: Blackwell.

Harris, P.L. (1994). The child's understanding of emotion: developmental changes and the family environment. *Journal of Child Psychology and Psychiatry*, **35**, 3–28.

Harris, P.L. (1999). Individual differences in understanding emotions: the role of attachment status and emotional discourse. *Attachment and Human Development*, **1**, 307–24.

Harris, P.L. (2005). Conversation, pretence, and theory of mind. In *Why language matters for theory of mind* (ed. J.W. Astington and J.A. Baird), pp. 70–83. Oxford University Press.

Harris, P.L., Guz, G., Lipian, M., and Man-Shu, Z. (1985). Insight into the time course of emotion among Western and Chinese children. *Child Development*, **56**, 972–88.

Harris, P.L., Donnelly, K., Guz, G., and Pitt-Watson, R. (1986). Children's understanding of the distinction between real and apparent emotion. *Child Development*, **57**, 895–909.

Harris, P.L., Johnson, C.N., Hutton, D., Andrews, G., and Cooke, T. (1989). Young children's theory of mind and emotion. *Cognition and Emotion*, **3**, 379–400.

Harris, P.L., de Rosnay, M., and Pons, F. (2005). Language and children's understanding of mental states. *Current Directions in Psychological Science*, **14**, 69–73.

Haviland, J. and Lelwica, J. (1987). The induced affect response: 10-week-old infants' responses to three emotion expression. *Developmental Psychology*, **23**, 97–104.

Hoffman, M.L. (1982). Development of prosocial motivation. In *The development of prosocial behavior* (ed. N. Eisenberg). Sydney: Academic Press.

Howes, C. and Espinosa, M.P. (1985). The consequences of child abuse for the formation of relationships with peers. *International Journal of Child Abuse and Neglect*, **9**, 397–404.

Hughes, C. and Dunn, J. (1998). Understanding mind and emotion: longitudinal associations with mental-state talk between young friends. *Developmental Psychology*, **34**, 1026–37.

Hughes, C. and Dunn, J. (2000). Hedonism or empathy? Hard-to-manage children's moral awareness and links with cognitive and maternal characteristics. *British Journal of Developmental Psychology*, **8**, 227–45.

Hughes, C. and Leekam, S. (2004). What are the links between theory of mind and social relations? Review, reflection and new directions for studies of typical and atypical development. *Social Development*, **13**, 590–619.

Hughes, C., Dunn, J., and White, A. (1998). Trick or treat? Uneven understanding of mind and emotion and executive dysfunction in 'hard-to-manage' preschoolers. *Journal of Child Psychology and Psychiatry*, **39**, 981–94.

Hughes, C., White, A., Sharpen, J., and Dunn, J. (2000). Antisocial, angry, and unsympathetic: 'hard-to-manage' preschoolers' peer problems and possible cognitive influences. *Journal of Child Psychology and Psychiatry*, **41**, 169–179.

Hughes, C., Cutting, A.L., and Dunn, J. (2001). Acting nasty in the face of failure? Longitudinal observations of 'hard-to-manage' children playing a rigged competitive game with a friend. *Journal of Abnormal Child Psychology*, **29**, 403–16.

Iannotti, R.J. (1985). Naturalistic and structured assessments of prosocial behavior in preschool children: the influence of empathy and perspective taking. *Developmental Psychology*, 21, 46–55.

Izard, C.E. (1971). *The face of emotion*. New York: Appleton–Century–Croft.

Izard, C.E. and Harris, P.L. (1995). Emotional development and developmental psychopathology. In *Developmental psychopathology*. Vol. I. *Theory and methods* (ed. D. Cohen and D.J. Cohen), pp. 467–503. New York: John Wiley.

Izard, C., Fine, S., Schultz, D., Mostow, A., Ackerman, B., and Youngstrom, E. (2001). Emotion knowledge as a predictor of social behavior and academic competence in children at risk. *Psychological Science*, 12, 18–23.

Jenkins, J.M. and Astington, J.W. (1996). Cognitive factors and family structure associated with theory of mind development in young children. *Developmental Psychology*, 32(1), 70–98.

Jenkins, J.M. and Astington, J.W. (2000). Theory of mind and social behavior: causal models tested in a longitudinal study. *Merrill-Palmer Quarterly*, 46, 203–20.

Jenkins, J.M. and Greenbaum, R. (1996). Metacognition about emotion and child psychopathology. In *Proceedings of the 9th Conference of the International Society for Research on Emotion* (ed. N. Frijda). Toronto: International Society for Research on Emotion.

Jenkins, J.M., Turrell, S.L., Kogushi, Y., Lollis, S., and Ross, S.H. (2003). A longitudinal investigation of the dynamics of mental state talk in families. *Child Development*, 74, 905–20.

Klimes-Dougan, B. and Kistner, J. (1990). Physically abused preschoolers' responses to peers' distress. *Developmental Psychology*, 25, 516–24.

Kupersmidt, J., Coie, J.D., and Dodge, K. (1990). The role of poor peer relations in the development of disorder. In *Peer rejection in childhood* (ed. S.R. Asher and J.D. Coie). Cambridge University Press.

Ladd, G.W. and Kochenderfer, B. (1996). Linkages between friendship and adjustment during early school transitions. In *The company they keep* (ed. W.M. Bukowski, A.F. Newcomb, and W.W. Hartup), pp. 322–45. Cambridge University Press.

Lagattuta, K. and Wellman, H. (2001). Thinking about the past: early knowledge about links between prior experience, thinking and emotion. *Child Development*, 72, 82–100.

Laible, D. and Thompson, R.A. (1998). Attachment and emotional understanding in preschool children. *Developmental Psychology*, 34, 1038–45.

Lalonde, C. and Chandler, M. (1995). False belief understanding goes to school: on the social emotional consequences of coming early or late to a first theory of mind. *Cognition and Emotion*, 9, 167–85.

Lewis, M. and Saarni, C. (1985). Culture and emotions. In *The socialization of emotions* (ed. M. Lewis and C. Saarni), pp. 1–17. New York: Plenum Press.

Light. P. (1979). *The development of social sensitivity*. Cambridge University Press.

McGuire, M. and Dunn, J. (1997). Friendships in early childhood, and social understanding. *International Journal of Behavioural Development*, 21, 669–86.

MacQuiddy, S.L., Maise, S.J., and Hamilton, S.B. (1987). Empathy and affective perspective-taking skills in parent-identified conduct-disordered boys. *Journal of Clinical Child Psychology*, 16, 260–8.

Main, M. and George, C. (1985). Responses of abused and disadvantaged toddlers to distress in agemates: a study in the day care setting. *Developmental Psychology*, 21, 407–12.

Main, M., Kaplan, N., and Cassidy, J. (1985). Security in infancy, childhood and adulthood: a move to the level of representation. *Monographs of the Society for Research in Child Development*, 50, 66–104.

Maughan, A. and Cicchetti, D. (2002). Impact of child maltreatment and interadult violence on children's emotion regulation abilities and socioemotional adjustment. *Child Development*, 73, 1525–42.

Meerum Terwogt, M. and Harris, P.L. (1993). Understanding of emotion. In *The development of social cognition: the child as psychologist* (ed. M Bennett, pp. 62–86. New York: Guilford Press.

Meins, E. (1997). *Security of attachment and the social development of cognition*. Hove: Psychology Press.

Meins, E., Fernyhough, C., Russell, J., and Clark-Carter, D. (1998). Security of attachment as a predictor of symbolic and mentalising abilities: a longitudinal study. *Social Development*, 7, 1–24.

Meins, E., Fernyhough, C., Wainwright, R., Das Gupta, M., Fradley, E., and Tuckey, M. (2002). Maternal mind-mindedness and attachment security as predictors of theory of mind understanding. *Child Development*, 73, 1715–26

Moore, C., Jarrold, C., Russell, J., and Lumb, A. (1995). Conflicting desire and the child's theory of mind. *Cognitive Development*, 10, 467–82.

Moses, L.J., Baldwin, D.A., Rosicky, J.G., and Tidball, G. (2001). Evidence for referential understanding in the emotions domain at twelve and eighteen months. *Child Development*, 72, 718–35.

Mostow, A.J., Izard, C.E., Fine, S., and Trentacosta, C.J. (2002). Modeling emotional, cognitive, and behavioral predictors of peer acceptance. *Child Development*, 73, 1775–87.

Nangle, D.W., Erdley, C.A., Newman, J.E., Mason, C.A., and Carpenter, E.M. (2003). Popularity, friendship quantity, and friendship quality: interactive influences on children's loneliness and depression. *Journal of Clinical Child and Adolescent Psychology*, 32, 546–55.

Nelson, K. (2005). Language pathways into the community of minds. In *Why language matters for theory of mind* (ed. J.W. Astington and J.A. Baird), pp. 26–49. Oxford University Press.

Olson, S.L., Smeroff, A.J., Kerr, N.L., and Wellman, H.M. (2005). Developmental foundations of externalizing problems in young children: the role of effortful control. *Development and Psychopathology*, 17, 25–45.

Ontai, L.L. and Thompson, R.A. (2002). Patterns of attachment and maternal discourse effects on children's emotion understanding from 3 to 5 years of age. *Social Develpment*, 11, 433–50.

Oppenheim, D., Koren-Karie, N., Etzion-Carasso, A., and Sagi-Schwartz, A. (2005). Maternal insightfulness but not infant attachment predicts 4 year olds' theory of mind. Presented at the biennial meeting of the Society for Research in Child Development, Atlanta, GA.

Pears, K.C. and Fisher, P.A. (2005). Emotion understanding and theory of mind among maltreated children in foster care. *Development and Psychopathology*, 17, 47–65.

Peterson, C.C. and Siegal, M. (2000). Insights into theory of mind from deafness and autism. *Mind and Language*, **15**, 123–45.

Peterson, C. and Slaughter, V. (2003). Opening widows into the mind: mothers' preference for mental state explanations and children's theory of mind. *Cognitive Development*, **18**, 399–429.

Peterson, C.C., Wellman, H.M., and Liu, D. (2005). Steps in theory-of-mind development for children with deafness or autism. *Child Development*, **76**, 502–17.

Pollak, S.D. and Sinha, P. (2003). Effects of early experience on children's recognition of facial displays of emotion. *Developmental Psychology*, **38**, 784–91.

Pollak, S.D., Klorman, R., Thatcher, J.E., and Cicchetti, D. (2001). P3b reflects maltreated children's reactions to facial displays of emotion. *Psychophysiology*, **38**, 267–74.

Pons, F., Lawson, J., Harris, P.L., and de Rosnay, M. (2003). Individual differences in children's emotion understanding: effects of age and language. *Scandinavian Journal of Psychology*, **44**, 347–53.

Pons, F., Harris, P.L., and de Rosnay, M. (2004). Emotion comprehension between 3 and 11 years: developmental periods and hierarchical organization. *European Journal of Developmental Psychology*, **2**, 127–52.

Putallaz, M. (1983). Predicting children's sociometric status from their behaviour. *Child Development*, **54**, 1417–26.

Raikes, H.A. and Thompson, R.A. (2006). Family emotional climate, attachment security, and young children's emotion knowledge in a high-risk sample. *British Journal of Developmental Psychology*, **24**, 89–104.

Reese, E. (2002). Social factors in the development of autobiographical memory: the state of the art. *Social Development*, **11**, 124–42.

Repacholi, B. and Slaughter, V. (2003). *Individual differences in theory of mind: implications for typical and atypical development*. New York: Psychology Press.

Rieder, C. and Cicchetti, D. (1989). An organizational perspective on cognitive control functioning and cognitive-affective balance in maltreated children. *Developmental Psychology*, **25**, 382–93.

Rieffe, C., Meerum Terwogt, M., Koops, W., Stegge, H., and Oomen, A. (2001). Preschoolers' appreciation of uncommon desires and subsequent emotions. *British Journal of Developmental Psychology*, **19**, 259–74

Rogosch, F.A., Cicchetti, D., and Aber, J.L. (1995). The role of child maltreatment in early deviations in cognitive and affective processing abilities and later peer relationship problems. *Development and Psychopathology*, **7**, 591–609.

Rose-Kransor, L. (1997). The nature of social competence: a theoretical review. *Social Development*, **6**, 111–35.

Rothenberg, B.B. (1970). Children's social sensitivity and the relationship to interpersonal competence, intrapersonal comfort, and intellectual level. *Developmental Psychology*, **2**, 335–50

Rubin, K.H. (1993). The Waterloo Longitudinal Project: the long term predictive 'outcomes' of passive-withdrawal in childhood. In *Social withdrawal, inhibition, and shyness in childhood* (ed. K.H. Rubin and J. Asendorpf), pp. 291–314. Hillsdale, NJ: Lawrence Erlbaum.

Ruffman, T. and Keenan T.R. (1996). The belief-based emotion of surprise: the case for a lag in understanding relative to false belief. *Developmental Psychology*, **32**, 40–9.

Ruffman, T., Slade, L., and Crowe, E. (2002). The relation between children's and mother's mental state language and theory-of-mind understanding. *Child Development*, 73, 734–51.

Ruffman, T., Slade, L., Rowlandson, K., Rumsey, C., and Garnham, A. (2003). How language relates to belief, desire, and emotion understanding. *Cognitive Development*, 18, 139–58.

Rutter, M. (2005). Multiple meanings of a developmental perspective on psychopathology. *European Journal of Developmental Psychology*, 2, 221–52.

Saarni, C. (1999). *The development of emotional competence*. New York: Guilford Press.

Saarni, C., Mumme, D., and Campos, J. (1998). Emotional development: action, communication, and understanding. In *Handbook of child psychology*. Vol. 3: *Social, emotional and personality development* (5th edn) (ed. N. Eisenberg), pp. 237–309. New York: John Wiley.

Schultz, D., Izard, C.E., Ackerman, B.P., and Youngstrom, E.A. (2001). Emotion knowledge in economically disadvantaged children: self-regulatory antecedents and relations to social difficulties and withdrawal. *Development and Psychopathology*, 13, 53–67.

Shipman, K and Zeman, J. (1999). Emotional understanding: a comparison of physically maltreating and nonmaltreating mother–child dyads. *Journal of Clinical Child Psychology*, 28, 407–17.

Slaughter, V., *et al*. (1999).

Slaughter, V., Dennis, M.J., and Pritchard, M. (2002). Theory of mind and peer acceptance in preschool children. *British Journal of Developmental Psychology*, 20, 545–64.

Smith, M. and Walden, T. (1999). Understanding feelings and coping with emotional situations: a comparison of maltreated and nonmaltreated preschoolers. *Social Development*, 8, 93–116.

Southam-Gerow, M.A. and Kendall, P.C. (2002). Emotion regulation and understanding: implications for child psychopathology and therapy. *Clinical Psychology Review*, 22, 189–222.

Sroufe, L.A. (1996). *Emotional development: the organization of emotional life in the early years*. Cambridge University Press.

Sroufe, L.A. and Rutter, M. (1984). The domain of developmental psychopathology. *Child Development*, 55, 17–29.

Steele, H., Steele, M., Croft, C., and Fonagy, P. (1999). Infant–mother attachment at one year predicts children's understanding of mixed emotions at six years. *Social Development*, 8, 161–78.

Stewart, R.B. and Marvin, R.S. (1984). Sibling relations: the role of conceptual perspective taking in the ontogeny of sibling caregiving. *Child Development*, 55, 1322–32.

Strayer, J. and Roberts, W. (2004). Empathy and observed anger and aggression in five-year-olds. *Social Development*, 13, 1–13.

Symons, D.K. (2004). Mental state discourse, theory of mind, and the internalization of self-other understanding. *Developmental Review*, 24, 159–88.

Termine, N.T. and Izard, C.E. (1988). Infants' responses to their mothers' expressions of joy and sadness. *Developmental Psychology*, 24, 223–9.

Thompson, R.A. (2000). The legacy of early attachments. *Child Development*, 71, 145–52.

Tronick, E.Z. (1989). Emotions and emotional communication in infants. *American Psychologist*, 44, 112–19.

Underwood, B. and Moore, B.S. (1982). The generality of altruism in children. *Psychological Bulletin*, **91**, 143–73.

van Tijen, N., Stegge, H., Meerum Terwogt, M., and van Panhuis, N. (2004). Anger, shame and guilt in children with externalizing problems: an imbalance of affects? *European Journal of Developmental Psychology*, **1**, 271–9.

Vygotsky, L. (1994). The problem of the environment. In *The Vygotski reader* (ed. R van der Veer and J Valsiner), pp. 338–354. Oxford, Blackwell (first published 1935).

Walden, T.A. and Field, T.M. (1990). Preschool children's social competence and production and discrimination of affective expressions. *British Journal of Developmental Psychology*, **8**, 65–76.

Watson, A.C., Nixon, C.L., Wilson, A., and Capage, L. (1999). Social interaction skills and theory of mind in young children. *Developmental Psychology*, **35**, 386–91.

Wellman, H.M. and Liu, D. (2004). Scaling of theory-of-mind tasks. *Child Development*, **75**, 523–41.

Wellman, H.M., Harris, P.L., Banerjee, M., and Sinclair, A. (1995). Early understanding of emotion: evidence from natural language. *Cognition and Emotion*, **9**, 117–49.

Youngblade, L.M. and Dunn, J. (1995). Individual differences in young children's pretend play with mother and sibling: links to relationships and understanding of other people's feelings and beliefs. *Child Development*, **66**, 1472–92.

Yuill, N. (1984). Young children's co-ordination of motive and outcome in judgments of satisfaction and morality. *British Journal of Developmental Psychology*, **2**, 73–81.

Zahn-Waxler, C., Radke-Yarrow, M., and King, R. (1982). Early altruism and guilt. *Academic Psychology Bulletin*, **5**, 247–59.

Zahn-Waxler, C., Radke-Yarrow, M., Wagner, E., and Chapman, M. (1992). Development of concern for others. *Developmental Psychology*, **28**, 126–36.

Zahn-Waxler, C., Cole, P.M., Welsh, J.D., and Fox, N.A. (1995). Psychophysiological correlates of empathy and prosocial behaviors in preschool children with behavior problems. *Development and Psychopathology*, **7**, 27–48.

13
Social cognition and genetics
Thomas G. O'Connor and Cathy Creswell

Social cognition is a variegated clinical and developmental concept which underlies many psychological processes. Indeed, it has been appreciated for some time that impairments in social cognition are central to psychiatric disorders and symptoms as diverse as autism, conduct disorder, and paranoia. Furthermore, clinical assessments often focus on social cognitions, particularly in work with young people, and a number of intervention models which view altering distorted social cognitions as an essential component of treatment success have been designed. Normal developmental research also attends to multiple definitions of social cognition when considering how, for example, the effects of parental sensitivity towards an infant are carried forward in development or how individuals learn to understand the reasons for others' behaviour. Therefore understanding the origins and developmental course of social cognitions is essential for understanding normal and abnormal development, with applications from the childcare setting to the school to the clinic.

The aim of this chapter is to articulate how our understanding of social cognition may be informed by a behavioural genetics perspective. It is important to emphasize the focus on how behavioural genetics *may* be important social cognitive research because, as the research reviewed below will illustrate, there are too few behavioural genetic studies of social cognition *per se* to support firm conclusions. This is notable, given the wealth of research on intelligence, psychopathology, language, and social behaviour, i.e. phenotypes that are at least partly 'social' or have to do with one or other aspect of 'cognition'.

The hypothesis that genetic factors might underlie individual differences in social cognition is important for at least two obvious reasons. The first is general: so many other developmental and clinical constructs have been shown to be under genetic influence that it would be unusual if this were not the case for social cognition. To be sure, 'because most other relevant phenotypes also show genetic influence' is not a sufficiently compelling rationale to launch an extensive research programme. However, it would be unusual if social cognition were an exception to an emerging rule about genetic mediation of psychological phenotypes, although that needs to be assessed directly.

And, if there were a genetic influence on social cognitive processes, there would be enormous implications for developmental theory and there could also be practical applications. That is the second and more conceptual motivation for pursuing a behavioural genetics perspective on social cognition. Thus, there are a number of exquisite strategies for describing the ways in which some forms of social cognition emerge in infancy (Gergely *et al.* 1995; Nichols *et al.* 2001; Tomasello and Carpenter 2007; see also Chapter 11, this volume). There is recognition that these processes have biological correlates, and even evolutionary value, but the hypothesis that individual differences arise because of heritable rather than experiential factors has been neglected. There are many areas of developmental and clinical research in which basic questions of aetiology have been up-ended or substantially altered, including parent–child relationships (Reiss *et al.* 2000). Whether this may also be the case for models of social cognition in infancy and childhood and in later life are uncertain, and resolving that matter may be of more than academic interest, a matter to which we will return.

Our aims in this chapter are, first, to review some of the major tenets of genetics research, secondly, to consider why a behavioural genetics perspective on social cognition is needed, and, thirdly, to review available data on genetic influences on social cognition, including constructs which may involve social cognitive processes. Throughout, we seek to piece together a set of developmental and clinical models which incorporate the largely distinct fields of social cognition and genetics. We also set several parameters for this chapter. Congruent with the developmental psychopathology theme of this volume (see Chapter 1), we prioritize developmental thinking with application to clinical conditions. Additionally, because much of the emphasis in the social cognition literature is on infants and children, we prioritize studies in this age group. Furthermore, we avoid those segments of the literature that are not easily linked to behavioural genetic perspectives, for example studies not particularly concerned with aetiology. There are, of course, very many studies assessing social cognition in numerous clinical groups; we address these findings only insofar as they may be directly germane to behavioural genetics hypotheses. Several other chapters in this volume review broader segments of this diverse research literature.

13.1 **Behavioural genetics: hypotheses and strategies**

There are many reviews of the conceptual and methodological strengths and weakness of behavioural genetics research (Rutter *et al.*1999; Plomin *et al.* 2003). Given the rise of behavioural genetics research in the past 10–20 years in the developmental literature, we presume that most readers are familiar with the accoutrements of behavioural genetics research and so only an abbreviated discussion is presented.

The essential aim and strength of behavioural genetic methodology is that it provides an alternative hypothesis, or set of hypotheses, for examining aetiology. In the case of behavioural genetics research, testing the hypothesis of genetic influence requires particular research designs rather than a measure or measures of genetics; in other words, behavioural genetic studies do not index 'genetics' directly. Instead, behavioural genetics researchers infer a degree of genetic influence according to patterns of similarity in groups of individuals with different degrees of biological relatedness. For example, if monozygotic (MZ) twins (identical twins), whose genetic make-up is identical, are more similar on a measure of hostile attribution bias or joint attention than dizygotic (DZ) twins (fraternal twins), who on average have only half their genes in common, one plausible explanation is that this greater similarity among MZ twins, on average, is due to their greater genetic resemblance. There may be non-genetic reasons why MZ twins may be more similar to one another than DZ twins, including the possibility that they are exposed to more similar environments. Nevertheless, the basic logic is simple and straight forward. However, the simplicity and elegance of the method is not without detractors.

There are good methodological concerns of which readers of the behavioural genetic literature need to be aware. These include the lower birthweight and higher rate of prematurity in twins, which may be particularly relevant for assessing social and cognitive abilities in young infants. There is also the matter of the equal environments assumption, i.e. the assumption that MZ and DZ twins are similarly correlated in their exposure to environmental factors that are causally related to the phenotype being investigated. Empirical reports of violations of the equal environment assumption are uncommon, i.e. it is usually upheld (e.g. Cronk *et al.* 2002), but the matter remains unsettled. There are also concerns about sample generalizability, particularly with respect to adoption design, because adoptive families tend to be low risk and that may alter the estimate of environmental variance (Stoolmiller 1998). To some extent this can be addressed by the use of sampling strategies that include a wide array of genetically informative pairs, including halfsiblings and unrelated siblings in stepfamilies (O'Connor *et al.* 1995; Cleveland *et al.* 2000; Deater-Deckard *et al.* 2002) but that also needs further investigation.

Twin, adoptee, and related genetically informative designs are examples of a 'natural experiment', or an experiment that occurs in nature and may prove valuable for testing hypotheses and elucidating mechanisms in development. Twin and adoption designs are 'experimental' insofar as they allow researchers to estimate genetic influence on development. Thus, comparing similarity of MZ and DZ twins, or of full, half-, or unrelated siblings, is a way of testing the hypothesis of genetic influence. A key feature to keep in mind is that these genetically informative designs do not 'separate' the influence of genes and environments (i.e. contrast nature with nurture)—no design can do that. However, they do make it possible to test the hypothesis that outcomes or processes are partly genetically mediated, and that is why they are valuable.

There are then a set of concerns about the models used for taking correlations between, for example, MZ and DZ twins, and yielding estimates of heritability or the percentage of phenotype variance that is accounted for by genetics. This set of concerns is both esoteric and substantive, and is at the root of the fully grown resistance in some audiences to behavioural genetic findings. One point of consensus in this debate is that heritability is a population parameter derived from a particular sample using particular measures at a particular time. There is no single 'real' answer, just as there is no 'real' answer to how predictive hostile parenting is of children's hostile attribution bias. It is worth noting that the literature is filled with examples of how heritability is moderated by the methodology used, such as sample, source of reporting, and type of measure used. Some published reports even suggest that the range of heritabilities is extremely wide, almost covering the range of possible values.

More controversial is how well behavioural genetic analyses model genetic influence in development. A basic criticism is that the analytical models are insensitive to the dynamic nature of genetic processes. For example, neither the nature of gene expression nor the way in which genes interact with other genes and the environment (very broadly defined) are encapsulated in the models used to compared heritability—'shared' or 'non-shared' environmental variance (Partridge 2005). That is so, and perhaps inevitable, although gene–environment interplay is a topic that is receiving a good deal of attention, and some creative, if partial, strategies have been posed. Perhaps the more important lesson is not to confuse the analytical models with the research design. To be sure, there is tremendous difficulty in modelling epistasis or the other complex ways in which genes might influence behavioural phenotypes. Nevertheless, the formidable task does not render the adoption or twin design scientifically uninformative about genetics, as some authors have suggested. Instead, it seems more likely that behavioural genetics methods are indeed instrumental, but that they can only go so far in identifying mechanisms in development, and that research studies using twin or adoption designs are fairly blunt instruments. Rather than getting into the details of the more nuanced aspects of behavioural genetic analyses, which in any event may not carry additional illustrative value, our review of findings merely emphasizes patterns of similarity between groups who differ in genetic resemblance; we make only passing reference to heritabilities.

13.1.1 'Environmental' hypothesis testing

Behavioural genetic designs such as twin or adoption studies are powerful for testing genetic hypotheses *and* environmental hypotheses. In fact, some of the strongest evidence for environmental mediation is based on adoption studies. For example, the significant link between quality of parent–child relationships and adoptee child psychological adjustment (McGue *et al.* 1996) is one of the most rigorous forms of evidence that the two are environmentally connected; that is, because the genetic confound has been eliminated (the finding that the associations are stronger in biologically related families attests to the additional influence of genetic mediation). A further example of the environmentally informative nature of twin and adoption studies comes from the impressive work of Duyme *et al.* (1999). They capitalized on a 'cross-fostering' study in which adoptive parents of high and low socio-economic status (SES) adopted children who were born into high- and low-SES families. Duyme *et al.* reported that low-SES children adopted into high-SES families exhibited a higher IQ than children who were adopted into low-SES families; the difference was about half a standard deviation, and the gain was found even for late-adopted children. By incorporating the adoption design, albeit not for testing genetic hypotheses, the researchers provide some of the strongest evidence that the home environment may have a causal influence on children's intellectual ability. A third example, with perhaps even greater relevance to social cognition, is recent attachment studies showing that the concordance of twins in their attachment classification differs trivially between MZ and DZ twins (O'Connor and Croft 2001; Bokhorst *et al.* 2003). Moreover, Dozier *et al.* (2001) found that the link between parental attachment based on the Adult Attachment Interview and infant attachment classification from the Strange Situation was high in infants in foster care (i.e. non-biologically related), and no less than what is found in biologically related parent–infant dyads. The above set of findings shows how behavioural genetic methods can be a foundation for some of the strongest evidence of environmental influence in developmental science. Thus even those who are uninterested in genetics have reason to employ behavioural genetic research designs.

13.1.2 Gene–environment interplay

A central aim of current psychological research using behavioural genetic methodology is to examine how genetic factors may be involved in psychosocial adjustment and psychosocial risk. In other words, there has been a shift away from asking if there is a role of genetic factors to a more biologically and developmentally sophisticated model which seeks to incorporate the dynamic unfolding link between genetic factors and environmental mechanisms in development. Indeed, even among the most active critics of behavioural genetics methods there is acceptance of the general premise that genetic influences are important for very many psychological or behavioural phenotypes; the criticism has changed from doubting the pervasive genetic influence to criticizing the adequacy of the analytical approaches.

A substantial step forward in this line of research is the move towards assessing gene–environment interplay, a model that is being increasingly used as a framework for reviewing existing studies and designing new ones (Moffitt 2005). Of particular importance are studies documenting genotype–environment correlations. The basic notion here is that genes and environments which may be of particular importance for a given outcome or process are not independent. Genotype–environment correlations arise in several forms and require a variety of research designs (Plomin *et al.* 1977). 'Passive' genotype–environment correlations exist because parents provide both genes and environments for their children. The correlation is termed 'passive' because children play no direct role in creating this overlap. This form of genotype–environment correlation means that the interpretation of environmental effects is dubious in studies that rely solely on biologically related parents and children. Adoptive designs are the most obvious way to estimate passive genotype–environment correlations. If, in adoptive families, the association between, for example, parental sensitivity and child mentalizing is weaker than that found in biologically related parent–child dyads, then some degree of genetic mediation, in the form of passive genotype–environment correlation, is implied.

Another pervasive form of genotype–environment correlation is evocative or active. Evocative or active genotype–environment correlations arise because individuals are active agents in seeking out and evoking experiences and reactions from their environment, including relationships with caregivers, teachers, and siblings (Bell and Harper 1977; Anderson *et al.* 1986). In other words, environments and experiences are not randomly distributed in the population. The concept of active or evocative genotype–environment correlation suggests that individual characteristics that are correlated with experiences are themselves partly genetically mediated. The research literature from the past decade offers many examples of active or evocative genotype–environment correlations.

One replicated example concerns the way in which individual child characteristics that evoke negative or harsh parenting are themselves under genetic influence (Ge *et al.* 1996; O'Connor *et al.* 1998). And, as Plomin (1994) and others have shown, most measures of the 'environment' can be shown to be partly genetically influenced when subjected to a behavioural genetics design. The lesson here is that genotype–environment correlations are pervasive in development.

Just as important, and perhaps as pervasive, are genotype–environment interactions. Although largely dismissed until recently in the human literature, genotype–environment interactions are now at the forefront of research in behavioural genetics. The general notion of the interaction is that there is genetic control over sensitivity to the environment and/or environmental moderation of heritable characteristics (Kendler and Eaves 1986). This may be why there is wide variation among individuals in response to adversity. Several empirical examples of genotype–environment interaction have been reported using a range of designs, including both behavioural and molecular genetic approaches (Cadoret *et al.* 1995; Kendler *et al.* 1995; Bohman 1996; Caspi *et al.* 2002; O'Connor *et al.* 2003; Tienari *et al.* 2004). 'Main effects' models, in which a certain phenotype is associated with a particular candidate gene, are no longer seen as developmentally or biologically plausible, and have given way to a more complex developmental model which examines the joint effects of genetic influence and environment exposure across development.

13.1.3 Molecular genetic research

There is a logical, and large, step from the behavioural genetic evidence of genetic influence to molecular genetic studies identifying which genes may be involved. Indeed, psychological research on many phenotypes, including cognition, personality, and psychopathology, is making use of molecular genetic techniques, and it is now clear that psychological research needs to be equipped with this knowledge and skill (Plomin and Crabbe 2000). As noted above, molecular genetic research is playing a major role in understanding gene–environment interplay. Of course, the usual set of caveats continue to be important, and it is worth noting that many examples of non-replication continue to be reported, as in the case of disorganized attachment in infants (Lakatos *et al.* 2000; Bakermans-Kranenburg and van Ijzendoorn 2004). Interestingly, however, itis possible that failures to replicate main effects might be explicable when genotype–environment interactions are considered (Bakermans-Kranenburg and van Ijzendoorn 2006); this means that studies which fail to include sensitive environmental measures are unlikely to make real headway in understanding genetics.

13.1.4 Implications for intervention

One of the least well-understood aspects of the wealth of behavioural genetic findings is their practical value, i.e. what influence they should have on clinical intervention or social policy. On the one hand, most open-minded readers of the literature would conclude that extreme positions concerning the deterministic or irrelevant nature of genetics or of psychosocial processes can be dismissed. However, there are virtually no good examples of if and how genetic influence might pertain to treatment. What is clear is that studies showing modest or no 'shared' environment say nothing about how effective psychosocial interventions might be. This is because conclusions about genetic influence and the impact of psychosocial interventions are based on completely different research designs, and findings between these designs are not readily transferable. Thus we know that antisocial behaviour is strongly influenced by genetics, but parenting interventions are (nevertheless) effective in reducing antisocial behaviour (Scott *et al.* 2001). The application to the particular case of social cognition is even more uncertain.

13.1.5 Summary

Ultimately, the point of subjecting a construct to a twin or adoption study methodology is to begin to address questions about gene–environment interplay. There is no doubt that experiments in nature used in behavioural genetics designs, such as a twin or adoption study, cannot definitely rule in or rule out the involvement of genetics, just as these studies are unable to point to the specific genes that may be giving rise to the phenotypic patterns of resemblance. What the behavioural genetics methods offer is a set of powerful alternative hypotheses which deserve serious conceptual consideration.

13.2 Arguments, strategies, and methodologies for studying the genetics of social cognition

It is notable that the topic of social cognition has received very little research attention from a behavioural genetic perspective. Why that is so, and what the limited available findings suggest are addressed in the next sections. In this section the aim is to articulate why behavioural genetic perspectives on social cognition are needed, and how that might be obtained.

13.2.1 Intergenerational transmission

Probably the most compelling reason why a behavioural genetics perspective is needed is that it offers a set of alternative hypotheses to the presumption of environmental influence that is almost pervasive in studies of social attributions, mentalizing, theory of mind, and most other illustrations of social cognitive processes. In fact, behavioural geneticists have made a habit of raising contrary hypotheses to explain why, for example, parents' reading to children might not be causally linked with the child's IQ or why smoking in pregnancy might not cause antisocial behaviour in the child. We offer a case example in the area of social cognition.

Many studies have explored the hypothesis that social cognitions associated with vulnerability to psychopathology are transmitted intergenerationally. One of the better examples of this research is in the area of anxiety (Barlow 1988; Barrett *et al.*1996). Cross-sectional and longitudinal studies report significant parent–child resemblance for distinct categories of anxious cognitions, including attribution style and dysfunctional attitudes (Seligman *et al.* 1984; Brewin *et al.* 1996; Stark *et al.* 1996; Alloy *et al.* 2001; Creswell and O'Connor 2006; Creswell *et al.* 2006). Parental modelling is a strong possible explanation, and anxious parents are also known to anticipate (perhaps wrongly) that their children will have trouble managing situations. There is ample evidence that these processes occur and may provide a basis for intergenerational transmission (Turk and Bry 1992; Cobham *et al.* 1999; Garber and Flynn 2001; Turner *et al.* 2003). But that may not be so. A standard reasonable critique from a behavioural genetics perspective is that because the studies are based on biologically related parents and children, it is equally possible that this transmission is genetic. Thus there may be a genetic origin to anxiety and the social cognitive processes that underlie it; moreover, the observation that parents and children resemble one another may be evidence of genetic rather than psychological/environmental transmission. The more important point is that most of the studies reported so far are unable to rule out the genetic account, and cannot rule in modelling or other favoured explanations.

The behaviour genetic alternative hypothesis may have a practical application—for example, if genetic accounts were correct and that parents' modelling of anxious cognitions was an epiphenomenon of the genetic transmission. In that instance, interventions seeking to alter parental cognitions to improve child outcomes would be misguided. Fortunately for social accounts of the transmission hypothesis, there are other designs that do provide leverage for testing environmental/social transmission hypotheses directly. Chief among these are intervention designs. Using the power of an intervention design, Creswell *et al.* (2005), found that both children's and mothers' level of threat interpretation were significantly reduced following treatment. Even if there is a strong genetic basis for child and parent anxious social cognitions, the finding that they are both responsive to treatment implies that (a) there may be an environmentally mediated link between the two, and (b) behavioural genetic studies will always need to be complemented by intervention studies.

Other research groups have also shown how the manipulation of the family environment, including the alteration of parental cognitions, may be causally linked to child psychological adjustment (Barrett *et al.* 1996). These intervention studies tackle questions of environmental (albeit not genetic) aetiology in ways that are valuable to mental health professionals. What is needed now is a dialogue between research findings from experimental interventions and observational studies using behavioural genetic designs.

13.2.2 Neuroscience models of social cognition

In addition to testing presumed models of environmental transmission, behavioural genetic studies of social cognition may also help to spur research into the neuroscience basis of social cognition. Behavioural genetic designs are not synonymous with biological models, but they do signal an interest in biological mechanisms, and that is much needed. Towards that end, it is useful to consider some of the neuroscience findings on social cognition.

The neuroscience of social cognition in humans is an area of study just now developing its set of paradigms and conceptual–biological models. It is too soon to identify which paradigms may be of particular value or which might most closely approximate 'real-life' social cognitive processes and interpersonal transactions. However, the experimental animal data provide some good targets for study, and some interesting findings are emerging. For example, one set of investigators (Kirsch *et al.* 2005) focused on the neuropeptide oxytocin, a molecule shown to play substantial roles in several forms of affiliative, attachment, and bonding behaviours in animals. Using a double-blind cross-over design in which 15 adult male subjects were given an intranasal injection of oxytocin or placebo, the authors found that oxytocin reduced both activation of the amygdala and coupling of the amygdala to brainstem regions associated with fear. It is not clear whether the findings have relevance to normative social cognitions or to disorders in which there are deficits in social cognition. Nevertheless, this is one line of research that is likely to receive increased attention. A question for behavioural genetic researchers (of both humans and animals) is to examine, for example, the origins of individual differences in the physiology of oxytocin receptors, and to link that work to genetic work on phenotypes of particular interest to social cognition researchers (e.g. Wu *et al.* 2005).

In addition, systematic study of genetic hypotheses of social cognition needs to be placed alongside studies seeking to settle the neuroscience basis of social cognition using imaging and related techniques. In fact, there is already a great deal of imaging data on social cognition, although, as with most imaging studies, samples are small and questions remain about the appropriateness of comparison groups, the specificity of the findings, and the adequacy of the measures used *in situ*. One study of eight males suggested that theory of mind may be particularly associated with neural activity in the anterior cingulate cortex, left temporopolar cortex, and right prefrontal cortex (Vogeley *et al.* 2004). Another study of 13 males indicated that, compared with measures of empathy, measures of theory of mind were particularly associated with increased activations in lateral orbitofrontal cortex, middle frontal gyrus, cuneus, and superior temporal gyrus (Vollm *et al.* 2006). A possible direction for behavioural genetics research is to use the sort of designs that have proved useful in imaging studies, notably the study of twins discordant for social cognitive impairments or for clinical conditions closely connected with certain forms of social cognitive disturbances of theory of mind or attributional processes that are involved in pervasive developmental disorders, personality disorders, or major mental illness.

13.2.3 Summary

Research into the aetiology and developmental course of social cognition, in its variety of forms, emphasizes both normal maturational processes and the ways in which experience shapes individual variability. It is this latter feature which provides a way into considering behavioural genetic hypotheses, which are focused on the sources of individual differences. Social cognition research based in early childhood may be particularly targeted for future behavioural genetic research because of its emphasis on intergenerational transmission. Indeed, why it is that children and their parents resemble each other in the tendency to appraise ambiguous stimuli as threatening is a question that requires behavioural genetic methods.

13.3 Research findings on the genetics of social cognition

Whereas there are numerous sound studies assessing cognition from a behavioural genetics perspective (Spinath *et al.* 2003), the number of studies assessing *social* cognition from behavioural genetics studies is minimal. No doubt there are many reasons for this. The more important matter may be whether or not the findings on cognition (by which we might infer general intelligence, although there are of course a number of studies using a variety of cognitive indicators, such as reaction time) apply to social cognition; that is not yet certain, at any age. It is also worth considering whether genetic influence on activity (Saudino and

Eaton 1991) and social behaviours (Goldsmith *et al.*1999) might shape infants' and children's performance on social cognitive measures. It may be, for instance, that individual differences in joint attention and engagement—core features of social cognition research with infants—may be modulated, in part, by genetic influences on behaviours that compose part of the social cognitive assessment. Similarly, genetic findings on language and communication might influence social cognitive performance to the extent that social cognition incorporates language and communication from a social pragmatic perspective. Although these questions remain speculative, fortunately there are a number of measures of social cognition that have been subjected to behavioural genetic methods.

13.3.1 Theory of mind

The theory of mind (ToM) literature has only recently emphasized individual differences and the role of psychosocial experience. To date, however, most of the interest in experiential (versus maturational) processes is limited to structural features of the family or sibship. The more recent work which seeks to elucidate the role that sensitive parenting may play in ToM-related outcomes is an important step forward (Fonagy and Target 1997; Fonagy *et al.* 1997; Humfress *et al.* 2002; Meins *et al.* 2002; Fonagy and Bateman 2006; Sharp *et al.* 2006). Research of that kind may also connect ToM research with the rich collection of studies on parent–child relationship quality that has its own track record in the behavioural genetics area.

To date, very limited data that have examined specific and conventional measures of ToM are available. One study of 119 pairs of MZ and DZ twins who were approximately 42 months old found intraclass correlations of 0.66 for identical twins and 0.32 for fraternal twins (Hughes and Cutting 1999). This implied that 67 per cent of the phenotypic variability was genetically mediated. There was no evidence that similarity between twin siblings in their ToM was associated with environmental factors; rather, to the extent that there were environmental influences, they appeared to make siblings different from one another. On the other hand, a very contrary conclusion concerning genetic factors on similar ToM measures was suggested in a much larger study of over 1000 twins who were 60 months of age (Hughes *et al.* 2005). Indeed, it was striking that the correlation between twins in that study was identical for MZ and DZ twins ($r = 0.53$), nullifying any genetic hypothesis. The age difference between the samples may account for this difference; if this is so, it would imply that environmental factors have more influence on individual differences in ToM later in development. Alternatively, it may be that the contrasting findings represent random variation (the correlations for MZ and

DZ twins in the later study falls between those observed in the earlier study), although the medium to large sample sizes in the two studies make this explanation unlikely. In any event, these findings leave open a largely genetic or wholly environmental account of ToM in young children. The hypothesis that there are genetic influences on individual differences in ToM is far from settled.

Another study which examined a possible genetic influence on ToM used the sibling study design. Dorris *et al.* (2004) compared 27 siblings of an autistic child with 27 non-clinic comparison children, matched for age, sex, and verbal comprehension, on a measure that required participants to indicate what a person was thinking or feeling based only on a photograph of the eyes; the measure is thought to index one feature of social cognition. They found that siblings of autistic children were significantly poorer on the test than the matched controls. This implies that social cognition is a possible endophenotype, and that would imply some degree of genetic influence. However, quite the opposite conclusion was reached by another group of investigators (Shaked *et al.* 2006) who compared 24 siblings of autistic children with 24 normally developing children; the average age was about 41/2 years. A variety of ToM tasks were used, such as false-belief tasks. None of the ToM tasks differed between the groups. Other investigators failed to find differences in ToM ability in siblings of autistic individuals compared with siblings of learning disabled child (Ozonoff *et al.* 1993). On the other hand, another group assessing parents of children with Asperger syndrome did find evidence of familial resemblance in a measure of reading emotion/mind from photographs of the eyes (Baron-Cohen and Hammer 1997). The mixed set of findings may be due to variation in methodology across studies, but it is also possible that there is no clear signal to detect.

A small but intensive study (Yirmiya *et al.* 2006) examined precursors of ToM by examining social engagement and communication in a sample of siblings of autistic individuals and normally developing children at 4 and 14 months of age. Modest and scattered differences between groups were obtained, although these may have been due to a particular subset of siblings of autistic individuals. The study is helpful, but the findings are too preliminary to make firm conclusions. Of course, neither family history nor sibling studies distinguish between genetic and environmental explanations.

13.3.2 Attributional style

Attributional style has a firm conceptual and empirical position in the social cognition literature, particularly as a risk factor for depression. Individuals who attribute negative events to internal (versus external), stable (versus non-persistent), and global (versus idiosyncratic) causes are at risk for depression (Abramson *et al.* 1978). This model has been translated and modified in many ways to address many clinical problems in a wide age range of individuals.

As in the case of ToM, few studies have assessed specific and conventional measures of attribution in genetically informative designs. Schulman *et al.* (1993) studied attributional style in adults using the Attributional Style Questionnaire. In their sample of 115 MZ twin pairs and 27 DZ twin pairs, they obtained intraclass correlations of 0.48 for MZ twins and zero for DZ twins, implying a strong genetic influence. The small sample size, extremely disproportionate percentage of MZ twins, and the zero correlation in the DZ twins are all unusual features of the method and findings. This raises a number of concerns about the generalizability of the findings.

In their study of attributional style in 12–19-year-old twins, Lau *et al.* (2006) used adolescent self-reports on questionnaires of attributional style. They found that the correlation was 0.35 for MZ male twins and 0.34 for DZ male twins, which implies no genetic influence. However, the correlations for female twins were more discrepant: 0.47 for MZ twins and 0.28 for DZ twins. The authors reported that 13–49 per cent of the variability in attributional style was mediated by genetic factors. What was less clear was the extent to which the genetic mediation of attributional style covaried with the genetic influence on depression. In fact, even in the large sample of over 3000 individuals it was not possible to decipher clearly whether the correlation between depression and attributional style was mediated by genetic or shared environmental factors.

13.3.3 Empathy and its converse

The construct of empathy is another operationalization of social cognition that has a substantial conceptual basis and clinical history. In a study of approximately 200 twin pairs aged 14 months, Emde and colleagues (Emde *et al.* 1992; Zahn-Waxler *et al.* 1992) reported some of the only data available on empathy. In this study, the inventive measure of empathy was based on observer ratings of the infant's behaviour to several stimuli thought to elicit an empathic response (e.g. sound of a child's cry, a stranger feigning hurting herself). The results (Emde *et al.* 1992) showed that the correlation was 0.42 for MZ twins and −0.03 for DZ twins, implying genetic influence. Detailed analyses of several subtypes of empathic behaviour at age 14 months (Zahn-Waxler *et al.* 1992) showed that this pattern was observed for several behaviours, including prosocial acts and empathic concern. Interestingly, observed unresponsive/indifference showed as strong a genetic influence as the other empathic behaviours (the correlation for MZ twins was 0.33 compared with 0.08 for DZ twins). However, the pattern was far less robust at 20 months, with only empathic concern showing the anticipated greater resemblance for MZ than for DZ twins. Quite what that means is not certain.

There is an equally limited, but perhaps important, literature on psychopathy, the putative opposite of empathy. In one study, based on a selected sample of extreme groups of 7-year-olds, teacher reports of callous–unemotional traits (e.g. 'Does not show feelings or emotions') were compared for MZ and DZ twin pairs (Viding *et al.* 2005). Using an extremes group analysis (DeFries and Fulker 1988), the authors estimated that two-thirds of the difference between the extreme callous—unemotional children and the population of children could be accounted for by genetic factors. Another study (Larsson *et al.* 2006), based on a sample of over 2000 twins aged 16–17 years, used a self-report measure to assess several aspects of psychopathy (e.g. callousness: 'When other people have problems it is often their own fault; therefore one should not help them'). Across several scales of psychopathy, correlations between MZ twins range from 0.44 to 0.61; for same-sex DZ twins, the correlations ranged from 0.17 to 0.31 (correlations were still lower among opposite sex twins). These correlations yielded heritabilities that were approximately 50 per cent. A further study of 626 pairs of 17-year-old male and female twins from the community examined psychopathic traits using the Multidimensional Personality Questionnaire (Blonigen *et al.* 2005). Results again showed that dimensions that index psychopathy (e.g. 'fearless dominance') were under some degree of genetic influence, suggested by the stronger correlation of MZ than DZ twins (e.g. for fearless dominance, the correlations were .44 and .20, respectively).

A consistent suggestion of genetic influence is suggested across a range of different operationalizations of empathy in studies that vary widely in ages and settings. This is the sort of robustness that implies that a genetic influence might be 'real', although how it is that genetics influences social behaviour as complex as empathy cannot be determined from these studies.

13.3.4 Indirect indicators of social competence

The current review suggests that direct evidence of genetic influence on social cognition is limited. However, it is possible that there are findings on other constructs which might inform our search for genetic accounts of social cognition. That is, another place to look would be to outcomes or processes that might reflect individual differences in social cognition. Quality of peer relationships is one obvious place to look. The reason is that there is bountiful evidence that an admixture of social cognitive abilities underlie competence with peers, including social attributional bias and empathy (Dodge 1986).

The hypothesis that children's peer relationships might show genetic influence has attracted some attention, with one set of studies assessing group affiliation (Iervolino *et al.* 2002), another examining relationship quality (O'Connor *et al.* 2001), and yet another examining peer influence on substance use and related outcomes (Walden *et al.* 2004). Perhaps predictably, findings from studies using contrasting measures of peer influence and sample characteristics yield no clear conclusion, apart from the prosaic one that there is scattered evidence for both genetic and environmental influence.

13.3.5 Summary

One of the difficulties in linking research on social cognition with behavioural genetic hypotheses is that social cognition has typically examined in terms of developmental differences (e.g. When does joint attention or ToM emerge?) and much less in terms of individual differences (e.g. Why is there variation among children in their tendency to see others as acting in a hostile manner?). In fact, for many indicators of social cognition, there is a paucity of research on the origins of individual differences, which is a starting point for testing behavioural genetic hypotheses.

There was a familiar pattern to the findings for certain forms of social cognition, such as empathy and its converse, psychopathy. For other indicators of social cognition there were either too few studies (e.g. attributional processes) or the findings were mixed—and even quite contrary, as in the case for ToM measures. There was also a suggestion that genetic explanations were being discussed in studies that used inadequate research designs (e.g. sibling or family studies). Furthermore, given the primitive state of behavioural genetics research into social cognition, it is hardly surprising that more advanced questions such as developmental change and gene–environment interplay have attracted virtually no attention. Even so, there is not yet evidence that the interest in the neuroscience of social cognition is being taken up in behavioural genetics studies—it needs to be.

13.4 Conclusion and future directions

We conclude by making several observations about the field of social cognition and identifying challenges for integrating research and devising syncretic models across paradigms and conditions. The first point is that few 'developmental lines' are evident in the research on social cognition. Thus we know little about the extent to which social cognition operationalized as joint attention in infancy carries through to an analogue of joint attention in preschoolers. Neither is it yet evident that performance on measures of ToM in the key developmental window of around 4 years has much to do with ToM or mentalizing in older individuals. Although it is now apparent that attributional biases can be observed in young children, it has not yet been demonstrated that these biases are stable and grow into the sort of distortions that are measured in adolescents and adults. There are several implications of this uncertainty about the developmental continuity of social cognition constructs. From a behavioural genetic perspective, one concern is that the nature of the phenotype is restricted to a narrow developmental window. Inevitably, this will mean that findings will be of limited use, and one should prepare for discrepant findings, as even modest study differences in age or measure could mean that the studies are assessing qualitatively different phenomena. The problem here is not only a lack of long-term developmental research, but also a lack of a broader conceptual model for understanding the range of social cognition constructs.

A second limitation of past research and need for future research concerns the integration of developmental differences (how 3- and 5-year-olds differ in mentalizing) and individual differences (why some 5-year-olds seem to be particularly skilled at reading others' minds and some have great difficulty). To a considerable extent, the former has been conceived as a process of maturation. This is changing somewhat, but how one might conceptualize individual differences in normal maturational processes has been left underexamined. For example, are individual differences in (the onset of) ToM assessed at age 4 of long-term significance? That is, are the individual differences in the age at which these skills emerge developmentally important (aside from particular clinical conditions such as autism)?

A third factor needing more attention concerns the distinction that Carpenter et al. (1998) refer to as 'understanding that' versus 'understanding what' (see also Chapters 1 and 14, this volume). The former precedes the latter developmentally. That distinction was applied to a study of nine 15-month-olds, but parallel distinctions emerge in studies of later-emerging social cognitive abilities. For example, children around 4 years of age develop a ToM, or show the ability to differentiate their own mind/perspective from that of another (a sort of 'understanding that'). Apparently, not long after, children also develop the ability not only to attribute thoughts and feelings to others, but also to mislabel or misread thoughts and feelings of others (showing a '[mis]understanding what'). However, the capacity to mentalize and the accuracy of the mentalizing are typically studied as separate phenomena. Whether it is profitable for these paradigms to be brought together is unclear. For example, 'understanding that' forms of social cognition may be normal developmental processes with merely transient individual differences, in which case the role of behavioural genetic research will be limited. On the other hand, 'understanding what' forms of social cognition may be more profitably researched from an individual differences perspective, which is more amenable to behaviour genetic models and hypotheses.

In this regard, it is noteworthy that there is growing evidence that individual differences in social cognition subserving behavioural/emotional problems may be evident in very young children. One of the better pieces of evidence suggesting this comes from a careful detailed study of 5-year-olds by Murray *et al.* (2001). They reported that higher rates of spontaneously expressed negative cognitions during an experimentally manipulated card game with a friend were observed in children whose mothers were or had been depressed. In that study, negative social cognitions were defined as hopelessness or low self-worth. Particularly intriguing was the observation that differences between the children of depressed and non-depressed mothers were seen only when the children were losing in the card game, suggesting that cognitive distortions do not operate in a trait-like manner, even in 5-year-olds.

Other studies similarly imply that even early emerging social cognitive biases may be formed from the early rearing environment (see Chapters 10 and 11, this volume). For example, compared with securely attached children, 3-year-olds with an insecure attachment relationship were more likely to recall negative emotions in a recall test paradigm (Belsky *et al.* 1996). Problems in social cognition may also be found in understanding emotions and how they influence feelings and behaviour in the self and others (Denham *et al.* 1994; Cutting and Dunn 1999;). For example, one study of children aged between 2 and 6 1/2 years found that insecurely attached children showed poorer understanding of negative emotions than securely attached children (Laible and Thompson 1998). In other words, insecurely attached children had more difficulty in explaining or making sense of negative emotions.

Finally, as also pointed out in Chapter 1 of this volume, we note that one of the obstacles to researching the aetiology of social cognition, both genetic and non-genetic, is the variability with which the term has been defined. This is obvious when social cognition is considered an umbrella construct incorporating many different skills with differing developmental trajectories. However, problems in definition and development are seen even when one specific skill is considered. Indeed, in the case of joint attention, some researchers have suggested evidence as early as 2 months (Scaife and Bruner 1975), whereas others suggest 6 months (Butterworth and Jarrett 1991), and yet others suggest 12–13 months (Carpenter *et al.* 1998). There are perhaps understandable reasons behind these discrepancies, attributable to both varying methodologies and a different threshold for interpreting joint attention.

Nevertheless, if the phenotype is variously defined, then behavioural genetic methods will offer little clarity on aetiology.

In this chapter we have sought to collate findings on a newly emerging area of research—social cognition and genetics. What has resulted is a sort of a bricolage built from an admixture of findings on diverse models of social cognition that do not relate to one another in an obvious way. Perhaps the only strong conclusion that can be made is that the research base is too limited to make strong statements about the aetiology of social cognition. Nonetheless, the argument for devising programmatic research into social cognition using behavioural genetics methods and hypotheses is strong, and there are indeed important hypotheses that require the input of behavioural genetics methods.

References

Abramson, L.Y., Seligman, M.E., and Teasdale, J.D. (1978). Learned helplessness in humans: critique and reformulation. *Journal of Abnormal Psychology*, **87**, 49–74.

Alloy, L.B., Abramson, L.Y., Tashman, N.A., et al. (2001). Developmental origins of cognitive vulnerability to depression: parenting, cognitive, and inferential feedback styles of the parents of individuals at high and low cognitive risk for depression. *Cognitive Therapy and Research*, **25**, 397–423.

Anderson, K.E., Lytton, H., and Romney, D.M. (1986). Mothers' interactions with normal and conduct disordered boys. Who affects whom? *Developmental Psychology*, **22**, 604–9.

Bakermans-Kranenburg, M.J. and van Ijzendoorn, M.H. (2004). No association of the dopamine D4 receptor (DRD4) and −521 C/T promoter polymorphisms with infant attachment disorganization. *Attachment and Human Development*, **6**, 211–18.

Bakermans-Kranenburg, M.J. and van Ijzendoorn, M.H. (2006). Gene–environment interaction of the dopamine D4 receptor (DRD4) and observed maternal insensitivity predicting externalizing behavior in preschoolers. *Developmental Psychobiology*, **48**, 406–9.

Barlow, D.H. (1988). *Anxiety and its disorders: the nature and treatment of panic and anxiety*. New York: Guilford Press.

Baron-Cohen, S. and Hammer, J. (1997). Parents of children with Asperger syndrome. What is the cognitive phenotype? *Journal of Cognitive Neuroscience*, **9**, 548–54.

Barrett, P.M., Rapee, R.M., Dadds, M.M., and Ryan, S.M. (1996). Family enhancement of cognitive style in anxious and aggressive children. *Journal of Abnormal Child Psychology*, **24**, 187–203.

Bell, R.Q. and Harper, L.V. (1977). *Child effects on adults*. Lincoln, NB: University of Nebraska Press.

Belsky, J., Spritz, B., and Crnic, K. (1996). Infant attachment security and affective-cognitive information processing at age 3. *Psychological Science*, **7**, 111–14.

Blonigen, D.M., Hicks, B.M., Krueger, R.F., Patrick, C.J., and Iacono, W.G. (2005). Psychopathic personality traits: heritability and genetic overlap with internalizing and externalizing psychopathology. *Psychological Medicine*, **35**, 637–48.

Bohman, M. (1996). Predisposition to criminality: Swedish adoption studies in retrospect. In *Genetics of criminal and antisocial behavior* (ed. G.R. Bock and J.A. Goode), pp. 99–114. Chichester: John Wiley.

Bokhorst, C.L., Bakermans-Kranenburg, M.J., Fearon, R.M., *et al.* (2003). The importance of shared environment in mother-infant attachment security: a behavioral genetic study. *Child Development*, 74, 1769–82.

Brewin, C.R., Andrews, B., and Furnham, A. (1996). Intergenerational links and positive self-cognitions: parental correlates of optimism, learned resourcefulness, and self-evaluation. *Cognitive Therapy and Research*, 20, 247–63.

Butterworth, G.E. and Jarrett, N.L. (1991). What minds have in common is space: spatial mechanisms for perspective-taking in infancy. *British Journal of Developmental Psychology*, 9, 55–72.

Cadoret, R.J., Yates, W.R., Troughton, E., Woodworth, G., and Stewart, M.A. (1995). Genetic-environmental interaction in the genesis of aggressivity and conduct disorders. *Archives of General Psychiatry*, 52, 916–24.

Carpenter, M., Nagell, K., and Tomasello, M. (1998). Social cognition, joint attention, and communicative competence from 9 to 15 months of age. *Monographs of the Society for Research in Child Development*, 63, 1–143.

Caspi, A., McClay, J., Moffitt, T.E., *et al.* (2002). Role of genotype in the cycle of violence in maltreated children. *Science*, 297, 851–4.

Cleveland, H.H., Wiebe, R.P., van den Oord, E.J., and Rowe, D.C. (2000). Behavior problems among children from different family structures: the influence of genetic self-selection. *Child Development*, 71, 733–51.

Cobham, V.E., Dadds, M.M., and Spence, S.H. (1999). Anxious children and their parents. What do they expect? *Journal of Clinical Child Psychology*, 28, 220–31.

Creswell, C. and O'Connor, T.G. (2006). 'Anxious cognitions' in children: an exploration of associations and mediators. *British Journal of Developmental Psychology*, 24, 761–6.

Creswell, C., Schniering, C.A., and Rapee, R.M. (2005). Threat interpretation in anxious children and their mothers: comparison with nonclinical children and the effects of treatment. *Behaviour Research and Therapy*, 43, 1375–81.

Creswell, C., O'Connor, T.G., and Brewin, C.R. (2006). A longitudinal investigation of maternal and child anxious cognitions. *Cognitive Therapy and Research*, 30, 135–47.

Cronk, N.J., Slutske, W.S., Madden, P.A., Bucholz, K.K., Reich, W., and Heath, A.C. (2002). Emotional and behavioral problems among female twins: an evaluation of the equal environments assumption. *Journal of the American Academy of Child and Adolescent Psychiatry*, 41, 829–37.

Cutting, A.L. and Dunn, J. (1999). Theory of mind, emotion understanding, language, and family background: individual differences and interrelations. *Child Development*, 70, 853–65.

Deater-Deckard, K., Dunn, J., O'Connor, T.G., Davies, L., Golding, J., and the ALSPAC Study Team (2002). Using the step-family genetic design to examine gene–environment processes in family functioning. *Marriage and Family Review*, 33, 131–56.

DeFries, J. and Fulker, D.W. (1988). Multiple regression analysis of twin data: etiology of deviant scores versus individual differences. *Acta Geneticae Medicae et Gemellologiae: Twin Research*, 37, 205–16.

Denham, S.A., Zoller, D., and Couchoud, E.A. (1994). Socialisation of preschoolers emotion understanding. *Developmental Psychology*, **30**, 928–36.

Dodge, K.A. (1986). A social information processing model of social competence in children. In *Minnesota Symposium on Child Psychology*, Vol. 18 (ed. M. Perlmutter), pp. 75–127. Hillsdale, NJ: Lawrence Erlbaum.

Dorris, L., Espie, C.A., Knott, F., and Salt, J. (2004). Mind-reading difficulties in the siblings of people with Asperger's syndrome: evidence for a genetic influence in the abnormal development of a specific cognitive domain. *Journal of Child Psychology and Psychiatry*, **45**, 412–18.

Dozier, M., Stovall, K.C., Albus, K.E., and Bates, B. (2001). Attachment for infants in foster care: the role of caregiver state of mind. *Child Development*, **72**, 1467–77.

Duyme, M., Dumaret, A.C., and Tomkiewicz, T.C. (1999). How can we boost IQs of 'dull children'? A late adoption study. *Proceedings of the National Academy of Sciences of the USA*, **96**, 8790–4.

Emde, R.N., Plomin, R., Robinson, J., *et al.* (1992). Temperament, emotion, and cognition at fourteen months: the MacArthur Longitudinal Twin Study. *Child Development*, **63**, 1437–55.

Fonagy, P. and Bateman, A.W. (2006). Mechanisms of change in mentalization-based treatment of BPD. *Journal of Clinical Psychology*, **62**, 411–30.

Fonagy, P. and Target, M. (1997). Attachment and reflective function: their role in self-organization. *Development and Psychopathology*, **9**, 679–700.

Fonagy, P., Redfern, S., and Charman, T. (1997). The relationship between belief-desire reasoning and a projective measure of attachment security (SAT). *British Journal of Developmental Psychology*, **15**, 51–61.

Garber, J. and Flynn, C. (2001). Predictors of depressive cognitions in young adolescents. *Cognitive Therapy and Research*, **25**, 353–76.

Ge, X., Conger, R.D., Cadoret, R.J., *et al.* (1996). The developmental interface between nature and nurture: a mutual influence model of child antisocial behavior and parent behaviors. *Developmental Psychology*, **32**, 574–89.

Gergely, G., Nadasdy, Z., Csibra, G., and Biro, S. (1995). Taking the intentional stance at 12 months of age. *Cognition*, **56**, 165–93.

Goldsmith, H.H., Lemery, K.S., Buss, K.A., and Campos, J. (1999). Genetic analyses of focal aspects of infant temperament. *Developmental Psychology*, **35**, 972–85.

Hughes, C. and Cutting, A.L. (1999). Nature, nurture, and individual differences in early understanding of mind. *Psychological Science*, **10**, 429–32.

Hughes, C., Jaffee, S.R., Happé F., Taylor, A., Caspi, A., and Moffitt, T.E. (2005). Origins of individual differences in theory of mind: from nature to nurture? *Child Development*, **76**, 356–70.

Humfress, H., O'Connor, T.G., Slaughter, J., Target, M., and Fonagy, P. (2002). General and relationship-specific models of social cognition: explaining the overlap and discrepancies. *Journal of Child Psychology and Psychiatry*, **43**, 873–83.

Iervolino, A., Pike, A., Manke, B., Reiss, D., Hetherington, E.M., and Plomin, R. (2002). Genetic and environmental influences in adolescent peer socialization: evidence from two genetically sensitive designs. *Child Development*, **73**, 162–74.

Kendler, K.S. and Eaves, L.J. (1986). Models for the joint effect of genotype and environment on liability to psychiatric illness. *American Journal of Psychiatry*, **143**, 279–89.

Kendler, K.S., Kessler, R.C., Walters, E.E., et al. (1995). Stressful life events, genetic liability, and onset of an episode of major depression in women. *American Journal of Psychiatry*, 152, 833–42.

Kirsch, P., Esslinger, C., Chen, Q., et al. (2005). Oxytocin modulates neural circuitry for social cognition and fear in humans. *Journal of Neuroscience*, 25, 11489–93.

Laible, D.J. and Thompson, R.A. (1998). Attachment and emotional understanding in preschool children. *Developmental Psychology*, 34, 1038–45.

Lakatos, K., Toth, I., Nemoda, Z., Ney, K., Sasvari-Szekely, M., and Gervai, J. (2000). Dopamine D4 receptor (DRD4) gene polymorphism is associated with attachment disorganization in infants. *Molecular Psychiatry*, 5, 633–7.

Larsson, H., Andershed, H., and Lichtenstein, P. (2006). A genetic factor explains most of the variation in the psychopathic personality. *Journal of Abnormal Psychology*, 115, 221–30.

Lau, J.Y., Rijsdijk, F., and Eley, T.C. (2006). I think, therefore I am. A twin study of attributional style in adolescents. *Journal of Child Psychology and Psychiatry*, 47, 696–703.

McGue, M., Sharma, A., and Benson, P. (1996). The effect of common rearing on adolescent adjustment: evidence from a U.S. adoption cohort. *Developmental Psychology*, 32, 604–13.

Meins, E., Fernyhough, C., Wainwright, R., Das, G.M., Fradley, E., and Tuckey, M. (2002). Maternal mind-mindedness and attachment security as predictors of theory of mind understanding. *Child Development*, 73, 1715–26.

Murray, L., Woolgar, M., Cooper, P., and Hipwell, A. (2001). Cognitive vulnerability to depression in 5-year-old children of depressed mothers. *Journal of Child Psychology and Psychiatry*, 42, 891–9.

Nichols, K., Gergely, G., and Fonagy, P. (2001). Experimental protocols for investigating relationships among mother-infant interaction, affect regulation, physiological markers of stress responsiveness, and attachment. *Bulletin of the Menninger Clinic*, 65, 371–9.

Moffitt, T.E. (2005). The new look of behavioral genetics in developmental psychopathology: gene–environment interplay in antisocial behaviors. *Psychological Bulletin*, 131, 533–54.

O'Connor, T.G. and Croft, C.M. (2001). A twin study of attachment in pre-school children. *Child Development*, 72, 1501–11.

O'Connor, T.G., Hetherington, E.M., Reiss, D., and Plomin, R. (1995). A twin-sibling study of observed parent–adolescent interactions. *Child Development*, 66, 812–29.

O'Connor, T.G., Deater-Deckard, K., Fulker D.W., Rutter, M., and Plomin, R. (1998). Genotype–environment correlations in late childhood and early adolescence: antisocial behavioral problems and coercive parenting. *Developmental Psychology*, 34, 970–81.

O'Connor, T.G., Jenkins, J.M., Hewitt, J., DeFries, J.C., and Plomin, R. (2001). Longitudinal connections between parenting and peer relationships in adoptive and biological families. *Marriage and Family Review*, 33, 251–71.

O'Connor, T.G., Caspi, A., DeFries, J.C., and Plomin, R. (2003). Genotype–environment interactions in children's adjustment to parental separation. *Journal of Child Psychology and Psychiatry*, 44, 849–56.

Ozonoff, S., Rogers, S.J., Farnham, J.M., and Pennington, B.F. (1993). Can standard measures identify subclinical markers of autism? *Journal of Autism and Developmental Disorders*, 23, 429–41.

Partridge, T. (2005). Are genetically informed designs genetically informative? Comment on McGue, Elkins, Walden, and Iacono (2005) and quantitative behavioral genetics. *Developmental Psychology*, **41**, 985–8.

Plomin, R. (1994). *Genetics and experience*. Newbury Park, CA: Sage.

Plomin, R. and Crabbe, J. (2000). DNA. *Psychological Bulletin*, **126**, 806–28.

Plomin, R., DeFries, J.C., and Loehlin, J.C. (1977). Genotype–enviroment interaction and correlation in the analysis of human behavior. *Psychological Bulletin*, **84**, 309–22.

Plomin, R., DeFries, J.C., Craig, I.W., and McGuffin, P. (2003). *Behavioral genetics in the postgenomic era*. Washington, DC: American Psychological Association.

Reiss, D., Neiderhiser, J.M., Hetherington, E.M., and Plomin, R. (2000). *The relationship code: deciphering genetic and social influences on adolescent development*. Cambridge, MA: Harvard University Press.

Rutter, M., Silberg, J., O'Connor, T., and Simonoff, E. (1999). Genetics and child psychiatry. I: Advances in quantitative and molecular genetics. *Journal of Child Psychology and Psychiatry*, **40**, 3–18.

Saudino, K.J. and Eaton, W.O. (1991). Infant temperament and genetics: an objective twin study of motor activity level. *Child Development*, **65**, 1167–74

Scaife, M. and Bruner, J.S. (1975). The capacity for joint visual attention in the infant. *Nature*, **253**, 265–6.

Schulman, P., Keith, D., and Seligman, M.E. (1993). Is optimism heritable? A study of twins. *Behavior Research and Therapy*, **31**, 569–74.

Scott, S., Spender, Q., Doolan, M., Jacobs, B., and Aspland, H. (2001). Multicentre controlled trial of parenting groups for child antisocial behaviour in clinical practice. *British Medical Journal*, **323**, 194–8.

Seligman, M.E.P, Peterson, C., Kaslow, N.J., Tanenbaum, R.L., Alloy, L.B., and Abramson, L.Y. (1984). Attributional style and depressive symptoms among children. *Journal of Abnormal Psychology*, **93**, 235–8.

Shaked, M., Gamliel, I., and Yirmiya, N. (2006). Theory of mind abilities in young siblings of children with autism. *Autism*, **10**, 173–87.

Sharp, C., Fonagy, P., and Goodyer, I.M. (2006). Imagining your child's mind: psychosocial adjustment and mothers' ability to predict their children's attributional response styles. *British Journal of Developmental Psychology*, **24**, 197–214.

Spinath, F.M., Ronald, A., Harlaar, N., Price, T., and Plomin, R. (2003). Phenotypic 'g' early in life: on the etiology of general cognitive ability in a large population sample of twin children aged 2 to 4 years. *Intelligence*, **31**, 195–210.

Stark, K.D., Schmidt, K.L., and Joiner, T.E. (1996). Cognitive triad: relationship to depressive symptoms, parents' cognitive triad, and perceived parental messages. *Journal of Abnormal Child Psychology*, **24**, 615–31.

Stoolmiller, M. (1998). Correcting estimates of shared environmental variance for range restriction in adoption studies using a truncated multivariate normal model. *Behavior Genetics*, **28**, 429–41.

Tienari, P., Wynne, L.C., Sorri, A., et al. (2004). Genotype–environment interaction in schizophrenia-spectrum disorder: long-term follow-up study of Finnish adoptees. *British Journal of Psychiatry*, **184**, 216–22.

Tomasello, M. and Carpenter, M. (2007). Shared intentionality. *Developmental Science*, **10**, 121–5.

Turk, E. and Bry, B.H. (1992). Adolescents' and parents' explanatory styles and parents' causal explanations about their adolescents. *Cognitive Therapy and Research*, **16**, 349–57.

Turner, S.M., Beidel, D.C., Roberson-Nay, R., and Tervo, K. (2003). Parenting behaviors in parents with anxiety disorders. *Behaviour Research and Therapy*, **41**, 541–54.

Viding, E., Blair, J.R., Moffitt, T.E., and Plomin, R. (2005). Evidence for substantial genetic risk for psychopathy in 7-year-olds. *Journal of Child Psychology and Psychiatry*, **46**, 592–7.

Vogeley, K., Bussfeld, P., Newen, A., *et al.* (2004). Mind reading: neural mechanisms of theory of mind and self-perspective. *NeuroImage*, **14**, 170–81.

Vollm, B.A., Taylor, A.N., Richardson, P., *et al.* (2006). Neuronal correlates of theory of mind and empathy: a functional magnetic resonance imaging study in a nonverbal task. *NeuroImage*, **29**, 90–8.

Walden, B., McGue, M., Iacono, W.G., Burt, S.A., and Elkins, I. (2004). Identifying shared environmental contributions to early substance use: the respective roles of peers and parents. *Journal of Abnormal Psychology*, **113**, 440–50.

Wu, S., Jia, M., Ruan, Y., *et al.* (2005). Positive association of the oxytocin receptor gene (OXTR) with autism in the Chinese Han population. *Biological Psychiatry*, **58**, 74–7.

Yirmiya, N., Gamliel, I., Pilowsky, T., Feldman, R., Baron-Cohen, S., and Sigman, M. (2006). The development of siblings of children with autism at 4 and 14 months: social engagement, communication, and cognition. *Journal of Child Psychology and Psychiatry*, **47**, 511–23.

Zahn-Waxler, C., Robinson, J., and Emde, R.N. (1992). The development of empathy in twins. *Developmental Psychology*, **28**, 1038–47.

14

Treatment outcome of childhood disorders: the perspective of social cognition

Peter Fonagy and Carla Sharp

14.1 Introduction

It is beyond the scope of a final chapter to review the entire body of literature on the outcome of treatments for childhood disorders in relation to issues of social cognition. The review presented here will necessarily be selective and, as ever, will focus on areas where the literature is at its most comprehensive and implications as well as issues of contention are clearest. Comprehensive reviews of the outcome of psychosocial treatments with children's disorders are available (Fonagy *et al.* 2002; Kazdin 2004; Target and Fonagy 2005; Weisz *et al.* 2005).

We have also decided to use this chapter to provide a preliminary summary and integration of some of the ideas concerned with the causation of psychological disorders that have been reviewed in this book. We feel comfortable in suggesting that treatment outcomes should be reviewed concurrently with a general consideration of the role of social cognition in a range of childhood disorders. A number of influential reviewers of the psychosocial treatment outcomes literature, especially Kazdin (2000, 2003, 2004), have insisted that concerted efforts should be made to bring knowledge concerning treatment processes into alignment with what is known about disease mechanisms in the case of all mental disorders, an aim that is probably most realistic in the case of the distortion of developmental processes in childhood disorders. This orientation lies at the heart of the developmental psychopathology approach (Cicchetti and Cohen 2006), to which all the contributors to this volume subscribe.

Social cognition deficits represent one such disease mechanism and it is possible to review much of what is known about psychosocial treatment outcomes in relation to the findings and models elucidating social cognition that have been presented in this volume. Following a brief introduction to the current status of evidence-based psychosocial treatments, this chapter will be divided into five sections. Each section corresponds to one of five different contexts in which problems of social cognition may be seen to contribute to creating childhood mental disorders: (1) lacking the ability to represent other minds (as in childhood autism or psychopathy); (2) overactivation and distorted use of mentalization (as in schizophrenia); (3) context-specific inhibition or decoupling of social cognitive capacities, such as the failure to mentalize in emotionally highly charged intimate interpersonal relationships and situations (as in borderline personality disorder); (4) dysfunctional mentalization processes resulting in distorted representations of the other's or self's mind states (as in anxiety and depression); (5) a failure of natural protection (resilience) normally provided by mentalization (as in disruptive behavior disorder). The first two of these headings correspond to research on conditions where the capacity for social cognition was the central question ('understanding that'). The fourth heading pertains to accuracy of mentalizing ('understanding what'), which must be defined by content rather than capacity. O'Connor and Creswell (Chapter 13) helpfully suggest that an individual differences paradigm may be more appropriate for 'understanding what' questions rather than 'understanding that' questions, because the latter tend to reflect transient differences in development rather than stable characteristics. The third and fifth groups are intermediate categories. The third concerns the interaction of 'what' and 'that'. In other words, are there contexts (defined by content) within which mentalizing capacity is more or less available? The final heading concerns the implications of individual differences in mentalization for the interpretation of the social context, a promising but not yet thoroughly elaborated field.

Obviously this categorization is idealistic rather than realistic and aims to be heuristic rather than systematizing. However, to some degree the developmental themes and disorders that have been reviewed in this volume do fit under one or more of these headings. As the treatment literature is also organized in terms of diagnostic categories, we have attempted to summarize some of the key theoretical claims of contributors to this volume at the same time as exploring the treatment literature in relation to these ideas.

14.2 **Evidence-based psychological therapy**

Our approach to reviewing psychosocial treatments will adopt a strictly evidence-based perspective. No one can doubt the massive progress that the field of child psychotherapy has made over the last 15 years in adopting some of the principles of evidence-based medicine (Evidence-Based Medicine Group 1992, Sackett *et al.* 2000, Strauss *et al.* 2005). Evidence-based medicine

(EBM) prevents reliance on rhetoric and removes the implicit assumption of authority from decision-making, requiring the professional to provide a reasoned argument for treatment choices. Before the shift towards EBM, doctors rarely researched the problems of individual patients. In sharp contrast with law practices, most doctors' offices did not have libraries. The intent behind EBM is to promote decision-making based on increased certainty in place of intuition and unsystematic clinical experience by generating data that strengthen the clinician's grasp of cause and effect relationships (enabling them to be confident that it is the specified therapy that leads to the change in status of the patient rather than extraneous uncontrolled factors). The clinician's main tool is the 'hierarchy of evidence' based essentially on the design of studies rather than on the quality of effort that went into their implementation (Miles *et al.* 2006). The balance of 'heart' and 'brain' in general medical care as well as in the application of psychosocial treatments has shifted from 'big heart–small brain' to an approach that combines intellectual rigour with compassion in equal measure.

In considering the current status of EBM we have to acknowledge that it has brought about radical positive change in almost all fields of health care where it has been applied: The approach has been influential in delivering the appropriate biological treatments in child psychiatry, for example in governing prescription patterns in the use of antidepressants for adolescent depression (Boylan *et al.* 2007). The meta-analysis by Bridge *et al.* (2007) demonstrated that fluoxetine and sertraline were relatively effective selective serotonin-reuptake inhibitors (SSRIs) for childhood and adolescent depression, but paroxetine, citalopram, venlafaxine, and nefazodone were not. Other studies which monitor prescription patterns are able to map prescribing to the evidence base and identify pertinent deviations between the two (e.g. Clavenna *et al.* 2007) and provide appropriate correction. No one is under any illusion that consistency with evidence provides a 'guarantee of quality'. As Goldenberg (2006) pointed out: 'While evidence-based approaches can improve de rigueur medical practice, "evidence-based" should not be understood to be synonymous with "best practice" in all relevant respects'.

14.3 Lacking the ability to represent other minds

The clearest case for considering the developmental psychopathology of social cognition comes from conditions where a comprehensive incapacity generates a total absence of concern with minds or some aspect of minds. Historically, a clinical concern with mentalization originated from consideration of such conditions at the MRC Developmental Psychology Unit at University College London (Baron *et al.*1985; Leslie 1987; Frith *et al.* 1991; Blair 1995). While our understanding of these deficits has become more sophisticated in the intervening years, the general approach identifying a 'deep deficit of social cognition' in autism and psychopathy has not altered.

14.3.1 Model of autism and autism spectrum disorders

Baron-Cohen and colleagues (Chapter 2) aim to describe the clinical phenomenon of an individual with a profoundly limited capacity for social cognition. Baron-Cohen's account of autistic spectrum disorders suggests a highly modularized structure where two modules, the theory of mind module (ToMM) and the empathy module (TESS), are respectively responsible for two categories of mental contents representations, M- and E-representations respectively. M-representations have the form of agent-attitude propositions (e.g. 'Mother believes that Johnny took the cookie') and E-representations are self-affect-state propositions (e.g. 'I feel sorry that Mum feels sad about the news in the letter'). It is particularly important to note that Baron-Cohen believes E-state propositions to be constrained in the direction of empathy, i.e. that representation of emotion in the other is always consistent with that of the self. There is something inherently wrong with the proposition 'I feel happy that you are in pain'. The module or processing system that generates E-representations is constrained by the experiences that the self can generate in relation to the presumed state in the other.

Individuals with autism spectrum conditions are assumed to have difficulties in recognizing more complex emotional and mental states. The problems in generating these representations may arise from difficulty in attending to the right cues, failure in integrating them, or under-connectivity of brain areas. Baron-Cohen and colleagues (Chapter 2) review a series of potential causes. One possible explanation may be an excess of synaptogenesis or a failure of synaptic pruning. Abnormalities in functioning and structure have been observed in social brain areas, at least in the amygdala and the orbital and medial-frontal cortex. The cause is assumed to be genetic, and it is as yet unclear to what extent early remedial intervention might reverse the cascade of developmental distortions which the disorder entails. However, the well-established heuristic of fractionation of theory of mind and emotion understanding provides a comprehensive description of autistic spectrum conditions.

14.3.2 Model of psychopathy

Blair and Baron-Cohen both suggest a partial deficit of representation of mental states in their accounts of psychopathy. Baron-Cohen suggests that self-affective state propositions are selectively absent in psychopathy, i.e. psychopaths have a relatively intact ToM but a dysfunctional empathizing system. Similarly, Blair makes a case for a dysfunction of emotional empathy where empathy is a translation of the communication of an emotional state by the observer. The responses of the amygdala provide reinforcement information in emotional learning. In this way Blair's model expands on that of Baron-Cohen. The absence of a representation of fearfulness, sadness, or pain deprives the individual with psychopathy of a component of a motivational system which may be crucial in the acquisition of moral reasoning.

A further property of the system proposed by Blair is a dual subcortical and cortical pathway to the amygdala, allowing for coarse-grained rapid stimulus-reinforcement learning alongside more fine-grained stimulus-encoding which mediates discrimination learning. Moral socialization occurs because most humans are predisposed to find distress of conspecifics aversive. Moral transgressions cause distress, and if the empathic experience of this distress is aversive, the transgression will be avoided. Thus the failure to represent self-affective propositions or the more immediate subcortical affective reactions (which are probably non-propositional) undermines the possibility of appropriate moral socialization in individuals with psychopathic tendencies.

As with autism, the analysis of psychopathy centres on genetic causation. Environmental factors such as abuse or exposure to violence do not lead to psychopathy, and neither does incompetent parenting. Socio-economic status and low IQ may be associated with psychopathy because both these factors restrict the range of prosocial strategies which give the individual access to social rewards.

14.3.3 Interventions with autism and psychopathy

Behavioural treatments have been shown to reduce some of the secondary problems associated with autism, but social and communicative abnormalities have proved more resistant to intervention (Anderson *et al.* 1987; Howlin and Rutter 1987; Lovaas 1987). In order to have an impact, interventions probably need to be intensive (e.g. offering a behavioural programme both at home and at school) and to involve both parents and teachers (Anderson *et al.* 1987; McEachin *et al.* 1993; Eikeseth *et al.* 2002). In at least some studies there is evidence of gains in IQ, improvements in daily living skills, communication, and the ability to socialize, and a decrease of behaviour problems. Studies have tended to focus on children under the age of 4 years at the time of commencing treatment, but it is unclear whether early commencement of treatment is a necessary condition for success.

Despite a variety of approaches there is no good evidence that individual social skills training significantly benefits autistic individuals. Lord and Rutter (1994) review school programmes which aim to encourage satisfactory vocational behaviours, such as task completion and self-management (e.g. Mesibov 1986; Dunlap et al. 1987). They conclude that these individuals respond best to a well-structured environment where the individual needs of each child are considered (Harris et al. 1990). For example, several case studies (Matson et al. 1990, 1993; Ingenmey and Van Houten 1991) have reported that spontaneous verbalizations can be increased using either time-delay or visual cue prompting (Charlop-Christy et al. 2002). Despite the fact that a number of studies have examined variants of social skills training, there is little evidence that this approach significantly benefits autistic individuals beyond the environment in which training takes place (Campbell et al. 1996; Matson and Swiezy 1994).

A potentially promising line of studies is exploring interventions related to specific deficits of social cognition assumed to underpin many other behavioural dysfunctions, including difficulty in engaging in a teaching–learning process. Trials have tried to teach social understanding rather than social skills (Howlin et al. 1999). Most promising results are reported to follow using a social understanding task which was broken down into a sequence of small steps, beginning with simpler skills that are learnt earlier in normal development. A series of studies (Hadwin et al. 1996, 1997) demonstrated that children with autism could be taught to understand emotions, belief, and pretence. A randomized controlled trial (RCT), designed to explore the effects of a computer-based method of training emotion recognition and prediction, established that autistic adolescents could improve on tasks calling for these abilities (Silver and Oakes 2001). However, no evidence was provided that these gains were carried over into real-life situations.

An innovative study investigated the value of behavioural training methods in teaching 'joint attention', a social capacity thought to be both developmentally fundamental and completely lacking in autistic children (Whalen and Schreibman 2003). There were substantial individual differences in the rate of acquisition of behaviours, but four of the five showed improvement in joint attention initiations and three in supported joint attention. However, the study also reported significant loss of gains from post-treatment to follow-up, suggesting that parents were not able to maintain these behaviours and that parent-training programmes might be a helpful addition. A conceptually linked study of parent training (Drew et al. 2002) focused on the development of joint attention skills and joint action routines. Young autistic children (mean age 23 months) were randomly assigned to either parent training or treatment as usual. Although at 1 year follow-up there were indications that language development was faster in the parent training group, this was based on parent report, which may have been biased.

Strategies for intervention with autistic children based on social cognitive models are in their infancy. A number of trials are currently attempting to explore improved understanding of specific components of the social cognitive deficits in order to build alternative neural-behavioural strategies which can compensate for cognitive processing limitations. The increased prevalence of autism spectrum disorders makes the development of effective strategies a priority. The promise of social cognition research for the effective treatment of autism spectrum disorders is yet to be realized.

The treatment implications of Blair's model of psychopathy (Chapter 7) are disheartening, but clear. Cognitive interventions will not be effective because there is no deficit in the mediation of M-representations. The deficit in E-representations is associated with dysfunctions of the amygdala and will need to be addressed in the light of the limitations imposed on moral development by the lack of feedback in relation to the emotional experience of others. Interventions will have to build on systems that function rather than those that do not respond in normal ways. Punishment will not affect behaviour. The only way out of antisocial behaviour associated with psychopathy will be reward. Admittedly, it is hard to find positive social reinforcers, gained legitimately, that will ever compare with those that can be achieved by selectively ignoring social convention and causing distress to others. This is the challenge to clinicians arising from improved understanding of this condition.

14.4 Overactivation and distorted use of social cognition

14.4.1 Model of schizophrenia

This book has not dealt with social cognition in psychosis (few such studies exist for child samples), but since interventions based on social cognitive deficits in schizophrenia are a very important part of the clinical implications of these psychological data for young people we shall summarize the core ideas here. A highly influential and persuasive line of thought has linked the presence of paranoid and delusional ideation to psychotic pathology, particularly schizophrenia (Frith 1992; Brune and Bodenstein 2005; Harrington *et al.* 2005). Frith argues that delusions of persecution and reference arise when the individual concerned knows that people have mental states that cannot be directly viewed but makes invalid attempts at inferring them. Delusions of reference may come about because actions are mislabelled as having intentions behind them, whilst persecutory delusions could arise because whilst the intentions behind people's actions appear opaque, an inference of a conspiracy is drawn from the experience of inaccessibility.

In all these cases both agent-attitude propositions and, to a lesser degree, self-affective state propositions are generated without adequate assessment of their relevance and accuracy, leading to incorrect judgments about others' intentions. Patients with schizophrenia appear to be significantly impaired in both cognitive and affective empathy compared with healthy control subjects (e.g. Shamay-Tsoory *et al.* 2007). The deficits are present in young people with first-episode psychosis (Bertrand *et al.* 2007). Corcoran *et al.* (1995) suggested that patients with negative symptoms and/or incoherence would be most impaired in theory of mind tasks because of their inability to represent mental states of others as well as themselves. Paranoid patients are assumed to have difficulty in monitoring other people's intentions, while patients in remission and those with passivity symptoms are expected to have normal mentalizing capacities (e.g. Pickup and Frith 2001).

In a meta-analysis of 32 studies, Sprong *et al.* (2007) reported a weighted mean effect size of −1.25 (95% CI −1.44, −1.07). In this meta-analysis the disorganised subgroup appeared to perform worse, closely followed by the paranoid symptoms group. Even patients in remission show a mentalization impairment with an effect size of −0.7. Reviewers of this literature suggest that, as with childhood autism, mentalizing deficit is a general impairment. The mentalizing deficit of patients in remission suggests that this is a trait rather than a state deficit (e.g. Herold *et al.* 2002). The trait argument is further supported by observations of mentalization deficit in individuals with genetic risk for schizophrenia (Wykes *et al.* 2001; Irani *et al.* 2006; Marjoram *et al.* 2006). A particularly interesting study of genetically high-risk children who would later develop schizophrenia spectrum disorders showed that these children had lower scores on role-taking tasks (Schiffman *et al.* 2004). A particularly pertinent study by Pickup (2006) showed that schizotypal traits analogous to positive symptoms of schizophrenia predicted poor mentalizing performance.

14.4.2 Interventions with schizophrenia

Social cognition has become a target of intervention research in schizophrenia (Couture *et al.* 2006), particularly since social cognition has a stronger relationship with functional outcome in schizophrenia than neuropsychological measures of cognitive deficits (Brune 2005; Pinkham and Penn 2006) and social skills training has very limited effect (Roth and Fonagy 2005). A number of studies have explored the impact of training in single aspects of social cognition such as emotion perception or theory of mind (Penn and Combs 2000;

Frommann *et al.* 2003; Silver *et al.* 2004; Wolwer *et al.* 2005; Choi and Kwon 2006; Kayser *et al.* 2006; Russell *et al.* 2006). These trials show promise, although generalization beyond the treatment context has not been demonstrated. One reported study (Combs *et al.* 2007) addressed three key aspects of social cognition in schizophrenia (emotion perception, attributional style, and theory of mind). Social Cognition and Interaction Training (SCIT) (D.L. Roberts, D.L. Penn, and D. Combs, unpublished) has been tested in an open trial where it was compared with coping skills training in 28 patients. Individuals who received SCIT improved in all social cognitive domains, reported better social relationships, and exhibited fewer aggressive behaviours on the ward. All the measures used in this trial were highly reactive. This small study suggests that social cognitive impairments can and should be directly addressed in treatment programmes, even if the extent to which this might generalize to wider symptomatic improvements is not yet known. Large-scale trials in this important area are sorely needed.

14.5 Context-specific facilitation and inhibition of social cognition

14.5.1 Models of developmental influence

Is it possible to arrive at a state where either agent-attitude propositions or self-affective state propositions are poorly represented, but only some of the time? This is a somewhat controversial issue and not all contributors to this volume appear to be of one mind. Sharp and Fonagy, in their chapter on personality disorder (Chapter 10), and Gergely and Unoka (Chapter 11), in their contribution on the developmental origins, advance a model that has the context specificity of social cognition at its core. Gergely and Unoka assume that the building of representation for mental states is not simply a maturational given but rather depends on necessary environmental input conditions in infancy. Emotional states are initially non-conscious stimulus-controlled procedural derivatives of an innate constitutional self. Representation-building and attention-socialization mechanisms work to establish cognitively accessible second-order representations of internal states. Early affective attachment interactions, including the caregiver's teaching stance towards the child and marked contingent interactions with her, serve to transfer relevant cultural knowledge about shared emotion categories. Gergely and Unoka suggest that whilst understanding other minds may indeed be a constitutional given, introspective mentalizing about one's own affective mental states and anticipated emotion-induced actions is fostered in the context of the attachment relationship. They argue that affect regulation critically depends on the extension of the innate ability to mentalize the other. Emotional self-regulation is then achieved through the anticipation and adaptive modification of emotion-induced action tendencies.

This developmental model is to a certain point consistent with O'Connor and Creswell's summary of the behaviour genetics literature (Chapter 13). They emphasize that studies showing modest or no shared environment effects say nothing about how effective psychosocial interventions are likely to be because the research design of genetic and randomized controlled studies are different and incommensurable. There are significant parent–child resemblances for distinct categories of anxious cognitions, including attribution style and dysfunctional attitudes (e.g. Murray *et al.* 2007). Similarities in patterns of social cognition may be genetically or socially mediated, or both. O'Connor and Creswell discuss the value of intervention designs in showing that treating the mother's anxiety, for example, reduces the child's threat interpretations (Creswell *et al.* 2005), suggesting that even if the link is genetic, it is environmentally mediated. On balance the behaviour genetic studies reviewed by O'Connor and Creswell suggest low genetic loading for theory of mind performance but high loading for attributional style and empathic concern, and a mixture of results for the complex set of capacities that might be reflected in quality of child peer relationships. Clearly, the lack of clear genetic influence, at least on the capacity for mentalization ('understanding that'), leaves room for exploration of contextual factors which might influence the development of that capacity or its use across settings and contexts.

Sharp and Fonagy (Chapter 10) extend the model of context-dependent mentalization to both other and self, and to both agent-attitude and self-affective state propositions. In their model of emergent personality disorder, early attachment experience as well as later trauma play central roles. Although in no way diminishing the importance of genetic influence, both these models are somewhat at variance with the modular frameworks suggested by Baron-Cohen and Blair. de Rosnay and colleagues (Chapter 12) also raise the question of what aspects of the child's early environment may be hypothesized to generate superior emotional understanding. In their cognitive model, linguistic competence and conversational interaction are the key drivers of precocious emotional understanding. Children treated as independent psychological agents within a family and those who have better psychological insight are, for example, more likely to negotiate conflict in ways that minimize the opportunity for aggression and are able to maintain amicable friendship relations. What we see in these instances is a virtuous cycle of social growth. It seems that emotion understanding plays a role in keeping a child out of conflict, which in turn creates an environment more conducive to the development of social cognition. Mind-minded socialization practices lead to a fuller elaboration of psychological understanding, which in turn provides the child with resources that enable them to respond appropriately to complex social interactions.

The impact of positive context is more evident than the detrimental effect of negative experience on social cognition. Sharp and Fonagy (Chapter 10) and de Rosnay and colleagues (Chapter 12) offer slightly different appraisals of this literature. Emotion understanding is likely to be delayed, but at least for de Rosnay and colleagues (Chapter 12) no specific patterns emerge. Sharp and Fonagy are more impressed by findings which suggest that maltreatment and trauma cause elevated limbic outflow, which has the potential to disrupt cognitive processes that normally recruit prefrontal cortical areas (Cicchetti and Curtis 2005). In relation to theory of mind or agent-attitude propositions, de Rosnay and colleagues express considerable scepticism about the evidence base for delay in theory of mind acquisition associated with maltreatment. Following a comprehensive review of studies of maltreatment in childhood, they assert that effects were negligible once verbal IQ was appropriately controlled for. Sharp and Fonagy are more persuaded by the processing bias that many studies report in relation to maltreated children, particularly the increased reactions to anger and hostility. Further, studies of older children, including those who experienced maltreatment in adolescence, appear to offer some evidence of theory of mind deficit, at least as measured by the Reading the Mind in the Eyes test (Baron-Cohen et al. 2001; Dorris et al. 2004). The suggestion that when children are engaged in causally coherent psychological discourse the development of social cognition will benefit is generally accepted. This general explanation encompasses findings concerning the beneficial effects of mind-mindedness or reflective function of the primary caregiver, conversational interactions, the quality of attachment relationship, the beneficial effects of play, and more generally the emotional climate of the family (for a comprehensive review of this literature, see Sharp and Fonagy (in press)).

14.5.2 Interventions with maltreatment

The proposition that the development of social cognition depends on family atmosphere and parent–child relationship has important treatment implications, in particular for indicating a way to address parent–child relations where there is early maltreatment. To illustrate, the work of the Mount Hope Family Center shows how the demonstration of a relationship-specific social cognitive deficit can lead to the formulation of a treatment protocol. There was evidence from the work of Toth and her colleagues that maltreated children have relationship-specific deficits in social cognition. In a study of 80 maltreated preschoolers, Macfie et al. (1999) showed clear limitations in the representation of social cognition in a story stem completion task, where the story stem called for the relief of distress principally from the mother. In a further study (Macfie et al. 2001), maltreated children, especially physically or sexually abused children, were shown to manifest more dissociation as measured by a coding system for the MacArthur Story Stem Narratives. Maltreated children showed disruptions of identity and incoherence of parental representations, which may be seen as indicators of a failure of mentalizing or meta-cognitive capacities. A more detailed report (Toth et al. 2000) points to an important developmental perspective in that the capacity for social cognition, particularly the complexity of the representation of the parent in conflict-imbued settings, decreased with development while the children's representation of themselves became increasingly simplified and exaggerated.

A randomized controlled intervention study where preschooler parent psychotherapy was offered to 23 maltreating families was reported by Toth et al. (2002). This 12-month intervention aimed at elaborating and modifying the relationship between parents and child by linking current maternal conceptualization of relationships to the mother's childhood caregiving response. Social cognitive measures of outcome favoured this group, in contrast with psychoeducational home visitation or treatment as usual, in a range of domains including degree of maladaptiveness of maternal representation and the quality of self and mother–child relationship representation. An impressive large-scale replication of this study was reported recently by Toth et al. (2006). Mothers who had experienced depression since their child's birth were recruited ($n = 130$) and randomized to toddler–parent psychotherapy (DI) or a control group (DC). Higher rates of insecure attachment relative to a normal control group were present in both the DI and the DC groups at baseline. Post-intervention, at age 36 months, insecure attachment continued to predominate in the DC group. In contrast, the rate of secure attachment had increased substantially in the DI group and was higher than that for the normal controls. A similar dyadic narrative-oriented therapeutic approach has been demonstrated to be effective for toddlers of depressed mothers (Cicchetti et al. 1999, 2000; Toth et al. 2006) and maltreating families with insecurely attached children (Cicchetti et al. 2006). In all, recent work from the Mount Hope Family Center is consistent with the assumption of profound impairment of social cognition associated with maltreatment. It also reinforces the potential for reducing this impairment through a relationship-focused intervention which takes the aspect of the relationship that may impede social cognitive development as a focus.

14.5.3 Interventions with borderline personality disorder

The theoretical model of emerging borderline personality disorder advanced by Sharp and Fonagy (Chapter 10) assumes that contextual influences are powerful for both the development and the performance of social cognition. Reduced to its essentials, they suggest that individuals whose early experiences left them with a less robustly established set of social cognitive capacities (for example, as described by Gergely and Unoka in Chapter 11) may be less resilient in the face of trauma and may be more likely to respond to that trauma by a functional decoupling of mentalizing capacities. They further suggest that emotional arousal, particularly the activation of the attachment system, may be specifically potent in undermining social cognition. The clinical implications of this model for psychological therapy are of course profound in that generic psychotherapy is unlikely to be helpful for these individuals, as the absence of an adequate capacity to mentalize will undermine their ability to make use of an initiative to improve their self-understanding, or indeed their understanding of others, at either a cognitive or an emotional level. Similarly, the deficit in social cognition will not be apparent under most circumstances, unlike with schizophrenia, autism spectrum conditions, or psychopathy, but will emerge only when emotional arousal or the activation of attachment feelings undermine mentalization. On the basis of a brief review of what is a largely adult literature, we argue that, to be effective, treatment has to focus on enhancing mentalization in the context of attachment relationships.

The treatment outcome literature is consistent with this proposition. Although there are no trials focused on adolescent emerging borderline personality disorder, trials on young adults suggest that short-term cognitive treatments appear to be marginally effective, ineffective, or frankly iatrogenic with this group of patients (Tyrer *et al.* 2004). In this large study ($n = 480$) brief manual-assisted cognitive therapy slightly increased the likelihood of self-harm relative to treatment as usual with PD patients and in BPD it increased the costs associated with ongoing treatment (Tyrer *et al.* 2004). In a more recent randomized controlled trial of borderline personality disorder with longer treatment (up to 30 sessions) from therapists trained in advance, there was significant benefit on suicidal behaviour ($n = 104$), but a non-significant increase in emergency presentations in those allocated to cognitive behaviour therapy (Davidson *et al.* 2006a,b).

In contrast, a number of relatively long-term treatments are highly efficacious. The widespread adoption of dialectical behaviour therapy (DBT) (Linehan 1993) is a tribute not just to the first RCT with BPD women ever reported (Linehan et al. 1991, 1993) but also to the energy and charisma of its founder, Marsha Linehan, and to the attractiveness of the treatment, with its combination of acceptance and change, skills training, excellent manualization, and a climate of opinion that is willing and able to embrace this multifaceted approach (Swenson 2000). A recent replication of the original study with very similar findings gives further support to its effectiveness (Linehan et al. 2006). In this replication, treatment as usual was performed by therapists who were thought to be experts in their practice of non-DBT therapy, and despite their level of expertise, the results of this study duplicate the results of the 1991 study quite closely. It is not clear which are the active elements of DBT (individual psychotherapy, skills training, phone consultation, therapist consultation team) (Lynch et al. 2006). Two process studies investigated the process of change in DBT by focusing on the possible influence of validation (Shearin and Linehan 1992; Linehan and Heard 1993; Linehan et al. 2002), but the results are inconclusive. What we know thus far is that adding a DBT skills training group to ongoing outpatient individual non-DBT psychotherapy does not seem to enhance treatment outcomes. Given that DBT is described as primarily a skills training approach (Koerner and Linehan 1992), this finding might indicate that the central skills training component of DBT may not be of primary importance. It is possible to argue that a key aspect of DBT lies in the capacity of this multifaceted treatment to enhance social cognitive capacities, particularly those relating to the reduction of impulsivity and the improvement of affect regulation (Fonagy and Bateman 2006).

More recently, investigations have shown that patients with BPD respond to a range of therapies including schema-focused therapy (Giesen-Bloo et al. 2006), transference-focused psychotherapy (Clarkin et al. 2007), and mentalization-based treatment (Bateman and Fonagy 1999, 2001). In addition, non-randomized studies have claimed effectiveness for cognitive analytical therapy (Ryle and Golynkina 2000), group psychotherapy (Wilberg et al. 1998), and therapeutic community-based treatments (Lees et al. 1999). It may be argued that a therapeutic approach with these individuals will be effective to the extent that they are able to enhance their capacity to mentalize, but this may be achieved by a wide variety of therapeutic strategies, not necessarily an approach directly focused on social cognition (Allen et al. 2008). This common factor approach may be increasingly important as psychosocial treatment trialists and reviewers try to make sense of the increasingly complex pattern of outcome studies becoming available from multisite studies around the world.

14.6 Reality-distorting dysfunctional mentalization processes

Distorted representation of mind states in self and others appears to be a core feature of most of the disorders considered in this volume. Clearly, dysfunctional mentalization processes are responsible for profound distortions of the representation of mind states in schizophrenia and in borderline personality disorder. However, in the case of three of the most important disorders—depression, anxiety, and conduct problems—the distortion in representation of mental states (what Sharp (2000) and Sharp et al. (2007) refer to as 'distorted' or 'biased mentalizing') has been a primary focus of enquiry as well as, in some instances, the primary target of interventions. In the case of psychosis, borderline personality disorder, autism, or even psychopathy, it is not specific categories or themes of cognitions but the dysfunctional mechanisms which give rise to these that are considered as central for interventions related to social cognition. By contrast, in the case of depression, particular styles of social cognitive thought have been a focus of both aetiological models and interventions, whilst with anxiety disorders the particular situations and social cognitions associated with these have been the focus of inquiry. In the case of conduct problems attributional biases in social information processing models have dominated both the treatment and the intervention literature. Mize and Pettit (Chapter 6) have helpfully outlined the six steps of social information processing (encoding or selective attention, interpretation or attribution, the identification of goals, accessing response or response construction, response decision, and response enactment) with knowledge schemas influencing all these. Studies in this context have primarily concerned themselves with the 'understanding what' question (O'Connor and Creswell, Chapter 13) of the accuracy of social cognition.

14.6.1 Childhood and adolescent depression

Psychosocial treatment of depression

Assuming that a focus on social cognition forms an integral part of cognitive behavioural therapy (CBT) for depression, it would follow that most work on social cognition is probably reported in relation to childhood depression. Therefore it is perhaps fitting to start with a brief review of CBT treatment effectiveness studies in relation to youth depression. A useful meta-analysis of childhood and adolescent psychotherapy treatment trials was reported by

Weisz et al. (2006b). They identified 35 trials performed between 1980 and 2004, and reported an average weighted mean effect size (ES) of 0.34 (95% CI: 0.21, 0.47). This effect size is significantly smaller (about half) than those observed in earlier meta-analyses (Reinecke et al. 1998; Michael and Crowley 2002) and in studies of other childhood and adolescent conditions treated psychotherapeutically (Weisz et al. 2005). For 20 studies the control group received no treatment (ES: 0.41) while in 15 studies there was active treatment (ES: 0.24). The significantly lower mean ES for the latter studies is largely accounted for by the fact that cases were clinically referred. There was a correlation between the follow-up time lag and ES ($R = -0.50$; 95% CI: 0.06, 0.78) indicating that follow-up of more than 6 months suggested small, if any, treatment effects. Neither gender nor age appeared to be associated with outcome. Group and individual studies had similar outcomes and treatment duration was also unrelated to effect size.

Turning to the different types of treatments evaluated in these studies, three types of treatment have been most commonly tested. The most extensively tested approach is Lewinsohn's Coping With Depression course for adolescents which directly addresses socio-cognitive deficits, attempting to treat depression by addressing cognitive, behavioural, and affective skills deficits. Young people are instructed on how emotions and cognitions interact to produce actions in interpersonal contexts. They also learn to identify social stimuli and activities that elevate their mood, identify unrealistic negative thoughts, and learn to interrupt these to defend themselves from being stuck in unproductive ruminations. CBT appears to be effective, whether provided individually or in a group (Lewinsohn et al. 1994, 1996; Kroll et al. 1996; Wood et al. 1996; Brent et al. 1998; Clarke et al. 1999). Providing longer courses of CBT (or booster sessions) in cases of non-response to a standard length of treatment improved recovery and reduced relapse (Kroll et al. 1996; Clarke et al. 1999).

Recent studies have confirmed that referred depressed adolescents are more difficult to treat successfully than recruited cases, even when severity is comparable (Brent et al. 1999; Birmaher et al. 2000). In a trial of CBT including 96 depressed adolescents (Lewinsohn et al. 1994, 1996) best results were found for those with less severe symptoms and better initial adaptation. When compared with pill placebo administered to a clinical sample of adolescent cases, CBT was initially found to be slightly less effective than placebo, although in combination with medication it produced greater reduction than medication alone, with the added benefit of moderating the increased suicidality associated with fluoxetine (March et al. 2004, 2006; Glass 2005; Emslie et al. 2006;). Results after 36 weeks have shown CBT to 'catch up' with medication and in combination with medication to continue to be helpful in limiting the increase in suicidality associated with SSRIs (March *et al.* 2007). However, the limited effectiveness of CBT relative to fluoxetine in a moderately to severely depressed group of adolescents was confirmed in a large UK multi-centre study which contrasted fluoxetine alone and a fluoxetine plus CBT condition (Goodyer *et al.* 2007). Adolescents who received CBT in addition to fluoxetine did no better on any indicator, including suicidality, than those who received fluoxetine alone. The differences between CBT and control conditions have been observed to effectively disappear at follow-up (Wood *et al.* 1996; Brent *et al.* 1999; Birmaher *et al.* 2000). Family factors such as maternal depression and family discord can apparently reduce treatment response to CBT (e.g. Brent *et al.* 1998).

An alternative evidence-based approach to the psychotherapeutic treatment of depression is interpersonal therapy for adolescents (IPT-A) (Moreau *et al.* 1991; Mufson *et al.* 1994). IPT-A is based on the assumption that an improved understanding of the interpersonal context of the individual and assistance in the negotiation of that context will assist recovery from depression. There is always a focus (or a maximum of two foci) to the therapeutic work such as loss, role disputes, interpersonal deficits, role transitions, etc. The therapy begins with psychoeducation linking the symptoms of depression to interpersonal processes in the adolescent's mind, followed by the creation of an inventory of the youth's interactions with important others, identifying gratifying and frustrating/unsatisfactory aspects. The contract for the treatment identifies key problematic areas to be worked on over the course of the treatment, during which the adolescent monitors his/her symptoms, links affect to interpersonal events, explores conflicts and ways of communicating, and uses a range of strategies to experiment with alternative ways of managing things. The end of treatment includes an attempt to equip the young person to anticipate and rehearse strategies in relation to future stressors. Two small early clinical RCTs have been reported (Mufson *et al.* 1999; Rosselló and Bernal 1999). The Mufson trial included 48 referred adolescents with major depressive disorder (MDD), of whom 32 completed the protocol. The majority of dropouts came from the control condition, which was 'clinical monitoring'. An intent-to-treat analysis showed that 75 per cent of patients assigned to IPT-A recovered, as judged by Hamilton Rating Scale scores, compared with 46 per cent of those in the control group. This compares with 80 per cent recovery rate at 36 weeks following CBT (March *et al.* 2007).

A more direct comparison of IPT and CBT was provided by Rosselló and Bernal (1999) who studied 71 Puerto Rican adolescents meeting criteria for MDD. The study showed that while both IPT and CBT reduced depressive symptoms (Children's Depression Inventory and Child Behavior Checklist), IPT was more effective in improving self-esteem (Piers–Harris Children's Self-Concept Scale) and social adaptation (Social Adjustment Scale for Children and Adolescents) (Rosselló and Bernal 1999). This study was the first to compare IPT and CBT, but needs to be replicated with other cultural groups since the treatments were manualized to be specifically appropriate to Puerto Rican society. Santor and Kusumakar (2001) reported a controlled study comparing 12 weeks of IPT with sertraline in the treatment of 49 moderately to severely impaired adolescents with MDD. The 25 IPT cases were compared with 24 who had previously been treated using sertraline in an open trial. Outcomes were compared on the Beck Depression Inventory, the Children's Global Assessment Scale, and an index of clinical recovery. Both treatments led to significant improvement, but IPT was superior across all three measures. A more recent trial (Mufson et al. 2004) was performed a school-based health clinic and compared IPT-A with treatment as usual (TAU) in a 16-week randomized clinical trial. Adolescents who met DSM-IV criteria and were randomly assigned to IPT-A ($n = 34$) showed greater symptom reduction and improvement in overall functioning than those receiving TAU ($n = 29$) on the Hamilton Depression Rating Scale and a range of social functioning measures including the Clinical Global Impressions scale.

Perhaps somewhat surprisingly, several studies have found that relaxation training alone produces significant relief from depression (Reynolds and Coats 1986; Kahn et al. 1990). In this intervention youths learn to tense and relax muscle groups progressively until they feel calm and relaxed. They also learn to use relaxation as a coping strategy when facing sudden stressful situations.

Although there is ample evidence of the importance of the family context and parental psychological problems in relation to child and adolescent depression (for a clear description see Asarnow et al. (2001)), there is little evidence of the effectiveness of family therapy for depression. One study without a no-treatment control condition reported substantial remission in moderate to severe depression in a relatively young sample following a relatively long course (26 weeks) of systemic family therapy (Trowell et al. 2007). Family therapy or parent work in parallel with individual treatment for the child has been included as a comparison condition in four RCTs (e.g. Brent et al. 1997), and has generally been found to be of less benefit than the experimental condition. However, Brent et al. (1997) employed systemic-behavioural family therapy as a control condition, and found that this form of family therapy was beneficial, especially in cases where the mother was perceived to be controlling. Recently an RCT conducted by Diamond et al. (2002) evaluated the impact of 'attachment-based family therapy' in comparison with waiting list. Family therapy was associated with significantly greater reduction in depression scores on the Beck Depression Inventory and the Hamilton Rating Scale for Depression, and with greater likelihood of remission by the end of treatment. This new model of therapy deserves further evaluation in comparison with active treatments.

Childhood depression from a social cognitive perspective

Kyte and Goodyer (Chapter 8) have reviewed the literature on social cognition in adolescence. In outlining social information processing (SIP) theory, they have demonstrated deficits and distortions in social information processing in depressed youths at most stages of SIP—attending, encoding, interpreting, retrieval, and response evaluation. The empirical data, admittedly mostly from adult subjects, strongly supports the idea of distorted knowledge structures (stable negative self-schema) biasing information processing in the direction of negative explanations or interpretations (Gotlib *et al.* 2004a). Selective focus on or attention to negative content has been demonstrated for adults (Gotlib *et al.* 2004b; Koster *et al.* 2005) although not so reliably in young people (Neshat-Doost *et al.* 2000; Kyte *et al.* 2005). There is ample evidence for the presence of negative attributional style in depressed youths (e.g. Voelz *et al.* 2003). In addition, we know that response style (the retrieval of effective responses) is impaired, leading to frequent chronic rumination which in turn engenders depressed mood (e.g. Nolen-Hoeksema 2000; Park *et al.* 2004). We have seen that brooding-type rumination is associated with a range of difficulties in social cognition, including over-general autobiographical memories and deficits in interpersonal problem-solving. The evidence points to a general failure of the memory system which, nevertheless, may be amenable to modification (Watkins *et al.* 2000). Emotional avoidance, deliberately redirecting attention from depressive thoughts, provides an immediate escape but undermines the possibility of arriving at alternative constructions (Watkins and Teasdale 2004). In terms of response evaluations, adolescents appear to make decisions which produce desired outcomes but allocate inappropriately large resources to unfavourable outcomes (Kyte *et al.* 2005). Deficits in social decision-making account for the apparent impulsivity but may also be related to the propensity to see social situations as uncontrollable.

Kyte and Goodyer (Chapter 8) speculate that the maturation of brain structures underpinning social cognition 'come on stream' only in adolescence, and it is for this reason that abnormalities of social cognition which arguably underpin depression do not become apparent until adolescence. They offer the intriguing suggestion that abnormalities associated with normal and pathological emotional states are mood state dependent while other abnormalities such as those linked to orbital and medial prefrontal cortex functions are anatomical (Drevets 2000) and would be expected to persist following recovery. This might explain some aspects of the complex pattern of results which have emerged from studying adult patients' social cognitions after recovery (e.g. Evans *et al.* 2005). In their sophisticated aetiological model, Kyte and Goodyer see a genetically linked deficit in social cognition mediated via limbic and prefrontal structures as generating susceptibility to specific types of environmental experiences including adversity, attachment history, parenting style, peer relationships, etc. These linked aetiological factors generate the distorted knowledge structures, processing impairments and depressogenic behavioural responses which produce depression as a clinical phenomenon.

Implications of the social cognitive perspective for treatment

The coherent statement of aetiology and mediating function which arises from SIP theories of depression suggests that a close connection should exist between SIP and treatment process and outcome. As we have seen, for the most part interventions with adolescents have been strongly influenced by the literature on social cognition, and most interventions that have been evaluated aim to address one or other aspect of the sophisticated and strongly evidence-based SIP model outlined by Kyte and Goodyer. However, if we turn to the outcomes literature we see a more complex picture emerging. While CBT has been shown to be effective in treating depression in both clinical and non-clinical contexts, ESs associated with CBT trials have been variable. Some meta-analyses have indicated powerful effects associated with CBT (Lewinsohn and Clarke 1999; Michael and Crowley 2002), yet meta-analyses have not succeeded in demonstrating that treatments involving an emphasis on change in social cognition were any more effective than treatments that were non-cognitive. In the meta-analysis performed by Weisz *et al.* (2006a) cognitive treatments had an ES of 0.35 whereas non-cognitive treatments had an ES of 0.47. Whilst the observed slight superiority of non-cognitive treatments in reducing young people's depression scores is not significant, one might expect that directly addressing the psychological processes that underpinned a pathology would generate greater and more frequent changes than a treatment such as relaxation which does not obviously involve SIP. Further, and contrary to expectations based on the theory underpinning SIP, it is not more effective in cases where there are greater cognitive distortions, and its benefits are apparently not explained by a reduction in such cognitions (Lewinsohn *et al.* 1990; Brent *et al.* 1998).

How does this affect our understanding of the implications of social cognitive models for the treatment of adolescent depression? In the adult literature the superiority of CBT to alternative treatments is somewhat better established (Roth and Fonagy 2005). However, even in this literature simple links between changes in SIP and depressive symptoms associated with treatment are notoriously elusive. Before concluding that the treatment literature does not bear out the emphasis on social cognition advocated by all the authors in this volume, we should consider a number of alternative explanations for the observed pattern of outcomes. First, many of the trials contributing to the small effect size are relatively recent. In fact plotting effect sizes of trials against date of publication in this field reveals a substantial downward trend ($R = 0.53$) (see Figure 14.1). In the late 1990s much attention was given to the challenges of generalizing from RCTs of psychosocial treatments because RCTs mirrored real life so poorly (Hoagwood *et al.* 1995; Lambert and Ogless 2004). For example, Weisz *et al.* (2006a), reviewing the entire child psychotherapy outcomes literature of 236 studies, found that only 13 per cent of study samples were clinically referred, only 19 per cent of studies employed at least one practising clinician, and in only 4 per cent of studies was treatment provided in an actual service setting separate from the research. Combining these indicators we find that only 1 per cent of studies included at least one practising clinician, clinically referred children, and some treatment carried out in a service setting.

It is also possible that CBT differs less from other treatments in its focus than might at first appear and that in fact all treatments in the final analysis may turn out to work with social cognition (Allen *et al.* 2008).

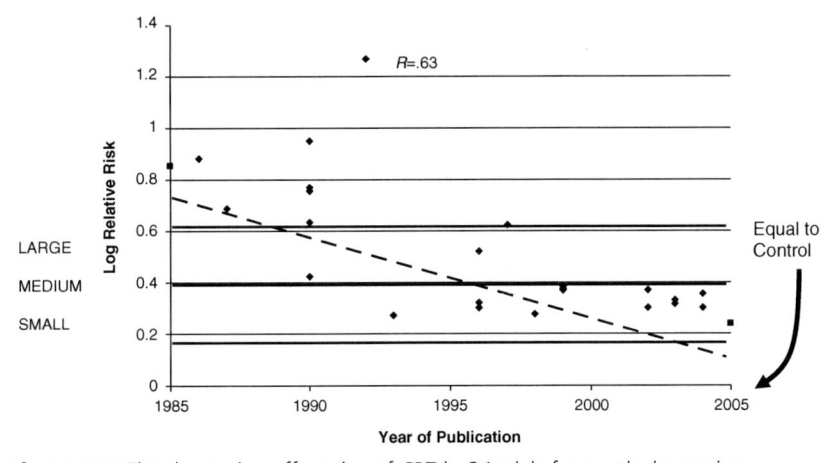

Figure 14.1 The decreasing effect size of CBT in 24 trials for youth depression.

An analysis of the components of evidence-based treatments of adolescent depression suggested that this indeed may be the case (McCarty and Weisz 2007). All therapies aim to promote competency and nearly all involve self-monitoring (89 per cent) and addressing relationship skills (89 per cent). Two-thirds include communication training (67 per cent), psychoeducation (67 per cent), some form of problem-solving training (67 per cent) and cognitive restructuring (67 per cent) as part of the treatment protocol. Even apparently specialized interventions, such as improving parent–child relationships or relaxation, are shared by nearly half the trialled approaches (44 per cent). It could be argued that IPT-A involves a large proportion of social-cognition-oriented interventions. For example, helping adolescents to understand the nature of their interactions with others would inevitably entail a meta-cognitive review of social information processing strategies. Equally, linking changes in intensity of symptomatology to interpersonal events will help to address distortions in attribution as well as biases in attention. In the adult literature there is evidence that suggests that the more IPT resembles a CBT approach, the more effective it is (Ablon and Jones 2002). However, the argument that all therapies of adolescent depression fundamentally aim at social cognition falters in the face of the evidence in relation to the effectiveness of relaxation as a therapy for depression. It should also be made clear that this argument is separate from one we shall discuss later which might attribute the mediation of non-specific common factors across all therapies to changes in social cognition.

A third possible explanation for the relative limitations of psychosocial interventions specifically focused on social cognition may build on the case for age specificity of depression outlined by Kyte and Goodyer in Chapter 8. There has been considerable excitement in the literature concerning the late maturation of the brain, a spurt in the creation of synaptic connections and their subsequent pruning, specifically linked with adolescence (Giedd *et al.* 1999; Thompson *et al.* 2000). There are both behavioural and fMRI indications that this reorganization is real and specific to adolescence (Blakemore and Choudhury 2006). For example, the development of social perspective-taking appears to undergo a kind of perturbation during puberty in parallel with the discontinuous processes of brain maturation (Choudhury *et al.* 2006). The capacity to decide whether words match emotion expression, which implies both working memory and decision-making, declines in speed and accuracy with onset of puberty by about 10–20 per cent (McGivern *et al.* 2002). Adolescents also take longer to make judgements about risk (Baird *et al.* 2005). Brain reorganization is suggested by the developmental shift in the pattern of recruitment of brain areas by this task. Adults show greater activation of insula and right fusiform face area compared with adolescents during thinking about 'not good ideas', while adolescents show greater activation of the dorsolateral prefrontal cortex. Responses to risky scenarios may be efficient in adults because they are driven by mental images of possible outcomes and visceral response to those images in line with the somatic marker hypothesis (Damasio 1999). These results have to be placed side by side with indications that amygdala activation in response to pictures of faces expressing emotion is significantly greater in adolescents than adults (Monk *et al.* 2003).

The implication here is that the very same brain changes specific to adolescents which might make them vulnerable to depression after the onset of puberty might also in some way make it harder for them to engage in the kind of therapeutic relationship which CBT requires. For example, the study by Monk *et al.* (2003) showed that when attention was drawn away from the emotional content of the face towards specific non-emotion-related features ('How afraid does it make you feel' versus 'How wide is the nose') part of the orbitofrontal cortex was activated in adults but not in adolescents. These areas where selective engagement and disengagement were detected to the same stimuli under differing attentional demands in a population of healthy young adults may be crucial to implementing a comprehensive CBT programme. They may be functioning less than efficiently in adolescents, particularly in those with a problem of moderate to severe major depression. This differential pattern of activation was not evident in adolescents whose activation patterns did not vary by attentional condition. This difference probably reflects maturation within the cognitive-regulatory node of the Social Information Processing Network (Monk *et al.* 2003)—a maturation that could be a prerequisite of directly addressing social cognitions in these individuals.

14.6.2 **Anxiety and related conditions**

Psychosocial treatment of anxiety

The methods and rationale of behavioural treatments for childhood anxiety are fully described by King and Ollendick (King and Ollendick 1997; Ollendick and King 1998), who also give a clear and comprehensive overview of studies of the cognitive behavioural treatment of childhood phobias. The effectiveness of these treatments has been reviewed by Target and Fonagy (2005a) and a meta-analysis based on a systematic review is also available (Cartwright-Hatton *et al.* 2004). There have been 22 RCTs using behavioural or cognitive behavioural techniques to treat young people with anxiety disorders prior to 2004. Three different treatment approaches are particularly strongly supported by evidence. One of these is **modelling**, an approach which was designed to disrupt the self-sustaining cycle where avoidance is employed to obtain relief from the aversive arousal generated by anxious thoughts about the feared object. Observing a model who violates the assumptions of fear (e.g. by holding the spider) generates emulation, teaching the child that adverse consequences do not follow. Participation with the model appears to be required as only this ensures that observation is accompanied by exposure in the company of a confident partner (Ollendick and King 1998). Modelling normally starts at low intensity and increases incrementally in terms of distance and/or duration. A second well-established approach is **reinforced exposure** where taking steps towards the feared object is rewarded. Here the consequences of the behaviour are altered (Ollendick and King 1998), so that the intervention is a carefully sculpted contingency management intervention using praise or concrete incentives as rewards (Muris et al. 1998). Exposure has been assumed to be a central aspect of the efficacy of CBT, but two well-designed studies of the treatment of school phobia found that therapeutic support without exposure was equally effective (Last et al. 1998; Silverman et al. 1999).

The most complex and frequently evaluated treatment implementations address multi-symptom disorders using **multi-component CBT**. Examples are the Coping Cat programme (Kendall et al. 1990) and the Transfer of Control approach (Silverman and Kurtines 1996). These complex implementations include psychoeducation concerning the nature of anxiety, learning behavioural strategies for coping with anxious feelings, and devising behavioural plans to meet anxious feelings (e.g. STOP: recognize being **S**cared, identify anxious **T**houghts, refute them with **O**ther more realistic ideas, and **P**raise yourself). They are designed to address the more complex disorders such as generalized anxiety disorder, separation anxiety, and social phobia of childhood. Children work with the therapist to identify and rank the feared situation (Albano et al. 1995). Family anxiety management programmes take a similar approach to address youth anxiety disorders through sessions with the parent and child together and then separate sessions with the parents as a couple (Barrett et al. 1996). Anxiety symptoms associated with sexual trauma have been addressed similarly with both individual (child-focused) and mother-focused (mother as therapist) strategies (Deblinger and Lippman 1996; Deblinger et al. 1999).

Ten trials have compared CBT with no treatment. Four of these were conducted by one research group (Barrett et al. 1996; Dadds et al. 1997; Barrett 1998; Flannery-Schroeder and Kendall 2000; Shortt et al. 2001) and three by another (Kendall 1994; Kendall et al. 1997; Flannery-Schroeder and Kendall 2000). Children randomized to receive CBT had a 56.5 per cent chance of remission of their anxiety (225/398), compared with a 34.8 per cent chance of remission (73/210) in the wait list group. The odds of recovery in the treatment group relative to the controls was 3.27 (95% CI: 1.92, 5.55; $p < 0.001$). However, there is significant bias of these estimates from small studies ($n < 30$ per arm), with odds ratios dropping substantially when small n (unrepresentative) studies are excluded.

These results should not yet be taken to indicate that CBT is well established as a treatment for anxiety disorders, as the effectiveness of CBT compared with other available treatments is not yet known. Many of the studies use extensive exclusion criteria and recruit their participants from non-clinical settings. Only a handful of studies have compared CBT with another active treatment. Bernstein et al. (2000) found CBT plus imipramine to be significantly better than CBT plus placebo for anxiety-based school refusal in terms of school attendance, but not in terms of anxiety symptoms. Beidel et al. (2000) found CBT to be more effective at ameliorating social anxiety symptoms than an educational support intervention (study skills and an element of exposure). There is accumulating evidence that CBT for childhood anxiety disorders can be delivered in a group as successfully as in an individual format (Flannery-Schroeder and Kendall 2000; Manassis et al. 2002). A number of early trials have shown that CBT which includes a family component is more successful than CBT alone (e.g. Cobham et al. 1998; Mendlowitz et al. 1999; Shortt et al. 2001). In a small open trial of parent–child group CBT for preadolescent children with anxiety disorders (Toren et al. 2000), the children whose mothers met criteria for an anxiety disorder (half the sample) did better than those whose mothers were not anxious, even though the anxious mothers' own anxiety levels were not reduced during treatment. Adding a family component to CBT may well be beneficial for younger children (Creswell and Cartwright-Hatton 2007) or for families where parental anxiety is also high (Barrett et al. 1996; Howard and Kendall 1996; Cobham et al. 1998; Mendlowitz et al. 1999).

Modifying anxious cognitions and confronting phobic assumptions via exposure have also been applied to obsessive compulsive symptoms with the added component of response prevention which prevents the child from engaging in the compulsions that reduce obsession-triggered distress (Barrett et al. 2004). March et al. (2001) have described the rationale and effective elements of CBT for childhood obsessive–compulsive disorder (OCD) and summarized the outcome literature. Outcome studies suggest that OCD can be improved in some cases, although generally not eliminated, by a CBT approach (March 1995; March and Mulle 1995; March and Leonard 1996; March et al. 2001). This approach has so far mostly been evaluated with concurrent medication (e.g. Neziroglu et al. 2000), but there is some evidence that

CBT makes a distinctive contribution (DeVeaugh-Geiss et al. 1992; March et al. 1994). In practice, some patients will not comply with behavioural treatments, and parents claim that clinicians are inadequately trained in CBT procedures. From a practical stance it seems wise to maintain more than one psychosocial treatment approach to provide options in cases where the child or family does not comply. It is also important to ensure that treatment manuals and procedures are well adapted to children so that compliance is more likely.

There is limited evidence for the effectiveness of other modalities of intervention for anxiety problems (Target and Fonagy 2005). There is only very preliminary evidence that psychodynamic psychotherapy may be effective (Target and Fonagy 1994). In this chart review study, over 85 per cent of 299 children with anxiety and depressive disorders no longer suffered any diagnosable emotional disorder after an average of 2 years' treatment. Phobias ($n = 48$), separation anxiety disorders ($n = 58$) and overanxious disorder ($n = 145$) were resolved in around 86 per cent of cases. OCD was more resistant, ceasing to meet diagnostic criteria in only 70 per cent of cases. Children with severe or pervasive symptomatology, such as generalized anxiety disorder, or multiple comorbid disorders required more frequent therapy sessions, whereas more circumscribed symptoms, such as phobias (even if quite severe), improved comparably with once-weekly sessions. Muratori et al. (2001) examined the efficacy, among 58 children with depression and anxiety, of 11 sessions of psychodynamic therapy based on the parent–child model involving work with the parents for six of the 11 sessions contrasted with treatment as usual in the community. At 2-year follow-up only 34 per cent of the treated group were in the clinical range on symptomatic measures compared with 65 per cent of the controls. Unusually for trials of psychotherapy, treatment effects increased during the 2-year follow-up period (the so-called 'sleeper effect') (Muratori et al. 2003). A very small RCT ($n = 30$) of adolescents showed a surprisingly strong statistically significant benefit from 10 sessions of psychodynamic psychotherapy in a school setting in India. The vast majority of young people improved with psychodynamic psychotherapy (over 90 per cent; reported ES, 1.8) (Sinha and Kapur 1999).

No studies so far have examined the effectiveness of family therapy for childhood anxiety disorders. One recent study compared Brief Strategic Family Therapy (BSFT) with a routine community treatment, in which the results for adolescents with conduct disorder were compared with those for adolescents with anxiety disorders (Coatsworth et al. 2001). The results for the families with anxious youngsters were quite poor, although they engaged well with treatment, with few children making reliable improvements even if they stayed in treatment either in the BSFT condition or in the community clinic setting (23 per cent in both cases).

Anxiety from a social cognitive perspective

The findings of the social cognition literature in relation to anxiety were comprehensively summarized by Banerjee in Chapter 9. Social cognitive processes as depicted in cognitive theories of anxiety (Clark *et al.* 1994; Steer *et al.* 1994, 1995; Beck and Clark 1997) are distorted at all three stages of processing in anxious individuals: over-vigilant to threat in automatic registration, a constriction or narrowing of cognitive processing in preparing a response to threat, and a distorted evaluation of one's general capacities in relation to the threat. Thus social cognition in children with anxiety disorders is characterized by hyper-vigilance to threat, bias towards threatening and negative interpretation of social events, and negative appraisal of past encounters, including bias favouring recollections of negative (autobiographical) events. Banerjee (Chapter 9) summarizes evidence broadly consistent with all these expectations. The multistage model accounts well for finding both hyper-vigilance and avoidance in anxious individuals (Vassilopoulos 2005). However, the experimental effects are generally relatively small and could be related to general emotional distress and not specifically to anxiety. The studies of biased information processing do not include control groups of non-anxious equally distressed children (e.g. youths with depression without anxiety). As Banerjee points out, programmes such as Coping Cat were specifically designed to restructure or remediate automatic negative cognitions, biases in the interpretations of social events, and distortions of self-evaluations, while enhancing response strategies to improve problem-solving (Velting *et al.* 2004).

What aspect of social understanding is impaired in anxiety? It is not a general difficulty in understanding mental states, but rather a specific difficulty in understanding and effectively managing social situations involving multiple mental states and potential social evaluative threat. Indeed, there may be a deficit in anxious children in the performance of tasks requiring emotion understanding. Banerjee summarizes important evidence concerning the connections between mentalizing skills and social functioning. Concern about positive self-presentation is found to be associated with low responsiveness to preferences of the social partner and the combination of the two was found to predict social anxiety in a longitudinal study.

Implications of the social cognitive perspective for treatment

Does this mean that CBT is effective because it modifies social cognitions? A recent meta-analysis of 38 studies (Spielmans *et al.* 2007) demonstrated that while CBT interventions are undoubtedly more efficacious than non-bona fide psychotherapies in treating childhood anxiety (and depression), there is no evidence to suggest that they are more efficacious than other bona fide treatments.

Bona fide non-CBT treatments appear to be roughly equivalent in efficacy. Dismantling studies indicate that children receiving full CBT treatments derive no significant benefit relative to youngsters who receive only a component treatment (Spielmans *et al.* 2007). This report is consistent with findings in the adult psychotherapy outcomes literature (e.g. Ahn and Wampold 2001). When effect sizes are compared with a view to establishing subsets of therapies that produce homogenous effects it emerges that specific ingredients prescribed by various therapies for childhood anxiety do not relate to differing outcomes as long as the comparisons are restricted to bona fide therapies (Wampold 2001; Wampold *et al.* 2002). These appear to be nearly equivalent in efficacy (Spielmans *et al.* 2007). Thus the current corpus of comparison studies does not support specificity for the treatment elements unique to any intervention including CBT.

As noted by Banerjee (Chapter 9), findings concerning cognitive biases in anxious children are often inconsistent (Alfano *et al.* 2002) because cognitive processes considered pertinent to anxiety are poorly specified and are assessed by divergent methods. Assuming that the information processing bias is domain general in nature (Muris *et al.* 2000) may not be helpful from a treatment development standpoint. The deficit may *appear* to be generic but this does not mean that it is context independent, and its context dependence is critical in the context of achieving effective intervention. For example, if self-evaluation of performance is interactive with skill in socially anxious children (e.g. video-feedback worsens the self-evaluations of poorly performing socially anxious youngsters, Morgan and Banerjee 2006), addressing bias independent of performance is unlikely to be effective.

To summarize, it is clear that behavioural and cognitive behavioural approaches represent the first line of treatment for anxiety problems and that these interventions have been inspired by research on the social cognitive distortions of mental representations readily identified in this group. However, the connection between model and treatment protocol has been harder to establish than might have been expected. Again, as with depression, this does not cast doubt on the centrality of problems of social cognition to the anxiety. It is far more likely that social cognitive abnormalities create distorted expectations that trigger somatic responses which need to be addressed directly, principally by exposure and habituation (Marks 2002; Grandi *et al.* 2006; Mataix-Cols and Marks 2006).

14.6.3 Conduct problems in children

Psychosocial treatment of conduct problems

Parent management training is a highly effective intervention for young children with conduct problems. A meta-analysis of 37 trials (Dretzke *et al.* 2005) concluded that parent training programmes were both effective and potentially cost-effective therapy for children with conduct problems. The parent training model is based on the assumption that ODD and CD reflect parental difficulty in adequately reinforcing socially appropriate forms of conduct as well as a tendency to maintain inappropriate behaviour through coercive interactions (Patterson 1982; Miller and Prinz 1990; Kazdin 1995). Although programmes vary in terms of the exact syllabus and methods of delivery, in all programmes dyadic instruction is accompanied by other aids to learning, such as role playing, behavioural rehearsal, and structured homework exercises. Evidence that changing families' interaction patterns has the power to alter the child's behaviour is very strong (Forehand and Long 1988; Long *et al.* 1994; Nye *et al.* 1995; Webster-Stratton and Hammond 1997; Patterson and Chamberlain 1988; Schuhmann *et al.* 1998; Ducharme *et al.* 2000; Webster-Stratton and Reid 2003; Nixon *et al.* 2003). There is accumulating evidence that parent training programmes generally may be applied in a wide range of conduct problems and effectively delivered in various settings, including clinical populations (Cunningham *et al.* 1995; Bradley *et al.* 1999; Scott *et al.* 2001). The best evaluated programme (Webster-Stratton 1996b; Webster-Stratton and Reid 2003) comprises three complementary training curricula, known as the *Incredible Years Training Series*, targeted at parents, teachers, and children aged 2–8 years. There have been six controlled trials with children with ODD/CD at the University of Washington (Webster-Stratton 1981, 1982, 1984, 1990, 1994, 1998; Webster-Stratton and Hammond 1997; Webster-Stratton *et al.* 1988, 1989) and two independent replications (Taylor *et al.* 1998; Scott *et al.* 2001).

Parent training shows greater efficacy (fewer dropouts, greater gains, and better maintenance) where children are younger, where the disturbance of conduct is less severe, and there is less comorbidity and socio-economic disadvantage in the family (McMahon *et al.* 1981; Holden *et al.* 1990; Kazdin *et al.* 1992), the parents are together (Dumas and Albin 1986; Farmer *et al.* 2002), parental discord and stress are low (McMahon *et al.* 1981; Dumas and Albin 1986; Dadds *et al.* 1987; Kazdin *et al.* 1992; Webster-Stratton 1996a), social support is high, and there is no parental history of antisocial behaviour. There are also findings which indicate that single-parent status (Dumas and Albin 1986), only one parent attending (Farmer *et al.* 2002), and maternal insecurity of attachment (Routh *et al.* 1995) may undermine progress, but these associations are not sufficiently consistent across studies. Failure to benefit is associated with parental psychiatric difficulties (such as substance abuse, depression, and personality difficulties). Programmes increasingly attempt to meet the challenge of comorbidity, severity, and parental psychopathology and social disadvantage. These interventions have evolved to become longer, and include children and teachers, and this appears to improve generalization. There are indications that barriers such as parental stresses need to be managed specifically for programmes to show benefit. A particular clinical challenge is posed by parents who do not initiate treatment themselves, or who do not perceive the need for an intervention. Further research is required on the impact of parent training programmes on the quality of life of children with CD and their parents/carers, as well as on longer-term child outcomes.

The Oregon model of parent training, designed for 6–10 year olds, has been extended to adolescents by targeting risk behaviours for delinquency (such as class attendance, affiliation with antisocial peers, or drug use), enhancing parental monitoring, and replacing time-out procedures with more radical punishments (such as restriction of free time and restitution of stolen property). A Cochrane review (Woolfenden *et al.* 2002, 2003) identified eight trials of parent training and multisystemic therapy (which includes parent training). Essentially, both concluded that family and parenting interventions for juvenile delinquents have beneficial effects in reducing time spent in institutions and the frequency of arrests. However, the effectiveness of this procedure appears limited (Patterson and Forgatch 1987; Forgatch and Patterson 1989; Bank *et al.* 1991). In addition, a controlled trial (Dishion and Andrews 1995) found that instituting this approach in a group format was associated with particularly poor outcomes, possibly due to peer influence. Further studies show more positive benefit with children in foster care, where it appears to reduce behaviour problems as well as recidivism (Chamberlain and Rozicky 1995; Chamberlain and Reid 1998), perhaps because of a higher level of motivation in the foster parents.

Functional family therapy (a form of behavioural family therapy) has been shown to be effective in reducing recidivism in adolescents who have multiply offended. Nine studies carried out between 1973 and 1997 report an improvement of 25–80 per cent in recidivism, out-of-home placement, or future offending by siblings of the treated youths (Fonagy and Kurtz 2002). Although a promising treatment, it has not yet been widely applied. There is less work on structural family therapy, mostly on Hispanic children, where it has been shown to be effective in youths with conduct problems (Szapocznik *et al.* 1989; Santisteban *et al.* 2003; Coatsworth *et al.* 2001). Multisystemic therapy (MST) is a home-based approach provided by one therapist, who potentially offers a range of techniques, dependent on the clinical picture. These include marital and family therapies, parent training, behavioural and cognitive approaches, supportive therapy, and case management (which may involve liaison with outside agencies). A number of good-quality RCTs of this approach suggest that it is the most effective treatment for delinquent adolescents in reducing recidivism and improving individual and family pathology (Henggeler *et al.* 1986, 1992, 1993, 1996a; Borduin 1999). It is substantially more effective than individual treatment even for quite troubled and disorganized families (Borduin *et al.* 1995). MST shares a particular strength with other systemic family approaches in reducing attrition rates in this highly volatile group (Henggeler *et al.* 1996b) and maintenance of outcomes at long-term follow-up (Henggeler *et al.* 2002).

Mild conduct problems are also ameliorated with the help of social skills and anger management coping skills training (reviewed by Quinn *et al.* 1999; Beelmann and Losel 2006). In a school-based coping skills intervention (Lochman *et al.* 1993) children rated aggressive and socially rejected benefited from this package in terms of reduced aggression (ES = 0.85) and social acceptance (ES = 0.89), but those who were aggressive but not socially rejected did not. However, attrition was high at 45 per cent. There is no evidence for the use of social skills and anger management coping skills training approaches on their own with more chronic and severe cases (Fonagy *et al.* 2002).

Problem-solving skills training (PSST) is the most rigorously investigated and effective of cognitive-behavioural approaches, perhaps because this helps children to develop alternative strategies to resolve problems that cause disruptive behaviour (rather than attempting to regulate it). Its effectiveness in combination with parent training has been demonstrated by two independent studies (Kazdin *et al.* 1992; Kazdin and Wasser 2000) and it seems to be the treatment of choice for conduct problems in school aged children (8–12). In a trial contrasting relationship therapy (RT) with (a) PSST, and (b) PSST and *in vivo* practice outside the treatment setting, PSST produced improvements with the milder or moderate severity outpatient group, as well as with the inpatient group. Children with more severe conduct disturbance (in terms of either frequency or intensity) were more likely to drop out or have negative outcomes (Kazdin *et al.* 1994), and there is some indication that ethnic minority status may be associated with relatively poorer outcomes (Kazdin 1996). Of 242 children aged 3–14 years referred to a specialist outpatient unit for treatment for oppositional, aggressive, and antisocial behaviour, 39.9 per cent dropped out (Kazdin *et al.* 1997), and a similar proportion was lost in an uncontrolled study of 250 children and families treated over 22 weeks (Kazdin and Wasser 2000). These individuals were more likely to be from minority groups, from single-parent families, on public assistance, to have adverse child-rearing practices, to be of low SES, and to have another child with a history of antisocial behaviour. Families who dropped out had higher levels of stressors and obstacles which competed with treatment, including conflict with a significant other about coming to treatment, problems with other children, and treatment being seen as adding to other stressors. Those terminating early also perceived the treatment as less relevant to the child's problems and appeared to have poorer relationships with the therapist. Helping parents deal with stress independently improves the outcome of already potent combinations of parent management training and PSST (Kazdin and Nock 2003).

Conduct problems from a social information processing perspective

There is a remarkably rich history of high-quality research on social information processing abnormalities associated with conduct problems elegantly summarized by Mize and Pettit (Chapter 6). These authors outlined the nature of the distortions, due to biased and/or deficient processing, commonly observed in aggressive children at each of the six steps of social information processing.

1. They seek and receive less information and obtain less relevant detail, fail to shift away from aggressive presentations, but also suppress aggressive stimuli.
2. They interpret ambiguous stimuli as threatening and attribute malevolent hostile states of mind to others.
3. They endorse more instrumental goals aimed at the dominance or control of others and care less if others retaliate or reject them;
4. They are able to access fewer responses and select ineffective and/or manipulative, aggressive strategies.
5. They select aggressive response options about which they have unrealistically positive expectations and which they consider acceptable and likely to lead to positive outcomes including stopping others' unpleasant behaviour and generating an experience of success.

SIP anomalies account for about 10 per cent of the variance in aggression. Mize and Pettit point out that the social information processing perspective is not, at root, a developmental model, as few hypotheses are offered about how SIP changes with development. Their exploration of developmental aspects of SIP is remarkable in highlighting many extant complexities and inconsistencies previously not dealt with adequately by the model. They point to a number of the major conceptual questions arising from developmental findings, such as the confounding of encoding measures by verbal skills, how increased sophistication in interpreting the intention behind actions independent of their effects (increasing mentalizing capacity with age) impacts on the levels of aggression, or how contextual effects on the development of cognitive mechanisms might influence SIP. They raise further methodological issues such as poor test–retest reliability of SIP measures in younger age groups and, related to this, measurement issues with SIP parameters such as encoding and attributional bias. The lack of stability in SIP in younger age groups may be associated with the greater malleability of young children or (more likely) the greater influence of stable situational determinants such as peer groups. They also point to the importance of the excessive use of self-report and hypothetical scenario type assessments which create a confound between conscious awareness and SIP assessment. They point out that as reactive aggression, in particular, is based on extremely rapid impulsive reactions which have not been thought through, unconsciously encoded and processed stimuli may have important motivational and cognitive effects, and motives for actions may not fall into the conscious purview of the actor (see e.g. Pessiglione *et al.* (2007) and Frith (2007) for the neuroscientific underpinnings of such unconsciously constructed reactions).

Although the evidence supporting SIP in relation to conduct problems is the richest of all the conditions considered in this volume, there are important unanswered questions related to this body of work. Some developmental findings are inconsistent across studies. For example, while some findings reviewed suggest that younger children are more likely to attribute hostility to peers, other studies find that hostile attributions increase with age. Mize and Pettit (Chapter 6) make the ingenious suggestion that underlying such contradictory observations may be a U-shaped curve in children's perception and approval of aggression. Parents' influence on social cognition wanes with development as the influence of peers grows. As children become more aware of the power of aggression, threat, and intimidation, they also become more sensitive to the opinions of age-mates and friends. During preschool and elementary school years they learn to think in increasingly complex and accurate ways about the intentions underlying others' behaviour and acquire superior capacities for regulating aggression. Thus early approval of aggression is driven by 'ignorance' and later approval is down to self-interest and peer influence overriding increased mentalization of the impact of violence. Of course, this model is only partially consistent with the emerging data on the trajectories of violence which show partial desisting from violence with the emergence of social cognition. This downward trend does not characterize about 10 per cent of physically aggressive children who remain violent individuals (Broidy *et al.* 2003; Tremblay *et al.* 2004; Cote *et al.* 2006). However, the model is consistent with the emergence of adolescent specific conduct disorder as suggested by Moffitt (e.g. Moffitt *et al.* 2002). The SIP mechanisms of non-desisters may be immune in some way to social influence, a suggestion consistent with Blair's model (Chapter 7). Clearly, what is required is a trajectory analysis of SIP in conjunction with measures of change in aggression.

An important limitation of SIP identified by Mize and Pettit (Chapter 6) relates to the situational specificity of SIP. There is considerable intra-individual variation of SIP, and so even the most violent individual is unlikely to interpret every action by inferring hostile intent. For example, the individual's state of arousal appears to be influential in determining whether the hostile attributional bias is likely to be triggered. Similarly, recent experiences and characteristics of the situation can prime goals unconsciously, and goals outside awareness may be more influential than the goals of which the child is aware.

Implications of the social cognitive perspective for treatment

Mize and Pettit (Chapter 6) cited some work which suggests that interventions designed to reduce hostile attributions might reduce aggression (in this instance as rated by the teacher) or that assisting children with response generation could lead to increased peer acceptance and increased use of classroom tuition. However, these are somewhat isolated instances. There appears to be a striking mismatch between the evidence-based treatments for conduct problems for children we have reviewed and the very substantial literature on SIP. While research over the past 25 years has established beyond doubt the social cognitive bias associated with conduct problems, particularly aggression, therapeutic interventions which appear to have strong effect sizes are either non-cognitive in focus (e.g. parent training) or cognitive but addressing only one component of SIP (response generation) assisting with problem-solving rather than comprehensively addressing the child's pervasive social information processing deficits. The evidence for therapies that aim to address cognitive distortions directly is relatively less compelling. Mild conduct problems are ameliorated with the help of social skills and anger management coping skills training (reviewed by Quinn et al. 1999) in adolescents, and social skills and social problem-solving approaches lead to desirable short-term changes in younger conduct-disordered children, but do not appear to generalize well across settings or engender lasting improvements (Huey and Rank 1984; Feindler et al. 1984; Guerra and Slaby 1990). Individual treatment approaches in general appear to be less effective than family-based approaches, and if individual approaches are implemented, these are better focused on proximal causes for delinquent behaviour rather than more distal underlying problems. The most effective programmes, particularly, for adolescents are skills oriented.

There are a number of reasons why focusing on attributional bias or encoding deficit or other steps within the social information processing paradigm may be less effective as a focus of treatment than is the case for anxiety or even depression. First, although these biases are consistently found in study after study, they are also quite highly correlated and the overall effect sizes are relatively low. The correlation with aggressive behaviour rarely yields $R > 0.3$. In this sense addressing a single component step of SIP (e.g. response generation) may be more sensible than using the SIP model to guide a six-step treatment programme. Secondly, some of the bias in information processing may be the consequence rather than the cause of aggressive behaviour. Dodge (2006) argued that attributional biases were normative early in life, because at this age causes are assumed to match outcomes. By age 4, when SIP studies tend to begin assessing children, attributional style already differentiates aggressive from non-aggressive children, and this difference increases as the child moves into adolescence. However, this pattern of findings is equally consistent with a reverse causality model, which suggests that aggressive behaviour, marked from as early as 2 years of age (NICHD Early Child Care Research Network 2004; Cote *et al.* 2007), distorts social cognition rather than the other way round. In other words, the growing attributional bias may be a reflection of the child's experience of others' reaction to his aggressive behaviour. If attributional bias is an epiphenomenon in relation to aggression, we cannot expect the modification of these interpersonal expectations to lead to substantive improvement in behaviour.

Thirdly, while it is very likely that SIP has an important causal role in setting a child on the path of aggression (it most probably has an important mediating role in relation to both biological and social aetiological factors, although, as Mize and Pettit (Chapter 6) show, this is not likely to be a straightforward story), the factors that maintain the child on this developmental path may be more important as foci for intervention. In this context behaviour genetic studies are particularly interesting (Reiss and Leve 2007). It is possible that most of the genetic effects related to aggression are environmentally mediated via evocatory effects. Aggressive behaviour is particularly powerful in eliciting strong negative reactions from family members and friends which could be the immediate generators of the maladaptive response. Hughes and Ensor (Chapter 5) report similar findings in relation to social cognition in hard-to-manage children. Thus, while SIP abnormalities accompany aggression, these effects are perhaps maintained by the reaction of the social environment rather than SIP. This would suggest that the social environment may be the most important context for intervention.

Fourthly, the SIP model implicitly includes family and attachment relationships as sources of distortion to information processing. Mize and Pettit (Chapter 6) consider evidence that family context is one source of SIP distortion. However, as we have emphasized, the family context may be a powerful source of the development of social cognition, especially in the early years

(Sharp and Fonagy, in press; Sharp and Fonagy, Chapter 10). Thus the family-focused interventions may owe some of their effectiveness to the potential of the family environment to generate greater awareness of mental states (see also de Rosnay and colleagues, Chapter 12). In this way family-based interventions may have an SIP as well as a contingency management and other behavioural control function. For example, Webster-Stratton's (1992) programme includes an important component of teaching parents to play with their children. Such joint (particularly pretend) play is known to facilitate of the development of mentalizing (Flavell *et al.* 1987; Lillard 1993; Rakoczy *et al.* 2005; Csibra and Gergely 2006). The prominence of family-based interventions for conduct problems is of course consistent with an emphasis on family influences on SIP.

The assumption of a developmental U-turn in aggressogenic social cognition fits well with the observed patterns of findings from RCTs. Interventions in young children draw their effectiveness from the parent's influence on social cognition, while in middle childhood a combination of problem-solving and parent training might be most effective. By adolescence, social cognitive patterns are so well established that only a combination of a number of systems is likely to shift the young person's social cognitive stance.

14.7 Mentalization as a protective factor

14.7.1 Disruptive behaviour disorders and social cognition in very young children

Hughes and Ensor (Chapter 5) review research that specifies the complex relation between findings of social cognition research and early disruptive behaviour disorders, particularly 'hard-to-manage' preschoolers. Certainly, there is considerable evidence that preschoolers with conduct problems have atypical social cognition. Indeed, children with conduct disorders have what Happé and Frith (1996) called a 'theory of nasty minds', while school bullies may even have superior social cognitive capacities (Sutton *et al.* 1999a,b). Children with attention deficit–hyperactivity disorder may not manifest either retardation or precocious development in this domain (Perner *et al.* 2002). However, Hughes and Ensor insightfully argue that within a dynamic model of development the impact of social cognitive problems may not be the same in early development as at school age. As we have seen in the case of the SIP model of conduct disorder, social cognitive capacities have different determinants and functions at different developmental stages. Hughes and Ensor discuss early intuitive mentalizing, what Tager-Flusberg (2001) called socio-perceptual awareness of mind, which may have independent predictive power from the results of the much more verbally keyed theory of mind tests. It is reasonable to argue that this kind of intuitive mentalizing (Frith 1989) could serve as a protective factor against social adversity in a range of contexts. In fact, we argued this position strongly some time ago in relation to the multifaceted concept of resilience (Fonagy et al. 1994). Genuinely identifying the mental states underpinning even hostile behaviour appears to reduce the impact of that experience on current functioning (Fonagy et al. 1991; Hesse 1999; Allen 2001; Slade 2005). Here we are aiming to link social cognition to a universal human tendency to 'turn around' passivity, helplessness, and lack of response and create (or re-create) activity, control, and human connection through accurately elaborating intentional states behind actions.

Hughes and Ensor (Chapter 5) report a number of findings pertinent to the notion of social cognition as a protective mechanism. To summarize, hard-to-manage preschoolers appeared to have less 'connectedness' in their conversation with their mothers where connectedness was thought of as each member of the dyad tuning into the other's thoughts, desires, or feelings. Theory of mind and emotion understanding in these hard-to-manage groups appeared to show a relationship with connectedness. Positive and negative maternal control showed the expected correlations with non-compliance—negative control predicting increased disruptiveness. From Hughes and Ensor's research, the deficit in social cognition appears to be a consequence rather than a cause of behavioural disorder. Executive functioning and peer problems, but not social cognition, appear to correlate with disruptive behaviour. However, this is not to say that social cognition is unimportant in the aetiology of the problems of hard-to-manage children.

Detailed video coding of mother–child play across settings and across measures yielded a robust index of harsh parenting. The video-based coding of non-compliance, emotion dysregulation, and maternal rating of attention and hyperactivity problems strongly correlated with the measure of parenting negativity. However, this correlation was strongest amongst children whose social cognitive capacities were most limited. The suggestion here is that social cognition can provide an important barrier to help the child counteract the influence of parental negativity. Thus whilst Hughes and Ensor provide no evidence for social cognitive deficit as a cause of disruptive behaviour, they do suggest that social cognition may be a protective factor under conditions of some adversity.

14.7.2 Generic social cognitive interventions

As we have seen, many current interventions for young children with behavioural problems tend to focus on modifying parents' inclination to be critical, punitive, and sparse in positive reinforcement. Whilst the effects of these interventions are undoubtedly quite powerful, there are children who benefit less, particularly when other stressors make parents less available to parent training (Dretzke *et al.* 2005). In these cases it seems sensible to focus therapeutic efforts on the child (Kazdin 1997), in particular on enhancing the child's capacity to interpret the parent's behaviour in more mentalizing ways and thereby potentially reduce the impact of such negativity. It is possible that problem-solving training, when used in conjunction with parent training (Kazdin 1995), is so effective just because of its potential to enhance the social cognitive skills of the child. We might predict that improvements in social cognitive capacities associated with such intervention would bring greatest benefit when parenting training had least effect in altering or reducing parenting negativity. Considering the child's role in initiating episodes of harsh parenting, it is also possible that enhancing mentalization may reduce exposure to harsh parenting by improving the child's ability to anticipate parents' reactions and pre-empt negative cycles of family interaction.

A further treatment implication concerns a focus of family therapy. Given the role that family discourse and parental attitudes might have in the development of social cognition (Sharp and Fonagy, Chapter 10; Gergely and Unoka, Chapter 11; de Rosnay and colleagues, Chapter 12), it can be argued that focusing treatment on precisely this aspect of family life may bring about improvements through the mediation of enhanced social cognition. This is precisely the logic underlying SMART (Short-Term Mentalization and Relational Therapy) (Fearon *et al.* 2006). This is a model of systemic family therapy aimed specifically at enhancing mentalization within a family system. It is assumed that all behavioural–emotional problems of children are both a reflection of biological vulnerability and/or adversity and an effort to cope and adapt (identity, safety, control, gratification, attachment). 'Turning off' mentalizing—doing rather than thinking—can create an illusion of control and safety. Non-mentalizing behaviour (coercive, non-psychological) evokes non-mentalizing responses leading to self-perpetuating and self-reinforcing cycles (coercive cycles or impasses).

This resilience enhancing has four key aims:

(1) to help families shift from coercive non-mentalizing cycles (impasses) to mentalizing discussions that can promote trust, security, and attachment;

(2) to promote parents' sense of competence in general and, in particular, in helping their children develop mentalizing skills and attitudes;

(3) to practice mentalizing in the specific areas in which mentalizing has become inhibited;

(4) to initiate virtuous cycles within the family, with peers, and in school which reinforce mentalizing, communication, and mutually supportive solutions to problems.

In sum, the protocol aims to help the family make sense of what feelings are experienced by each family member, what thoughts are connected with these feelings, how these feelings are communicated within the family, and ways in which miscommunication or misunderstanding (or lack of understanding) of these feelings leads to interactions that maintain family problems.

There are several key characteristics of the intervention:

(1) to model the inquisitive stance of not knowing about mental states as these are genuinely opaque;

(2) encouraging family members to learn something new or remind them of something forgotten about the inner experience of oneself or others;

(3) using techniques aimed at confronting mechanisms used by family members to avoid thinking about each others' subjective experience (inhibitory cycles, noticing non-mentalizing fillers, identifying blocking anxiety);

(4) adapting specific mentalizing games to provide a context in which to learn about and become more comfortable with taking the inquisitive stance.

The evaluation of this treatment approach is in its infancy, but we mention it here as it builds on the type of connection between psychiatric disorder and social cognition identified by Hughes and Ensor. There are as yet no RCT data to support the effectiveness of SMART. It is possible that other systemic interventions that are known to be helpful in the treatment of childhood conduct problems have part of their impact through their potential to enhance social cognition in the child, and this may help them to withstand the pressures of relatively harsh parental environments.

Some have argued that enhancing social cognition is the key common factor across psychosocial treatments as dissimilar as individual psychodynamic therapy and trauma focused cognitive behaviour therapy (Allen *et al.* 2008). We may not wish to go that far in this context. However, in the course of this chapter we have come to see that probably all childhood psychiatric disorders involve a dysfunction of social cognition; inevitably there is misinterpretation of self and others and maladaptive non-mentalizing perceiving, feeling, thinking, behaving, coping, and relating to others. Whether this entails a persistent neurobiological deficit, the prototype being childhood autism, or an increased disposition to mentalize, as might be the case in a socially phobic child contemplating risks associated with an encounter with others, or the inhibition of mentalization associated with the activation of fight-or-flight either episodically as in depression or bipolar disorder or intermittently as in trauma within a specific context, it may be helpful to take as at least one focus of therapy the child's ability to perceive others as well as him/herself as a thinking and feeling being and to extend this systematically to his/her family and perhaps even the wider school and peer environment.

14.8 Conclusion

In this chapter we have reviewed the social cognitive models described in preceding chapters and taken on the ambitious task of delineating a taxonomy of social cognition by which models can be classed, while concurrently reviewing the treatment outcome literature associated with each approach to social cognition. We have delineated five classes of social cognition that map onto aetiological models of childhood disorders:

(1) lacking the ability to represent other minds, such as the case of autism-spectrum disorders or psychopathy;

(2) over-activation and distorted use of social cognition (schizophrenia);

(3) context-specific facilitation and inhibition of social cognition in the case of, for example, borderline personality disorder and victims of maltreatment;

(4) reality-distorting dysfunctional mentalization processes as found in depression, anxiety, and conduct problems;

(5) mentalization or social cognition as a protective factor as suggested for disruptive behaviour disorders in preschoolers.

Clearly, there is a role for social cognition in both the conceptualization and treatment of childhood disorders, either as disease mechanism (e.g. as suggested by Baron-Cohen and colleagues in Chapter 2) or as epiphenomenon (e.g. as suggested earlier in this chapter for attributional biases in conduct disorder). Either way, social cognition should be considered in all treatment of childhood disorders and in some cases should be the main focus of treatment. Of course, one can argue, as do Allen *et al.* (2008), that most treatment approaches lead to improvement in mentalization anyway. Whilst psychotherapeutic interventions have many goals, it is true that most disorders of childhood (and adulthood) affect individuals' capacity to connect to others in meaningful ways. Whether explicitly focusing on improving mentalization (social cognition) or not, the positive outcome of intervention usually involves a restoration of the capacity for minding the minds of others. By fully integrating the developmental psychopathology of social cognition into the conceptualization and treatment of childhood disorder, we move away from an 'isolated mind metaphor' (Brothers 1997, p. xi) to a view that is thoroughly social. In addition, we honour the principle that psychotherapeutic interventions be tailored directly to psychological processes. We are, after all, 'homo psychologicus' (Humphrey 1984)—that is, naturally born psychologists with the capacity to reflect on the mental states of self and others in the service of human affiliation.

References

Ablon, J.S. and Jones, E.E. (2002). Validity of controlled clinical trials of psychotherapy: Findings from the NIMH Treatment of Depression Collaborative Research Program. *American Journal of Psychiatry*, **159**, 775–83.

Ahn, H. and Wampold, B.E. (2001). Where oh where are the specific ingredients? A meta-analysis of component studies in counseling and psychotherapy. *Journal of Counseling Psychology*, **48**, 251–7.

Albano, A.M., Marten, P.A., Holt, C.S., Heimberg, R.G., and Barlow, D.H. (1995). Cognitive-behavioral group treatment for social phobia in adolescents: a preliminary study. *Journal of Nervous and Mental Disease*, **183**, 649–56.

Alfano, C.A., Beidel, D.C., and Turner, S.M. (2002). Cognition in childhood anxiety: conceptual, methodological, and developmental issues. *Clinical Psychology Review*, **22**, 1209–38.

Allen, J.G. (2001). Traumatic relationships and serious mental disorders. Chichester: John Wiley.

Allen, J., Fonagy, P., and Bateman, A. (2008). *Mentalizing in clinical practice*. Washington, DC: American Psychiatric Press.

Anderson, S.R., Avery, D.L., Dipeitro, E.K., Edwards, G.L., and Christian, W.P. (1987). Intensive home based early intervention with autistic children. *Education and Treatment of Children*, **10**, 352–66.

Asarnow, J.R., Jaycox, L.H., and Tompson, M.C. (2001). Depression in youth: psychosocial interventions. *Journal of Clinical Child Psychology*, **30**, 33–47.

Baird, A.A., Veague, H.B., and Rabbitt, C.E. (2005). Developmental precipitants of borderline personality disorder. *Developmental Psychopathology*, **17**, 1031–49.

Bank, L., Marlowe, J.H., Reid, J.B., Patterson, G.R., and Weinrott, M.R. (1991). A comparative evaluation of parent-training interventions for families of chronic delinquents. *Journal of Abnormal Child Psychology*, **19**, 15–33.

Baron, J., Gruen, R., Asnis, L., and Lord, S. (1985). Familial transmission of schizotypal and borderline personality disorders. *American Journal of Psychiatry*, **142**, 927–34.

Baron-Cohen, S., Wheelwright, S., Hill, J., Raste, Y., and Plumb, I. (2001). The 'Reading the Mind in the Eyes' Test revised version: a study with normal adults and adults with Asperger syndrome or high-functioning autism. *Journal of Child Psychology and Psychiatry and Allied Disciplines*, **42**, 241–51.

Barrett, P.M. (1998). Evaluation of cognitive-behavioral group treatments for childhood anxiety disorders. *Journal of Clinical Child Psychology*, **27**, 459–68.

Barrett, P.M., Dadds, M.R., and Rapee, R.M. (1996). Family treatment for childhood anxiety: a controlled trial. *Journal of Consulting and Clinical Psychology*, **64**, 333–42.

Barrett, P., Healy, L., Piacentine, J., and March, J. (2004). Treatment of OCD in children and adolescents. In *Handbook of interventions that work with children and adolescents* (ed. P. Barrett and T. Ollendick), pp. 187–216. Chichester: John Wiley.

Bateman, A.W. and Fonagy, P. (1999). The effectiveness of partial hospitalization in the treatment of borderline personality disorder—a randomized controlled trial. *American Journal of Psychiatry*, **156**, 1563–9.

Bateman, A.W. and Fonagy, P. (2001). Treatment of borderline personality disorder with psychoanalytically oriented partial hospitalization: an 18-month follow-up. *American Journal of Psychiatry*, **158**, 36–42.

Beck, A.T. and Clark, D.A. (1997). An information processing model of anxiety: automatic and strategic processes. *Behavior Research and Therapy*, **35**, 49–58.

Beelmann, A. and Losel, F. (2006). Child social skills training in developmental crime prevention: effects on antisocial behavior and social competence. *Psicothema*, **18**, 603–10.

Beidel, D.C., Turner, S.M., and Morris, T.L. (2000). Behavioral treatment of childhood social phobia. *Journal of Consulting and Clinical Psychology*, **68**, 1072–80.

Bernstein, G.A., Borchardt, C.M., Perwien, A.R., *et al.* (2000). Imipramine plus cognitive-behavioral therapy in the treatment of school refusal. *Journal of the American Academy of Child and Adolescent Psychiatry*, **39**, 276–83.

Bertrand, M.C., Sutton, H., Achim, A.M., Malla, A.K., and Lepage, M. (2007). Social cognitive impairments in first episode psychosis. *Schizophrenia Research*, **95**, 124–33.

Birmaher, B., Brent, D.A., Kolko, D. *et al.* (2000). Clinical outcome after short-term psychotherapy for adolescents with major depressive disorder. *Archives of General Psychiatry*, **57**, 29–36.

Blair, R.J.R. (1995). A cognitive developmental approach to morality: investigating the psychopath. *Cognition*, **57**, 1–29.

Blakemore, S.J. and Choudhury, S. (2006). Development of the adolescent brain: implications for executive function and social cognition. *Journal of Child Psychology and Psychiatry*, **47**, 296–312.

Borduin, C.M. (1999). Multisystemic treatment of criminality and violence in adolescents. *Journal of the American Academy for Child and Adolescent Psychiatry*, **38**, 242–9.

Borduin, C.M., Mann, B.J., Cone, L.T., *et al.* (1995). Multisystemic treatment of serious juvenile offenders: Long-term prevention of criminality and violence. *Journal of Consulting and Clinical Psychology*, **63**, 569–78.

Boylan, K., Romero, S., and Birmaher, B. (2007). Psychopharmacologic treatment of pediatric major depressive disorder. *Psychopharmacology*, **191**, 27–38.

Bradley, S., Brody, J., Landy, S. *et al.* (1999). Brief psychoeducational parenting program: an evaluation. Presented at *46th Annual Meeting of the American Academy of Child and Adolescent Psychiatry*, Chicago.

Brent, D.A., Holder, D., Kolko, D., *et al.* (1997). A clinical psychotherapy trial for adolescent depression comparing cognitive, family and supportive therapy. *Archives of General Psychiatry*, **54**, 877–85.

Brent, D.A., Kolko, D., Birmaher, B., *et al.* (1998). Predictors of treatment efficacy in a clinical trial of three psychosocial treatments for adolescent depression. *Journal of the American Academy of Child and Adolescent Psychiatry*, **37**, 906–14.

Brent, D.A., Kolko, D., Birmaher, B., Baugher, M., and Bridge, J. (1999). A clinical trial for adolescent depression: predictos of additional treatment in the acute and follow-up phases of the trial. *Journal of the American Academy of Child and Adolescent Psychiatry*, **38**, 263–70.

Bridge, J.A., Iyengar, S., Salary, C.B., *et al.* (2007). Clinical response and risk for reported suicidal ideation and suicide attempts in pediatric antidepressant treatment:

a meta-analysis of randomized controlled trials. *Journal of the American Medical Association*, **297**, 1683–96.

Broidy, L.M., Nagin, D.S., Temblay, R.E., *et al*. (2003). Developmental trajectories of childhood disruptive behaviors and adolescent delinquency: a six-site, cross-national study. *Developmental Psychology*, **39**, 222–45.

Brothers, L. (1997). *Friday's footprint: how society shapes the human mind*. Oxford University Press.

Brune, M. (2005). Emotion recognition, 'theory of mind,' and social behavior in schizophrenia. *Psychiatry Research*, **133**, 135–47.

Brune, M. and Bodenstein, L. (2005). Proverb comprehension reconsidered—'theory of mind' and the pragmatic use of language in schizophrenia. *Schizophrenia Research*, **75**, 233–39.

Campbell, M., Schopler, E., Cueva, J.E., and Hallin, A. (1996). Treatment of autistic disorder. *Journal of the American Academy of Child and Adolescent Psychiatry*, **35**, 134–43.

Cartwright-Hatton, S., Roberts, C., Chitsabesan, P., Fothergill, C., and Harrington, R. (2004). Systematic review of the efficacy of cognitive behavior therapies for childhood and adolescent anxiety disorders. *Britesh Journal of Clinical Psychology*, **43**, 421–36.

Chamberlain, P. and Reid, J.B. (1998). Comparison of two community alternatives to incarceration for chronic juvenile offenders. *Journal of Consulting and Clinical Psychology*, **66**, 624–33.

Chamberlain, P. and Rozicky, J.G. (1995). The effectiveness of family therapy in the treatment of adolescents with conduct disorders and delinquency. *Journal of Marital and Family Therapy*, **21**, 441–59.

Charlop-Christy, M.H., Carpenter, M., Le, L., LeBlanc, L.A., and Kellet, K. (2002). Using the picture exchange communication system (PECS) with children with autism: assessment of PECS acquisition, speech, social-communicative behavior, and problem behavior. *Journal of Applied Behavior Analysis*, **35**, 213–31.

Choi, K.H. and Kwon, J.H. (2006). Social cognition enhancement training for schizophrenia: a preliminary randomized controlled trial. *Community Mental Health Journal*, **42**, 177–87.

Choudhury, S., Blakemore, S.J., and Charman, T. (2006). Social cognitive development during adolescence. *SCAN*, **1**, 165–74.

Cicchetti, D. and Cohen, D.J. (ed.) (2006). *Developmental psychopathology*, Vols 1, 2, 3. New York: John Wiley.

Cicchetti, D. and Curtis, W.J. (2005). An event-related potential study of the processing of affective facial expressions in young children who experienced maltreatment during the first year of life. *Developmental Psychopathology*, **17**, 641–77.

Cicchetti, D., Toth, S.L., and Rogosch, F.A. (1999). The efficacy of toddler–parent psychotherapy to increase attachment security in offspring of depressed mothers. *Attachment and Human Development*, **1**, 34–66.

Cicchetti, D., Rogosch, F.A., and Toth, S.L. (2000). The efficacy of toddler–parent psychotherapy for fostering cognitive development in offspring of depressed mothers. *Journal of Abnormal Child Psychology*, **28**, 135–48.

Cicchetti, D., Rogosch, F.A., and Toth, S.L. (2006). Fostering secure attachment in infants in maltreating families through preventive interventions. *Developmental Psychopathology*, **18**, 623–49.

Clark, D.A., Steer, R.A., and Beck, A.T. (1994). Common and specific dimensions of self-reported anxiety and depression: implications for the cognitive and tripartite models. *Journal of Abnormal Psychology*, **103**, 645–54.

Clarke, G.N., Rohde, P., Lewinsohn, P.M., Hops, H., and Seeley, J.R. (1999). Cognitive-behavioral treatment of adolescent depression: efficacy of acute group treatment and booster sessions. *Journal of the American Academy of Child and Adolescent Psychiatry*, **38**, 272–9.

Clarkin, J., Levy, K.N., Lenzenweger, M.F., and Kernberg, O.F. (2007). Evaluating three treatments for borderline personality disorder: a multiwave study. *American Journal of Psychiatry*, **164**, 922–8.

Clavenna, A., Rossi, E., Derosa, M., and Bonati, M. (2007). Use of psychotropic medications in Italian children and adolescents. *European Journal of Pediatrics*, **166**, 339–47.

Coatsworth, J.D., Santisteban, D.A., McBride, C.K., and Szapocznik, J. (2001). Brief Strategic Family Therapy versus community control: engagement, retention, and an exploration of the moderating role of adolescent symptom severity. *Family Process*, **40**, 313–32.

Cobham, V.E., Dadds, M.R., and Spence, S.H. (1998). The role of parental anxiety in the treatment of childhood anxiety. *Journal of Consulting and Clinical Psychology*, **66**, 893–905.

Combs, D., Adams, S.D., Penn, D.L., Roberts, D.L., Tiegreen, J., and Stern, P. (2007). Social Cognition and Interaction Training (SCIT) for inpatients with schizophrenia spectrum disorders: preliminary findings. *Schizophrenia Research*, **91**, 112–16.

Corcoran, R., Mercer, G., and Frith, C.D. (1995). The appreciation of visual jokes in people with schizophrenia: a study of 'mentalizing' ability. *Schizophrenia Research*, **24**, 319–27.

Cote, S.M., Vaillancourt, T., LeBlanc, J.C., Nagin, D.S., and Tremblay, R.E. (2006). The development of physical aggression from toddlerhood to pre-adolescence: a nation-wide longitudinal study of Canadian children. *Journal of Abnormal Child Psychology*, **34**, 68–82.

Cote, S.M., Boivin, M., Nagin, D.S., et al. (2007). The role of maternal education and nonmaternal care services in the prevention of children's physical aggression problems. *Archives of General Psychiatry*, **64**, 1305–12.

Couture, S.M., Penn, D.L., and Roberts, D.L. (2006). The functional significance of social cognition in schizophrenia: a review. *Schizophrenia Bulletin*, **32**, S44–63.

Creswell, C. and Cartwright-Hatton, S. (2007). Family treatment of child anxiety: outcomes, limitations and future directions. *Clinical Child Family Psychology Review*, **10**, 232–52.

Creswell, C., Schniering, C.A., and Rapee, R.M. (2005). Threat interpretation in anxious children and their mothers: comparison with non-clinical children and the effects of treatment. *Behavior Research and Therapy*, **43**, 1375–81.

Csibra, G. and Gergely, G. (2006). Social learning and social cognition: the case for pedagogy. In *Processes of change in brain and cognitive development* (ed. M.H. Johnson and Y.M. Munakata), pp. 249–74. Oxford University Press.

Cunningham, C.E., Bremner, R., and Boyle, M. (1995). Large group community-based parenting programs for family of preschoolers at risk for disruptive behavior disorders: utilization, cost-effectiveness and outcome. *Journal of Child Psychology and Psychiatry*, 36, 1141–59.

Dadds, M.R., Schwartz, S., and Sanders, M.R. (1987). Marital discord and treatment outcome in behavioral treatment of child conduct disorders. *Journal of Consulting and Clinical Psychology*, 55, 396–403.

Dadds, M.R., Spence, S.H., Holland, D.E., Barrett, P.M., and Laurens, K.R. (1997). Prevention and early intervention for anxiety disorders: a controlled trial. *Journal of Consulting and Clinical Psychology*, 65, 627–35.

Damasio, A. (1999). The feeling of what happens: body and emotion in the making of consciousness. New York: Harcourt Brace.

Davidson, K., Norrie, J., Tyrer, P., *et al.* (2006a). The effectiveness of cognitive behavior therapy for borderline personality disorder: results from the borderline personality disorder study of cognitive therapy (BOSCOT) trial. *Journal of Personality Disorders*, 20, 450–65.

Davidson, K., Tyrer, P., Gumley, A., *et al.* (2006b). A randomized controlled trial of cognitive behavior therapy for borderline personality disorder: rationale for trial, method, and description of sample. *Journal of Personality Disorders*, 20, 431–49.

Deblinger, E. and Lippman, J. (1996). Sexually abused children suffering posttraumatic stress symptoms: initial treatment outcome findings. *Child Maltreatment*, 1, 310–22.

Deblinger, E., Steer, R.A., and Lippman, J. (1999). Two-year follow-up study of cognitive behavioral therapy for sexually abused children suffering post-traumatic stress symptoms. *Child Abuse and Neglect*, 23, 1371–8.

DeVeaugh-Geiss, J., Moroz, G., Biederman, J., *et al.* (1992). Clomipramine in child and adolescent obsessive–compulsive disorder: a multicenter trial. *Journal of the American Academy of Child and Adolescent Psychiatry*, 31, 45–9.

Diamond, G.S., Reis, B.F., Diamond, G.M., Siqueland, L., and Isaacs, L. (2002). Attachment-based family therapy for depressed adolescents: a treatment development study. *Journal of the American Academy of Child and Adolescent Psychiatry*, 41, 1190–6.

Dishion, T.J. and Andrews, D.W. (1995). Preventing escalation in problem behaviors with high-risk young adolescents: immediate and 1-year outcomes. *Journal of Consulting and Clinical Psychology*, 63, 538–48.

Dodge, K.A. (2006). Translational science in action: hostile attributional style and the development of aggressive behavior problems. *Development and Psychopathology*, 18, 791–814.

Dorris, L., Espie, C.A., Knott, F., and Salt, J. (2004). Mind-reading difficulties in the siblings of people with Asperger's syndrome: evidence for a genetic influence in the abnormal development of a specific cognitive domain. *Journal of Child Psychology and Psychiatry*, 45, 412–18.

Dretzke, J., Frew, E., Davenport, C., *et al.* (2005). The effectiveness and cost-effectiveness of parent training/education programmes for the treatment of conduct disorder, including oppositional defiant disorder, in children. *Health Technology Assessment Reports*, 9, 1–233.

Drevets, W.C. (2000). Neuroimaging studies of mood disorders. *Biological Psychiatry*, 48, 813–29.

Drew, A., Baird, G., Baron-Cohen, S., *et al.* (2002). A pilot randomised control trial of a parent training intervention for pre-school children with autism: preliminary findings and methodological challenges. *European Child Adolescent Psychiatry*, **11**, 266–72.

Ducharme, J.M., Atkinson, L., and Poulton, L. (2000). Success-based, noncoercive treatment of oppositional behavior in children from violent homes. *Journal of the American Academy of Child and Adolescent Psychiatry*, **39**, 995–1004.

Dumas, J.E. and Albin, J.B. (1986). Parent training outcome. Does active parental involvement matter? *Behaviour Research and Therapy*, **24**, 227–30.

Dunlap, G., Koegel, R., Johnson, J., and O'Neill, R. (1987). Maintaining performance of autistic clients in community settings with delayed contingencies. *Journal of Applied Behaviour Analysis*, **20**, 185–91.

Eikeseth, S., Smith, T., Jahr, E., and Eldevik, S. (2002). Intensive behavioral treatment at school for 4- to 7-year-old children with autism: a 1-year comparison controlled study. *Behavior Modification*, **26**, 49–68.

Emslie, G., Kratochvil, C., Vitiello, B., *et al.* (2006). Treatment for Adolescents with Depression Study (TADS): safety results. *Journal of the American Academy of Child and Adolescent Psychiatry*, **45**, 1440–55.

Evans, J., Heron, J., Lewis, G., Araya, R., and Wolke, D. (2005). Negative self-schemas and the onset of depression in women: longitudinal study. *British Journal of Psychiatry*, **186**, 302–7.

Evidence-based Medicine Group (1992). Evidence-based medicine: a new approach to teaching the practice of medicine. *Journal of the American Medical Association*, **268**, 2420–5.

Farmer, E.M., Compton, S.N., Burns, B.J., and Robertson, E. (2002). Review of the evidence base for treatment of childhood psychopathology: externalizing disorders. *Journal of Consulting and Clinical Psychology*, **70**, 1267–1302.

Fearon, P., Target, M., Fonagy, P., *et al.* (2006). Short-Term Mentalization and Relational Therapy (SMART): an integrative family therapy for children and adolescents. In *Handbook of mentalisation based treatments* (ed. J. Allen and P. Fonagy). Chichester: John Wiley.

Feindler, E.L., Marriott, S.A., and Iwata, M. (1984). Group anger control training for junior high school delinquents. *Cognitive Therapy and Research*, **8**, 299–311.

Flannery-Schroeder, E.C. and Kendall, P.C. (2000). Group and individual cognitive-behavioral treatments for youth with anxiety disorders: a randomized controlled trial. *Cognitive Therapy and Research*, **24**, 251–81.

Flavell, J.H., Flavell, E.R., and Green, F.L. (1987). Young children's knowledge about the appearent-real and pretend-real distinction. *Developmental Psychology*, **23**, 816–22.

Fonagy, P. and Bateman, A. (2006). Progress in the treatment of borderline personality disorder. *British Journal of Psychiatry*, **188**, 1–3.

Fonagy, P. and Kurtz, A. (2002). Disturbance of conduct. In Fonagy, P., Target, M., Cottrell, D., Phillips, J., and Kurtz, Z. *What works for whom? A critical review of treatments for children and adolescents*. New York: Guilford.

Fonagy, P., Steele, H., Moran, G., Steele, M., and Higgitt, A. (1991). The capacity for understanding mental states: the reflective self in parent and child and its significance for security of attachment. *Infant Mental Health Journal*, **13**, 200–17.

Fonagy, P., Steele, M., Steele, H., Higgitt, A., and Target, M. (1994). Theory and practice of resilience. *Journal of Child Psychology and Psychiatry*, **35**, 231–57.

Fonagy, P., Target, M., Cottrell, D., Phillips, J., and Kurtz, Z. (2002). *What works for whom? A critical review of treatments for children and adolescents*. New York: Guilford Press.

Forehand, R. and Long, N. (1988). Outpatient treatment of the acting out child: procedures, long-term follow-up data, and clinical problems. *Advances in Behaviour Research and Therapy*, **10**, 129–77.

Forgatch, M.S. and Patterson, G.R. (1989). *Parents and adolescents living together*. Part 2: *Family problem solving*. Eugene, OR: Castalia.

Frith, C.D. (1992). *The cognitive neuropsychology of schizophrenia*. Hillsdale, NJ: Lawrence Erlbaum.

Frith, C.D. (2007). The social brain? Philosophical Transactions of the Royal Society of London. Series B: Biological Sciences, **362**, 671–8.

Frith, U. (1989). *Autism: explaining the enigma*. Oxford: Blackwell.

Frith, U., Morton, J., and Leslie, A.M. (1991). The cognitive basis of a biological disorder: autism. *Trends in Neuroscience*, **14**, 433–8.

Frommann, N., Streit, M., and Wolwer, W. (2003). Remediation of facial affect recognition impairments in patients with schizophrenia: a new training program. *Psychiatry Research*, **117**, 281–4.

Giedd, J.N., Blumenthal, J., Jeffries, N.O., *et al*. (1999). Brain development during childhood and adolescence: a longitudinal MRI study. *Nature Neuroscience*, **2**, 861–3.

Giesen-Bloo, J., Van Dyck, R., Spinhoven, P., *et al*. (2006). Outpatient psychotherapy for borderline personality disorder: randomized trial of schema-focused therapy vs transference-focused psychotherapy. *Archives of General Psychiatry*, **63**, 649–58.

Glass, R.M. (2005). Fluoxetine, cognitive-behavioral therapy, and their combination for adolescents with depression: Treatment for Adolescents with Depression Study (TADS) randomized controlled trial. *Journal of Pediatrics*, **146**, 145.

Goldenberg, M.J. (2006). On evidence and evidence-based medicine: lessons from the philosophy of science. *Social Science and Medicine*, **62**, 2621–32.

Goodyer, I., Dubicka, B., Wilkinson, P., *et al*. (2007). Selective serotonin reuptake inhibitors (SSRIs) and routine specialist care with and without cognitive behaviour therapy in adolescents with major depression: randomised controlled trial. *British Medical Journal*, **335**, 142.

Gotlib, I.H., Kasch, K.L., Traill, S., Joormann, J., Arnow, B.A., and Johnson, S.L. (2004a). Coherence and specificity of information-processing biases in depression and social phobia. *Journal of Abnormal Psychology*, **113**, 386–98.

Gotlib, I.H., Krasnoperova, E., Yue, D.N., and Joormann, J. (2004b). Attentional biases for negative interpersonal stimuli in clinical depression. *Journal of Abnormal Psychology*, **113**, 121–35.

Grandi, S., Fabbri, S., Panattoni, N., Gonnella, E., and Marks, I. (2006). Self-exposure treatment of recurrent nightmares: Waiting-list-controlled trial and 4-year follow-up. *Psychotherapy and Psychosomatics*, **75**, 384–8.

Guerra, N. and Slaby, R.G. (1990). Cognitive mediators of aggression in adolescent offenders. II: Intervention. *Developmental Psychology*, **26**, 269–77.

Hadwin, J., Baron-Cohen, S., Howlin, P., and Hill, K. (1996). Can we teach children with autism to understand emotions, belief, or pretence? *Development and Psychopathology*, **8**, 345–65.

Hadwin, J., Baron-Cohen, S., Howlin, P., and Hill, K. (1997). Does teaching theory of mind have an effect on the ability to develop conversation in children with autism? *Journal of Autism and Developmental Disorders*, **27**, 519–37.

Happé, F. and Frith, C.D. (1996). Theory of mind and social impairment in children with conduct disorder. *British Journal of Developmental Psychology*, **14**, 385–98.

Harrington, L., Siegert, R.J., and McClure, J. (2005). Theory of mind in schizophrenia: a critical review. *Cognitive Neuropsychiatry*, **10**, 249–86.

Harris, S.L., Handleman, J.S., Kristoff, B., Bass, L., and Gordon, R. (1990). Changes in language development among autistic and peer children in segregated and integrated pre-school settings. *Journal of Autism and Developmental Disorders*, **20**, 23–31.

Henggeler, S.W., Rodick, J., Borduin, C.M., Hanson, C., Watson, S., and Urey, J. (1986). Multisystemic treatment of juvenile offenders: effects on adolescent behavior and family interaction. *Developmental Psychology*, **22**, 132–41.

Henggeler, S.W., Melton, G.B., and Smith, L.A. (1992). Family preservation using multisystemic therapy: an effective alternative to incarcerating serious juvenile offenders. *Journal of Consulting and Clinical Psychology*, **60**, 953–61.

Henggeler, S.W., Melton, G.B., Smith, L.A., Schoenwald, S.K., and Hanley, J.H. (1993). Family preservation using multisystemic treatment: long-term follow-up to a clinical trial with serious juvenile offenders. *Journal of Child and Family Studies*, **2**, 283–93.

Henggeler, S.W., Cunningham, P.B., Pickrel, S.G., Schoenwald, S.K., and Brondino, M.J. (1996a). Multisystemic therapy: an effective violence prevention approach for serious juvenile offenders. *Journal of Adolescence*, **19**, 47–61.

Henggeler, S.W., Pickrel, S.G., Brondino, M.J., and Crouch, J.L. (1996b). Eliminating (almost) treatment dropout of substance abusing or dependent delinquents through home-based multisystemic therapy. *American Journal of Psychiatry*, **153**, 427–8.

Henggeler, S.W., Clingempeel, W.G., Brondino, M.J., and Pickrel, S.G. (2002). Four-year follow-up of multisystemic therapy with substance-abusing and substance-dependent juvenile offenders. *Journal of the American Academy of Child and Adolescent Psychiatry*, **41**, 868–74.

Herold, R., Tenyi, T., Lenard, K., and Troxler, M. (2002). Theory of mind deficit in people with schizophrenia during remission. *Psychological Medicine*, **32**, 1125–9.

Hesse, E. (1999). The Adult Attachment Interview: historical and current perspectives. In *Handbook of attachment: theory, research and clinical applications* (ed. J. Cassidy and P.R. Shaver). New York: Guilford Press.

Hoagwood, K., Hibbs, E., Brent, D., and Jensen, P. (1995). Introduction to the special section: efficacy and effectiveness in studies of child and adolescent psychotherapy. *Journal of Consulting and Clinical Psychology*, **63**, 683–7.

Holden, G.W., Lavigne, V.V., and Cameron, A.M. (1990). Probing the continuum of effectiveness in parent training: characteristics of parents and preschoolers. *Journal of Clinical Child Psychology*, **19**, 2–8.

Howard, B.L. and Kendall, P.C. (1996). Cognitive-behavioral family therapy for anxiety-disordered children: a multiple-baseline evaluation. *Cognitive Therapy and Research*, **20**, 423–43.

Howlin, P. and Rutter, M. (1987). *Treatment of autistic children*, New York: John Wiley.

Howlin, P., Baron-Cohen, S. and Hadwin, J. (1999). *Teaching children with autism to mind-read: a practical guide*. Chichester: John Wiley.

Huey, W.C. and Rank, R.C. (1984). Effects of counselor and peer-led group assertiveness training on black adolescent aggression. *Journal of Counseling Psychology*, **31**, 95–8.

Humphrey, N. (1984). *Consciousness regained*. Oxford University Press.

Ingenmey, R. and Van Houten, R. (1991). Using time delay to promote spontaneous speech in an autistic child. *Journal of Applied Behaviour Analysis*, **24**, 591–6.

Irani, F., Platek, S.M., Panyavin, I.S., et al. (2006). Self-face recognition and theory of mind in patients with schizophrenia and first-degree relatives. *Schizophrenia Research*, **88**, 151–60.

Kahn, J.S., Kehle, T.J., Jenson, W.R., and Clark, E. (1990). Comparison of cognitive-behavioral, relaxation, and self-modeling interventions for depression among middle-school students. *School Psychology Review*, **19**, 196–211.

Kayser, N., Sarfati, Y., Besche, C., and Hardy-Bayle, M.C. (2006). Elaboration of a rehabilitation method based on a pathogenetic hypothesis of 'theory of mind' impairment in schizophrenia. *Neuropsychological Rehabilitation*, **16**, 83–95.

Kazdin, A.E. (1995). *Conduct disorder in childhood and adolescence*. Thousand Oaks, CA: Sage.

Kazdin, A.E. (1996). Problem solving and parent management in treating aggressive and antisocial behaviour. In *Psychosocial treatments for child and adolescent disorders: empirically based strategies for clinical practice* (ed. E.S. Hibbs and P.S. Jensen). Washington, DC: American Psychological Association.

Kazdin, A.E. (1997). Practitioner review: psychosocial treatments for conduct disorder in children. *Journal of Child Psychology and Psychiatry and Allied Disciplines*, **38**, 161–78.

Kazdin, A.E. (2000). *Psychotherapy for children and adolescents: directions for research and practice*. Oxford University Press.

Kazdin, A.E. (2003). Psychotherapy for children and adolescents. *Annual Review of Psychology*, **54**, 253–76.

Kazdin, A.E. (2004). Psychotherapy for children and adolescents. In *Bergin and Garfield's handbook of psychotherapy and behavior change* (5th edn) (ed. M. Lambert). New York: John Wiley.

Kazdin, A.E. and Nock, M.K. (2003). Delineating mechanisms of change in child and adolescent therapy: methodological issues and research recommendations. *Journal of Child Psychology and Psychiatry*, **44**, 1116–29.

Kazdin, A.E. and Wasser, G. (2000). Therapeutic changes in children, parents and families resulting from treatment of children with conduct problems. *Journal of the American Academy of Child and Adolescent Psychiatry*, **39**, 414–20.

Kazdin, A.E., Siegel, T.C., and Bass, D. (1992). Cognitive problem-solving skills training and parent management training in the treatment of antisocial behavior in children. *Journal of Consulting and Clinical Psychology*, **60**, 733–47.

Kazdin, A.E., Mazurick, J.L., and Siegel, T.C. (1994). Treatment outcome among children with externalising disorder who terminate prematurely versus those who complete psychotherapy. *Journal of the American Academy of Child and Adolescent Psychiatry*, **33**, 549–57.

Kazdin, A.E., Holland, L., and Crowley, M. (1997). Family experience of barriers to treatment and premature termination from child therapy. *Journal of Consulting and Clinical Psychology*, **65**, 453–63.

Kendall, P.C. (1994). Treating anxiety disorders in children: results of a randomized clinical trial. *Journal of Consulting and Clinical Psychology*, **62**, 100–10.

Kendall, P.C., Kane, M., Howard, B., and Siqueland, L. (1990). *Cognitive-behavioural therapy for anxious children*. Philadelphia, PA: Temple University.

Kendall, P.C., Flannery-Schroeder, E., Panichelli-Mindel, S.M., Southam-Gerow, M.A., Henin, A., and Warman, M. (1997). Therapy for youths with anxiety disorders: a second randomized clinical trial. *Journal of Consulting and Clinical Psychology*, **65**, 366–80.

King, N.J. and Ollendick, T.H. (1997). Annotation: treatment of childhood phobias. *Journal of Child Psychology and Psychiatry*, **38**, 389–400.

Koerner, K. and Linehan, M.M. (1992). Integrative therapy for borderline personality disorder: dialectical behaviour therapy. In *Handbook of psychotherapy integration* (ed. M.R. Goldfried and J.C. Norcross). New York: Basic Books.

Koster, E.H., De Raedt, R., Goeleven, E., Franck, E., and Crombez, G. (2005). Mood-congruent attentional bias in dysphoria: maintained attention to and impaired disengagement from negative information. *Emotion*, **5**, 446–55.

Kroll, L., Harrington, R., Jayson, D., Fraser, J., and Gowers, S. (1996). Pilot study of continuation cognitive-behavioral therapy for major depression in adolescent psychiatric patients. *Journal of the American Academy of Child and Adolescent Psychiatry*, **35**, 1156–61.

Kyte, Z.A., Goodyer, I.M., and Sahakian, B.J. (2005). Selected executive skills in adolescents with recent first episode major depression. *Journal of Child Psychology and Psychiatry*, **46**, 995–1005.

Lambert, M. and Ogless, B.M. (2004). The efficacy and effectiveness of psychotherapy. In *Bergin and Garfield's handbook of psychotherapy and behavior change* (5th edn) (ed. M. Lambert). New York: John Wiley.

Last, C.G., Hansen, C., and Franco, N. (1998). Cognitive-behavioral treatment of school phobia. *Journal of the American Academy of Child and Adolescent Psychiatry*, **37**, 404–11.

Lees, J., Manning, N., and Rawlings, B. (1999). *Therapeutic community effectiveness. A systematic international review of therapeutic community treatment for people with personality disorders and mentally disordered offenders*. CRD Report 17, NHS Centre for Reviews and Dissemination, University of York.

Leslie, A.M. (1987). Pretense and representation: the origins of 'theory of mind'. *Psychological Review*, **94**, 412–26.

Lewinsohn, P.M. and Clarke, G.N. (1999). Psychosocial treatments for adolescent depression. *Clinical Psychology Review*, **19**, 329–42.

Lewinsohn, P.M., Clarke, G.N., Hops, H., and Andrews, J. (1990). Cognitive-behavioural treatment for depressed adolescents. *Behaviour Therapy*, **21**, 385–401.

Lewinsohn, P.M., Clarke, G.N., and Rohde, P. (1994). Psychological approaches to the treatment of depression in adolescents. In *Handbook of depression in children and adolescents* (ed. W.M. Reynolds and H.F. Johnston). New York: Plenum Press.

Lewinsohn, P.M., Clarke, G.N., Rohde, P., Hops, H., and Seeley, J.R. (1996). A course in coping: a cognitive-behavioral approach to the treatment of adolescent depression.

In *Psychosocial treatments for child and adolescent disorders: empirically based strategies for clinical practice* (ed. E.D. Hibbs and P.S. Jensen). Washington, DC: American Psychological Association.

Lillard, A.S. (1993). Pretend play skills and the child's theory of mind. *Child Development*, **64**, 348–71.

Linehan, M.M. (1993). The skills training manual for treating borderline personality disorder. New York: Guilford Press.

Linehan, M.M. and Heard, H. (1993). Impact of treatment accessibility on clinical course of parasuicidal patients: reply. *Archives of General Psychiatry*, **50**, 157–8.

Linehan, M.M., Armstrong, H.E., Suarez, A., Allmon, D., and Heard, H. (1991). Cognitive-behavioural treatment of chronically parasuicidal borderline patients. *Archives of General Psychiatry*, **48**, 1060–64.

Linehan, M.M., Heard, H.L., and Armstrong, H.E. (1993). Naturalistic follow-up of a behavioral treatment for chronically parasuicidal borderline patients. *Archives of General Psychiatry*, **50**, 971–4.

Linehan, M.M., Dimeff, L.A., Reynolds, S.K., et al. (2002). Dialectical behavior therapy versus comprehensive validation therapy plus 12-step for the treatment of opioid dependent women meeting criteria for borderline personality disorder. *Drug Alcohol Dependence*, **67**, 13–26.

Linehan, M.M., Comtois, K.A., Murray, A.M., et al. (2006). Two-year randomized controlled trial and follow-up of dialectical behavior therapy vs therapy by experts for suicidal behaviors and borderline personality disorder. *Archives of General Psychiatry*, **63**, 757–66.

Lochman, J.E., Coie, J.D., Underwood, M.K., and Terry, R. (1993). Effectiveness of a social relations intervention program for aggressive and nonaggressive, rejected children. *Journal of Consulting and Clinical Psychology*, **61**, 1053–8.

Long, P., Forehand, R., Wierson, M., and Morgan, A. (1994). Moving into adulthood: does parent training with young noncompliant children have long-term effects? *Behaviour Research and Therapy*, **32**, 101–7.

Lord, C. and Rutter, M. (1994). Autism and pervasive developmental disorders. In *Child and adolescent psychiatry: modern approaches* (3rd edn) (ed. M. Rutter, E. Taylor, and L. Hersov). Oxford: Blackwell Scientific.

Lovaas, O.I. (1987). Behavioral treatment and normal educational/intellectual functioning in young autistic children. *Journal of Consulting and Clinical Psychology*, **55**, 3–9.

Lynch, T.R., Chapman, A.L., Rosenthal, M.Z., Kuo, J.R., and Linehan, M.M. (2006). Mechanisms of change in dialectical behavior therapy: theoretical and empirical observations. *Journal of Clinical Psychology*, **62**, 459–80.

McCarty, C.A. and Weisz, J.R. (2007). Effects of psychotherapy for depression in children and adolescents. What we can (and can't) learn from meta-analysis and component profiling. *Journal of the American Academy of Child and Adolescent Psychiatry*, **46**, 879–86.

McEachin, J.J., Smith, T., and Lovaas, O.I. (1993). Long-term outcome for children with autism who received early intensive behavioral treatment. *American Journal of Mental Retardation*, **97**, 359–72.

Macfie, J., Toth, S.L., Rogosch, F.A., Robinson, J., Emde, R.N., and Cicchetti, D. (1999). Effect of maltreatment on preschoolers' narrative representations of responses to relieve distress and of role reversal. *Developmental Psychology*, **35**, 460–5.

Macfie, J., Cicchetti, D., and Toth, S.L. (2001). The development of dissociation in maltreated preschool-aged children. *Development and Psychopathology*, **13**, 233–54.

McGivern, R.F., Andersen, J., Byrd, D., Mutter, K.L., and Reilly, J. (2002). Cognitive efficiency on a match to sample task decreases at the onset of puberty in children. *Brain and Cognition*, **50**, 73–89.

McMahon, R.J., Forehand, R., Griest, D.L., and Wells, K.C. (1981). Who drops out of treatment during parent behavioural training? *Behavioural Counseling Quarterly*, **1**, 79–95.

Manassis, K., Mendlowitz, S.L., Scapillato, D., et al. (2002). Group and individual cognitive-behavioral therapy for childhood anxiety disorders: a randomized trial. *Journal of the American Academy Child and Adolescent Psychiatry*, **41**, 1423–30.

March, J.S. (1995). Cognitive-behavioral psychotherapy for children and adolescents with OCD: a review and recommendations for treatment. *Journal of the American Academy of Child and Adolescent Psychiatry*, **34**, 7–18.

March, J.S. and Leonard, H.L. (1996). Obsessive–compulsive disorder in children and adolescents: a review of the past 10 years. *Journal of the American Academy of Child and Adolescent Psychiatry*, **35**, 1265–73.

March, J.S. and Mulle, K. (1995). Behavioral psychotherapy for obsessive–compulsive disorder: a preliminary single-case study. *Journal of Anxiety Disorders*, **9**, 175–84.

March, J.S., Mulle, K., and Herbel, B. (1994). Behavioral psychotherapy for children and adolescents with obsessive–compulsive disorder: an open trial of a new protocol-driven treatment package. *Journal of the American Academy of Child and Adolescent Psychiatry*, **33**, 333–41.

March, J.S., Franklin, M., Nelson, A., and Foa, E. (2001). Cognitive-behavioral psychotherapy for pediatric obsessive–compulsive disorder. *Journal of Clinical Child Psychology*, **30**, 8–18.

March, J., Silva, S., Petrycki, S., et al. (2004). Fluoxetine, cognitive-behavioral therapy, and their combination for adolescents with depression: Treatment for Adolescents With Depression Study (TADS) randomized controlled trial. *Journal of the American Medical Association*, **292**, 807–20.

March, J., Silva, S., and Vitiello, B. (2006). The Treatment for Adolescents with Depression Study (TADS): methods and message at 12 weeks. *Journal of the American Academy of Child and Adolescent Psychiatry*, **45**, 1393–1403.

March, J.S., Silva, S., Petrycki, S., et al. (2007). The Treatment for Adolescents With Depression Study (TADS): long-term effectiveness and safety outcomes. *Archives of General Psychiatry*, **64**, 1132–43.

Marjoram, D., Miller, P., Mcintosh, A.M. Cunningham Owens, D.G., Johnstone, E.C., and Lawrie, S. (2006). A neuropsychological investigation into 'theory of mind' and enhanced risk of schizophrenia. *Psychiatry Research*, **144**, 29–37.

Marks, I.M. (2002). The maturing of therapy: some brief psychotherapies help anxiety/depressive disorders but mechanisms of action are unclear. *British Journal of Psychiatry*, **180**, 200–4.

Mataix-Cols, D. and Marks, I.M. (2006). Self-help with minimal therapist contact for obsessive–compulsive disorder: a review. *European Psychiatry*, **21**, 75–80.

Matson, J.L. and Swiezy, N. (1994). Social skills training with autistic children. In *Autism in children and adults: etiology assessment and intervention*. (ed. J.L.Matson). Pacific Grove, CA: Brooks–Cole.

Matson, J.L., Sevin, J.A., Fridley, D., and Love, S.R. (1990). Increasing spontaneous language in three autistic children. *Journal of Applied Behavioural Analysis*, **23**, 227–34.

Matson, J.L., Sevin, J.A., Box, M.L., and Francis, K.L. (1993). An evaluation of two methods for increasing self-initiated verbalisations in autistic children. *Journal of Applied Behaviour Analysis*, **26**, 389–98.

Mendlowitz, S.L., Manassis, K., Bradley, S., Scalpillato, D., Miezitis, S., and Shaw, B.F. (1999). Cognitive-behavioral group treatments in childhood anxiety disorders: the role of parental involvement. *Journal of the American Academy of Child and Adolescent Psychiatry*, **38**, 1223–9.

Mesibov, G.B. (1986). A cognitive program for teaching social behaviours in verbal autistic adolescents and adults. In *Social behaviour in autism* (ed. E. Schopler and G.B. Mesibov). New York: Plenum Press.

Michael, K.D. and Crowley, S.L. (2002). How effective are treatments for child and adolescent depression? A meta-analytic review. *Clinical Psychology Review*, **22**, 247–69.

Miles, A., Polychronis, A., and Grey, J.E (2006). The evidence-based health care debate–2006. Where are we now? *Journal of Evaluation in Clinical Practice*, **12**, 239–47.

Miller, G.E. and Prinz, R.J. (1990). The enhancement of social learning family interventions for childhood conduct disorders. *Psychological Bulletin*, **108**, 291–307.

Moffitt, T.E., Caspi, A., Harrington, H., and Milne, B.J. (2002). Males on the life-course-persistent and adolescence-limited antisocial pathways: follow-up at age 26 years. *Developmental Psychopathology*, **14**, 179–207.

Monk, C.S., McClure, E.B., Nelson, E.E., *et al.* (2003). Adolescent immaturity in attention-related brain engagement to emotional facial expressions. *NeuroImage*, **20**, 420–8.

Moreau, D., Mufson, L., Weissman, M.M., and Klerman, G.L. (1991). Interpersonal psychotherapy for adolescent depression: description of modification and preliminary application. *Journal of the American Academy of Child and Adolescent Psychiatry*, **30**, 642–51.

Morgan, J. and Banerjee, R. (2006). Social anxiety and self-evaluation of social performance in a nonclinical sample of children. *Journal of Clinical Child Adolescent Psychology*, **35**, 292–301.

Mufson, L., Moreau, D., Weissman, M.M., and Wickramaratne, P. (1994). Modification of interpersonal psychotherapy with depressed adolescents. *Journal of the American Academy of Child and Adolescent Psychiatry*, **33**, 695–705.

Mufson, L., Weissman, M.M., Moreau, D., and Garfinkel, R (1999). Efficacy of interpersonal psychotherapy for depressed adolescents. *Archives of General Psychiatry*, **56**, 573–9.

Mufson, L., Dorta, K.P., Wickramaratne, P., Nomura, Y., Olfson, M., and Weissman, M.M. (2004). A randomized effectiveness trial of interpersonal psychotherapy for depressed adolescents. *Archives of General Psychiatry*, **61**, 577–84.

Muratori, F., Picchi, L., Casella, C., Tancredi, R., Milone, A., and Patarnello, M.G. (2001). Efficacy of brief dynamic psychotherapy for children with emotional disorders. *Psychotherapy and Psychosomatics*, **71**, 28–38.

Muratori, F., Picchi, L., Bruni, G., Patarnello, M., and Romagnoli, G. (2003). A two-year follow-up of psychodynamic psychotherapy for internalizing disorders in children. *Journal of the American Academy of Child and Adolescent Psychiatry*, **42**, 331–9.

Muris, P., Merckelbach, H., Holdrinet, I., and Sijsenaar, M. (1998). Treating phobic children: effects of EMDR vs. exposure. *Journal of Consulting and Clinical Psychology*, **66**, 193–8.

Muris, P., Luermans, J., Merckelbach, H., and Mayer, B. (2000). 'Danger is lurking everywhere'. the relation between anxiety and threat perception abnormalities in normal children. *Journal of Behavior Therapy and Experimental Psychiatry*, **31**, 123–36.

Murray L, Cooper, P., Creswell, C., Schofield, E., and Sack, C. (2007). The effects of maternal social phobia on mother-infant interactions and infant social responsiveness. *Journal of Child Psychology and Psychiatry*, **48**, 45–52.

Neshat-Doost, H.T., Moradi, A.R., Taghavi, M.R., Yule, W., and Dalgleish, T. (2000). Lack of attentional bias for emotional information in clinically depressed children and adolescents on the dot probe task. *Journal of Child Psychology and Psychiatry*, **41**, 363–8.

Neziroglu, F., Yaryura-Tobias, J.A., Walz, J., and McKay, D. (2000). The effect of fluvoxamine and behavior therapy on children and adolescents with obsessive–compulsive disorder. *Journal of Child and Adolescent Psychopharmacology*, **10**, 295–306.

NICHD Early Child Care Research Network (2004). Trajectories of physical aggression from toddlerhood to middle childhood: predictors, correlates, and outcomes. *Monographs of the Society for Research in Child Development*, **69**, 1–129.

Nixon, R.D., Sweeny, L., Erickson, D.B., and Touyz, S.W. (2003). Parent–child interaction therapy: a comparison of standard and abbreviated treatments for oppositional defiant preschoolers. *Journal of Consulting and Clinical Psychology*, **71**, 251–60.

Nolen-Hoeksema, S. (2000). The role of rumination in depressive disorders and mixed anxiety/depressive symptoms. *Journal of Abnormal Psychology*, **109**, 504–11.

Nye, C.L., Zucker, R.A., and Fitzgerald, H.E. (1995). Early intervention in the path to alcohol problems through conduct problems: treatment involvement and child behaviour change. *Journal of Consulting and Clinical Psychology*, **63**, 831–40.

Ollendick, T.H. and King, N.J. (1998). Empirically supported treatments for children with phobic and anxiety disorders. *Journal of Clinical Child Psychology*, **27**, 156–67.

Park, R.J., Goodyer, I.M., and Teasdale, J.D. (2004). Effects of induced rumination and distraction on mood and overgeneral autobiographical memory in adolescent major depressive disorder and controls. *Journal of Child Psychology and Psychiatry*, **45**, 996–1006.

Patterson, G.R. (1982). *Coercive family processes*, Eugene, OR: Castalia.

Patterson, G.R. and Chamberlain, P. (1988). Treatment process: a problem at three levels. In *The state of the art in family therapy research: controversies and recommendations* (ed. L.C. Wynne). New York: Family Process Press.

Patterson, G.R. and Forgatch, M.S. (1987). *Parents and adolescents living together. Part 1. The basics*. Eugene, OR, Castalia.

Penn, D.L. and Combs, D. (2000). Modification of affect perception deficits in schizophrenia. *Schizophrenia Research*, **46**, 217–29.

Perner, J., Kain, W., and Barchfield, P. (2002). Executive control and higher-order theory of mind in children at risk of ADHD. *Infant and Child Development*, **11**, 141–58.

Pessiglione, M., Schmidt, L., Draganski, B., *et al.* (2007). How the brain translates money into force: a neuroimaging study of subliminal motivation. *Science*, **316**, 904–6.

Pickup, G.J. (2006). Theory of mind and its relation to schizotypy. *Cognitive Neuropsychiatry*, **11**, 177–92.

Pickup, G.J. and Frith, C.D. (2001). Theory of mind impairments in schizophrenia: symptomatology, severity and specificity. *Psychological Medicine*, **31**, 207–20.

Pinkham, A.E. and Penn, D.L. (2006). Neurocognitive and social cognitive predictors of interpersonal skill in schizophrenia. *Psychiatry Research*, **143**, 167–78.

Quinn, M.M., Kavale, K.A., Mathur, S.R., Rutherford, R.B., and Forness, S.R. (1999). A meta-analysis of social skill interventions for students with emotional or behavioral disorders. *Journal of Emotional and Behavioral Disorders*, **7**, 54–64.

Rakoczy, H., Tomasello, M., and Striano, T. (2005). On tools and toys: how children learn to act on and pretend with 'virgin objects'. *Development Science*, **8**, 57–73.

Reinecke, M.A., Ryan, N.E., and Dubois, D.L. (1998). Cognitive-behavioral therapy of depression and depressive symptoms during adolescence: a review and meta-analysis. *Journal of the American Academy of Child and Adolescent Psychiatry*, **37**, 26–34.

Reiss, D. and Leve, L. (2007). Genetic expression outside the skin: clues to mechanisms of Genotype × Environment interaction. *Development and Psychopathology*, **19**, 1005–27.

Reynolds, W.M. and Coats, K.I. (1986). A comparison of cognitive-behavioural therapy and relaxation training for the treatment of depression in adolescents. *Journal of Consulting and Clinical Psychology*, **54**, 653–60.

Rosselló, J. and Bernal, G. (1999). The efficacy of cognitive-behavioral and interpersonal treatments for depression in Puerto Rican adolescents. *Journal of Consulting and Clinical Psychology*, **67**, 734–45.

Roth, A. and Fonagy, P. (2005). *What works for whom? A critical review of psychotherapy research*. New York: Guilford Press.

Roth *et al.* (2002).

Routh, C.P., Hill, J.W., Steele, H., Elliott, C.E., and Dewey, M.E. (1995). Maternal attachment status, psychosocial stressor and problem behaviour: follow-up after parent training course for Conduct Disorder. *Journal of Child Psychology and Psychiatry*, **36**, 1179–98.

Russell, T.A., Chu, E., and Phillips, M.L. (2006). A pilot study to investigate the effectiveness of emotion recognition remediation in schizophrenia using the micro-expression training tool. *British Journal of Clinical Psychology*, **45**, 579–83.

Ryle, A. and Golynkina, K. (2000). Effectiveness of time-limited cognitive analytic therapy of borderline personality disorder: factors associated with outcome. *British Journal of Medical Psychology*, **73**, 197–210.

Sackett, D.L., Richardson, W.S., Rosenberg, W.M., and Haynes, R.B. (2000). *Evidence-based medicine: how to practice and teach EBM*. Edinburgh: Churchill Livingstone.

Santisteban, D.A., Perez-Vidal, A., Coatsworth, J.D., *et al.* (2003). The efficacy of brief strategic family therapy in modifying Hispanic adolescent behavior problems and substance use. *Journal of Family Psychology*, **17**, 121–33.

Santor, D.A. and Kusumakar, V. (2001). Open trial of interpersonal therapy in adolescents with moderate to severe major depression: effectiveness of novice IPT therapists. *Journal of the American Academy Child and Adolescent Psychiatry*, **40**, 236–40.

Schiffman, J., Lam, C.W., Jiwatram, T., Ekstrom, M., Sorensen, H., and Mednick, S. (2004). Perspective-taking deficits in people with schizophrenia spectrum disorders: a prospective investigation. *Psychological Medicine*, **34**, 1581–6.

Schuhmann, E.M., Foote, R.C., Eyberg, S.M., Boggs, S.R., and Algina, J. (1998). Efficacy of parent–child interaction therapy: interim report of a randomized trial with short-term maintenance. *Journal of Clinical Child Psychology*, **27**, 34–45.

Scott, S., Spender, Q., Doolan, M., Jacobs, B., and Aspland, H. (2001). Multicentre controlled trial of parenting groups for childhood antisocial behaviour in clinical practice. *British Medical Journal*, **323**, 194–8.

Shamay-Tsoory, S.G., Shur, S., Harari, H., and Levkovitz, Y. (2007). Neurocognitive basis of impaired empathy in schizophrenia. *Neuropsychology*, **21**, 431–8.

Sharp, C. (2006). Mentalizing problems in childhood disorders. In *Handbook of mentalization-based treatments* ((ed. J.G. Allen and P. Fonagy.), pp. 201–12. Chichester: John Wiley.

Sharp, C. and Fonagy, P. The parent's capacity to treat the child as a psychological agent: constructs, measures and implications for developmental psychopathology. *Social Development*, in press.

Sharp, C., Croudace, T.J., and Goodyer, I.M. (2007). Biased mentalising in children aged 7–11: latent class confirmation of response styles to social scenarios and associations with psychopathology. *Social Development*, **16**, 181–202.

Shearin, E. and Linehan, M.M. (1992). Patient-therapist ratings and relationship to progress in dialectical behaviour therapy for borderline personality disorder. *Behaviour Therapy*, **23**, 730–41.

Shortt, A.L., Barrett, P.M., Dadds, M.R., and Fox, T.L. (2001). The influence of family and experimental context on cognition in anxious children. *Journal of Abnormal Child Psychology*, **29**, 585–96.

Silver, H., Goodman, C., Knoll, G., and Isakov, V. (2004). Brief emotion training improves recognition of facial emotions in chronic schizophrenia: a pilot study. *Psychiatry Research*, **128**, 147–54.

Silver, M. and Oakes, P. (2001). Evaluation of a new computer intervention to teach people with autism or Asperger syndrome to recognize and predict emotions in others. *Autism*, **5**, 299–316.

Silverman, W.K. and Kurtines, W.M. (1996). Transfer of control: a psychosocial intervention model for internalizing disorders in youth. In *Psychosocial treatments for child and adolescent disorders: empirically based strategies for clinical practice* (ed. E.D. Hibbs and P.S. Jensen). Washington, DC: American Psychological Association.

Silverman, W.K., Kurtines, W.M., Ginsburg, G.S., Weems, C.F., Rabain, B., and Serafini, L.T. (1999). Contingency management, self-control, and education support in the treatment of childhood phobic disorders: a randomized clinical trial. *Journal of Consulting and Clinical Psychology*, **67**, 675–87.

Sinha, U.K. and Kapur, M. (1999). Psychotherapy with emotionally disturbed adolescent boys: Outcome and process study. *NIMHANS Journal*, **17**, 113–30.

Slade, A. (2005). Parental reflective functioning: an introduction. *Attachment and Human Development*, **7**, 269–81.

Spielmans, G.I., Pasek, L.F., and McFall, J.P. (2007). What are the active ingredients in cognitive and behavioral psychotherapy for anxious and depressed children? A meta-analytic review. *Clinical Psychology Review*, **27**, 642–54.

Sprong, M., Schothorst, P., Vos, E., Hox, J., and Van Engeland, H. (2007). Theory of mind in schizophrenia: meta-analysis. *British Journal of Psychiatry*, **191**, 5–13.

Steer, R.A., Clark, D.A., and Ranieri, W.F. (1994). Symptom dimensions of the SCL-90-R: a test of the tripartite model of anxiety and depression. *Journal of Personality Assessment*, **62**, 525–36.

Steer, R.A., Clark, D.A., Beck, A.T., and Ranieri, W.F. (1995). Common and specific dimensions of self-reported anxiety and depression: a replication. *Journal of Abnormal Psychology*, **104**, 542–5.

Strauss, S.E., Richardson, W.S., Glasziou, P., and Haynes, R.B. (2005). *Evidence-based medicine: how to practice and teach EBM*. New York: Elsevier.

Sutton, J., Smith, P.K., and Swettenham, J. (1999a). Bullying and 'theory of mind': a critique of the 'social skills deficit' view of anti-social behaviour. *Social Development*, **8**, 117–27.

Sutton, J., Smith, P.K., and Swettenham, J. (1999b). Social cognition and bullying: social inadequacy or skilled manipulation? *British Journal of Developmental Psychology*, **17**, 435–50.

Swenson, C. (2000). How can we account for DBT's widespread popularity. *Clinical Psychology Science and Practice*, **7**, 87–91.

Szapocznik, J., Rio, A., Murray, E., *et al.* (1989). Structural family versus psychodynamic child therapy for problematic Hispanic boys. *Journal of Consulting and Clinical Psychology*, **57**, 571–8.

Tager-Flusberg, H. (2001). A re-examination of the theory of mind hypothesis of autism. In *The development of autism: perspectives from theory and research* (ed. J. Burack, T. Charman, N. Yirmiya, and P. Zelazo). Mahwah, NJ: Lawrence Erlbaum.

Target, M. and Fonagy, P. (1994). The efficacy of psychoanalysis for children with emotional disorders. *Journal of the American Academy of Child and Adolescent Psychiatry*, **33**, 361–71.

Target, M. and Fonagy, P. (2005). The psychological treatment of child and adolescent psychiatric disorders. In *What works for whom? A critical review of psychotherapy research* (2nd edn) (ed. A. Roth and P. Fonagy). New York: Guilford Press.

Taylor, T.K., Schmidt, F., Pepler, D., and Hodgins, C. (1998). A comparison of eclectic treatment with Webster-Stratton's Parents and Children Series in a children's mental health center: a randomized controlled trial. *Behavior Therapy*, **29**, 221–40.

Thompson, P.M., Giedd, J.N., Woods, R.P., Macdonald, D., Evans, A.C., and Toga, A.W. (2000). Growth patterns in the developing brain detected by using continuum mechanical tensor maps. *Nature*, **404**, 190–3.

Toren, P., Wolmer, L., Rosental, B., *et al.* (2000). Case series: brief parent–child group therapy for childhood anxiety disorders using a manual-based cognitive-behavioral technique. *Journal of the American Academy of Child and Adolescent Psychiatry*, **39**, 1309–12.

Toth, S.L., Cicchetti, D., Macfie. J., Maughan, A., and Vanmeenen, K. (2000). Narrative representations of caregivers and seld in maltreated pre-schoolers. *Attachment and Human Development*, **2**, 271–305.

Toth, S.L., Maughan, A., Manly, J.T., Spagnola, M., and Cicchetti, D. (2002). The relative efficacy of two interventions in altering maltreated preschool children's representational models: implications for attachment theory. *Developmental Psychopathology*, **14**, 877–908.

Toth, S.L., Rogosch, F.A., Manly, J.T., and Cicchetti, D. (2006). The efficacy of toddler-parent psychotherapy to reorganize attachment in the young offspring of mothers with major depressive disorder: a randomized preventive trial. *Journal of Consulting and Clinical Psychology*, **74**, 1006–16.

Tremblay, R.E., Nagin, D.S., Seguin, J.R., et al. (2004). Physical aggression during early childhood: trajectories and predictors. *Pediatrics*, **114**, e43–50.

Trowell, J., Joffe, I., Campbell, J., et al. (2007). Childhood depression: a place for psychotherapy: an outcome study comparing individual psychodynamic psychotherapy and family therapy. *European Child and Adolescent Psychiatry*, **16**, 157–67.

Tyrer, P., Tom, B., Byford, S., et al. (2004). Differential effects of manual assisted cognitive behavior therapy in the treatment of recurrent deliberate self-harm and personality disturbance: the POPMACT study. *Journal of Personality Disorders*, **18**, 102–16.

Vassilopoulos, S. (2005). Social anxiety and the vigilance–avoidance pattern of of attentional processing. *Behavioural and Cognitive Psychotherapy*, **33**, 13–24.

Velting, O., Setzer, N., and Albano, A, (2004). Update on and advance in assessment and cognitive-behavioral treatment of anxiety disorders in children and adolescents. *Professional Psychology: research and Practice*, **35**, 42–54.

Voelz, Z.R., Haeffel, G.J., Joiner, T.E., Jr., and Dineen Wagner, K. (2003). Reducing hopelessness: the interation of enhancing and depressogenic attributional styles for positive and negative life events among youth psychiatric inpatients. *Behaviour Research and Therapy*, **41**, 1183–98.

Wampold, B.E. (2001). The great psychotherapy debate: models, methods, and findings. Hillsdale, NJ: Lawrence Erlbaum.

Wampold, B.E., Minami, T., Baskin, T.W., and Callen Tierney, S. (2002). A meta-(re)analysis of the effects of cognitive therapy versus 'other therapies' for depression. *Journal of Affective Disorders*, **68**, 159–65.

Watkins, E. and Teasdale, J.D. (2004). Adaptive and maladaptive self-focus in depression. *Journal of Affective Disorders*, **82**, 1–8.

Watkins, E., Teasdale, J.D., and Williams, R.M. (2000). Decentring and distraction reduce overgeneral autobiographical memory in depression. *Psychological Medicine*, **30**, 911–20.

Webster-Stratton, C. (1981). Modification of mothers' behaviours and attitudes through a videotape modelling group discussion programme. *Behaviour Therapy*, **12**, 634–42.

Webster-Stratton, C. (1982). Teaching mothers through videotape modelling to change their children's behaviour. *Journal of Pediatric Psychology*, **7**, 279–94.

Webster-Stratton, C. (1984). Randomized trial of two parent-training programmes for families with conduct-disordered children. *Journal of Consulting and Clinical Psychology*, **52**, 666–78.

Webster-Stratton, C. (1990). Enhancing the effectiveness of self-administered videotape parent training for families with conduct-problem children. *Journal of Abnormal Child Psychology*, **18**, 479–92.

Webster-Stratton, C. (1992). The Incredible Years: a trouble-shooting guide for parents and children aged 3–8. Toronto: Umbrella Press.

Webster-Stratton, C. (1994). Advancing videotape parent training: a comparison study. *Journal of Consulting and Clinical Psychology*, **62**, 583–593.

Webster-Stratton, C. (1996a). Early-onset conduct problems: does gender make a difference? *Journal of Consulting and Clinical Psychology*, **64**, 540–51.

Webster-Stratton, C. (1996b). Early intervention with videotape modelling: programmes for families of children with oppositional defiant disorder or conduct disorder. In In *Psychosocial treatments for child and adolescent disorders: empirically based strategies for clinical practice* (ed. E.S. Hibbs and P.S. Jensen). Washington, DC: American Psychological Association.

Webster-Stratton, C. (1998). Preventing conduct problems in Head Start children: strengthening parenting competencies. *Journal of Consulting and Clinical Psychology*, **66**, 715–30.

Webster-Stratton, C. and Hammond, M. (1997). Treating children with early-onset conduct problems: a comparison of child and parent training interventions. *Journal of Consulting and Clinical Psychology*, **65**, 93–109.

Webster-Stratton, C. and Reid, M.J. (2003). The incredible years parents, teachers and children training series. In *Evidence-based psychotherapies for children and adolescents* (ed. A.E. Kazdin and J.R. Weisz). New York: Guilford Press.

Webster-Stratton, C., Kolpacoff, M., and Hollinsworth, T. (1988). Self-administered videotape therapy for families with conduct problem children: comparison of two cost-effective treatments and a control group. *Journal of Consulting and Clinical Psychology*, **57**, 550–3.

Webster-Stratton, C., Hollinsworth, T., and Kolpacoff, M. (1989). The long-term cost effectiveness and clinical significance of three cost-effective training programs for families with conduct problem children. *Journal of Consulting and Clinical Psychology*, **57**, 550–3.

Weisz, J.R., Doss, A.J., and Hawley, K.M. (2005). Youth psychotherapy outcome research: a review and critique of the evidence base. *Annual Review of Psychology*, **56**, 337–63.

Weisz, J.R., Jensen-Doss, A., and Hawley, K.M. (2006a). Evidence-based youth psychotherapies versus usual clinical care: a meta-analysis of direct comparisons. *American Psychologist*, **61**, 671–89.

Weisz, J.R., McCarty, C.A., and Valeri, S.M. (2006b). Effects of psychotherapy for depression in children and adolescents: a meta-analysis. *Psychological Bulletin*, **132**, 132–49.

Whalen, C. and Schreibman, L. (2003). Joint attention training for children with autism using behavior modification procedures. *Journal of Child Psychology and Psychiatry*, **44**, 456–68.

Wilberg, T., Friis, S., Karterud, S., Mehlum, L., Urnes, O., and Vaglum, P. (1998). Outpatient group psychotherapy: a valuable continuation treatment for patients with borderline personality disorder treated in a day hospital? A 3-year follow-up study. *Nordic Journal of Psychiatry*, **52**, 213–22.

Wolwer, W., Fromann, N., Halfmann, S., Piaszek, A., Streit, M., and Gaebel, W. (2005). Remediation of impairments in facial affect recognition in schizophrenia: efficacy and specificity of a new training program. *Schizophrenia Research*, **80**, 295–303.

Wood, A.J., Harrington, R.C., and Moore, A. (1996). Controlled trial of a brief cognitive-behavioural intervention in adolescent patients with depressive disorders. *Journal of Child Psychology and Psychiatry*, **37**, 737–46.

Woolfenden, S.R., Williams, K., and Peat, J.K. (2002). Family and parenting interventions for conduct disorder and delinquency: a meta-analysis of randomised controlled trials. *Archives of Disease in Childhood*, **86**, 251–6.

Woolfenden, S.R., Williams, K., and Peat, J.K. (2003). Family and parenting interventions in children and adolescents with conduct disorder and delinquency aged 10–17 (Cochrane Review). Cochrane Library, Issue 4. Chichester: John Wiley.

Wykes, T., Hamid, S., and Wagstaff, K. (2001). Theory of mind and executive function in the non-psychotic siblings of patients with schizophrenia. *Schizophrenia Research*, **49**, 148.

Index

abuse
  aggression development 185, 186
  distress response 343
  Williams syndrome 72–3
acute stress disorder 240
adoption studies 389–91, 392
affective labelling 354
agent-affective state-proposition 32
aggression
  abuse 185, 186
  approval of 145–6
  attention 150
  attributions 151–4
  autonomic arousal 159–60
  behavioural genetics 445
  biology 159–61
  cortisol 159
  cost/benefit 158
  criminality 141
  electrodermal response 159
  emotion understanding 370
  encoding deficits 148–51
  experiential influences 161–2
  fear–dysfunction hypothesis 160
  goal clarification 154–5
  heterogeneous construct 148
  hostile bias 151–4
  interpretation 151–4
  intervention 162–3
  parenting 185–6
  perception of 145–6
  proactive 148
  reactive 148
  representation 151–4
  response evaluation
    and decision 157–9
  response generation 156–7
  resting heart rate 159
  schemas 144
  social information
    processing 147–59
  socialization 161–2
  stability 146–7
  stimulation-seeking 160
  threat exposure 185, 186
  threat perception 153, 160–1
agoraphobia 240
amygdala 9, 37, 38, 39–40, 178, 179–80, 182, 220, 396, 415, 433

anger management training 441
animal
  mentalizing 310
  psychopathy model 188
anterior cingulate 9, 36, 37, 219, 220, 397
antidepressants 413, 426–7
Antisocial Process Screening Device 176
anxiety 239–69
  assessment and diagnosis 240–1
  attentional biases 245–6
  avoidance 245–6
  cognitive behavioural therapy 258–61, 433–6, 437–8
  cognitive theories 243–5
  depression and 19, 20, 241–3
  encoding 245–9
  environmental factors 257–8
  facial expression recognition 253–4
  family factors 257, 261
  family therapy 436
  genetics 256
  hyper-arousal 20, 242, 243, 245
  information processing 243–4, 246, 257, 259–60
  intergenerational transmission 395–6
  life experiences 258
  major types 240
  memory 248–9
  mentalizing 251–3
  modelling 433–4
  negative cognition 248, 249, 254–5
  parenting 257–8
  problem-solving 249–50
  psychodynamic psychotherapy 436
  reinforced exposure 434
  self-presentation 250–4
  social information processing 243–9, 254–5
  social skills 254–5, 260
  theory of mind 250–4
  threat perception 245–7, 258
  treatment 258–61, 433–8
  tripartite model 242, 243
aphasia 91
arousal
  aggression 159–60
  autism 39
  hyper-arousal in anxiety 20, 242, 243, 245
Asperger's syndrome 29, 34, 35, 100
associative network theory 206

attachment 20, 271
  borderline personality disorder 279–80
  disorganized 271, 279–80, 360
  emotion regulation 314
  emotion understanding 357, 359–60
  mentalizing 273–4, 306–11
  negative emotions 404
  theory of mind 273–4, 309
attention 145
  aggression 150
  anxiety 245–6
  depression 208, 214–15
  infants 325
  joint 30, 31, 37, 131, 404, 416–17
attention deficit–hyperactivity disorder (ADHD) 115, 119, 446
attributions/attributional style
  aggression 151–4
  behavioural genetics 399–400
  depression 209–11
auditory processing, autism 101–2; *see also* vocal emotion recognition
autism and autism spectrum conditions (ASC) 29–56
  arousal 39
  auditory processing 101–2
  behavioural training 415–17
  brain abnormalities 37–40
  comorbidity 41
  diagnosis 29
  emotion recognition 34–5, 42–4
  empathy 34
  epilepsy 38
  event-related potentials 39
  facial expression recognition 34–5, 37
  false belief 31
  genetics 40–2
  head circumference 38
  high-functioning 34, 35, 100
  interventions 42–4, 415–17
  IQ 29
  joint attention 131, 416–17
  language 17, 29, 100–3
  mental state recognition 35
  mindreading 34–6, 414
  molecular genetics 40–2
  shared attention 31
  sibling risk 40
  social brain 39–40
  social isolation 1
  social skills training 416
  social understanding training 416
  synaptic function 40–1
  theory of mind 15, 16, 71, 100–3
  training programmes 42–4, 415–17
  twin studies 40
  vocal emotion recognition 35
autobiographical memory 212–13

automatic processes 9
autonomic arousal 159–60
avoidance
  anxiety 245–6
  depression 214, 216

babbling 83
basal ganglia 9
basic emotions 32, 34, 311–13
behavioural automatisms 312
behavioural genetics 22, 387–410, 420
  aggression 445
  attributional style 399–400
  biological mechanisms 396–7
  empathy 400–1
  environmental factors 391
  gene–environment interplay 392–3
  hypotheses and strategies 388–91
  intergenerational transmission 394–6
  intervention 394, 395–6
  molecular genetics 393
  peer relationships 401–2
  psychopathy 401
  social cognition 397–402
  social competence 401–2
  theory of mind 398–9
behavioural inhibition 256
behavioural phenotypes 57, 58
behavioural training, autism 415–17
behaviour disorders, *see* disruptive behaviour disorders
biased mentalizing 425
biological factors 7–8
  aggression 159–61
  behavioural genetics 396–7
blindness
  affective information 32
  joint attention 31
  language development 17, 93–7
  theory of mind 98–100
borderline personality disorder
  aetiological model 285–7
  attachment 279–80
  cognitive therapy 423
  definition 272–3
  dialectical behaviour therapy 424
  facial expression recognition 277
  genetic factors 287
  interventions 287–92, 423–5
  mentalization-based treatment (MBT) 289–92
  mentalizing 277–9
  nature–nurture interaction 287
  parenting 280–5
  psychotherapy 423
  self-regulation 277
  social cognition 277–85

brain
    autism 37–40
    behavioural genetics 396–7
    C-system 9
    depression 220–2, 429–30, 433
    emotional empathy 178–80, 182
    empathy 36, 39, 189
    face processing 37, 68, 220
    gaze direction 36
    joint attention 37
    mindreading 36–7
    social cognition 219–20
    sympathy 36
    theory of mind 36, 397
    X-system 9
brainstem 37, 38
brooding 213
bullies 119, 446

callous–unemotional traits 158, 160, 176, 177, 184
care-based morality 181–2
catastrophising 6
caudate nucleus 37
causal contingency detection mechanism 314–16, 326–7
cerebellum 37–8
cerebral palsy 93
cingulate cortex 9, 36, 37, 219, 220, 221, 397
CNTNAP2 41
cochlear implants 85, 93
cognitive behavioural therapy 258–61, 425–7, 430–1, 433–6, 437–8
cognitive biases 20, 208, 245–9
cognitive constructs 2
cognitive empathy 177
cognitive therapy 423
cognitive triad 207
comorbidity 19, 20, 41, 115, 202–3, 241–3
computer-based training 42–3
conditioning 179
conduct disorder 115, 141
    anger management training 441
    family therapy 440–1
    multisystemic therapy 440–1
    'nasty minds' 119
    parent training 438–40
    problem-solving skills training 441–2
    SMART 449
    social information processing 442–6
    social skills training 441
    treatment 438–46, 449
conflict management 369–70
CONLERN 180
connectedness 122, 128, 447
conscience 182
CONSPEC 180

constitutional self 311–13, 324–5
constructs 4–5
contactin-associated protein-like 2 (CNTNAP2) 41
contingency detection mechanism 314–16, 326–7
controllable events 216
controlled processes 9
conversation ability
    blindness 95, 96–7
    emotion understanding 357, 358–9
    evolutionary process 81
    theory of mind 62, 81, 90, 92–3, 103
    Williams syndrome 60, 73
Coping Cat 434, 437
Coping Power Program 163
Coping With Depression 426
corpus callosum 38
cortisol 159
creativity 2
criminality 141
C-system 9
cuneus 397

deafness
    cochlear implants 85, 93
    language acquisition 17, 83–5, 86–7
    theory of mind 88–9, 92
decision making, depression 215–16
deep structure 8–9
deficit approach 6, 16
delusions 417–18
depression 201–37
    across the lifespan 203–4
    age specificity 432–3
    antidepressants 413, 426–7
    anxiety and 19, 20, 241–3
    attention 208, 214–15
    attributional style 209–11
    avoidance 214, 216
    brain 220–2, 429–30, 433
    brooding 213
    chronicity 218
    cognitive behavioural therapy 425–7, 430–1, 433
    comorbidity 202–3
    control 216
    cortical thickness 221
    decision making 215–16
    diagnosis 201–2
    differential activation hypothesis 206–7
    distraction 211–12, 213–14
    enactment 216–17
    encoding 208
    environmental factors 217–18
    family therapy 428–9
    gene–environment interaction 217–18

depression (*cont.*)
  hopefulness 209–10
  hopelessness 209
  impulsivity 216
  interpersonal therapy for adolescents (IPT-A) 427–8
  knowledge structures 206–8, 217–18
  learned helplessness 209
  locus of control 216
  memory 212–13
  negative schemas 206–8
  neural model 222, 223
  reflection 213
  relaxation training 428
  representations 208–11
  response accessing 211–15
  response evaluation 215–16
  rumination 211–13, 214
  social information processing 19, 205–17, 429
  symptoms 202–3
  treatment 425–33
  tripartite model 242, 243
depressogenic attributional style 209–11
developmental disorders 15–17
dialectical behaviour therapy 424
differential activation hypothesis 206–7
disorganized (disoriented) attachment 271, 279–80, 360
disruptive behaviour disorders 17–18, 115–39, 141, 446–7
  emotion understanding 125, 126
  environmental factors 162
  executive function 120, 129–30
  family influences 132
  interventions 132–3, 447–9
  maternal interactions 126–8
  parenting 119–21
  social cognition 119–21, 128–9
  theory of mind 119, 125, 126
  verbal ability 120
distorted mentalizing 425
distortion approach 6
distraction 211–12, 213–14
distress response 131, 181–2, 343–4
domain-generality 20, 246–7
domain-specificity 20
dorsal cingulate 9, 219
dorsolateral prefrontal cortex 220
dorsomedial prefrontal cortex 220
Down syndrome 68
dyadic representations 30, 31, 32

elastin 58
electrodermal response 159
Embedded Figures Task 39
embedding 30

emotion
  basic 32, 34, 311–13
  folk theories 352–3
  second-order representations 323–31
emotional competence 344, 345, 372–3
emotional deficits 6
emotional empathy 18–19, 177
  brain activity 178–80, 182
  care-based morality 181–2
  development 180–1
  psychopathy 178, 182–3
emotional self-states 323–7
emotion appraisal system 348, 351, 374
emotion attributional system 348, 351, 374
emotion control 314, 318–23, 331–2
Emotion Detector, The (TED) 31–2, 35–6
emotion matching 64
emotion processing tasks 12
emotion recognition 346
  anxiety 253–4
  autism 34–5, 42–4
  borderline personality disorder 277
  emotion understanding 353–4, 356, 374
  empathy 374
  maltreatment 361–3
  training 42–4
emotion representations 316–18, 323–31
emotion understanding 21–2, 343–85
  aggression 370
  attachment 357, 359–60
  components 350, 354
  conflict management 369–70
  conversations 357, 358–9
  development 349–52
  developmental precursors and correlates 357–65
  developmental psychopathology 345, 365, 373
  distress response 131
  emotional expressions 353–4, 356, 374
  family environment 357
  foundations 346–9
  hard-to-manage children 125, 126, 370
  language 347, 357, 358–9
  likeability 367, 372
  maltreatment 282, 360–4, 368
  maternal mind-mindedness 357, 359
  maternal reflective function 357
  measurement 353–5
  mental 350, 354
  organizational approach 375
  play 357
  prosocial behaviour 366–8, 372, 375
  public 350, 354
  reflective 350, 354
  situational 350, 354
  socio-emotional competence 365–73

tasks 10, 11, 13, 118
  theory of mind 351–2
Empathizing SyStem, The (TESS) 16, 32, 33, 35–6
empathy
  autism 34
  behavioural genetics 400–1
  brain activity 36, 39, 189
  cognitive 177
  emotion expression recognition 374
  individual differences 33–4
  motor 177
  psychopaths 35–6, 415
  schizophrenia 418
  see also emotional empathy
enactment 142, 205
  depression 216–17
encoding 142, 144, 204
  aggression 148–51
  anxiety 245–9
  depression 208
  tasks 11
  unconscious 150
environmental factors 7
  anxiety 257–8
  behavioural genetics 391
  depression 217–18
  disruptive behaviour 162
  psychopathy 184–6
  theory of mind 120, 287
  see also gene–environment interplay
E-representation 33, 414
event-related potentials 39, 102
evidence-based medicine 412–13
evocative genotype–environment correlations 392–3
executive function
  behaviour problems 120, 129–30
  social cognition 2
  tests 117–19
  theory of mind 130
experiential influences, aggression 161–2
explicit processes 9
externalizing disorders 17–19
Eye Direction Detector (EDD) 30, 36

facial expression recognition 346
  anxiety 253–4
  autism 34–5, 37
  borderline personality disorder 277
  emotion understanding 353
  maltreatment 361–2
  two-system model 180
face processing
  brain activity 37, 68, 220
  self-training 70
  typical development 67–8
  Williams syndrome 68–70

false belief
  autism 31
  blindness 99–100
  language growth 90
  parenting practices 274–5
  social competence 131–2
  testing theory of mind 30, 61–2, 87, 117, 309
family environment
  anxiety 257, 261
  behaviour problems 132
  emotion understanding 357
  social cognition 2
  theory of mind 120
family therapy
  anxiety 436
  behaviour problems 448–9
  conduct disorder 440–1
  depression 428–9
fantasy 2
Fast Track 163
faux pas 251, 252
fear
  aggression 160
  amygdala 396
  moral development 182
fluoxetine 413, 426–7
FMR1 40
FMRP 40
folk theories of emotion 352–3
fragile X syndrome 40, 57
friendships 366
frontal cortex 36, 37, 39, 70
functional family therapy 440–1
fusiform gyrus 37, 68, 70, 220

GABRB3 41
gaze monitoring 30
gene–environment interplay 22
  behavioural genetics 392–3
  depression 217–18
  maltreatment 162
  molecular genetics 393
generalized anxiety disorder 240
genetic factors 22
  anxiety 256
  autism 40–2
  borderline personality disorder 287
  psychopathy 184
  theory of mind 120
  Williams syndrome 74
  see also behavioural genetics
genotype–environment correlations 392–3
genotype–environment interactions 393
gestural communication 83–4, 87
goal clarification 12, 142, 154–5
grammar 8, 82, 89, 90, 91
grey matter 38

GRIK2 41
GRIN2A 41

hard-to-manage children 121–32, 370, 446–7
harsh parenting 120, 132
head circumference 38
heart rate 159
helplessness 209
hierarchy of evidence 413
high-functioning autism 34, 35, 100
hippocampus 37, 38
homo psychologicus 450
hopefulness 209–10
hopelessness 209
hostile attributional bias 144–5, 151–4
hostile goals 155
5-HTTLPR 188
hyperacusis 58
hyper-arousal 20, 242, 243, 245
hypersociability 60

imitation 32
implicit processes 9
impulsivity 216
Incredible Years Training Series 439
individual differences
  empathy 33–4
  social behaviour 128–9
  social cognition 1–2, 16, 404
  theory of mind 120
inferior frontal cortex 36
inferior frontal gyrus 36
information processing 6, 145
  anxiety 243–4, 246, 257, 259–60
  see also social information processing (SIP)
inhibitory control 119
instrumental goals 155
insula 179
Integrated Emotions Systems model 181
Intentionality Detector (ID) 29, 30, 36
interactions 21, 72, 126–8, 306–11
intergenerational transmission 394–6
internalizing disorders 19–20
internal working model 357
interpersonal characteristics 5–6
interpersonal therapy for
  adolescents (IPT-A) 427–8
interpretation 142, 144, 204
  aggression 151–4
  tasks 11
intersubjectivity 323
interventions
  aggression 162–3
  autism 42–4, 415–17
  behavioural genetics 394, 395–6
  behaviour problems 132–3, 447–9
  borderline personality disorder 287–92, 423–5

maltreatment 421–3
schizophrenia 418–19
social information processing 162–3
speech and language therapy 73
Williams syndrome 73
see also treatment
intrapersonal characteristics 5–6
introspective emotion recognition 325
intuitive mentalizing 131
IQ 29, 58, 186
isolated mind metaphor 450
joint attention 30, 31, 37, 131, 404, 416–17
knowledge structures 143, 205, 206–8, 217–18

language
  acquisition 82–7
  autism 17, 29, 100–3
  blindness 17, 93–7
  deafness 17, 83–5, 86–7
  deep structure 8
  emotion understanding 347, 357, 358–9
  evolutionary process 81
  innate linguistic structure 86
  social cognition 2, 16–17
  social experience 86
  socio-emotional competence 372
  theory of mind 81, 89–93
  Williams syndrome 59, 60, 72, 73
lateral parietal cortex 9
lateral prefrontal cortex 9
lateral temporal cortex 9
learned helplessness 209
learning disabilities, classification 57; *see also* Williams syndrome
left inferior frontal gyrus 36
left medial prefrontal cortex 37
left temporopolar cortex 397
life experiences 258
likeability 367, 372
limbic–cortical–striatal–pallidal–thalamic (LCSPT) circuit 222
limbic–thalamic–cortical (LTC) circuit 222
linguistic structure 86
locus of control 216

macrocephaly 38
macroparadigm 3
main effects models 393
major depressive disorder, *see* depression
maltreatment
  distress response 343
  emotion expression recognition 361–3
  emotion understanding 282, 360–4, 368
  gene–environment interplay 162
  interventions 421–3
  mentalization 282–3
  psychopathology risk 358
  theory of mind 283–4, 363–4, 421

manual babbling 83
MAOA 162, 188
'markedness' 327, 329–31
maternal interactions 126–8, 306–7
maternal mentalizing 2
maternal mind-mindedness 274, 276
  emotion understanding 357, 359
  social cognition 2
maternal reflective function 2, 274, 357
measurement of social cognition 10–14
MeCP2 41
medial frontal cortex 39
medial parietal cortex 9
medial prefrontal cortex 9, 36, 37, 430
medial temporal lobe 9
memory
  anxiety 248–9
  depression 212–13
mental emotion understanding 350, 354
mentalization-based treatment (MBT) 289–92, 448–9
mentalizing 21
  animals 310
  anxiety 251–3
  attachment 273–4, 306–11
  biased/distorted 425
  borderline personality disorder 277–9
  emotional self-control 331–2
  maltreated children 282–3
  maternal 2
  parents 13, 274–6
  secondary cognitive reappraisal 331–2
  tasks 13
  treatment outcomes 413–17
mental representation 142, 204
  aggression 151–4
  depression 208–11
mental states
  recognition in autism 35
  relationships 30–1
  social cognition 2
MET 41
middle frontal gyrus 397
mindful self-awareness 214
'mindless' parenting 280–5
mind-mindedness 274, 276
  emotion understanding 357, 359
  social cognition 2
Mind Reading 43
mindreading 16, 29–37, 414
minicolumns 38–9
mirroring 324, 326, 327
mirror neurons 36, 178
modelling 395, 433–4
molecular genetics 40–2, 188, 393
monoamine oxidase A 162, 188
moral socialization 181–2, 183–4
mother–child interactions 126–8, 306–7

motherese 32
motor empathy 177
M-representations 33, 414
multi-component CBT 434
multisystemic therapy 440–1

narcissism 176
'nasty minds' 119, 446
nature–nurture interaction 8, 287
necessity index 316
negative cognition 248, 249, 254–5
negative emotions 404
negative schemas 206–8
neurexin-1 41
neurocognitive systems 9
neuroligin genes 41
neurotic disorders 19
neurotoxins 162
NF1 41
NLGN3/NLGN4 41
NRXN1 41

obsessive–compulsive disorder 240, 435–6
oppositional defiant disorder 115, 141
orbitofrontal cortex 39, 220, 397, 430
ostensive communication 328–31
other-to-self causal emotion schemes 317–18
outcome expectations 157
outcome values 157
oxytocin 396

panic disorder 240
parents and parenting
  aggression 185–6
  anxiety 257–8
  behaviour disorders 119–21, 132
  borderline personality disorder 280–5
  false beliefs 274–5
  harsh parenting 120, 132
  mentalization 13, 274–6
  'mindless' 280–5
  modelling 395
  parent training for conduct problems 438–40
  theory of mind 398
  see also maternal headings
parietal cortex 9, 37, 38
passive genotype–environment correlations 392
pedagogy 328–9
peer relationships
  behavioural genetics 401–2
  behaviour bias 145
  emotion understanding 367
  social cognition 2
  Williams syndrome 60
perspective-taking 343–4, 354
physical abuse 185, 186

play 357
  pretend play 30, 61, 89, 91, 98
posterior superior temporal sulcus 36–7
post-traumatic stress disorder 240
poverty of the stimulus 81, 85
Prader–Willi syndrome 63–4
pragmatics 97
prefrontal cortex 9, 36, 37, 220, 397, 430
pretend play 30, 61, 89, 91, 98
prevention, usefulness of social cognitive constructs 15
primary response inhibition 318–20
problem-solving
  anxiety 249–50
  skills training 163, 441–2, 448
processing speed 145
prosocial behaviour 366–8, 372, 375
protodeclarative pointing 30
psychodynamic psychotherapy 436
psychopathy
  aetiology 184–6
  animal model 188
  antisocial behaviour 176
  assessment 175–6, 177, 186–7
  behavioural genetics 401
  emotional dysfunction 176
  emotional empathy 178, 182–3
  empathy 35–6, 415
  environmental factors 184–6
  genetics 184
  molecular genetics 188
  moral socialization/reasoning 183–4
  three-factor structure 176
  treatment 189, 417
  two-factor structure 176
Psychopathy Checklist (PCL/PCL-R) 175–6, 177
psychotherapy 422, 423, 436
PTEN 41
public emotion understanding 350, 354
Purkinje cells 38

recursion 30
referential knowledge manifestation 328–9
reflection 213
reflective emotion understanding 350, 354
reflective function 2, 274, 357
reinforced exposure 434
reinforcers 179
relational schemas 143
relaxation training 428
representation 142, 204
  aggression 151–4
  depression 208–11
representational affective self 311–23
response accessing 142, 204
  depression 211–15
response construction 142

response decision 142
  aggression 157–9
response evaluation 12, 157, 204–5
  aggression 157–9
  depression 215–16
response generation 12, 142
  aggression 156–7
response inhibition 318–20
response selection 142, 157
response substitution 320–1
Rett syndrome 41
right prefrontal cortex 36, 397
rostral cingulate 9, 219, 220, 221
rule-shifting 118–19
rumination 211–13, 214

Sally–Anne task 87
schemas 143, 144
  depression 206–8
schizophrenia 417–19
SCIT 419
scripts 143
secondary cognitive appraisal 321–3, 331–2
second-order belief attribution 63–4
second-order configural processing 69–70
second-order emotion representations 323–31
seeing-leads-to-knowing principle 31
self-efficacy 157
self-narrative 278
self-presentation 250–4
self-regulation 277
self-to-other causal emotion schemes 317
sentence complementation 90–1
separation anxiety disorder 240
sertraline 413
sex differences, empathy 33–4
sexual abuse 185, 186
SHANK3 41
Shared Attention Mechanism (SAM) 30, 31, 32, 37
sharing 123
Short-term Mentalizing and Relational Therapy (SMART) 289–92, 448–9
siblings
  autism 40
  social cognition 2
  studies 399
sign language 83, 84–5, 89
situated goals 154
situational emotion understanding 350, 354
SLC6A4 41
SMART 289–92, 448–9
Smarties task 87
sociability 59–60
social anxiety 240, 250–4, 256
social brain 39–40

social cognition
  approaches 6–7
  automatic/controlled 9
  constructs 4–5
  content definitions 6
  deficit approach 6
  definition 1, 6
  distortion approach 6
  domain–general/domain-specific 20
  emotional approach 6
  implicit/explicit 9
  individual differences 1–2, 16, 404
  interpersonal/intrapersonal 5–6
  language 2, 16–17
  measurement 10–14
  neurocognitive system 9
  ontogeny 7–9
  tasks 12, 13
  definition 4–6
Social Cognition and Interaction
    Training (SCIT) 419
social cognitive information processing
    approach 6, 141; see also social
    information processing (SIP)
social competence
  behavioural genetics 401–2
  false belief 131–2
  social cognition 2
  see also social skills
social goals 155
social information processing (SIP) 18, 141,
    142–3, 204–5
  aggression 147–59
  anxiety 243–9, 254–5
  conduct problems 442–6
  depression 19, 205–17, 429
  developmental changes 143–7
  interventions 162–3
social isolation 1
socialization
  aggression 161–2
  psychopathology 349
social mirroring 324, 326, 327
social neuroscience 7–8
social outcome 2
social phobia 240
social problem-solving 249–50
social referencing 32
social skills
  anxiety 254–5, 260
  theory of mind 61–2, 72
  training 42–3, 73, 416, 418–19, 441
  see also social competence
social stories technique 73
social understanding training 416
socio-economic status 2, 186
socio-emotional competence 365–73
solutions, see response generation

specific phobia 240
speed of processing 145
stimulation-seeking hypothesis 160
STOP 434
Strange Situation Test 271
Strange Stories Test 35, 72
strategies, see response generation
subgenual cingulate 219
subjective sense of emotional state 323–7
subjective value 186
sufficiency index 316
superior temporal gyrus 36, 39, 397
superior temporal sulcus 36–7, 39, 220
sympathy
  brain activity 36
  TESS 33
synaptic abnormalities 40–1
systemizing 34

temporal cortex 9
temporo-parietal junction 36
The Emotion Detector (TED) 31–2, 35–6
The Empathizing SyStem (TESS) 16, 32, 33,
    35–6
theory of mind 3
  anxiety 250–4
  aphasia 91
  attachment 273–4, 309
  autism 15, 16, 71, 100–3
  behavioural genetics 398–9
  blindness 98–100
  brain activity 36, 397
  conversation 62, 81, 90, 92–3, 103
  deaf children 88–9, 92
  disruptive behaviour 119, 125, 126
  emotion understanding 351–2
  environmental factors 120, 287
  executive function 130
  expanding construct 5
  family variables 120
  genetics 120
  grammar 89, 90, 91
  individual differences 120
  language 81, 89–93
  maltreatment 283–4, 363–4, 421
  parenting 398
  selection processor 88
  sentence complements 91
  social-cognitive component 67
  social interactions 61–2, 72
  social-perceptual component 67
  socio-emotional competence 369
  tests 10, 11, 12, 13, 87, 117, 118
  typical development 60–2, 87–8
  vocabulary 89, 90
  Williams syndrome 62–7, 71–2
Theory of Mind Mechanism (ToMM) 30, 31,
    32–3, 35–6

therapy, *see* treatment
thought pictures 87
threat exposure 185, 186
threat perception
  aggression 153, 160–1
  anxiety 245–7, 258
training
  autism 42–4, 415–17
  problem-solving 163, 441–2, 448
  self-training of face processing 70
  social skills 42–3, 73, 416, 418–19, 441
  Williams syndrome 73
Transfer of Control 434
treatment 411–70
  anxiety 258–61, 433–8
  borderline personality disorder 287–92, 423–5
  conduct problems 438–46, 449
  depression 425–33
  evidence-based 412–13
  mentalization 413–17
  psychopathy 189, 417
  schizophrenia 418–19
  usefulness of social cognitive constructs 15
  see also interventions
triadic representations 30, 32
tripartite model 242, 243
TSC1/TSC2 41
twin studies 40, 120, 389–91, 398–9, 400–1

uncontrollable events 216
understanding that and understanding what 403–4, 420

ventrolateral prefrontal cortex 220
ventromedial prefrontal cortex 9, 220
Violence Inhibition Mechanism 181
vocabulary development 89, 90, 95–7
vocal emotion recognition 35, 353–4, 361

white matter 38
Williams syndrome 16
  abuse 72–3
  behavioural phenotype 58
  characteristics 58–9
  cognitive profile 59
  conversational ability 60, 73
  description 58–60
  elastin 58
  exploitation 72–3
  face processing 68–70
  genetic variations 74
  hypersociability 60
  interventions 73
  language abilities 59, 60, 72, 73
  mental retardation 58
  peer relationships 60
  personality traits 59
  sociability 59–60
  social cognition 60, 70–1
  social interaction training 73
  sound sensitivity 58
  theory of mind 62–7, 71–2
withdrawal schemas 144
working memory tasks 118–19
working models of relationships 143

X-system 9